Clinical Atlas of Skin Tumors

Can Baykal • K. Didem Yazganoğlu

Clinical Atlas of Skin Tumors

With contributions by
Nesimi Büyükbabani, MD

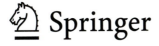

Can Baykal, MD
Department of Dermatovenereology
Istanbul Medical Faculty
Istanbul University
Istanbul
Turkey

K. Didem Yazganoğlu, MD
Department of Dermatovenereology
Istanbul Medical Faculty
Istanbul University
Istanbul
Turkey

Contributor Author
Nesimi Büyükbabani, MD
Department of Pathology
Dermatopathology Section
Istanbul Medical Faculty
Istanbul University
Istanbul
Turkey

ISBN 978-3-642-40937-0   ISBN 978-3-642-40938-7   (eBook)
DOI 10.1007/978-3-642-40938-7
Springer Heidelberg New York Dordrecht London

Library of Congress Control Number: 2014930572

© Springer-Verlag Berlin Heidelberg 2014

This work is subject to copyright. All rights are reserved by the Publisher, whether the whole or part of the material is concerned, specifically the rights of translation, reprinting, reuse of illustrations, recitation, broadcasting, reproduction on microfilms or in any other physical way, and transmission or information storage and retrieval, electronic adaptation, computer software, or by similar or dissimilar methodology now known or hereafter developed. Exempted from this legal reservation are brief excerpts in connection with reviews or scholarly analysis or material supplied specifically for the purpose of being entered and executed on a computer system, for exclusive use by the purchaser of the work. Duplication of this publication or parts thereof is permitted only under the provisions of the Copyright Law of the Publisher's location, in its current version, and permission for use must always be obtained from Springer. Permissions for use may be obtained through RightsLink at the Copyright Clearance Center. Violations are liable to prosecution under the respective Copyright Law.

The use of general descriptive names, registered names, trademarks, service marks, etc. in this publication does not imply, even in the absence of a specific statement, that such names are exempt from the relevant protective laws and regulations and therefore free for general use.

While the advice and information in this book are believed to be true and accurate at the date of publication, neither the authors nor the editors nor the publisher can accept any legal responsibility for any errors or omissions that may be made. The publisher makes no warranty, express or implied, with respect to the material contained herein.

Printed on acid-free paper

Springer is part of Springer Science+Business Media (www.springer.com)

Preface

Skin tumors are undoubtedly one of the most important topics in dermatologic practice. Due to the variety of tissues present in normal skin, these tumors have numerous types and subtypes. The incidence of benign skin tumors is not low at all. The elderly, especially, may have hundreds of benign skin tumors. Some benign tumors have important implications as they may be the first markers of a syndrome and they may also lead to functional or cosmetic problems. On the other hand, underdiagnosis of malignant types may be the cause of mortality. Thus, the importance of recognizing these tumors cannot be disregarded. Prevention, early detection, and treatment of skin cancers are mainly related with the physician's appropriate knowledge and management skills, as well as expertise, in this area.

This comprehensive and useful atlas provides a practical guide on neoplastic skin diseases accompanied by concise text. Featuring 1774 images, it most likely provides one of the richest collections of clinical images on skin tumors. Almost all photos in this book have been taken by two authors working in the same Dermatovenereology department and thus reflect the experience of a single university hospital. We aimed to select photos of a variety of clinical presentations of most skin tumors. Moreover, images related to the evolution and follow-up of tumors were also included. As a result, we tried to tell the "whole story" of the skin tumors with supporting images.

The atlas is arranged in two main parts according to the benign or malignant biological behavior of the tumors, and chapters of each part are organized according to the origin of the tumor. The text includes detailed information about clinical features of the tumors, with special emphasis on diagnostic clues. Advanced diagnostic techniques of skin tumors such as dermoscopy and confocal microscopy are not within the scope of this book. Histopathology of the tumors has been carefully summarized by an experienced dermatopathologist, Professor Nesimi Büyükbabani, who also contributed to the diagnosis of challenging cases. However, advanced pathologic information and histopathologic pictures have not been used.

It is not the purpose of this atlas to outline therapies but considerations for management are provided simply in short summaries. Therefore, this book should not be used as a single reference for therapeutic decisions. The organization and arrangement of the figure legends are planned to give rapid clues for clinical practice. Furthermore, in the third part of the book, all skin tumors are listed according to the predilection for distinct body areas in order to be helpful in localization based quick prediagnosis.

We believe that the *Clinical Atlas of Skin Tumors* will be helpful to dermatovenereologists and also to other physicians in allied specialties such as Plastic Surgery and Oncology.

Istanbul, Turkey Can Baykal, MD
Istanbul, Turkey K. Didem Yazganoğlu, MD

Acknowledgements

We would like to thank our colleagues in the Dermatovenereology Department of Istanbul Medical Faculty for their contributions to the diagnosis of challenging cases included in this book.

Image Contributors

Dr. Özlem Dicle (Akdeniz Medical Faculty)	Figure 2.62
Dr. Soner Uzun (Akdeniz University Medical Faculty)	Figure 3.135
Dr. Ümmühan Kaya (Istanbul Leprosy Hospital)	Figure 5.22, 5.24
Dr. Zeynep Demirçay (Marmara University Medical Faculty)	Figure 7.45
Dr. Tülin Mansur (Haydarpaşa Numune State Hospital)	Figure 10.8
Dr. Cuyan Demirkesen (Cerrahpaşa Medical Faculty)	Figure 11.61
Dr. Erdem Güven (Istanbul Medical Faculty)	Figure 12.51
Dr. Selma Sönmez Ergün (Bezmialem University Hospital)	Figure 13.63
Dr. Alper Alyanak (Istanbul Medical Faculty)	Figure 13.64
Dr. Sergülen Dervişoğlu (Cerrahpaşa Medical Faculty)	Figure 13.66
Dr. Gökhan Demir (Bilim University Medical Faculty)	Figure 13.70
Dr. Gonca Gökdemir (Şişli Etfal State Hospital)	Figure 14.63

Four hundred and eighty-nine images appeared in "Dermatoloji atlası (Atlas of Dermatology), edn 3" by Can Baykal published previously in Turkish (in 2012).

Contents

Part I Benign Tumors

1 Benign Epidermal Tumors 3
   1.1   Benign Tumors of Keratinocytes.................................... 3
       1.1.1   Seborrheic Keratosis 3
       1.1.2   Variants of Seborrheic Keratosis 15
       1.1.3   Nevoid Hyperkeratosis of the Nipple and Areola 15
       1.1.4   Verrucal Keratosis (Transplantation Keratosis)................ 17
       1.1.5   Clear Cell Acanthoma 18
   1.2   Hamartomas with Epidermal Differentiation 18
       1.2.1   Epidermal Nevus 18
       1.2.2   Nevus Sebaceus (Organoid Nevus) 24
       1.2.3   Nevus Comedonicus 30
       1.2.4   Becker Nevus.. 32
   1.3   White Sponge Nevus.. 35
   Suggested Reading... 36

2 Epidermal Precancerous Lesions and In Situ Malignancies 37
   2.1   Actinic Keratosis (Solar Keratosis)............................... 37
   2.2   Bowen Disease 41
   2.3   Erythroplasia of Queyrat... 46
   2.4   Leukoplakia.. 47
   2.5   Actinic Cheilitis.. 51
   2.6   Cutaneous Horn (Cornu Cutaneum) 52
   2.7   Arsenical Keratosis 54
   2.8   Chronic Radiodermatitis 54
   2.9   Keratoacanthoma... 55
   2.10 Paget Disease of the Breast 59
   2.11 Extramammary Paget Disease...................................... 61
   Suggested Reading... 62

3 Nevomelanocytic Benign Tumors 63
   3.1   Melanotic Lesions 63
       3.1.1   Ephelides (Freckles)... 63
       3.1.2   Labial Melanotic Macule..................................... 64
       3.1.3   Penile Melanotic Macule 65
       3.1.4   Vulvar Melanosis 65
   3.2   Epidermal Melanocytic Tumors 65
       3.2.1   Lentigo Simplex... 65
       3.2.2   Segmental Lentiginosis 68
       3.2.3   Actinic Lentigo (Lentigo Senilis) 68
       3.2.4   Café-au-lait Macules 72

	3.3	Dermal Melanocytic Tumors	74
		3.3.1 Mongolian Spot	74
		3.3.2 Nevus of Ota	76
		3.3.3 Nevus of Ito	78
		3.3.4 Congenital Dermal Melanocytosis (Dermal Melanocytic Hamartoma)	79
		3.3.5 Blue Nevus	80
	3.4	Melanocytic Nevi (Nevus Cell Nevi)	84
		3.4.1 Common Acquired Melanocytic Nevus	84
		3.4.2 Mucosal Melanocytic Nevi	95
		3.4.3 Congenital Melanocytic Nevus	97
		3.4.4 Dysplastic Nevus (Atypical Nevus)	109
		3.4.5 Halo Nevus (Sutton Nevus)	112
		3.4.6 Spitz Nevus	114
		3.4.7 Reed Nevus (Pigmented Spindle Cell Nevus)	117
		3.4.8 Deep Penetrating Nevus	118
		3.4.9 Nevus Spilus (Speckled Lentiginous Nevus)	119
		3.4.10 Meyerson Nevus (Meyerson Phenomenon)	121
		3.4.11 Epidermolysis Bullosa Nevus	121
		3.4.12 Pseudomelanoma (Recurrent Melanocytic Nevus)	122
	Suggested Reading		123
4	**Cutaneous Cysts**		125
	4.1	Epidermoid Cyst (Infundibular Cyst)	125
		4.1.1 Milium	131
	4.2	Trichilemmal Cyst (Pilar Cyst)	134
	4.3	Proliferating Trichilemmal Cyst	135
	4.4	Steatocystoma Multiplex	136
	4.5	Eruptive Vellus Hair Cyst	137
	4.6	Digital Mucous Cyst (Mucoid Cyst, Myxoid Cyst)	138
	4.7	Mucocele (Mucous Cyst of Oral Mucosa)	140
	4.8	Auricular Pseudocyst	142
	4.9	Preauricular Cyst (Preauricular Sinus)	142
	4.10	Median Raphe Cyst	143
	Suggested Reading		143
5	**Skin Appendage Tumors**		145
	5.1	Sweat Gland Tumors	145
		5.1.1 Syringoma	145
		5.1.2 Chondroid Syringoma (Mixed Tumor of the Skin)	147
		5.1.3 Eccrine Hidrocystoma	147
		5.1.4 Poroma (Eccrine Poroma)	149
		5.1.5 Poroid Hidradenoma	150
		5.1.6 Tubulopapillary Hidradenoma (Papillary Tubular Adenoma)	150
		5.1.7 Cylindroma	151
		5.1.8 Spiradenoma	152
		5.1.9 Syringocystadenoma Papilliferum	153
		5.1.10 Apocrine Hidrocystoma (Cystadenoma)	155
		5.1.11 Hidradenoma Papilliferum	156
		5.1.12 Erosive Adenomatosis of the Nipple (Papillary Adenoma of the Nipple)	156
	5.2	Hair Follicle Tumors	156
		5.2.1 Trichoepithelioma	156
		5.2.2 Trichoblastoma	158
		5.2.3 Trichofolliculoma	158
		5.2.4 Trichilemmoma	159
		5.2.5 Pilomatricoma (Calcifying Epithelioma of Malherbe)	160

	5.3	Tumors of Sebaceous Glands	162
		5.3.1 Senile Sebaceous Hyperplasia	162
		5.3.2 Sebaceous Adenoma and Sebaceous Epithelioma	163
		5.3.3 Fordyce Spots	164
	5.4	Tumors of Smooth Muscles of Skin	165
		5.4.1 Leiomyoma	166
		5.4.2 Congenital Smooth Muscle Hamartoma	167
	Suggested Reading		168
6	**Vascular Anomalies**		**169**
	6.1	Benign Vascular Tumors	169
		6.1.1 Infantile Hemangioma (Capillary Hemangioma)	169
		6.1.2 Congenital Hemangioma	179
		6.1.3 Kaposiform Hemangioendothelioma	181
		6.1.4 Tufted Angioma	182
		6.1.5 Pyogenic Granuloma	182
		6.1.6 Senile Angioma (Cherry Angioma)	186
		6.1.7 Targetoid Hemosiderotic Hemangioma (Hobnail Hemangioma)	189
		6.1.8 Glomeruloid Hemangioma	189
		6.1.9 Angiolymphoid Hyperplasia with Eosinophilia	190
		6.1.10 Kimura disease	192
		6.1.11 Intravascular Papillary Endothelial Hyperplasia (Masson Hemangioma)	193
	6.2	Vascular Malformations	193
		6.2.1 Capillary Malformations	193
		6.2.2 Venous Malformations	216
		6.2.3 Glomus Tumor and Glomuvenous Malformation (Glomangioma)	220
		6.2.4 Lymphatic Malformation	222
		6.2.5 Arteriovenous Malformation	229
	Suggested Reading		230
7	**Neural Skin Tumors**		**231**
	7.1	Neurofibroma	231
		7.1.1 Dermal Neurofibroma	231
		7.1.2 Plexiform Neurofibroma	232
	7.2	Schwannoma (Neurilemmoma)	237
	7.3	Neuromas	239
		7.3.1 Multiple Mucosal Neuromas	240
		7.3.2 Cutaneous Neuroma	240
		7.3.3 Palisaded Encapsulated Neuroma	241
		7.3.4 Traumatic Neuroma	241
	7.4	Neurothekeoma	242
	7.5	Granular Cell Tumor (Granular Nerve Sheath Tumor)	243
	Suggested Reading		243
8	**Benign Fibrohistiocytic Tumors and Proliferations**		**245**
	8.1	Dermatofibroma (Histiocytoma)	245
	8.2	Fibrous Papule of the Nose	248
	8.3	Angiofibroma	249
		8.3.1 Tuberous sclerosis	250
	8.4	Periungual Fibroma (Koenen Tumor)	252
	8.5	Perifollicular Fibroma	254
		8.5.1 Birt-Hogg-Dubé Syndrome	254
	8.6	Oral Fibroma	255
	8.7	Acquired Digital Fibrokeratoma	256

	8.8	Epithelioid Cell Histiocytoma	258
	8.9	Infantile Digital Fibromatosis	259
	8.10	Infantile Myofibromatosis	260
	8.11	Juvenile Hyaline Fibromatosis	260
	8.12	Calcifying Aponeurotic Fibroma	261
	8.13	Fibromatoses	261
		8.13.1 Palmar Fibromatosis	262
		8.13.2 Plantar Fibromatosis	262
		8.13.3 Knuckle Pads	262
		8.13.4 Penile Fibromatosis (Peyronie Disease)	262
	8.14	Acrochordon (Skin Tag)	262
	8.15	Connective Tissue Nevus (Collagenoma)	266
		8.15.1 Tuberous Sclerosis	266
		8.15.2 Buschke-Ollendorff syndrome	267
		8.15.3 Proteus syndrome	267
		8.15.4 Familial Cutaneous Collagenoma	268
		8.15.5 Eruptive Collagenoma and Isolated Collagenoma	268
		8.15.6 Papular Elastorrhexis	269
	8.16	Keloid and Hypertrophic Scar	269
	8.17	Giant Cell Tumor of the Tendon Sheath	273
	8.18	Weathering Nodules of the Ear	273
	Suggested Reading		273
9	**Mastocytosis**		275
	9.1	Cutaneous Mastocytosis	275
		9.1.1 Urticaria Pigmentosa	275
		9.1.2 Diffuse Cutaneous Mastocytosis	278
		9.1.3 Isolated (Solitary) Mastocytoma	279
		9.1.4 Telangiectasia Macularis Eruptiva Perstans	281
	9.2	Adult Systemic Mastocytosis	281
	Suggested Reading		283
10	**Neoplasms of Subcutaneous Fat**		285
	10.1	Lipoma	285
	10.2	Nevus Lipomatosus Superficialis	287
	Suggested Reading		289

Part II Malignant Tumors

11	**Malignant Epithelial Tumors**		293
	11.1	Basal Cell Carcinoma	293
		11.1.1 Noduloulcerative (Nodular) Type	297
		11.1.2 Superficial Type	303
		11.1.3 Morphoeic (Sclerosing) Type	305
		11.1.4 Pigmented Type	307
		11.1.5 Fibroepithelial Type (Pinkus Tumor)	308
		11.1.6 Basosquamous Carcinoma (Metatypical Carcinoma)	308
		11.1.7 Recurrent Basal Cell Carcinoma	309
		11.1.8 Metastatic Basal Cell Carcinoma	310
		11.1.9 Hereditary Tumor Syndromes	311
	11.2	Squamous Cell Carcinoma	315
		11.2.1 Metastatic Squamous Cell Carcinoma	327

	11.3	Verrucous Carcinoma	328
		11.3.1 Oral Florid Papillomatosis (Aerodigestive Verrucous Carcinoma)	328
		11.3.2 Buschke-Löwenstein Tumor (Anogenital Verrucous Carcinoma)	329
		11.3.3 Carcinoma Cuniculatum	329
	11.4	Malignant Adnexal Tumors	330
		11.4.1 Sebaceous Carcinoma	330
		11.4.2 Primary Cutaneous Adenoid Cystic Carcinoma	331
		11.4.3 Microcystic Adnexal Carcinoma (Sclerosing Sweat Duct Carcinoma)	332
		11.4.4 Hidradenocarcinoma	332
		11.4.5 Porocarcinoma (Malignant Eccrine Poroma)	333
	11.5	Merkel Cell Carcinoma	333
	Suggested Reading		334
12	**Malignant Melanoma**		**335**
	12.1	Primary Cutaneous Malignant Melanoma	335
		12.1.1 Lentigo Maligna Melanoma	336
		12.1.2 Superficial Spreading Melanoma	339
		12.1.3 Acral Lentiginous Melanoma	342
		12.1.4 Nodular Malignant Melanoma	345
		12.1.5 Mucosal Melanoma	348
		12.1.6 Amelanotic Melanoma	349
		12.1.7 Desmoplastic Melanoma	350
		12.1.8 Spitzoid Melanoma	350
		12.1.9 Malignant Blue Nevus	351
	12.2	Metastatic Malignant Melanoma	351
	Suggested Reading		356
13	**Cutaneous Sarcomas**		**359**
	13.1	Kaposi Sarcoma	359
		13.1.1 Classic Kaposi Sarcoma	359
		13.1.2 Acquired Immunodeficiency Syndrome (AIDS)–Related (Epidemic) Kaposi Sarcoma	365
		13.1.3 Iatrogenic Kaposi Sarcoma	366
		13.1.4 Endemic (African) Kaposi Sarcoma	368
	13.2	Cutaneous Angiosarcoma	370
	13.3	Epithelioid Hemangioendothelioma	372
	13.4	Dermatofibrosarcoma Protuberans	373
	13.5	Atypical Fibroxanthoma	375
	13.6	Malignant Fibrous Histiocytoma	375
	13.7	Fibrosarcoma	376
	13.8	Liposarcoma	376
	13.9	Leiomyosarcoma	377
	13.10	Epithelioid Sarcoma	378
	13.11	Malignant Peripheral Nerve Sheath Tumor (Malignant Schwannoma, Neurofibrosarcoma)	378
	Suggested Reading		379
14	**Cutaneous Lymphomas**		**381**
	14.1	Primary Cutaneous Lymphomas	381
		14.1.1 Cutaneous T-cell Lymphomas	381
		14.1.2 Cutaneous B-cell Lymphomas	426
		14.1.3 Blastic Plasmacytoid Dendritic Cell Neoplasm	434

	14.2	Pseudolymphomas of the Skin	435
		14.2.1 Lymphocytoma Cutis (Pseudolymphoma of Spiegler-Fendt)	436
		14.2.2 Jessner's Lymphocytic Infiltration of the Skin (Jessner-Kanof Disease)	439
	14.3	The Skin Infiltration of Hematologic Neoplasms	442
		14.3.1 Leukemia Cutis	443
		14.3.2 Cutaneous Infiltration of Hodgkin Lymphoma	444
		14.3.3 Cutaneous Infiltration of Non-Hodgkin Lymphomas	445
		14.3.4 Cutaneous Infiltration of Plasma Cell Dyscrasia	446
	Suggested Reading		447

15 Histiocytoses ... 449

15.1	Langerhans Cell Histiocytosis	449
15.2	Non-Langerhans Cell Histiocytoses	454
	15.2.1 Juvenile Xanthogranuloma	454
	15.2.2 Benign Cephalic Histiocytosis	458
	15.2.3 Generalized Eruptive Histiocytosis	459
	15.2.4 Xanthoma Disseminatum	460
	15.2.5 Reticulohistiocytosis	462
	15.2.6 Necrobiotic Xanthogranuloma	464
	15.2.7 Sinus Histiocytosis with Massive Lymphadenopathy (Rosai-Dorfman Disease)	465
15.3	Indeterminate Cell Histiocytosis	466
Suggested Reading		466

16 Cutaneous Metastasis ... 467

16.1	Nodular Cutaneous Metastasis	468
16.2	Carcinoma Erysipeloides	471
16.3	Scleroderma-like Cutaneous Metastasis	474
16.4	Telangiectatic Metastatic Carcinoma	475
16.5	Erythema Annulare Centrifugum-like Metastasis	475
Suggested Reading		476

Part III Regional Differential Diagnosis of Skin Tumors

17 Predilection Sites of Skin Tumors ... 479

Index ... 491

Part I
Benign Tumors

Benign Epidermal Tumors

Epidermis—namely the epithelium of skin—consists of keratinocytes, melanocytes, Merkel cells, and Langerhans cells. In this chapter, only the benign tumors of keratinocytes (real proliferations) or hamartomas (non-neoplastic malformations) with epidermal differentiation will be discussed. However, epidermal tumors causing dysplasia and benign tumors with adnexal differentiation are not included in this chapter. Epidermal proliferations induced by Human papilloma virus (HPV) infection (verrucae) are also not included.

Seborrheic keratosis is the most common type of benign keratinocytic tumors. The rich clinical spectrum of this lesion, its distinctive variants and a few rare benign epidermal tumors that have clinicopathologic similarities with seborrheic keratosis will be discussed in the first part. All types of epidermal hamartomas may be associated with extracutaneous abnormalities, causing the so-called "epidermal nevus syndromes". These syndromes are detailed in the relevant subtitles according to the main type of hamartoma. White sponge nevus will also be included in this chapter.

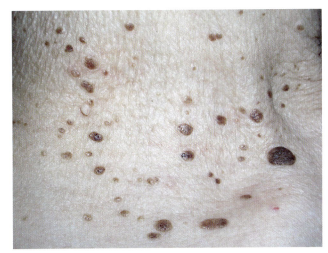

Fig. 1.1 Multiple seborrheic keratoses on the trunk

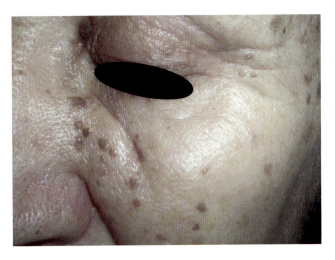

Fig. 1.2 Multiple small seborrheic keratoses on the face

1.1 Benign Tumors of Keratinocytes

1.1.1 Seborrheic Keratosis

Seborrheic keratosis is an epidermal cutaneous neoplasm that carries no risk of malignant degeneration. It is, undoubtedly, one of the most common benign tumors of adults. However, although rare, it may also be seen in childhood. The number of lesions increases with age, and many elderly people have numerous tumors. Classic lesions of seborrheic keratosis (other than dermatosis papulosa nigra) are rare in dark-skinned individuals. The great majority of patients, including the ones with hundreds of lesions, are usually otherwise healthy. The trunk is the most common location (see Fig. 1.1). The face (see Fig. 1.2), neck (see Fig. 1.3), and the upper parts of the limbs are other frequent sites, but any hair-bearing area of the body can be involved. Only palmoplantar areas and mucous membranes are spared. The underlying pathogenesis that causes proliferation of epidermal cells is not fully understood. Chronic sun exposure may be a triggering factor, as the lesions are more common in fair-skinned people and are rarely seen on the buttocks. However, on the contrary, intertriginous surfaces like the groin (see Fig. 1.4), axillae, and inframammary area (see Fig. 1.5) may sometimes be involved.

The clinical spectrum of seborrheic keratosis is wide. The lesions are observed in varying sizes, shapes, and colors. Although most lesions are 0.5 to 1.5 cm in diameter, tiny papules measuring 0.2 to 0.3 mm in diameter (see Fig. 1.6) or giant (>3 cm) plaques (see Fig. 1.7) can also occur. Especially the older lesions are relatively larger. Their shape is round (see Fig. 1.8), oval (see Fig. 1.9), or irregular (see Fig. 1.10). Tumors are generally light brown (see Fig. 1.11), yellow-brown (see Fig. 1.12), dark yellow (see Fig. 1.13), or black in color (see Figs. 1.14 and 1.15), but skin-colored (see Fig. 1.6)

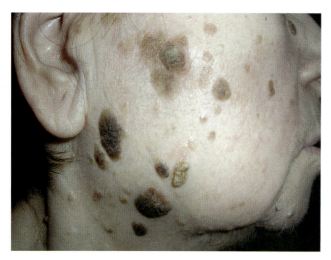

Fig. 1.3 Multiple seborrheic keratoses of different sizes and shapes on the face and neck

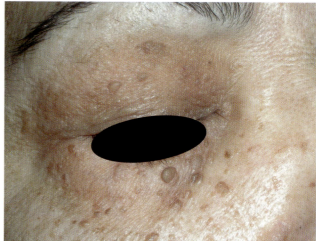

Fig. 1.6 Seborrheic keratoses presenting as multiple, skin-colored, tiny papules on the face

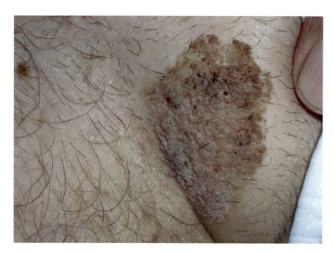

Fig. 1.4 Seborrheic keratosis on the groin. Large lesions may develop on intertriginous areas as seen in the figure

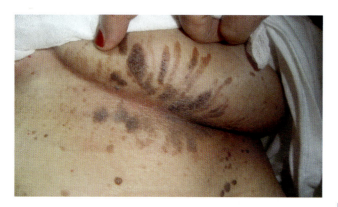

Fig. 1.5 Multiple seborrheic keratoses on the inframammary fold

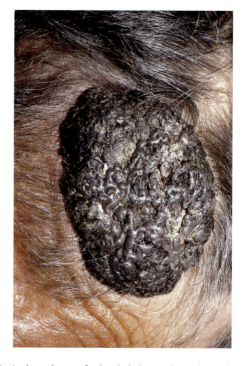

Fig. 1.7 A giant plaque of seborrheic keratosis on the scalp. Note the cerebriform appearance

1.1 Benign Tumors of Keratinocytes

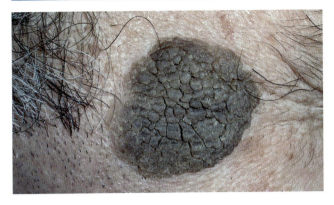

Fig. 1.8 Sharply demarcated, raised, round plaque with fine fissures on papillomatous surface; a typical presentation of seborrheic keratosis (solid type)

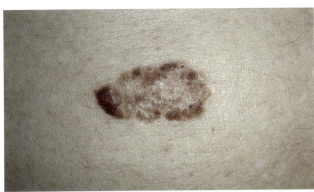

Fig. 1.11 Light brown seborrheic keratosis with an irregular surface

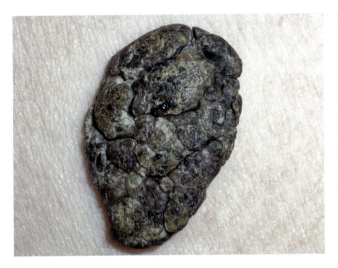

Fig. 1.9 Oval seborrheic keratosis showing deep cracks and greasy scaling on the surface

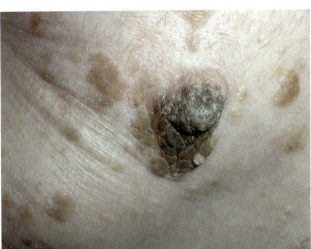

Fig. 1.12 Multiple seborrheic keratoses on the face. Note the large yellowish brown–colored one with an irregular surface

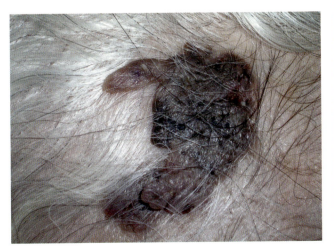

Fig. 1.10 Large irregular seborrheic keratosis on the scalp

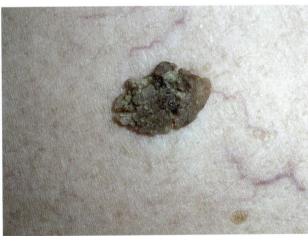

Fig. 1.13 Dark-yellow seborrheic keratosis. Yellow color causes "seborrheic" appearance, hence plays a role in the name of this keratinocyte tumor

or white lesions (*see* Fig. 1.16) may also be observed. The lesions may become darker with time. They may be flat (*see* Figs. 1.15 and 1.16) or raised (*see* Figs. 1.17 and 1.18), or flat lesions may become elevated in time. The surface of the lesions may become papillomatous (*see* Fig. 1.19). The whole mass of the classic solid type of seborrheic keratosis is above the skin surface (*see* Figs. 1.9 and 1.20). Sometimes two different components can be seen; namely, one or a few elevated papules or nodules over a relatively flat plaque (*see* Figs. 1.21 and 1.22). Some lesions may have a depressed center (*see* Fig. 1.23). The regions of the tumor may also appear in different colors (*see* Figs. 1.24, 1.25, and 1.26). Asymmetric lesions with two components should be distinguished from biphasic malignant melanoma in the invasive stage (*see* Fig. 12.23).

The lesions of seborrheic keratosis are typically well-circumscribed. Sometimes the border is notched (*see*

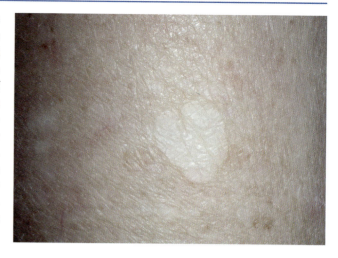

Fig. 1.16 A flat, white seborrheic keratosis is seen. The color of seborrheic keratosis may range from white to black

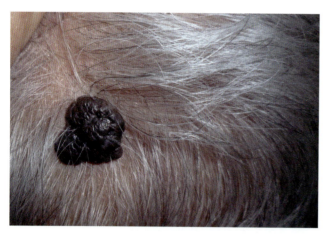

Fig. 1.14 Seborrheic keratosis with dense pigmentation. Dark lesions of this benign tumor have a particular importance as they may easily be misdiagnosed as malignant melanoma

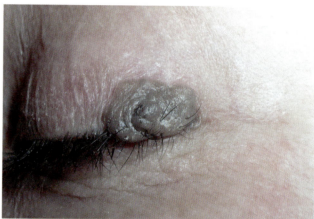

Fig. 1.17 Seborrheic keratosis presenting as a raised nodule on the eyelid

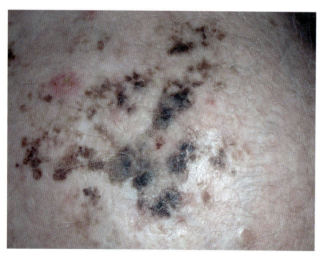

Fig. 1.15 Multiple, flat or slightly raised, irregularly distributed seborrheic keratoses on the scalp of an old bald man. Note the color variation with brown, grey, and black hue

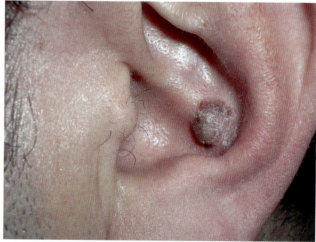

Fig. 1.18 Seborrheic keratosis as a raised hyperkeratotic lesion on the ear. Such a lesion may be confused with verrucae

1.1 Benign Tumors of Keratinocytes

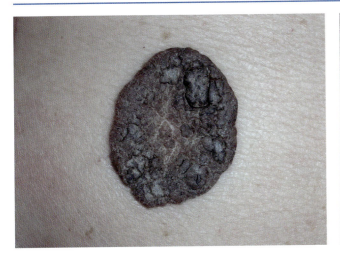

Fig. 1.19 Seborrheic keratosis with hyperkeratotic and papillomatous surface

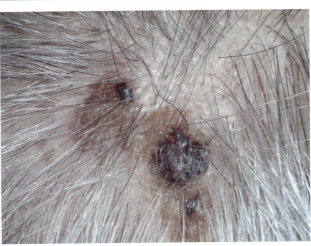

Fig. 1.22 Seborrheic keratosis with two components; dark-colored papulonodular lesions on the top of a light-colored flat plaque

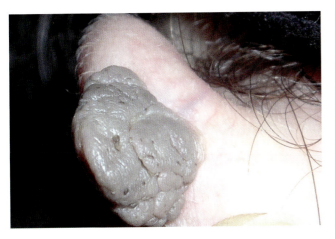

Fig. 1.20 Seborrheic keratosis presenting as a markedly elevated nodule on the ear

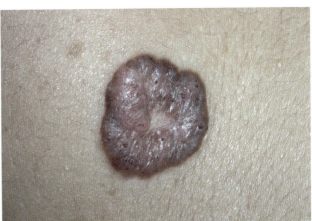

Fig. 1.23 Seborrheic keratosis with a depressed center

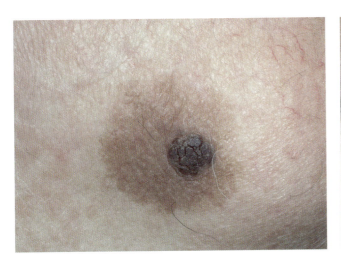

Fig. 1.21 Large seborrheic keratosis with two components; nodular part of the lesion is darker than the flat part

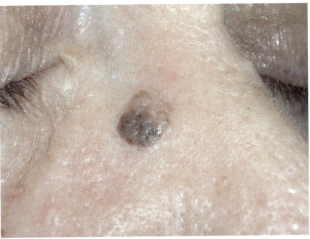

Fig. 1.24 Seborrheic keratosis showing light- and dark-colored regions concomitantly. Two-toned and asymmetric appearance may arouse suspicion of a malignant tumor

Fig. 1.27), simulating a superficial spreading melanoma (*see* Fig. 12.20). Polypoid (*see* Figs. 1.28 and 1.29), pedunculated (*see* Fig. 1.30), or pendulous (*see* Fig. 1.31) papules or nodules may be difficult to distinguish from acrochordon (*see* Fig. 8.72) and verruca filiformis. The surface characteristics are usually helpful for the diagnosis. White, yellow, or black tiny plugs of keratin (horn cysts, keratin pearls) embedded on the tumor (*see* Fig. 1.32) or slightly projecting from the velvety surface (*see* Fig. 1.33) are typical but are predominantly seen on elevated lesions. This finding is usually helpful in confirming the diagnosis and in distinguishing seborrheic keratosis from melanocytic nevus. Dermoscopic examination is also helpful in distinguishing seborrheic keratoses from benign melanocytic tumors and malignant melanoma. Some seborrheic keratoses show dense hyperkeratosis (*see* Fig. 1.34) and greasy scaling (*see* Fig. 1.9), leading to a misdiagnosis of

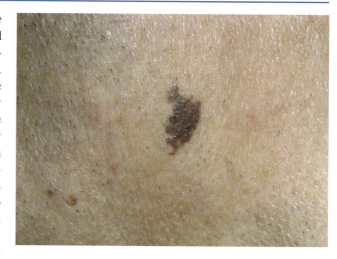

Fig. 1.27 Flat seborrheic keratosis with irregular and notched borders mimicking lentigo maligna

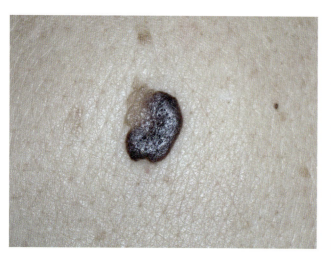

Fig. 1.25 Seborrheic keratosis with two components. Note that the small flat component is lighter (upper left) and the elevated larger component is darker

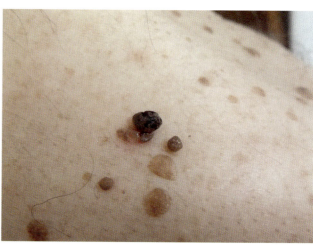

Fig. 1.28 Multiple seborrheic keratoses. Note the polypoid portion rising up from a papular lesion

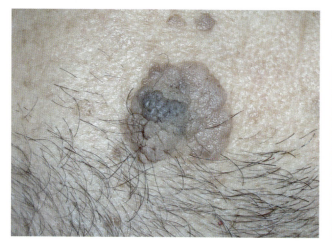

Fig. 1.26 Seborrheic keratosis with an asymmetric surface. Note a part of the lesion is more elevated and darker

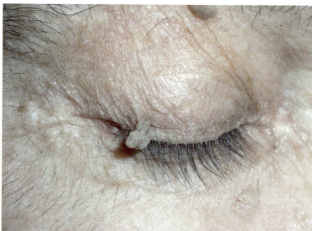

Fig. 1.29 Polypoid seborrheic keratosis on the eyelid

1.1 Benign Tumors of Keratinocytes

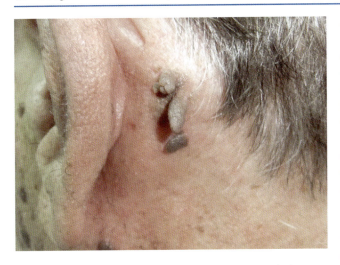

Fig. 1.30 Multiple seborrheic keratoses on the retroauricular area. Note that one of the lesions is pedunculated

epidermal nevus (*see* Fig. 1.70). Some tumors have a rough surface showing deep cracks (*see* Fig. 1.9). Cutaneous horn may overlie seborrheic keratoses (*see* Fig. 1.35). The tumor may occasionally diminish as a result of peel off but typically regrow later. Lesions presenting as plaques on the scalp (*see* Fig. 1.36) may be confused with nevus sebaceus, but the latter is typically hairless (*see* Fig. 1.99). Genital lesions may sometimes be hard to distinguish from condyloma acuminata. Lesions on the nipple (*see* Fig. 1.37) are considered in the differential diagnosis of nevoid hyperkeratosis of the nipple and areola (*see* Fig. 1.62).

A remarkably dark, flat, or thick seborrheic keratosis (*see* Figs. 1.14, 1.25, and 1.38) may also be challenging in the differential diagnosis of various melanocytic tumors. This type of seborrheic keratosis has been called "melanoacanthoma."

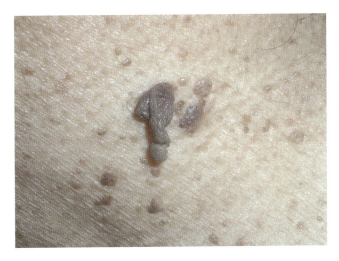

Fig. 1.31 Pendulous seborrheic keratosis. Multiple tiny dome-shaped lesions are also seen

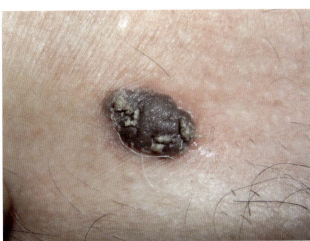

Fig. 1.33 Tiny horn cysts projecting from the surface of a dome-shaped seborrheic keratosis

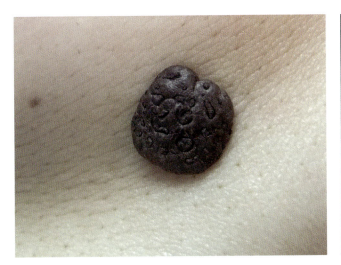

Fig. 1.32 Seborrheic keratosis with tiny horn cysts embedded in the surface, a distinctive feature

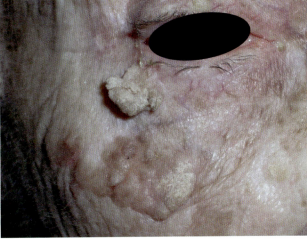

Fig. 1.34 A large flat plaque of seborrheic keratosis on the cheek seen concomitantly with a densely hyperkeratotic, pedunculated seborrheic keratosis located adjacent to the lower eyelid

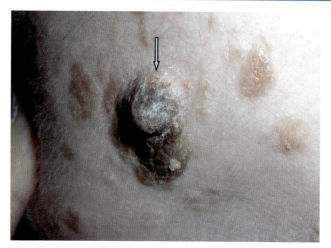

Fig. 1.35 Cutaneus horn (*arrow*) overlying seborrheic keratosis

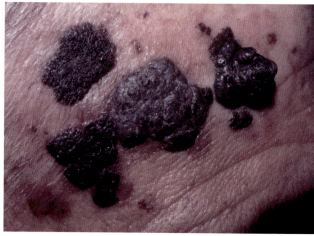

Fig. 1.38 Melanoacanthoma, the pigmented subtype of seborrheic keratosis. Multiple lesions are seen

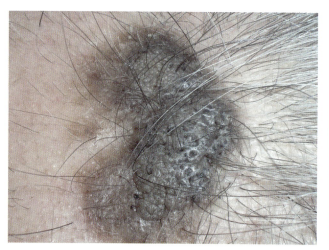

Fig. 1.36 Seborrheic keratosis on the scalp with papillomatous surface. Note that it is not associated with alopecia in contrast to the lesions of nevus sebaceus

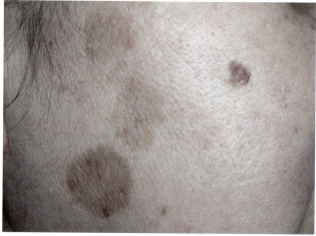

Fig. 1.39 Multiple, flat seborrheic keratoses on the face

There are other clinical presentations of seborrheic keratosis, mainly related to its localization. Flat lesions may be encountered more commonly on the face (*see* Fig. 1.39) and dorsum of the hands (*see* Fig. 1.40). These lesions are usually light brown in color (*see* Fig. 1.41) and often have a homogeneous appearance (*see* Fig. 1.42). Actinic lentigo is also considered among the clinical presentations of seborrheic keratoses. Multiple flat pigmented macules usually located on the upper back (*see* Fig. 1.43) and hands (*see* Fig. 1.44), namely, actinic lentigos, are thought to represent early stages of flat seborrheic keratoses. Macules of actinic lentigo and slightly elevated seborrheic keratoses may often be seen in the same area (e.g., the upper back). Facial flat seborrheic keratoses (*see* Figs. 1.45 and 1.46) can be confused with early lesions of lentigo maligna (*see* Fig. 12.9) and pigmented actinic keratosis (*see* Fig. 2.13). A papular component with different colors may overlie flat seborrheic keratoses (*see* Fig. 1.45). Extensive lesions may be seen in the elderly (see Fig. 1.47).

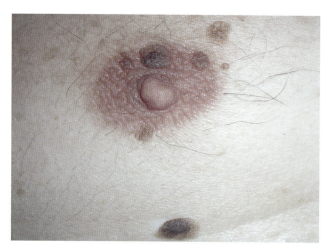

Fig. 1.37 Multiple seborrheic keratoses on and around the nipple

1.1 Benign Tumors of Keratinocytes

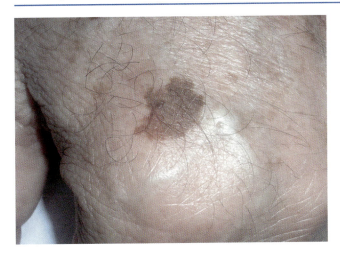

Fig. 1.40 Flat seborrheic keratosis on the dorsum of the hand

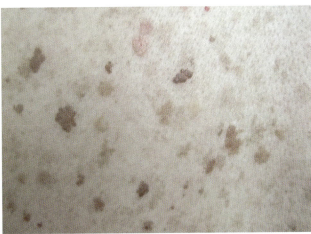

Fig. 1.43 Actinic lentigo is considered an early presentation of flat seborrheic keratosis. Note the macular and slightly elevated lesions located on the upper back representing early and late stages of the same benign tumor

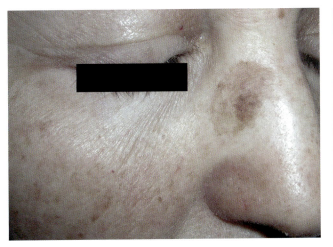

Fig. 1.41 Early lesion of flat seborrheic keratosis on the face (nose) with a typical light brown color

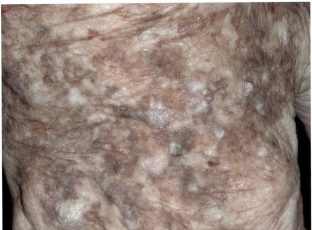

Fig. 1.44 Multiple lesions of actinic lentigo on the dorsum of the hand. Note the confluence of multiple lesions in an elder patient, a typical location

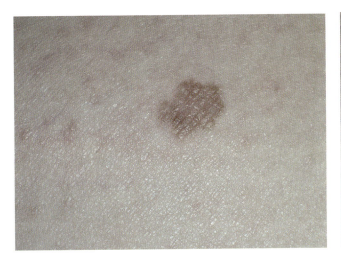

Fig. 1.42 A flat lesion of seborrheic keratosis with homogenous surface

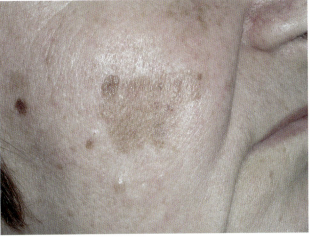

Fig. 1.45 Flat seborrheic keratosis on the cheek, a common location for this type of seborrheic keratosis. Note the papular component on one edge of the lesion

Multiple seborrheic keratoses on the back may show a "raindrop" pattern, appearing as small, slightly elevated, linear lesions in a parallel distribution (*see* Figs. 1.48 and 1.49). Coalescent and verrucous plaques of seborrheic keratoses may be observed on intertriginous surfaces (*see* Fig. 1.5). Different clinical presentations of seborrheic keratoses may be seen concomitantly in patients with multiple lesions (*see* Fig. 1.50).

Although they usually cause no symptoms, some seborrheic keratoses may be pruritic. Inflammation caused by trauma of clothings or rupture of a horn cyst can cause erythema, erosion (*see* Fig. 1.51), superficial ulceration, bleeding, crusting (*see* Fig. 1.52), and tenderness. These lesions, called "irritated seborrheic keratoses," may sometimes mimic basal cell carcinoma (*see* Fig. 11.13) or squamous cell carcinoma (*see* Fig. 11.122). Inflammation of irritated seborrheic keratoses regresses with the use of topical

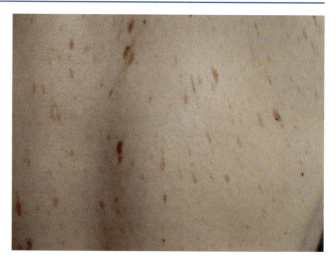

Fig. 1.48 Multiple seborrheic keratoses on the back. Note that most of them are linear in shape

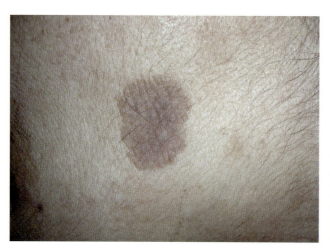

Fig. 1.46 A flat seborrheic keratosis with a slightly elevated morphology

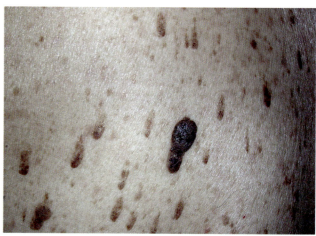

Fig. 1.49 Linear lesions of seborrheic keratosis in a parallel distribution. This distinctive appearance, called "rain drop pattern," is not rare

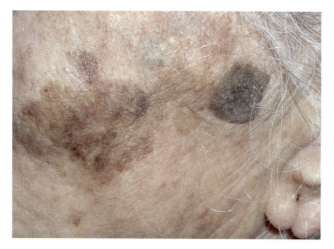

Fig. 1.47 A large flat seborrheic keratosis showing color variety and irregular borders on the cheek of an elder woman. There is also a classic raised solid type of seborrheic keratosis adjacent to the flat lesion

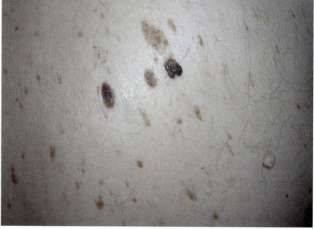

Fig. 1.50 Seborrheic keratoses of different morphologies are seen concomitantly on the back

1.1 Benign Tumors of Keratinocytes

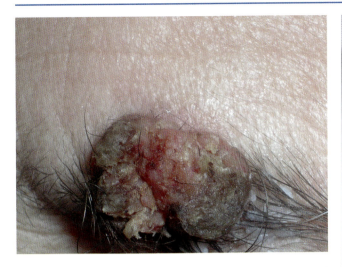

Fig. 1.51 Irritated seborrheic keratosis with severe inflammation and erosion. Note the lack of typical surface features in this situation

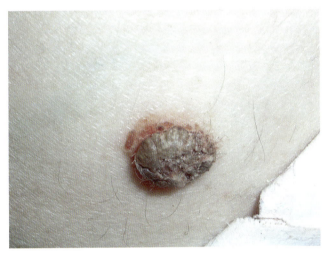

Fig. 1.52 Irritated seborrheic keratosis with central erosion and crusting

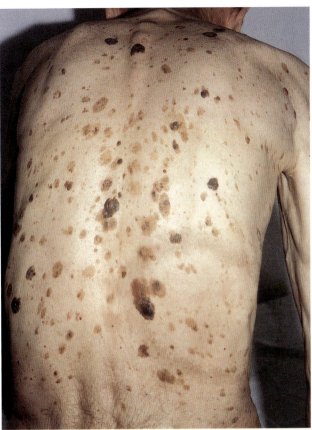

Fig. 1.53 Disseminated seborrheic keratoses on the back of an elderly. Rapid onset of numerous lesions may represent a rare paraneoplastic sign, called Leser-Trelat sign. However, this sign is not found in many elder patients

therapies in a few days; therefore there is no need for further treatment and prompt diagnostic intervention.

The Leser-Trélat sign is described as the sudden eruptive appearance and rapid increase in the size and number of seborrheic keratoses (*see* Fig. 1.53). It is considered a marker of internal malignancy, mainly adenocarcinoma of the gastrointestinal tract. However, the sudden development of numerous seborrheic keratoses only depends on the anamnesis, and most patients actually do not remember the exact time of onset of the lesions. A great majority of patients with numerous seborrheic keratoses are otherwise healthy. This is a very rare paraneoplastic sign. Therefore, a complete gastrointestinal evaluation of the patient, including endoscopic examination, is not commonly considered. It should be noted that pregnancy and erythroderma related with drug eruptions and inflammatory dermatoses like psoriasis and pityriasis rubra pilaris may also be associated with eruptive seborrheic keratoses.

Most seborrheic keratoses are diagnosed clinically but dermoscopy is also helpful. A punch biopsy may be indicated in lesions creating a diagnostic challenge. Histologically, seborrheic keratosis is mainly characterized by proliferation of small basaloid keratinocytes. The histopathologic appearance differs somewhat according to the type of the lesion. The most common hyperkeratotic type has a verruciform silhouette and a thickened keratin layer. In the acanthotic type, epidermal thickening, basaloid cell proliferation, and horn cysts (infoldings of surface keratin) are the main features. Irritated seborrheic keratosis is characterized by proliferation of larger keratinocytes resembling spinal layer cells, horn pearl formation, and an inflammatory infiltration. Differential diagnosis of this latter type from squamous cell carcinoma can sometimes be difficult. The exophytic structure and the presence of basaloid keratinocytes are helpful clues in favor of seborrheic keratosis.

Malignant tumors like basal cell carcinoma occuring within seborrheic keratosis is extremely rare and this seems to be an incidental phenomenon (*see* Fig. 1.54).

Management. Seborrheic keratosis is a benign tumor. Unless a suspicion of Leser-Trélat sign is present, further examination is not necessary. Although the number of tumors may increase in time, individual lesions do not usually enlarge after they reach a certain size. Spontaneous regression is not expected but may occur in exceedingly rare cases. An accurate diagnosis is important to prevent unnecessary aggressive surgery that may result in unsightly scars. Many patients do not request therapy if they are fully informed about the benign nature of the tumor. However, therapy can be performed for cosmetic reasons or if lesions become troublesome. Cryotherapy, electrocautery, carbon dioxide laser, or Er: YAG laser ablation and simple curettage are therapeutic options that are usually cosmetically helpful. Shave excision may be preferred as a surgical method. However, all these procedures may result in postinflammatory hypo- or hyperpigmentation (*see* Figs. 1.55 and 1.56).

Although it is not seen very often, lesions may recur after therapy. Recurrent lesions occur overlying the intervention area or on the border as one or several sharply demarcated papules (*see* Figs. 1.55, 1.56 and 1.57) or irregular confluent lesions (*see* Figs. 1.58). Routine follow-up of seborrheic keratoses is not necessary, but in patients with multiple

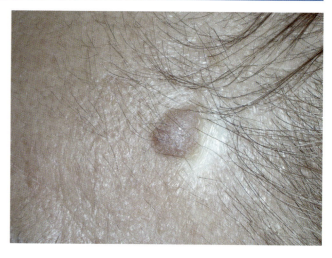

Fig. 1.56 A recurrent lesion of seborrheic keratosis presenting as a sharply demarcated nodule. Note the underlying hypopigmented, slightly atrophic scar on the site of cryotherapy

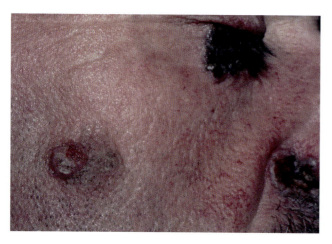

Fig. 1.54 Basal cell carcinoma arising on seborrheic keratosis on the cheek. The patient has also two other basal cell carcinomas on normal skin

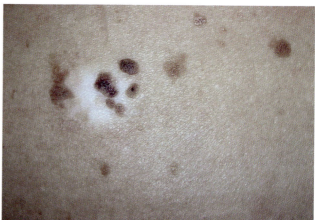

Fig. 1.57 Multiple recurrent small lesions arising on the scar area of formerly treated seborrheic keratosis

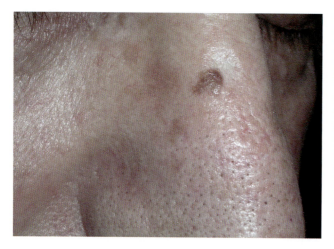

Fig. 1.55 Recurrent seborrheic keratosis developing on the border of a hypopigmented atrophic scar that has occurred on the site of a formerly treated lesion

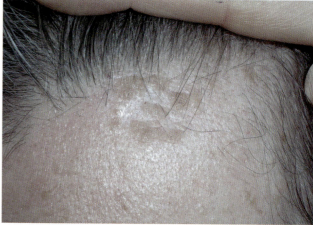

Fig. 1.58 Confluent seborrheic keratoses on a surgical scar. Though rare, even surgically treated seborrheic keratosis may recur

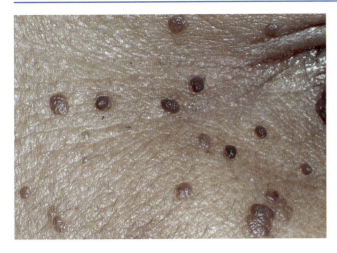

Fig. 1.59 Dermatosis papulosa nigra in an African-American patient. Note the small brown papules

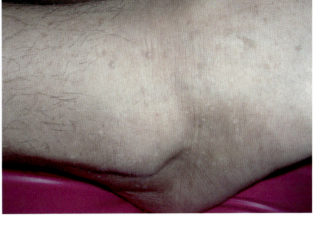

Fig. 1.60 Stucco keratoses around the ankle. Note the multiple small pale papules with rough surface

tumors, new occurrence of a different kind of pigmented or precancerous lesion may be confused with seborrheic keratosis, leading to a delay in consulting a dermatologist. Patients should be advised of the possibility of such a condition.

1.1.2 Variants of Seborrheic Keratosis

1.1.2.1 Dermatosis Papulosa Nigra

Dermatosis papulosa nigra is considered a variant of seborrheic keratosis or acrochordon that appears as numerous hyperpigmented small papules located on the mid-face of African-Americans. It may rarely be observed in other people with relatively dark skin. It shows a familial predisposition (autosomal dominant inheritance pattern) and occurs at younger ages than seborrheic keratosis. Typical lesions are multiple sessile or pedunculated papules measuring 1 to 5 mm in size that are symmetrically located on the cheeks and forehead of adults (*see* Fig. 1.59). Other areas of the face and trunk are infrequently affected. Hyperkeratosis is usually not prominent on the surface, unlike the classic lesions of seborrheic keratosis. The diagnosis is almost always clinical. Major histopathologic features are similar to those of seborrheic keratosis.

Management. These asymptomatic lesions can only be treated for cosmetic reasons. However, it should be kept in mind that destructive methods like cryotherapy may leave permanent postinflammatory hypopigmentation and therefore can cause a worse cosmetic appearance in dark-skinned individuals.

1.1.2.2 Stucco Keratosis

Stucco keratoses are benign hyperkeratotic lesions usually located on the lower legs. They are more frequent among adults, primarily men. Stucco keratoses are most commonly located around the ankles and dorsum of the feet (*see* Fig. 1.60). They may also be found on the dorsum of the hands and forearms. Lesions are usually multiple, asymptomatic, grayish keratotic papules measuring between 1 to 5 mm. Stucco keratosis is considered to be a variant of seborrheic keratosis. Typical location and small size are the differentiating features of stucco keratosis from the classic lesions of seborrheic keratosis. They can be clinically confused with acrokeratosis verruciformis of Hopf. The histologic appearance of stucco keratosis has a striking resemblance to the hyperkeratotic type of seborrheic keratosis. Prominent are orthokeratotic hyperkeratosis, papillomatosis, and verruciform acanthosis.

Management. Cryotherapy or curettage can be used to remove these small lesions. Topical emollients may be helpful in reducing the scales of the lesions.

1.1.2.3 Inverted Follicular Keratosis

Inverted follicular keratosis is a controversial entity. Whether it is a tumor of follicular infundibulum or a rare variant of seborrheic keratosis is a matter of debate. It is more commonly seen in patients after middle age. Most lesions are localized on the face, followed by the scalp and neck. It presents as a small, grey or pink, firm solitary papule, which may be crusted. It is clinically difficult to distinguish from irritated seborrheic keratosis or verruca. Histologically, it is typical to see an endophytic growth pattern, basaloid keratinocytes forming tumoral islands extending toward the dermis, and squamous eddy formation in its central part.

Management. The lesion does not have any risk of malignant transformation. The management is the same as that for seborrheic keratosis.

1.1.3 Nevoid Hyperkeratosis of the Nipple and Areola

Nevoid hyperkeratosis of the nipple and areola is a rare distinct entity with persistent localized hyperkeratotic lesions. The origin of this benign condition is not known, but clinical

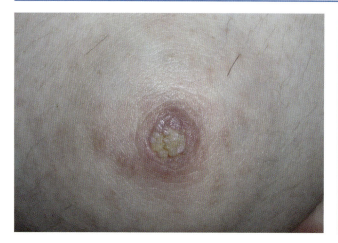

Fig. 1.61 Nevoid hyperkeratosis of the nipple and areola. Hyperkeratosis is restricted to the nipple in this young woman

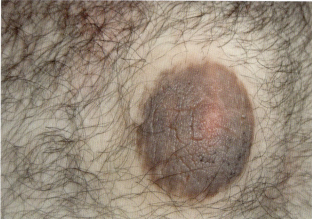

Fig. 1.63 Nevoid hyperkeratosis of the nipple and areola involving both the nipple and areola of a man

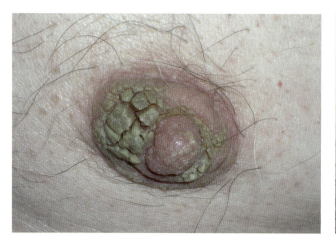

Fig. 1.62 Nevoid hyperkeratosis of the nipple and areola, prominent on the areola of a man. Diffuse involvement of the areola helps to distinguish it from seborrheic keratosis

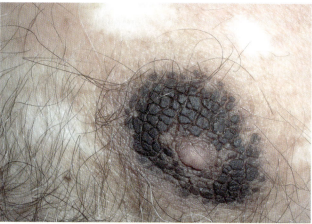

Fig. 1.64 Nevoid hyperkeratosis of the nipple and areola of a man with mycosis fungoides elsewhere

and histopathologic findings are typical. Lesions may be observed on the nipple (see Fig. 1.61), areola (see Fig. 1.62), or both (see Fig. 1.63). The distribution is predominantly bilateral. Women are more commonly affected, but it may also be found in men (see Fig. 1.63).

Nevoid hyperkeratosis of the nipple and areola is commonly acquired after puberty and is relatively common in women of childbearing age. It may also occur or exacerbate and become more verrucous during pregnancy. Thus, it has been suggested that hormones could play a role in the pathogenesis. It is not related to any systemic disease. The typical clinical lesions of nevoid hyperkeratosis of the nipple and areola are characterized by persistent verrucous thickening and dark brown pigmentation of the nipple and areola. There is no induration or discharge. Nevoid hyperkeratosis of the nipple and areola is usually asymptomatic. In some patients there may be mild pruritus or odor if the area is not properly cleaned. It may cause trouble in breast-feeding during the lactation period.

A similar clinical appearance may be observed in different diseases like ichthyoses, epidermal nevus, acanthosis nigricans, and mycosis fungoides (see Fig. 1.64). However, these diseases are usually not restricted to this region and they show specific histopathologic features. Seborrheic keratosis and verruca filiformis can also be considered in the clinical differential diagnosis. Seborrheic keratosis may occur on the nipple or the areola but, in contrast to diffuse involvement of nevoid hyperkeratosis of the nipple and areola, it is typically characterized by solitary or a few sharply demarcated papules or plaques (see Fig. 1.37). Paget disease beginning on the nipple (see Fig. 2.75) may be another differential diagnostic challange, but it is infiltrated and the surface may be eroded or crusted rather than hyperkeratotic.

Hyperkeratosis, acanthosis, papillomatosis, and keratin plugs are the main histopathologic features of nevoid hyperkeratosis of the nipple and areola. Anastomosing rete ridges and the striking filiform nature of papillomatosis are other important clues. Although histopathologic features may mimic those of epidermal nevus or acanthosis nigricans, there is no argument indicating a possible association with any systemic disease. Clinicopathologic correlation is important for the diagnosis.

Management. Nevoid hyperkeratosis of the nipple and areola is persistent if not treated, but there is no risk of malignant transformation. Patients with asymptomatic lesions may not seek medical attention. However, discomfort and serious cosmetic concern may be present in some patients, especially in young women. There is no standard therapy. Various therapeutic modalities have been used with varying success. Topically administered keratolytic agents (e.g., 6% salicylic acid, 12% lactic acid), calcipotriol, and topical retinoic acid (isotretinoin, tretinoin) can reduce hyperkeratosis in some cases. However, recurrence after discontinuation of topical therapy can be seen. Therefore, topical therapies can be applied intermittently to reduce recurrences. Cryotherapy and the carbon dioxide laser have also been used successfully. Curettage or surgical excision may be administered if patients are greatly disturbed by the cosmetic appearance.

1.1.4 Verrucal Keratosis (Transplantation Keratosis)

Hyperkeratotic papules and nodules without typical HPV-associated histologic features seen in organ transplant recipients are called verrucal keratosis or transplantation keratosis. The pathogenesis of these keratinocyte tumors is not understood. They are more common on the head and neck area, forearms, and dorsum of the hands, but they may occur anywhere. The lesions gradually increase in number. Some patients may have profuse lesions. The sizes of these pinkish to skin-colored, asymptomatic lesions vary between 2 and 10 mm (*see* Fig. 1.65). They may coalesce into plaques (*see* Figs. 1.66 and 1.67). Clinically, it is not easy to distinguish transplantation keratoses from viral warts (verruca), but typical epidermal changes seen in HPV infections are absent in the former. These keratoses, especially the ones on sun-exposed areas, may also be misdiagnosed as actinic keratoses. Malignant transformation of transplantation keratoses is not expected. However, as the risk of cutaneous malignancy development is increased in organ transplant patients, these keratoses may be confused with precancerous lesions and cutaneous malignancies. In addition, in the presence of multiple extensive lesions, dermatologic follow-up becomes more difficult and a risk of delay in the detection of squamous cell carcinoma arises. Multiple lesions on the face and hands may be cosmetically disturbing.

Management. Topical medications are usually ineffective. Curettage, electrocautery, or cryotherapy may be helpful for

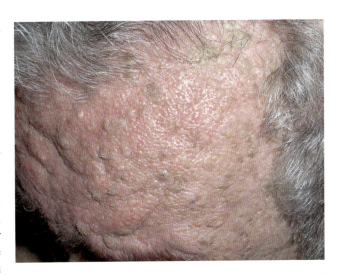

Fig. 1.66 Confluent verrucal keratoses on the forehead of a renal transplant recipient

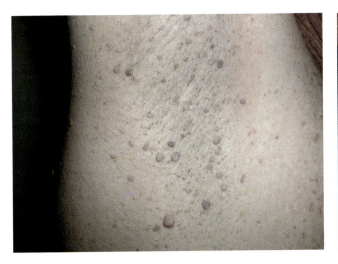

Fig. 1.65 Numerous verrucal keratoses presenting as verrucae-like or seborrheic keratosis-like papular lesions on the axilla of an organ transplant recipient

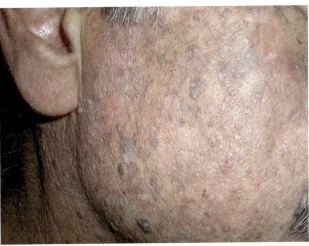

Fig. 1.67 Innumerable verrucal keratoses on the face of a renal transplant recipient. Though these lesions are benign, routine follow-up regarding the development of skin cancer is more difficult in these patients

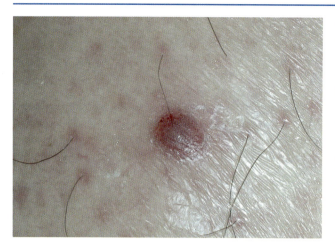

Fig. 1.68 Clear cell acanthoma manifesting as a solitary dome-shaped, pinkish papule

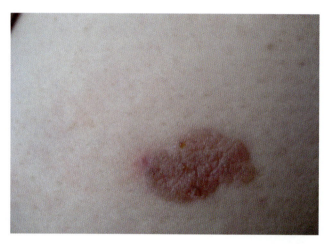

Fig. 1.69 Clear cell acanthoma presenting as a solitary large, slightly elevated plaque. Due to nonspesific clinical features the diagnosis can be established upon biopsy in most cases

discrete lesions. However, extensive lesions are hard to treat. Topical emollients may be used symptomatically.

1.1.5 Clear Cell Acanthoma

Clear cell acanthoma is a rare epidermal benign tumor predominantly seen on the legs of adults, mostly those in their fifties or sixties. It has also been suggested that this lesion is an inflammatory psoriasiform dermatosis. While it is mostly solitary, sometimes a few lesions may be seen. Pink-brown, slightly elevated, dome-shaped papules (*see* Fig. 1.68) or plaques (*see* Fig. 1.69) may have peripheral scales and erosion on the surface. It is difficult to differentiate this lesion clinically from irritated seborrheic keratosis (*see* Fig. 1.52), Bowen disease (*see* Fig. 2.20), pyogenic granuloma (*see* Fig. 6.42), amelanotic melanoma (*see* Fig. 12.57), and basal cell carcinoma (*see* Fig. 11.42). Diagnosis is always based on histopathologic examination. Epidermis with psoriasiform acanthosis containing large, pale (clear) keratinocytes

is the main histopathologic finding. A sharp demarcation from the surrounding epidermis is the rule.

Management. As the lesion is asymptomatic and malignant degeneration is not expected, therapy is mostly applied for cosmetic reasons. Destructive methods like cryotherapy or simple excision can be used. Recurrence is unusual after total removal of the tumor.

1.2 Hamartomas with Epidermal Differentiation

1.2.1 Epidermal Nevus

Epidermal nevus is a hamartomatous tumor composed of hyperkeratotic papules that often coalesce into plaques in different clinical patterns. There is only an alteration on the amount of the normal epidermal structures without any atypical cells. It is also called "keratinocytic epidermal nevus." It is seen approximately in 1 out of 1,000 population. It is mostly present at birth but may sometimes be noticed later when marked hyperkeratosis develops causing a verrucous surface and dark color. Lesions enlarge proportionally with the child's growth but some have a tendency to extend minimally over the adjacent areas of skin in years. The lesion persists throughout life, and it usually does not cause any subjective complaints. There is no increased risk of secondary cutaneous malignancy. It mostly presents as an isolated lesion or can rarely be associated with various abnormalities as a part of an epidermal nevus syndrome. Clinical subtypes of epidermal nevus have been described owing to the pattern of distribution, the extent, and the existence of an inflammatory component.

1.2.1.1 Nevus Verrucosus

Nevus verrucosus is mostly located on a single region of the body, and the size of the lesion is relatively small (*see* Fig. 1.70). Yellowish brown or dark brown warty plaque composed of grouped flat-topped or acrochordon-like papules is the typical appearance of this subtype of tumor (*see* Figs. 1.71 and 1.72). Erythema is absent or minimal. Some lesions are soft and have a velvety surface. There may be satellite papules and sometimes multiple lesions. Seborrheic keratosis (*see* Fig. 1.28) and papillomatous melanocytic nevus (*see* Fig. 3.127) can be considered in the differential diagnosis.

1.2.1.2 Nevus Unius Lateris

Epidermal nevus showing unilateral distribution and involving larger areas (*see* Fig. 1.73) is called nevus unius lateris. It is more common on the trunk and extremities. This subtype of epidermal nevus presents as linear streaks on the extremities and as swirls on the trunk due to the distribution along the lines of Blaschko (*see* Figs. 1.73 and 1.74). However, these streaks are not always continuous, as there are uninvolved sites in-between. Sometimes one half of the body—extending from the scalp to the face (*see* Figs. 1.75 and 1.76) and neck

1.2 Hamartomas with Epidermal Differentiation

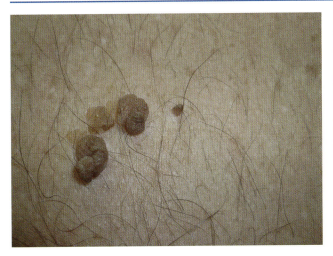

Fig. 1.70 Nevus verrucosus. A small lesion of epidermal nevus

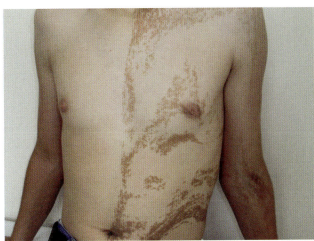

Fig. 1.73 Nevus unius lateris. Epidermal nevus with widespread lesions but distinctively restricted to one site of the body

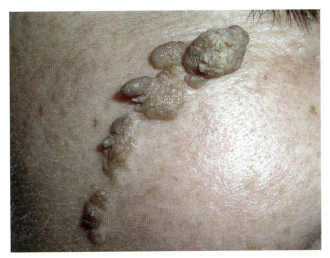

Fig. 1.71 Nevus verrucosus presenting as coalescing hyperkeratotic papules in a linear pattern

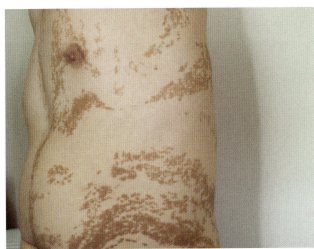

Fig. 1.74 Hyperkeratotic lesions forming swirls following the lines of Blaschko on one side of the trunk; a classical appearance of nevus unius lateris

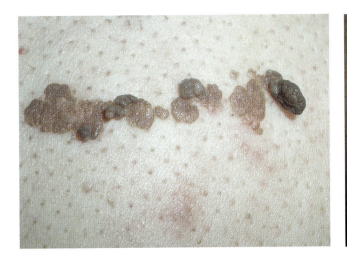

Fig. 1.72 Nevus verrucosus typically composed of linearly arranged acrochordon- or seborrheic keratosis-like lesions

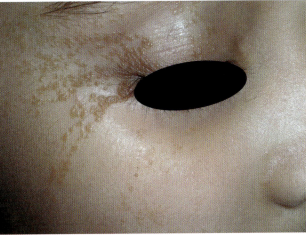

Fig. 1.75 Unilateral epidermal nevus on the face. Cosmetic concern is higher in this location

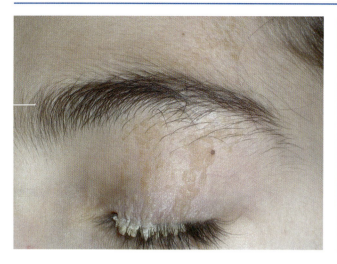

Fig. 1.76 Nevus unius lateris presenting with hyperkeratotic lesions extending from forehead to the upper eyelid on one side of the face

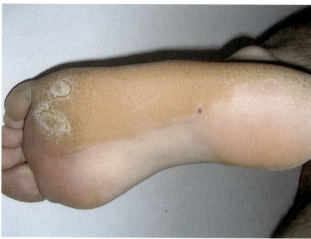

Fig. 1.78 Well-defined linear hyperkeratotic plaque on the sole. Palmoplantar presentation of epidermal nevus may be similar to palmoplantar keratoderma but the former one is mostly unilateral and limited to one part of the palm or sole

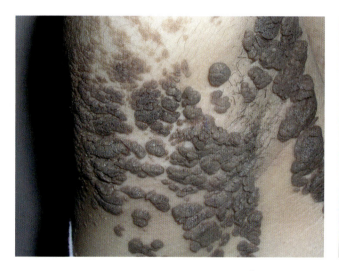

Fig. 1.77 Confluent hyperkeratotic papules on the axilla in nevus unius lateris; this is not an unusual location

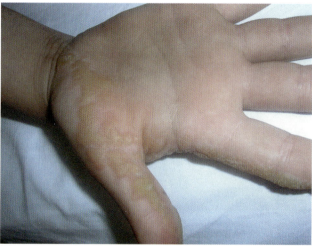

Fig. 1.79 Nevus unius lateris on the palm extending to the thumb and index finger

heading to the axilla (*see* Fig. 1.77), arm (*see* Fig. 1.73), hand, and foot—is involved without crossing the dorsal or ventral midline, thus showing a sharp demarcation line from the unaffected half of the body. In infants they may be flat and light-colored, but in the later period of childhood they may become elevated and more hyperpigmented. Lesions on the palmoplantar areas are usually more hyperkeratotic (*see* Figs. 1.78 and 1.79). The surface of epidermal nevus is hairless. However, angora hair nevus is a rare distinct variant of linear epidermal nevus with fine, white, long hairs.

1.2.1.3 Generalized Epidermal Nevus (Ichthyosis Hystrix)

Generalized epidermal nevus covers extensive areas of the trunk, extremities, and head bilaterally. The lesions are located along the lines of Blaschko, mostly symmetrically on both sides to a varying extent (*see* Figs. 1.80, 1.81, 1.82, 1.83 and 1.84) and typically stop sharply on the midline. Some lesions may be confluent (*see* Fig. 1.85). This subtype of the tumor is one of the most extensive benign tumors of the skin and causes serious cosmetic concern. Lesions on the intertriginous surfaces may sometimes be secondarily infected and malodorous. Large, unilateral or generalized epidermal nevi are usually diagnosed clinically. Generalized hyperkeratotic lesions in a similar pattern with generalized epidermal nevus may be observed in the early stage of incontinentia pigmenti, a rare genodermatosis. However, these lesions evolve into hyperpigmented macules, unlike the persistent hyperkeratotic lesions of epidermal nevus. Widespread lesions of epidermal nevus may rarely be a part of an epidermal nevus syndrome and in this case may be associated with involvement of other organs.

1.2 Hamartomas with Epidermal Differentiation

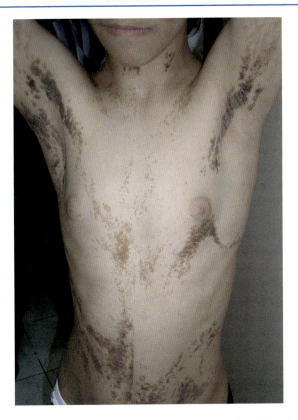

Fig. 1.80 Generalized epidermal nevus with typical bilateral involvement. Note the sharp demarcation on the midline

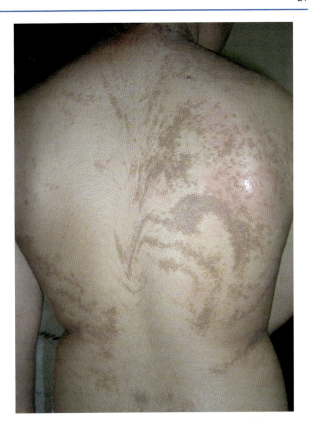

Fig. 1.82 Hyperkeratotic papular lesions forming swirls along the lines of Blaschko on the trunk, a characteristic feature of generalized epidermal nevus

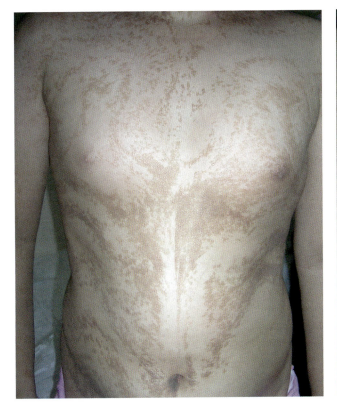

Fig. 1.81 Generalized epidermal nevus. Great majority of the trunk can be involved in some patients as seen in the figure

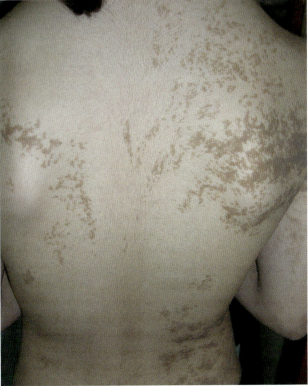

Fig. 1.83 Generalized epidermal nevus. The widely distributed lesions show linear configuration in some areas

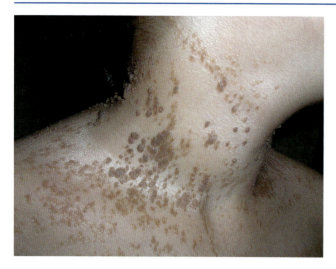

Fig. 1.84 Involvement of the neck in a patient with generalized epidermal nevus

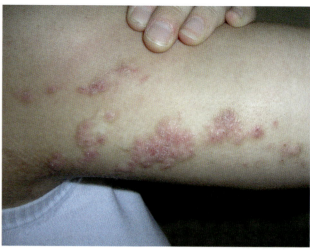

Fig. 1.86 ILVEN located on the arm. Erythematous, mild scaly plaques show a linear arrangement

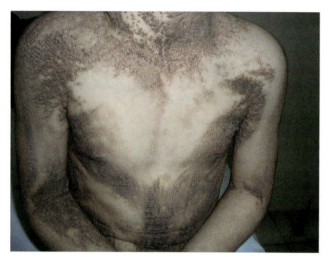

Fig. 1.85 Confluent dark-colored lesions of generalized epidermal nevus causing ichthyosis-like appearance in this case

Histopathologic features of epidermal nevus such as acanthosis, hyperkeratosis, and papillomatosis are not specific and are common in all clinical subtypes. There can be striking resemblance to seborrheic keratosis, acanthosis nigricans, or acrokeratosis verruciformis of Hopf. Clinicopathologic correlation confirms the diagnosis.

1.2.1.4 Inflammatory Linear Verrucous Epidermal Nevus (ILVEN)

A linear-shaped epidermal nevus with an inflammatory component is called ILVEN. This subtype of tumor is typically unilateral and mostly occurs on the extremities and the lower half of the body, especially the buttocks. It is more erythematous, scaly (see Fig. 1.86), and pruritic than classic (non-inflammatory) types of epidermal nevus. Thus, it can be misdiagnosed as some inflammatory disorders such as lichen striatus, psoriasis vulgaris, or lichen planus. Although these inflammatory dermatoses are mostly acquired, sometimes the distinction between these conditions can only be confirmed by histopathologic examination. Hyperkeratosis with alternating orto- and parakeratotic foci and psoriasiform epidermal hyperplasia are the main features of ILVEN. Scratching of the area may cause secondary bacterial infection. Lesions located on the acral region of the extremities may lead to destruction of the nails.

1.2.1.5 Epidermal Nevus Syndromes

Rarely an epidermal nevus may be a part of an epidermal nevus syndrome. The term epidermal nevus syndrome encompasses a heterogeneous group of syndromes characterized by epidermal or adnexal hamartomas associated with systemic involvement. Schimmelpenning-Feuerstein-Mims syndrome (see Figs. 1.87 and 1.88), Proteus syndrome (see Fig. 1.89), phacomatosis pigmentokeratotica, congenital hemidysplasia with ichthyosiform nevus and limb defects (CHILD) syndrome, angora hair nevus syndrome, nevus comedonicus syndrome, Becker nevus syndrome, and nevus sebaceus syndrome are classified under the term "epidermal nevus syndromes." Underlying genetic defects of some of these syndromes have been shown. It is well-known that classic (keratinocytic) epidermal nevi, especially nevus unius lateris and generalized epidermal nevus, may be associated with neurologic, skeletal, and other systemic manifestations. However, (keratinocytic) epidermal nevus syndrome is not accepted as a nosologic entity at this time. Epidermal nevus is among the well-known manifestations of Proteus syndrome, CHILD syndrome, and type II segmental Cowden disease.

Proteus syndrome is defined by skin tumors such as connective tissue nevus (plantar collagenoma), epidermal nevus, lipoma, vascular malformations, and overgrowth of

1.2 Hamartomas with Epidermal Differentiation

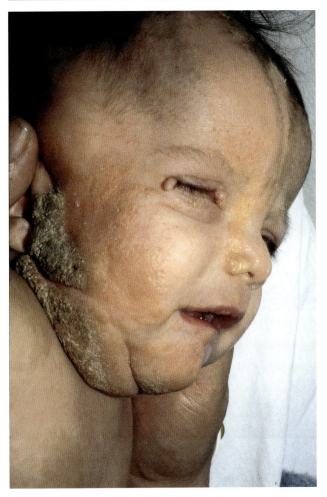

Fig. 1.87 Epidermal nevus syndrome of Schimmelpenning-Feuerstein-Mims syndrome type. The illustrated patient had unilateral facial lesions, showing clinically common features with epidermal nevus and nevus sebaceus, and additionally had neurologic and ocular findings

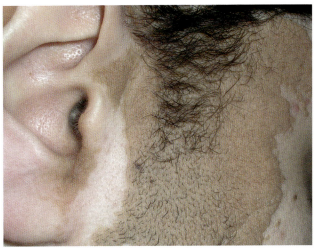

Fig. 1.88 Epidermal nevus syndrome of Schimmelpenning-Feuerstein-Mims syndrome type. Although partially hairy, the lesion was clinically typical for linear nevus sebaceus that was also confirmed with histopathologic examination

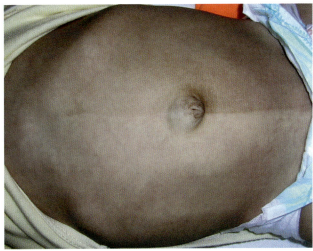

Fig. 1.89 Unilateral epidermal nevus on the trunk of a child with Proteus syndrome

multiple tissues. Epidermal nevus, which is seen in approximately 50 percent of cases, is soft and velvety (*see* Fig. 1.89).

CHILD (congenital hemidysplasia with ichthyosiform nevus and limb defects) syndrome is a very rare X-linked dominant disease characterized by ipsilateral hypoplasia of the limbs of varying severity and unilateral epidermal nevus. Inflammatory erythematous plaques are more commonly located on intertriginous areas and the vulva. Histologically, the epidermal nevus in CHILD syndrome shows psoriasis-like epidermal features and foamy lipid-laden histiocytes in the dermal papillae, a feature reminiscent of verruciform xanthoma. This nevus has a tendency to resolve spontaneously.

Type 2 segmental Cowden disease presents with a linear epidermal nevus, which is mostly thicker than classic lesions, shows a papillomatous surface, and is associated with focal segmental glomerulosclerosis.

Management. The size and location of the lesions are the major factors to be considered in the management of epidermal nevi. Although not associated with any serious complications, extensive lesions, especially those located on the face, neck, and extremities, can cause cosmetic distress. Destructive procedures including cryotherapy and electrocautery administered for epidermal nevus can lead to worse cosmetic results, and recurrence is possible on the intervention site (*see* Fig. 1.90). Only temporary improvement can be achieved by dermabrasion. Likewise, systemic retinoids have a temporary effect, with systemic side effects usually restricting their continuous use, especially in childhood.

Although radical surgery seems to be effective, full-thickness surgical excision is not feasible for large lesions, which can lead to undesirable scars and does not completely eliminate the risk of recurrence (*see* Fig. 1.91). Therefore, total excision can be performed only for small lesions and

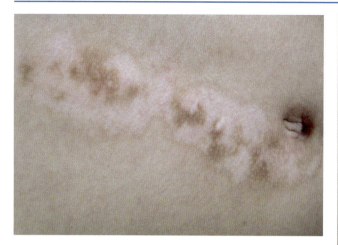

Fig. 1.90 Recurrence of epidermal nevus after cryotherapy. Note also the cryotherapy induced hypopigmentation

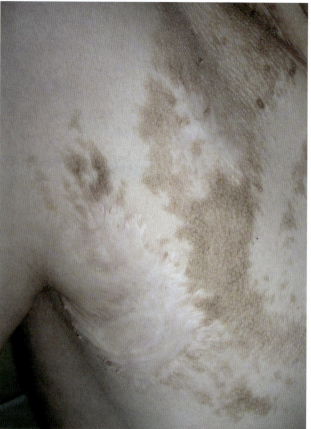

Fig. 1.92 Formation of scar on an area of previously excised epidermal nevus

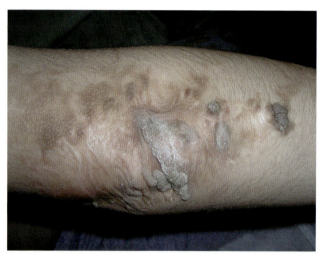

Fig. 1.91 Recurrence of epidermal nevus on site of previous excision

partial excision for the disturbing parts of the large tumors (*see* Fig. 1.92). Topical corticosteroids can be used for the relief of pruritus in ILVEN.

1.2.2 Nevus Sebaceus (Organoid Nevus)

Nevus sebaceus is a congenital hamartomatous lesion with concomitant abnormalities of the epidermis, hair follicles, sebaceous glands and sweat glands. It usually occurs sporadically and appears in less than 1 percent of neonates. It is primarily present at birth or appears in early childhood and follows a typical period of evolution. The initial presentation is usually a solitary round or oval, flat, smooth-surfaced yellowish or orange alopecic plaque of varying size (1 to 6 cm) (*see* Figs. 1.93, 1.94 and 1.95). Lesions may also be linear (*see* Figs. 1.96 and 1.97) or zosteriform (*see* Fig. 1.98)

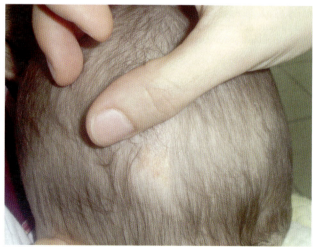

Fig. 1.93 Nevus sebaceus in early childhood. A quite flat, yellowish solitary alopecic plaque with smooth surface is seen

in configuration. The tumor most commonly occurs on the scalp (*see* Figs. 1.99 and 1.100) and face, especially on the frontotemporal region, cheeks (*see* Figs. 1.101 and 1.102), and retroauricular area (*see* Figs. 1.103 and 1.104). Other locations including the neck, sternal and interscapular

1.2 Hamartomas with Epidermal Differentiation

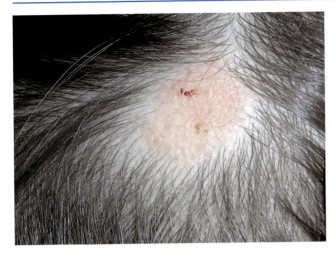

Fig. 1.94 Nevus sebaceus in childhood. A slightly elevated, round alopecic plaque with rough surface is seen

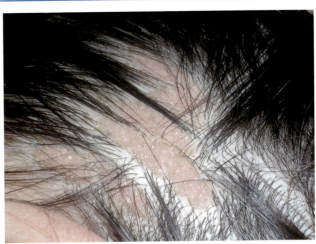

Fig. 1.97 Nevus sebaceus presenting as multiple linear plaques in a parallel distribution on the scalp

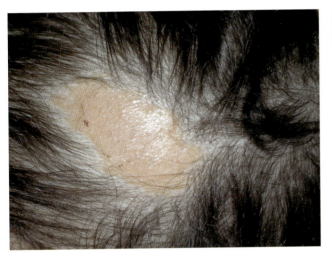

Fig. 1.95 Nevus sebaceus in childhood. A slightly elevated, oval-shaped, hairless plaque is seen

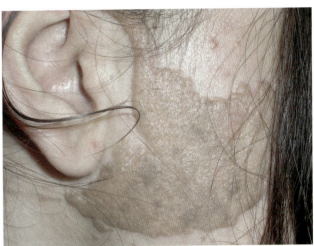

Fig. 1.98 Zosteriform nevus sebaceus extending from scalp to the cheek

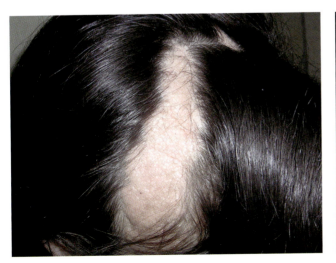

Fig. 1.96 A linear large alopecic plaque of nevus sebaceus

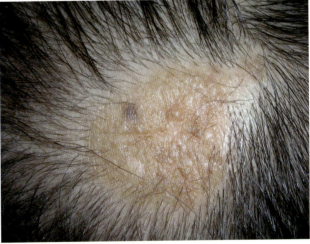

Fig. 1.99 A solitary yellowish plaque on the scalp measuring 2 to 3 cm; the most typical presentation of nevus sebaceus

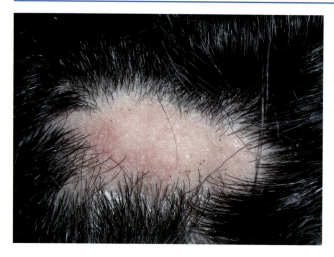

Fig. 1.100 Nevus sebaceus shown as a well-defined, yellowish, slightly elevated solitary plaque in an adult

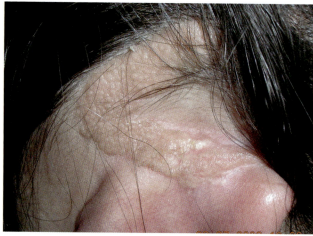

Fig. 1.103 Linear nevus sebaceus on the retroauricular area forming a V-shaped lesion

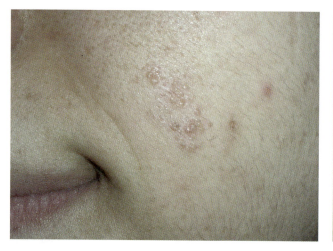

Fig. 1.101 Group of small yellow papules on the cheek. This is a kind of presentation of nevus sebaceus on the face

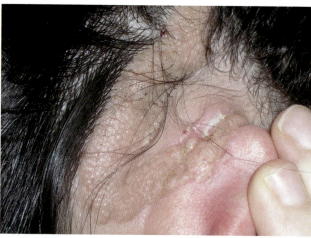

Fig. 1.104 Nevus sebaceus with a verrucous surface on the retroauricular area

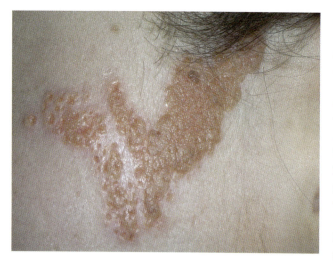

Fig. 1.102 Large linear nevus sebaceus on the face forming a V-shaped lesion

regions and the extremities are rare. Facial lesions may sometimes be observed as coalescing papules (see Fig. 1.105). Rarely, multiple lesions and plaques larger than 6 cm are observed. The size of the tumor grows proportionally with the child, and it may become elevated (see Fig. 1.106) at puberty, indicating sensitivity to androgens. The surface may become papillomatous, cobble-stoned, or sometimes verrucous (see Fig. 1.104). Lesions with a cerebriform appearance may rarely be encountered (see Fig. 1.107). Although asymptomatic, lesions may cause cosmetic concern. Moreover, scalp lesions may be disturbing when combing the hair.

A minority of patients, particularly those with extensive lesions, have epidermal nevus syndromes like nevus sebaceus syndrome or phacomatosis pigmentokeratotica. The characteristic of nevus sebaceus syndrome (Schimmelpenning-Feuerstein-Mims syndrome) is the linear

1.2 Hamartomas with Epidermal Differentiation

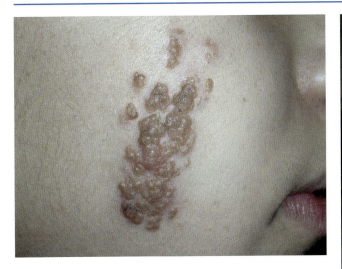

Fig. 1.105 Nevus sebaceus presenting as closely aggregated, dark yellow papules on the cheek

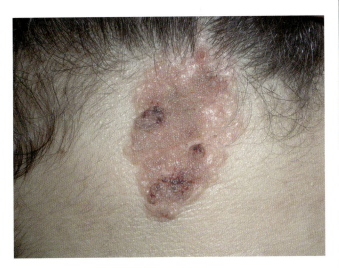

Fig. 1.106 Raised plaque of nevus sebaceus with an irregular surface

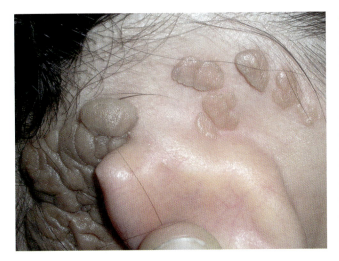

Fig. 1.107 Cerebriform nevus sebaceus on retroauricular area extending to the face; an unusual morphology

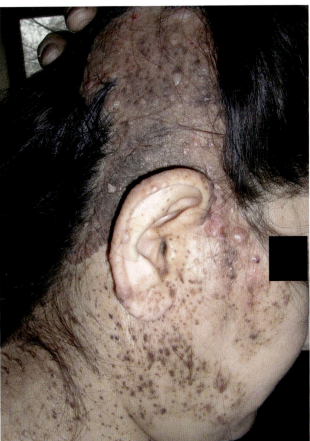

Fig. 1.108 Phakomatosis pigmentokeratotica. Extensive nevus sebaceus associated with nevus spilus is seen

pattern of nevus sebaceus that can be multiple or extensive. The large tumor is mostly located on the craniofacial area following Blaschko lines (see Figs. 1.87 and 1.88). Developmental abnormalities of the ocular, skeletal, neurologic, cardiovascular, and urinary system have been described as associated with this syndrome. Hemimegalencephaly with contralateral motor disease, seizures, developmental delay, and ocular anomalies (including lipodermoid of the conjunctiva and coloboma) are the main features. Vitamin D–resistant hypophosphatemic rickets may occur in these patients.

Phacomatosis pigmentokeratotica is characterized by nevus sebaceus associated with speckled lentiginous nevus (nevus spilus) of the papular type and systemic findings. Nevus sebaceus seen in the setting of phacomatosis pigmentokeratotica is commonly extensive and follows the lines of Blaschko (see Figs. 1.108 and 1.109); it is also associated with a high risk of development of basal cell carcinoma. The large nevus spilus usually shows a checkerboard pattern (see Fig. 3.226), and the darker or papular component may be absent in the infant age group. Neurologic findings such as segmental dysesthesia, seizures, hyperhidrosis in the area of nevus spilus, or musculoskeletal findings such as hemiatrophy with muscular weakness, scoliosis, or ocular abnormalities such as ptosis and strabismus

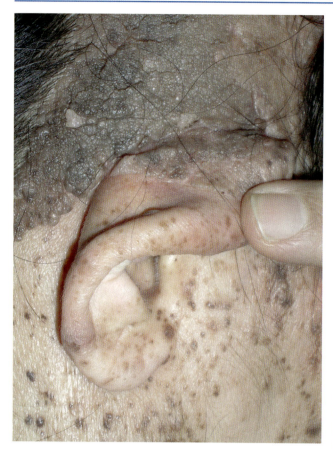

Fig. 1.109 Nevus sebaceus on the scalp and retroauricular area in a patient with phakomatosis pigmentokeratotica

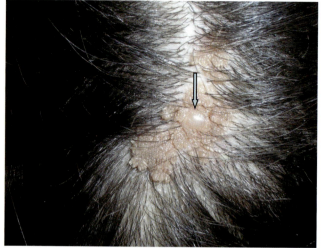

Fig. 1.110 Trichoblastoma arising on nevus sebaceus. Note the smooth-surfaced papule in the center of the mass of the nevus

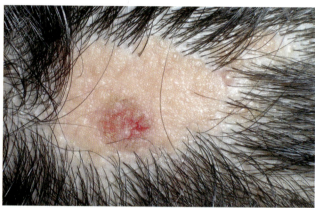

Fig. 1.111 Syringocystenoma papilliferum arising on nevus sebaceus. Note the nodule with verrucous surface in the center of the mass of the nevus

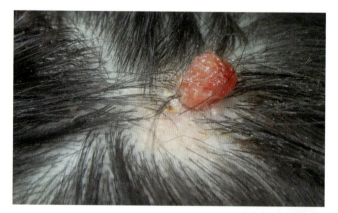

Fig. 1.112 A reddish exophytic tumor developing within nevus sebaceus. This lesion revealed both syringocystadenoma papilliferum and basal cell carcinoma on histopathological examination

are the extracutaneous manifestations of this rare syndrome. In rare instances, systemic findings are not present.

Aplasia cutis congenita, epidermal nevus, seborrheic keratosis (*see* Fig. 1.10), and verruca vulgaris may be considered in the differential diagnosis, but most lesions of nevus sebaceus are diagnosed clinically. Histopathology varies according to the age of the patient. In prepubertal patients acanthosis, papillomatosis, and abnormal pilosebaceous units are the main features. On post-pubertal biopsies epidermal changes become more prominent. Epidermal outgrowths are the result of striking acanthosis and papillomatosis. Prominent sebaceous lobules, and poorly formed pilar structures are closer to the epidermis, and numerous ectopic apocrine glands are also found.

Nevus sebaceus is frequently associated with numerous benign and malignant neoplasms. Secondary tumors occur, especially in adulthood. Trichoblastoma (*see* Fig. 1.110) and syringocystadenoma papilliferum (*see* Figs. 1.111 and 1.112) are the most common benign neoplasia reported to appear in nevus sebaceus. Other reported secondary benign tumors associated with nevus sebaceus are trichilemmoma, epidermoid cyst, melanocytic nevus, eccrine nevus, epidermal nevus, keratoacanthoma, acrochordon, syringoma, apocrine hydrocystoma, sebaceus adenoma, sebaceus epithelioma, spiradenoma, tubulopapillary hidradenoma, seborrheic keratosis (*see* Fig. 1.113), inverted follicular keratosis (*see* Fig. 1.114), and viral warts (*see* Figs. 1.115 and 1.116). Viral warts are usually in the form of filiform verruca and may be multiple. Sometimes more than one secondary tumor may be observed concomitantly on a nevus sebaceus (*see* Fig. 1.117).

1.2 Hamartomas with Epidermal Differentiation

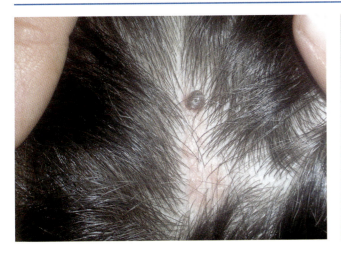

Fig. 1.113 Seborrheic keratosis arising on nevus sebaceus. Note the small pigmented papule on the upper part of the mass of the nevus

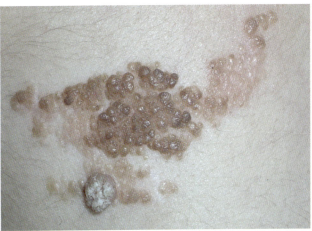

Fig. 1.116 Verruca filiformis arising on linear nevus sebaceus on the face. There is a solitary lesion on the lower part of the mass of the nevus

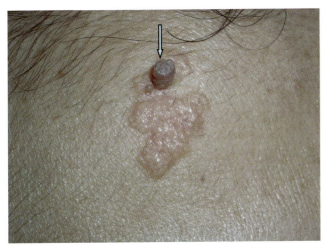

Fig. 1.114 Inverted follicular keratosis arising on nevus sebaceus. Note the small papule (*arrow*) on the upper part of the mass of the nevus

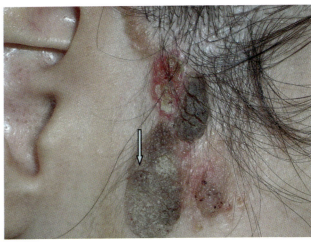

Fig. 1.117 Multiple secondary tumors may occur on the base of nevus sebaceus concomitantly. In the illustrated patient, seborrheic keratosis and trichoblastoma were diagnosed histopathologically. A typical seborrheic keratosis is seen at the left part of the lesion (*arrow*)

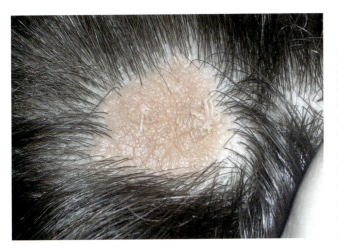

Fig. 1.115 Verruca filiformis developing within nevus sebaceus on the scalp. Irregularly distributed white filiform lesions are seen on the surface of the mass of the nevus

Malignant tumors arising in nevus sebaceus are rare. The most common malignant tumor developing on nevus sebaceus has generally been considered basal cell carcinoma (*see* Figs. 1.118 and 1.119). On the other hand, some trichoblastomas arising on nevus sebaceus may be misinterpreted as basal cell carcinomas. It may be difficult to differentiate trichoblastomas from basal cell carcinomas because both tumors have similar histopathologic features and may mimic each other clinically when they appear as pigmented papules or nodules (*see* Figs. 1.110, 1.118, and 1.119). Basal cell carcinomas on nevus sebaceus may sometimes be polypoid (*see* Fig. 1.119). Other reported malignancies associated with nevus sebaceus are squamous cell carcinoma, sebaceus carcinoma, apocrine carcinoma, porocarcinoma, trichilemmal carcinoma and malignant melanoma. Metastatic or locally aggressive carcinomas are very rare. The clinical features of secondary tumors

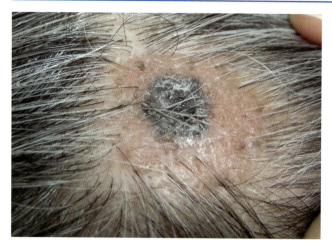

Fig. 1.118 Pigmented basal cell carcinoma arising on nevus sebaceus. Note centrally located pigmented nodule

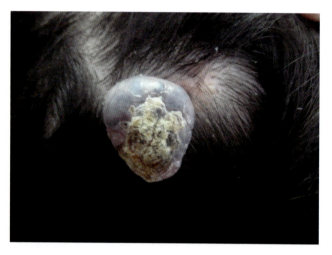

Fig. 1.119 A large polypoid basal cell carcinoma arising on nevus sebaceus in an adult patient. This is a rare morphology of basal cell carcinoma

on nevus sebaceus differ due to the variety of tumors. In general, asymmetric appearance should cause suspicion of a secondary neoplasm. Changes indicative of secondary tumors include hyperpigmented, hyperkeratotic, eroded, dome-shaped, filiform or pedunculated papules, nodules, erosions or ulcers. The distinction between the types of secondary tumors depends mainly on histopathologic examination.

Management. Routine examination of systemic involvement in nevus sebaceus patients is not indicated. However, when nevus sebaceus syndrome is suspected, especially in the presence of central nervous system findings, a complete physical examination and various investigations such as cranial/orbital magnetic resonance imaging, electroencephalogram, electrocardiogram, and ultrasonography of the abdomen and urinary system should be performed.

Nevus sebaceus can cause cosmetic disturbance when located on the face. Scalp tumors may be tolerated more easily. Although the risk is not very high, patients or parents of pediatric patients should be informed about the possibility of development of secondary malignant tumors. Destructive procedures like dermabrasion, electrocautery, cryotherapy, and ablative lasers cannot be considered as appropriate therapeutic alternatives for nevus sebaceus. While recurrence is common after these kinds of procedures, the risk of development of secondary tumors will still remain. Therefore complete surgical removal remains the single therapeutic alternative. However, cosmetic results may not be satisfactory in some cases, especially when lesions are located on the face.

Tumors that occur on nevus sebaceus are mostly benign, usually occur after adolescence, and can be detected during clinical follow-up. When considering the possibility of high morbidity related to excision in childhood, prophylactic excision of nevus sebaceus seems to be unnecessary in that age group. Likewise, the decision of removal of nevus sebaceus in adults is also uncertain unless the clinical signs are suggestive of malignant transformation. Patients with nevus sebaceus, especially adults, should be followed closely for above-mentioned clinical signs indicating the development of a secondary tumor on their nevi. However, even in the presence of such changes, it is still not easy to differentiate benign tumors from malignant ones. In such cases, an accurate diagnosis can be made after the histopathologic examination of an incisional biopsy specimen from the secondary tumor. When a secondary malignant tumor is diagnosed, nevus sebaceus should be excised totally. However, some secondary benign lesions like verrucae or seborheic keratosis can be treated with destructive modalities. On the other hand, the option of prophylactic excision of nevus sebaceus—although not considered to be urgent—should always be discussed with patients or parents.

1.2.3 Nevus Comedonicus

Nevus comedonicus is a hamartoma of the pilosebaceous unit characterized by dilated follicular openings containing keratin plugs that mimic comedones of acne. It is a rare type of benign epidermal tumor and is usually sporadic. It usually appears in childhood but may also be present at birth or arise during adulthood. It is most commonly located on the face, neck (*see* Fig. 1.120), and trunk. Other less common sites include the upper extremities, scalp (*see* Fig. 1.121), and palmoplantar region. Comedones containing darkly pigmented keratin coalesce to form irregularly shaped or linear plaques, sometimes with midline demarcation. There may be a single plaque or multiple plaques of nevus comedonicus affecting larger areas (*see* Fig. 1.122). In addition to comedones, inflammatory papules and larger cysts may also be observed (*see* Fig. 1.123). This tumor is usually asymptomatic but may be pruritic and painful if secondarily infected. In cases complicated by secondary bacterial infection and chronic inflammation, scarring is possible. Malignant degeneration is not seen. Epidermal nevus (*see* Fig. 1.75), nevus sebaceus

1.2 Hamartomas with Epidermal Differentiation

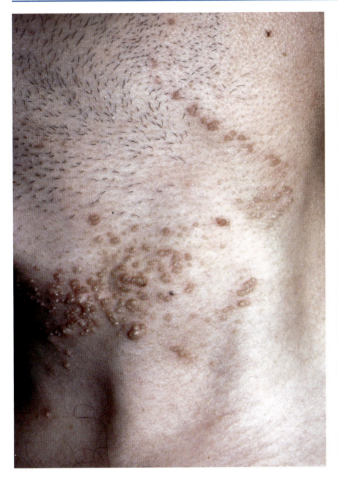

Fig. 1.120 Nevus comedonicus on the neck. Upper part of the lesion is linear in shape

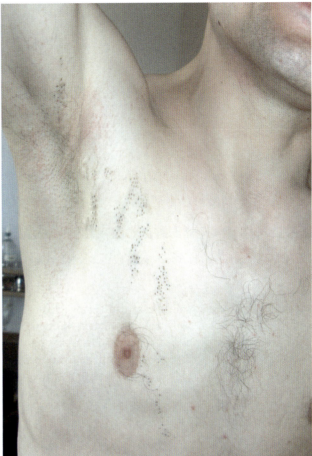

Fig. 1.122 Multiple plaques of nevus comedonicus on the chest and axilla

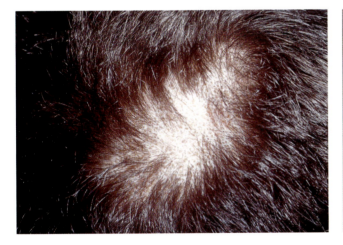

Fig. 1.121 Nevus comedonicus on the scalp. Note the comedones on the alopecic area

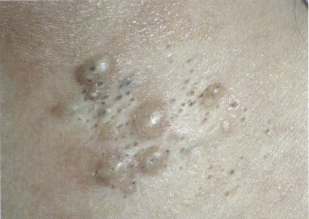

Fig. 1.123 Nevus comedonicus composed of grouped comedones and cysts

(*see* Fig. 1.102), basaloid follicular hamartoma, eruptive vellus hair cyst (*see* Fig. 4.56), and acneiform dermatoses may be considered in the differential diagnosis. Nevus comedonicus is mostly diagnosed clinically. Histologically, multiple dilated follicles, which are filled with keratin, are the main finding.

Nevus comedonicus syndrome, a very rare subtype of epidermal nevus syndromes, is characterized by nevus comedonicus associated with ipsilateral cataract, skeletal abnormalities such as hemivertebrae, and mental retardation.

Management. There is no satisfactory therapeutic alternative for nevus comedonicus. Topical keratolytic agents

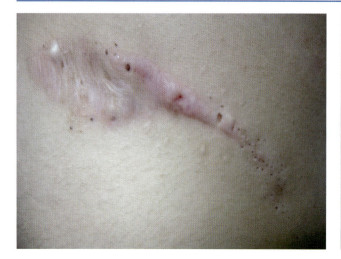

Fig. 1.124 Recurrence of nevus comedonicus on the excision site

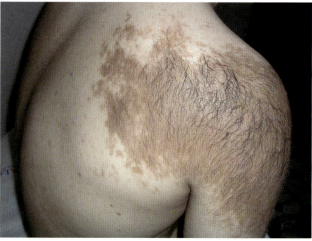

Fig. 1.125 Becker nevus located on the shoulder unilaterally

such as retinoids and salicylic acid or manual comedone extraction may provide only temporary relief. Systemic retinoids (isotretinoin) are also effective as long as they are continued, especially in the presence of inflammatory papules and cysts. Destructive methods may also be only temporarily effective. Therefore surgery remains the primary option. However, surgical removal of large lesions can be complicated by severe scarring, and local recurrence is quite possible (see Fig. 1.124).

1.2.4 Becker Nevus

Becker nevus is a hamartomatous lesion characterized by localized hyperpigmentation and hypertrichosis. The lesion is usually not noticed at birth. Faint hyperpigmentation at the outset becomes marked, together with the growth of hairs in puberty or in the second decade of life, possibly attributable to androgen sensitivity. Becker nevus is found in approximately 0.5 percent of young men and is about five times more frequent in males than in females. Occurrence is mostly sporadic but may sometimes be familial. This benign, asymptomatic, hamartomatous lesion typically appears on the upper half of the trunk or on the proximal upper extremities as a circumscribed brown patch associated with hypertrichosis (see Fig. 1.125). Most lesions are around the shoulder girdle (see Figs. 1.125 and 1.126). Lesions are typically localized on one site of the body but do not follow the lines of Blaschko (see Fig. 1.127). The size of the lesion is approximately 10 to 15 cm. The hyperpigmentation is uniform and sharply demarcated but has irregular outlines. The hairs are long and thick, especially in men. Acneiform lesions may occasionally appear within the nevus possibly related to local androgen sensitivity. Hyperpigmentation and hypertrichosis may overlap, but one of these components may be larger (see Fig. 1.128). Moreover, one of these features may

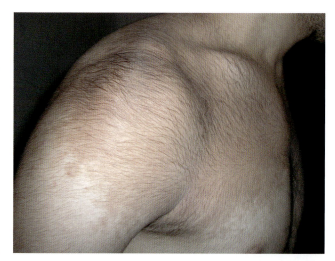

Fig. 1.126 Large brownish patch with hypertrichosis representing the typical appearance of Becker nevus

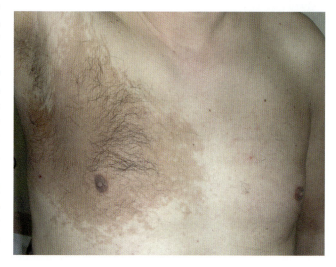

Fig. 1.127 Becker nevus unilaterally located on the chest. Note that the pigmented patch has an irregular outline

1.2 Hamartomas with Epidermal Differentiation

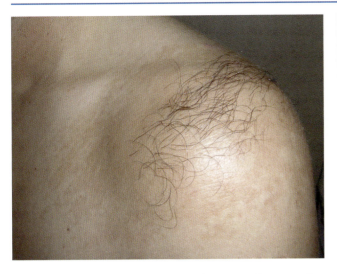

Fig. 1.128 Becker nevus. Hyperpigmentation covers a larger area than hypertrichosis in this patient

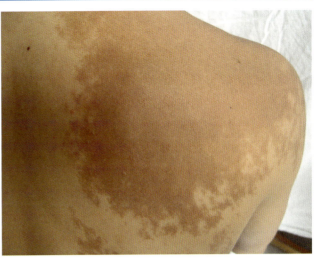

Fig. 1.130 Becker nevus presenting as hyperpigmented patch without hypertrichosis. Typical location of the lesion is helpful for diagnosis

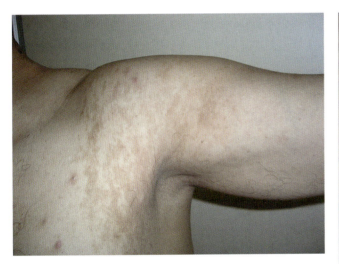

Fig. 1.129 Becker nevus without prominent hypertrichosis. Hypertrichosis may occur later than the macular component

sometimes appear later. If hypertrichosis is absent (see Figs. 1.129 and 1.130), Becker nevus may be confused with café-au-lait macules (see Fig. 3.34). Unlike large congenital melanocytic nevus (see Fig. 3.169), there is no palpable mass underlying the hairs.

All patients with Becker nevus do not present with the described classic features. Lesions may be seen at different locations, including the face, neck, lower trunk (see Fig. 1.131), and distal limbs (see Fig. 1.132). Although very rare, the nevus may be so giant that it may cause a serious cosmetic problem (see Figs. 1.133 and 1.134).

The typical clinical appearance is mostly sufficient for the diagnosis of Becker nevus. Histopathologic changes are subtle. There is mild acanthosis and elongation of rete ridges, accompanied by an increase in basilar melanin content. Melanocyte numbers are not increased.

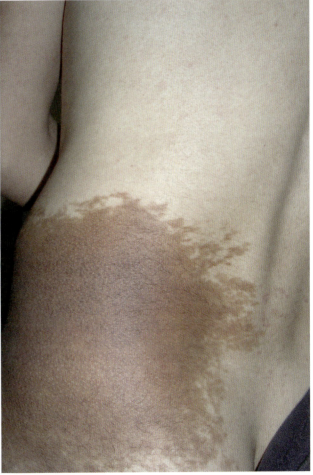

Fig. 1.131 Becker nevus on the flank, a relatively rare location

Becker nevus is usually not associated with any abnormalities or systemic disease. On the other hand, it may be associated with a smooth muscle hamartoma that can be

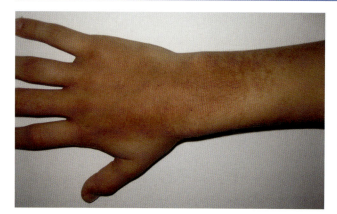

Fig. 1.132 Becker nevus on the lower arm. In this unusual location cosmetic concern may be higher

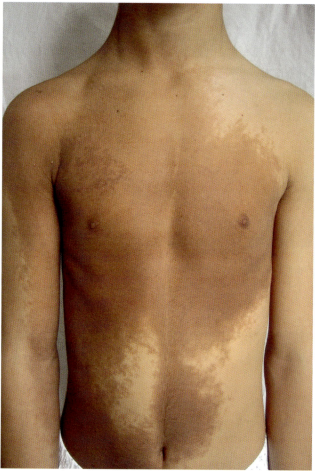

Fig. 1.134 Giant Becker nevus mainly located on one site of the trunk but also extending to the other site

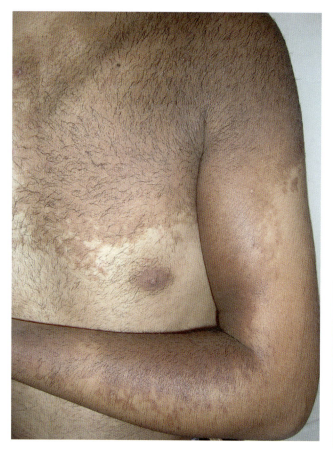

Fig. 1.133 Becker nevus unilaterally involving the chest and arm

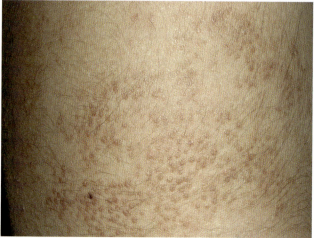

Fig. 1.135 Becker nevus associated with smooth muscle hamartoma. Tiny slightly hyperpigmented papules located on the upper arm are seen

observed as follicular papules on its surface (*see* Fig. 1.135). An increased number of smooth muscle fibers of the arrector pili may sometimes be observed only on histopathologic examination without causing any additional skin change.

Becker nevus syndrome is defined by Becker nevus associated with other anomalies of skin and muscular or skeletal defects. Ipsilateral hypoplasia of the breast is the most common anomaly, seen mostly in women. Skeletal anomalies including scoliosis, hypoplastic maxillofacial anomalies, and short limb are the main skeletal defects of this epidermal nevus syndrome. Ipsilateral shoulder girdle muscles may be hypoplastic.

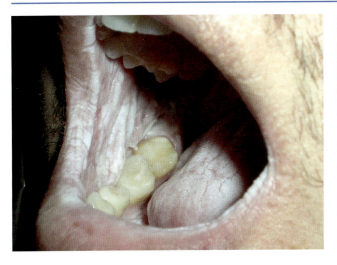

Fig. 1.136 White sponge nevus; typical diffuse white patch on the buccal mucosa. Patients are usually otherwise healthy

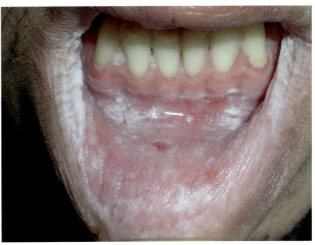

Fig. 1.137 White sponge nevus causing white patches on the labial mucosa and gingivae. The lesion developed from childhood onward

Management. Becker nevus does not have any malignant potential, and therapy is not obligatory. However, especially dense hairy lesions may bother some patients cosmetically and they may demand therapy. Classic surgical excision may cause unsightly scars and is not an alternative. Various methods, including simple shaving, epilation, lasers or bleaching, can be used in the management of hypertrichosis. Lasers (Er:YAG, Q-switched Ruby) can also be effective for hyperpigmentation.

1.3 White Sponge Nevus

White sponge nevus is an uncommon, autosomal-dominant inherited disorder restricted to the mucous membranes. Mutations in the keratin 4 and keratin 13 genes are possibly related to the development of the familial cases. However, a family history is not always present. The lesion may be present at birth or may appear in childhood or adolescence. The oral mucosa is predominantly involved, especially the buccal (*see* Fig. 1.136) and labial mucosae (*see* Fig. 1.137). However, the ventral surface of the tongue, floor of the mouth, and soft palate may also be involved. Lesions on the gingival margin and dorsal surface of the tongue (*see* Fig. 1.138) are rarer. White sponge nevus appears as white, patchy, or diffuse thick plaques that are spongy on palpation. Sometimes involvement of nearly the whole oral mucosa can be seen (*see* Fig. 1.139). Occasionally, nasal, laryngeal, esophageal, vaginal, and rectal mucosal surfaces are affected. However, extramucosal involvement or an association with other diseases is not seen. Although most lesions are asymptomatic, in some instances there may be a burning sensation, roughness, or dryness.

Clinical differential diagnosis of white sponge nevus includes various disorders of the oral mucosa that present with white lesions such as candidiasis, homogeneous

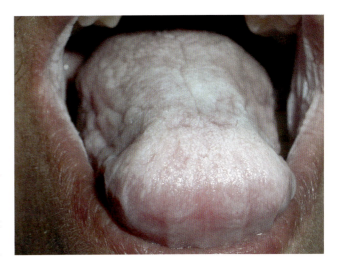

Fig. 1.138 Diffuse involvement of the tongue in a patient with white sponge nevus

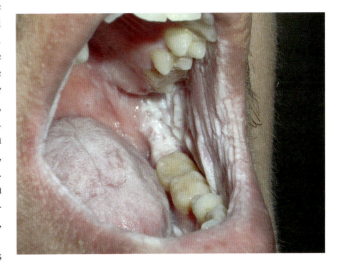

Fig. 1.139 White patches and plaques of white sponge nevus involved the oral mucosa in a diffuse pattern

leukoplakia (*see* Fig. 2.47), leukoedema, lichen planus, nicotine stomatitis, and frictional hyperkeratosis. Some hereditary conditions like dyskeratosis congenita (*see* Fig. 2.35), Howel-Evans syndrome (*see* Fig. 2.36), pachyonychia congenita (*see* Fig. 2.37), and hereditary benign intraepithelial dyskeratosis may also cause similar diffuse persistent white plaques on oral mucosa. Histologically the mucosal squamous epithelium is thickened and prominent intracellular edema gives the cytoplasm of keratinocytes a clear appearance. However, the characteristic histologic feature for the diagnosis is perinuclear eosinophilic cytoplasmic condensation. Among the above-mentioned disorders, the main clinical and histopathologic challenge is leukoedema. The typical distinguishing clinical feature of these two disorders is the clearance of leukoedema when the mucosal lesion is stretched. In contrast, lesions of white sponge nevus are persistent. Hereditary conditions can usually be differentiated by their accompanying skin lesions and systemic manifestations. Since malignant degeneration of white sponge nevus is not described, it is important to distinguish it from premalignant mucosal lesions like leukoplakia.

Management. When the diagnosis is certain following histopathologic examination, there is no need to search for any systemic findings. Therapy is not indicated for asymptomatic lesions. However, in symptomatic cases therapy is usually required. Although the mechanism of action is not definite, topical or systemic administration of antibiotics may be tried. Topical application of tetracycline or systemic administration of penicillin, ampicillin, amoxicillin, or tetracycline may be useful, especially in reducing the symptoms or in some instances causing clearance of the lesions. But recurrence is possible after cessation of therapy.

Suggested Reading

Al Aboud K, Al Hawsawi K. Becker nevus on the hand. Eur J Dermatol. 2002;12:588.

Alfadley A, Hainau B, Al Robaee A, Banka N. Becker's melanosis: a report of 12 cases with atypical presentation. Int J Dermatol. 2005;44:20–4.

Alpsoy E, Yilmaz E, Aykol A. Hyperkeratosis of the nipple: report of two cases. J Dermatol. 1997;24:43–5.

Bahcekapili D, Baykal C, Buyukbabani N, Saglik E. Nevus sabaceus associated with seborrheic keratosis. J Eur Acad Dermatol Venereol. 2006;20:875.

Baykal C, Buyukbabani N, Kavak A, Alper M. Nevoid hyperkeratosis of the nipple and areola: a distinct entity. J Am Acad Dermatol. 2002;46:414–8.

Baykal C, Buyukbabani N, Yazganoglu KD, Saglik E. Tumors associated with nevus sebaceous. J Dtsch Dermatol Ges. 2006;4:28–31.

Bayramgurler D, Bilen N, Apaydin R, Ercin C. Nevoid hyperkeratosis of the nipple and areola: treatment of two patients with topical calcipotriol. J Am Acad Dermatol. 2002;46:131–3.

Bolognia JL, Jorizzo JL, Schaffer JV. Dermatology, edn 3. London: Mosby; 2012.

Burgdorf WHC, Plewig G, Wolff HH, Landthaler M. Braun-Falco's dermatology, edn 3. Italy: Springer-Verlag; 2009.

Calonje JE, Brenn T, Lazar AJ, McKee PH. McKee's pathology of the skin, edn 4. China: Elsevier; 2012.

Caputo R, Tadini G. Atlas of genodermatoses. Spain: Taylor and Francis; 2006.

Chantorn R, Shwayder T. Phacomatosis pigmentokeratotica: a further case without extracutaneous anomalies and review of the condition. Pediatr Dermatol. 2011;28:715–9.

Cribier B, Scrivener Y, Grosshans E. Tumors arising in nevus sebaceus: a study of 596 cases. J Am Acad Dermatol. 2000;42:263–8.

Elder DE, Elenitsas R, Johnson BL, Murphy GF, Xu X. Lever's histopathology of the skin, edn 10. Philadelphia: Lippincott Williams and Wilkins; 2008.

Ferreira MJ, Bajanca R, Fiadeiro T. Congenital melanosis and hypertrichosis in bilateral distribution. Pediatr Dermatol. 1998;15:290–2.

Fink AM, Filz D, Krajnik G, et al. Seborrhoeic keratoses in patients with internal malignancies: a case–control study with prospective accrual of patients. J Eur Acad Dermatol Venereol. 2009;23: 1316–9.

Furue M, Kohda F, Duan H, et al. Spontaneous regression of multiple seborrheic keratoses associated with nasal carcinoma. Clin Exp Dermatol. 2001;26:705–9.

Glinick SE, Alper JC, Bogaars H, Brown JA. Becker's melanosis: associated abnormalities. J Am Acad Dermatol. 1983;9:509–14.

Happle R. The group of epidermal nevus syndromes, Part I. Well defined phenotypes. J Am Acad Dermatol. 2010;63:1–22.

Husain Z, Ho JK, Hantash BM. Sign and pseudo-sign of Leser-Trelat: case reports and a review of the literature. J Drugs Dermatol. 2013;12:e79–87.

James WD, Berger T, Elston D. Andrew's diseases of the skin: clinical dermatology, edn 11. China: Saunders Elsevier; 2011.

Jaqueti G, Requena L, Sánchez Yus E. Trichoblastoma is the most common neoplasm developed in nevus sebaceus of Jadassohn: a clinicopathologic study of a series of 155 cases. Am J Dermatopathol. 2000;22:108–18.

Krishnan RS, Angel TA, Roark TR, Hsu S. Nevoid hyperkeratosis of the nipple and/or areola: a report of two cases and a review of the literature. Int J Dermatol. 2002;41:775–7.

Lamey PJ, Bolas A, Napier SS, et al. Oral white naevus: response to antibiotic therapy. Clin Exp Dermatol. 1998;23:59–63.

Lim C. Seborrheic keratoses with associated lesions: a retrospective analysis of 85 lesions. Australas J Dermatol. 2006;47:109–13.

MacKie RM. Skin cancer: an illustrated guide to aetiology, clinical features, pathology and management of benign and malignant cutaneous tumors, edn 2. England: Martin Dunitz; 1996.

Miller CJ, Ioffreda MD, Billingsley EM. Sebaceous carcinoma, basal cell carcinoma, trichoadenoma, trichoblastoma, and syringocystadenoma papilliferum arising within a nevus sebaceus. Dermatol Surg. 2004;30(12 Pt 2):1546–9.

Miller CS, Craig RM Jr. White corrugated mucosa. J Am Dent Assoc. 1988;117:345–6.

Otley CC, Stasko T. Skin disease in organ transplantation. Hong Kong: Cambridge University Press; 2008.

Otobe IF, de Sousa SO, Matthews RW, et al. Successful treatment with topical tetracycline of oral white spongy nevus occurring in a patient with systemic lupus erythematosus. Int J Dermatol. 2006;45: 1130–1.

Patil K, Mahima VG, Srikanth HS. White spongy nevus: a nonhereditary presentation. J Indian Soc Pedod Prev Dent. 2008;26:125–7.

Regezi JA, Sciubba JJ, Jordan RCK. Oral pathology. Clinical pathologic correlations, edn 4. St. Louis: Saunders; 2003.

Shah KR, Boland CR, Patel M, et al. Cutaneous manifestations of gastrointestinal disease: part I. J Am Acad Dermatol. 2013;68: 189.e1–21.

Sugarman JL. Epidermal nevus syndromes. Semin Cutan Med Surg. 2007 ;26:221–30.

Warnke PH, Hauschild A, Schimmelpenning GW, et al. The sebaceous nevus as part of the Schimmelpenning-Feuerstein-Mims syndrome—an obvious phacomatosis first documented in 1927. J Cutan Pathol. 2003;30:470–2.

Weedon D. Weedon's skin pathology, edn 3. China: Elsevier; 2010.

Yazganoglu KD, Erbudak E, Buyukbabani N, Baykal C. Tanınız nedir?: Beyaz süngersi nevus. Turk J Dermatol. 2010;4:114–6.

Epidermal Precancerous Lesions and In Situ Malignancies

The main topic of this chapter is the skin and mucosal lesions that mainly show histologic epithelial dysplasia and have the potential of evolving into keratinocytic epidermal malignancies. Different clinical presentations include actinic keratosis, Bowen disease, erythroplasia of Queyrat, leukoplakia, and actinic cheilitis. All are accepted as in situ carcinomas and possible precursors of squamous cell carcinoma.

In addition, arsenical keratosis may evolve into lesions showing epithelial dysplasia. Chronic radiodermatitis is another precancerous lesion affecting both the epidermis and dermis histologically. Keratoacanthoma, another topic of this chapter, is a tumor that can be considered between benign and malignant. Paget disease and extramammary Paget disease may be accepted as intraepidermal metastases and are included in this chapter. However, their morbidity is not associated with cutaneous involvement but related to the underlying malignancies. Cutaneous horn is a benign lesion developing as a result of increased keratin. Because it may overlie precancerous lesions and malignant skin tumors, it may be a marker of underlying cutaneous malignancy. In summary, a large spectrum of skin diseases is discussed in this chapter.

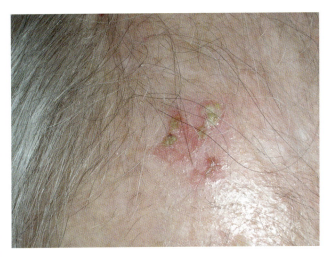

Fig. 2.1 Actinic keratosis on the forehead. Sun-exposed areas of the face are predilection sites

2.1 Actinic Keratosis (Solar Keratosis)

Actinic keratosis is a very common problem of fair-skinned individuals and has low malignant potential. Cumulative sun damage is the main underlying cause. Therefore, it is more common in individuals with outdoor occupations and who live in sunny climates. Typically, patients also show other features of ultraviolet-related skin changes such as telangiectasia and actinic lentigo.

Sunlight-exposed areas, especially the face, the V of the neck and dorsum of the hands are more commonly involved. The forehead (*see* Fig. 2.1), cheeks (*see* Fig. 2.2), and nose (*see* Fig. 2.3) are typical locations on the face. The upper part of the helix is the preferred site on the ears. The scalp of bald men is another common area of actinic keratosis (*see* Fig. 2.4). Involvement of the lower lip is relatively common in women.

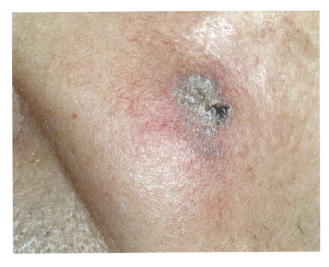

Fig. 2.2 Actinic keratosis on the cheek. This lesion was palpable

Lesions generally begin after middle age and their frequency increases with age. However, in patients with xeroderma pigmentosum, actinic keratoses begin to occur in childhood.

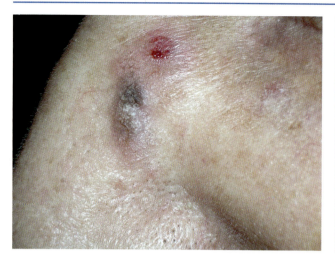

Fig. 2.3 Actinic keratosis on the nose, a predilected site

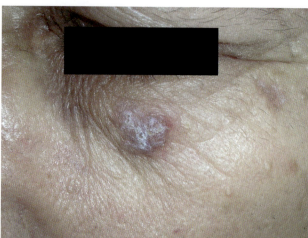

Fig. 2.5 Actinic keratosis presenting as a slightly elevated lesion measuring 1 cm located on the cheek

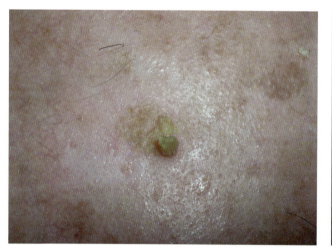

Fig. 2.4 Multiple actinic keratoses on the sun-damaged scalp of a bald man. An overlying cutaneous horn is also noticeable

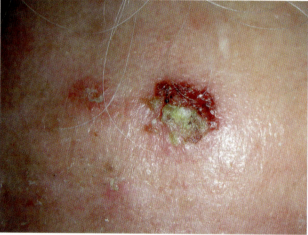

Fig. 2.6 Small and large actinic keratoses are seen concomitantly on scalp

Patients frequently have multiple lesions, but solitary lesions may also be seen. The size of the tumor is variable. Erythematous or flesh-colored, discrete, flat, or slightly elevated lesions that measure 3 to 10 mm in diameter (*see* Figs. 2.5 and 2.6) are more common, but larger lesions (*see* Fig. 2.7) or plaques (*see* Fig. 2.8) may also be found. Actinic keratoses may have yellow- or brown-colored, hard, adherent scales on their surfaces (*see* Fig. 2.9). Very early lesions may show no other features but a rough surface that can be felt on palpation. Borders of the lesions may be sharply demarcated (*see* Fig. 2.10) or indistinct (*see* Fig. 2.11). Lesions may be extensive in some anatomic areas and show confluence, causing eczema-like clinical appearance (*see* Fig. 2.12).

Some lesions may be brown-colored and called pigmented actinic keratosis (*see* Fig. 2.13). They may be clinically confused with actinic lentigo (*see* Fig. 3.18), a flat type of seborrheic keratosis, and lentigo maligna (*see* Fig. 12.8) but show no different biological behavior than nonpigmented actinic keratoses. Lesions may be thicker, especially on the forearms, lower legs, and hands (*see* Fig. 2.14). They are called hypertrophic actinic keratosis and may be confused with seborrheic keratosis (*see* Fig. 1.39) and verrucae. Sometimes a cutaneous horn may develop on the lesion.

Discoid lupus erythematosus is a differential diagnostic consideration, especially in the presence of scaly lesions. Disseminated superficial actinic porokeratosis presents as multiple sharply demarcated lesions on the sun-exposed sites and can also be considered in the differential diagnosis of multiple actinic keratoses. Some actinic keratoses can be mistaken for Bowen disease (*see* Fig. 2.22). Actinic keratoses on the face may also be confused with facial lesions of superficial basal cell carcinoma (*see* Fig. 11.51).

Actinic keratoses are usually persistent, and spontaneous regression is rare. Rapid enlargement, induration, pronounced

2.1 Actinic Keratosis (Solar Keratosis)

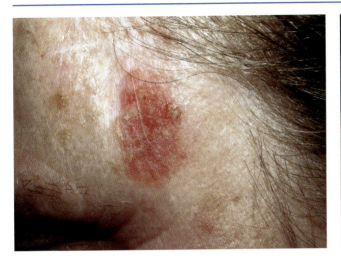

Fig. 2.7 A large lesion of actinic keratosis on the forehead

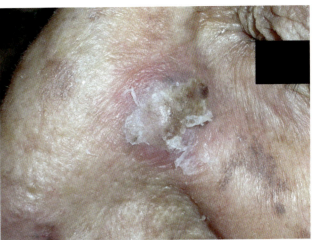

Fig. 2.9 Actinic keratosis presenting with thick adherent scales on a reddish base

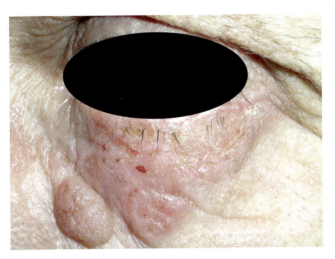

Fig. 2.8 Actinic keratosis as a plaque on the lower eyelid. A seborrheic keratosis on the adjacent area is also seen

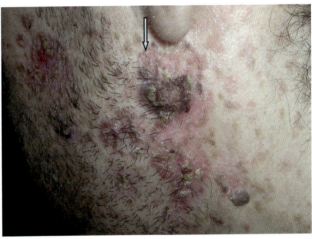

Fig. 2.10 Multiple sharply demarcated lesions of actinic keratosis. Note that one of them is slightly elevated (*arrow*)

hyperkeratosis, nodularity, erosion, and ulceration may be signs of malignant degeneration (*see* Fig. 2.15) that necessitate histopathologic confirmation. Biopsy can be performed to rule out other diseases causing diagnostic confusion or to eliminate invasive squamous cell carcinoma. Irregular acanthotic epidermis with epithelial dysplasia showing nuclear atypia and dyskeratosis is the main histologic picture of actinic keratosis. Alternating orthokeratotic hyperkeratosis and parakeratosis are also typical findings. The clinically normal tissue surrounding the lesion may also be histologically abnormal which has been described as "field cancerization".

Management. Although the exact risk and timing of malignant degeneration of actinic keratosis are not clear, the risk of invasive squamous cell carcinoma cannot be disregarded; therefore, it should be treated. In addition, as it is a marker of sun damage, patients should also be evaluated and followed for other ultraviolet-induced skin neoplasia.

Transplant recipients and other patients on immunosuppressive therapy such as cyclosporine have a higher risk of malignant transformation of actinic keratosis. Sun protection prevents the occurrence of new actinic keratoses and is mandatory for all patients with actinic keratoses.

The therapy is planned either for individual lesions or for "field cancerization", namely clearance of subclinical lesions. The number of lesions is important in determining the therapy. Topical medications are mostly used in patients with multiple lesions. Mild to moderate local adverse effects such as inflammatory erythema (*see* Fig. 2.16a) or erosion and crusting (*see* Fig. 2.17a) may occur during therapy with imiquimod cream, an immune response modifier. Topical 5-fluorouracil, a cytostatic agent, may cause an intense inflammatory reaction of the lesions and the surrounding skin. These inflammatory changes resolve after cessation of therapy (*see* Fig. 2.16b and 2.17b). Both topical

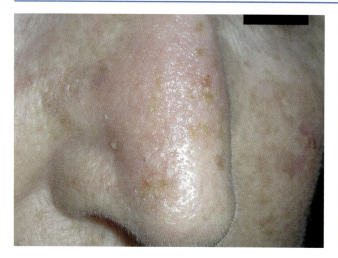

Fig. 2.11 Multiple ill-defined flat lesions of actinic keratosis on the nose

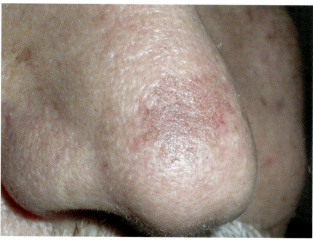

Fig. 2.13 Pigmented actinic keratosis

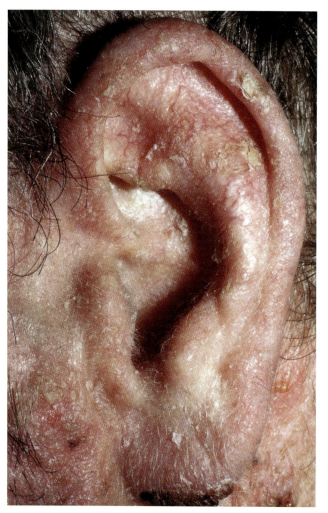

Fig. 2.12 Multiple actinic keratoses showing tendency to confluence on the auricle

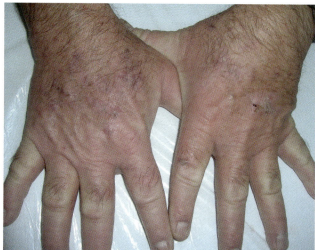

Fig. 2.14 Multiple actinic keratoses on the dorsum of the hands in a patient with severe sun-damage

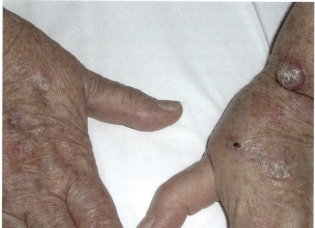

Fig. 2.15 Extensive actinic keratoses on the dorsum of the hands and a squamous cell carcinoma (dome-shaped nodule) on the wrist (*right*) are seen concomitantly

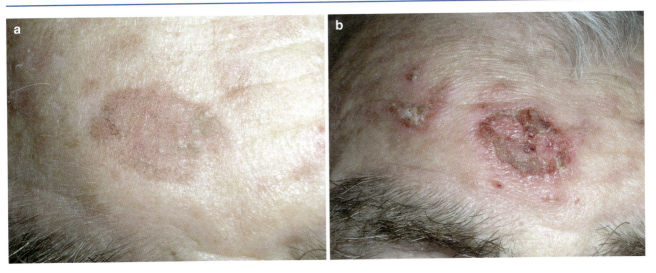

Fig. 2.16 (a) A large actinic keratosis on the forehead. (b) Lesion showed erosion and crusting during therapy with imiquimod cream (*right*). Note the formerly inconspicuous lesions have become noticeable after therapy (*left*)

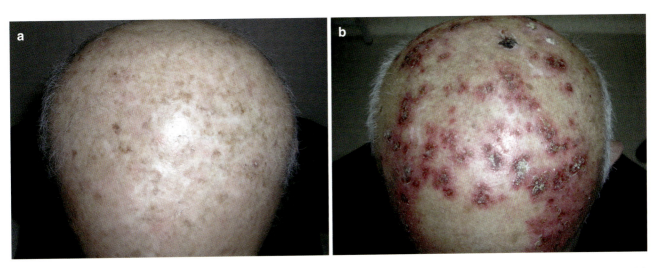

Fig. 2.17 (a) Extensive actinic keratoses on the scalp of a bald man. (b) Severe perilesional inflammatory erythema occurred during therapy with imiquimod cream (*right*)

imiquimod and topical 5-fluorouracil may also delineate lesions that were formerly unobserved (see Fig. 2.16a and b). Diclofenac, a nonsteroidal anti-inflammatory drug, can also be used topically mostly in mild lesions. Duration of therapy with ingenol mebutate, a plant derivate, is generally shorter than other topical drugs. Resiquimod, a toll-like receptor 7 and 8 agonist may be another option for field cancerization in addition to imiquimod and 5-fluorouracil. A DNA repair enzyme, T4 endonuclease 5 may be applied topically in liposomes to prevent the development of actinic keratoses in the setting of xeroderma pigmentosum.

Destructive methods are used when there is no doubt about the diagnosis. Cryotherapy is the most preferred one in patients with few small lesions. However, dyspigmentation may be observed on lesion sites after therapy. Photodynamic therapy and curettage combined with electrocautery can be other alternatives for multiple lesions. Carbondioxide laser is preferred for a single lesion.

Surgery is not a first-line therapeutic option of actinic keratosis and is usually preferred for solitary and therapy-resistant lesions. However, it also allows for a histopathologic examination. Sometimes various methods are combined. There is a risk of development of new lesions after all therapeutic methods, so patients should be followed for life.

2.2 Bowen Disease

Bowen disease is an in situ carcinoma of the skin, usually presenting as a slow-growing solitary lesion. It is derived from the epidermal or adnexal keratinocytes. In addition to the epidermis it may also involve the full depth of the hair follicle,

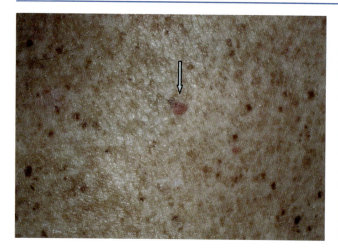

Fig. 2.18 Bowen disease presenting as an erythematous papule (*arrow*) on the trunk of a patient treated long term with PUVA. Note also the associated PUVA lentigines

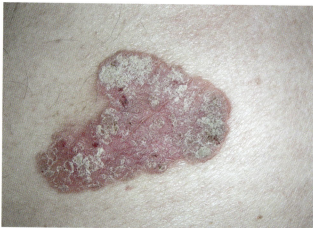

Fig. 2.20 Typical solitary plaque of Bowen disease on the trunk

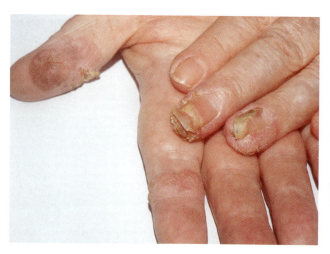

Fig. 2.19 Polydacytlous Bowen disease; involvement of multiple fingers and periungual areas are shown

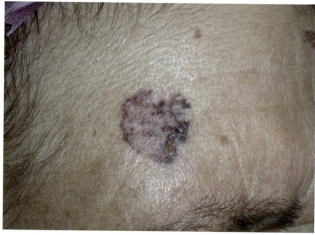

Fig. 2.21 Solitary plaque of Bowen disease on the face showing focal hyperpigmentation and crusting

creating a therapeutic challenge. It invades the underlying dermis, namely shows carcinomatous transformation only in a small subset of cases. It is more common in fair-skinned patients and seen preferentially on the sun-exposed areas of the skin. It may be seen together with other signs of actinic damage. Long-term use of PUVA (psoralen + ultraviolet A) therapy may also induce Bowen disease (*see* Fig. 2.18). On the other hand, Bowen disease may occur on covered sites, including the genitalia. High-risk types of HPV may play a role in the etiology of genital lesions. These types of HPV may also be associated with lesions on periungual areas (*see* Fig. 2.19). Chronic arsenic ingestion is a well-known cause of multiple lesions, especially located on the palms, soles, and non–sun-exposed areas of the body except for the genitalia. Although it has been formerly suggested that Bowen disease is a possible marker of visceral malignancies, this claim has not been confirmed later.

Bowen disease is a tumor of adulthood, predominantly seen in the elderly population. It may occur anywhere on the skin but is seen more commonly on the trunk (*see* Fig. 2.20), head (*see* Fig. 2.21), neck, and lower legs. Hands (*see* Fig. 2.22), fingers (*see* Fig. 2.23), and the palmoplantar area (*see* Fig. 2.24) may also be involved. Typically a solitary lesion is found, but multiple tumors may also be observed. A slightly elevated, sharply demarcated, pink or reddish, thin plaque with an irregular outline measuring 1 to 4 cm in diameter is usually observed at the time of the diagnosis (*see* Fig. 2.25). The surface of the lesion may show foci of mild scaling, crusting, fissures, or dyspigmentation. Less commonly Bowen disease may manifest as erythematous persistent papules (*see* Fig. 2.18). Most lesions are asymptomatic. Bowen disease may rarely be hyperpigmented (*see* Figs. 2.21 and 2.26), mimicking melanoma (*see* Fig. 12.18). Lesions of bowenoid papulosis on the

2.2 Bowen Disease

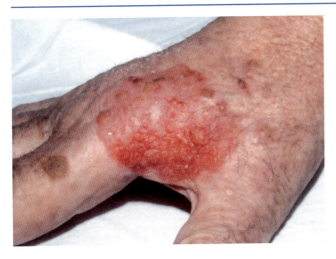

Fig. 2.22 Bowen disease on the back of the hand

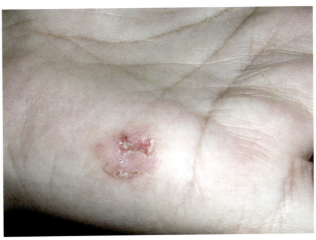

Fig. 2.24 Palmar plaque due to Bowen disease; a rare presentation

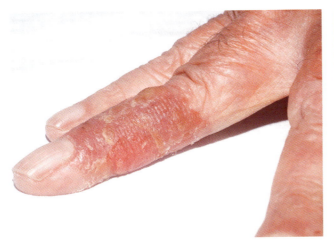

Fig. 2.23 Solitary sharply demarcated erythematous plaque of Bowen disease on the finger

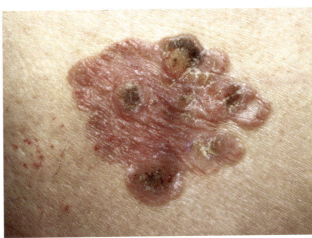

Fig. 2.25 Sharply demarcated reddish plaque with irregular outline; a classic appearance of Bowen disease

genital area, which are mostly hyperpigmented, may be considered as lesions between genital warts and Bowen disease (see Figs. 2.27 and 2.28).

The clinical presentation of the lesions may show differences depending on the location. Bowen disease found on intertriginous locations such as the axillae, interdigital area, perianal area (see Fig. 2.29a), and perigenital area may be moist, macerated, and nonscaly. Presentation of anogenital lesions may be erythroplasia-like, verrucous (see Figs. 2.30 and 2.31), or polypoid. It should also be kept in mind that even verrucous plaques of Bowen disease may only show intra-epidermal dysplasia histologically.

The lesions with prominent scales may be initially misdiagnosed as an inflammatory dermatosis such as psoriasis vulgaris or nummular eczema. Hyperkeratotic and verrucous lesions may mimic seborrheic keratosis (see Fig. 1.11) and

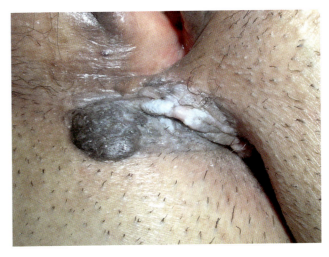

Fig. 2.26 Hyperpigmented Bowen disease on the perigenital area

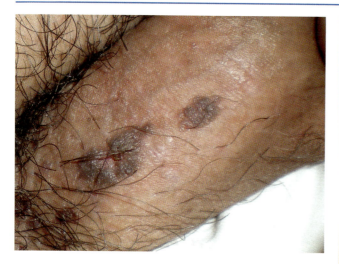

Fig. 2.27 Bowenoid papulosis presenting as hyperpigmented papules on the shaft of the penis

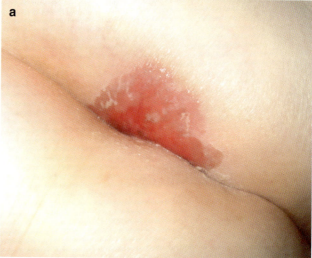

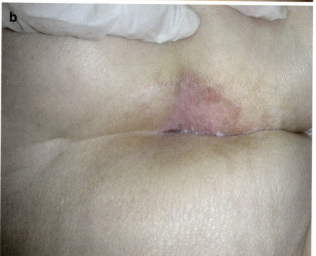

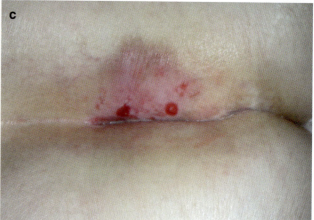

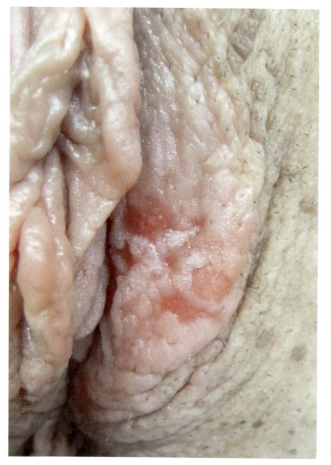

Fig. 2.28 Bowenoid papulosis on the vulva in an immune-suppressed patient. Note the multiple hyperpigmented papules and secondary erosions

Fig. 2.29 (**a**) Perianal Bowen disease; an eroded, non-scaly plaque is seen. (**b**) Regression with topical imiquimod therapy. (**c**) Recurrence as small papules in months after cessation of therapy

2.2 Bowen Disease

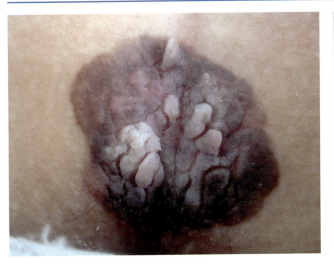

Fig. 2.30 Perianal Bowen disease presenting as a hyperpigmented verrucous plaque

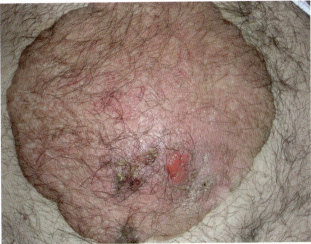

Fig. 2.32 Extensive plaque of Bowen disease. Note the raised nodule with eroded surface representing squamous cell carcinoma developing within the plaque of Bowen disease

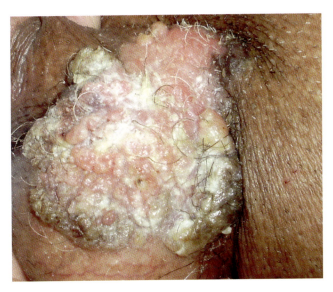

Fig. 2.31 Verrucous plaque on the scrotum due to Bowen disease

verruca vulgaris. Other differential diagnostic challenges are hypertrophic actinic keratosis (*see* Fig. 2.7), superficial basal cell carcinoma (*see* Fig. 11.57), superficial spreading melanoma (*see* Fig. 12.19), amelanotic melanoma (*see* Fig. 12.56), Paget disease of the breast (*see* Fig. 2.76), extramammary Paget disease (*see* Fig. 2.80), and pagetoid reticulosis.

Bowen disease may rarely involve periungual and subungual skin. These lesions may be strikingly different in appearance. Involvement of fingernails (*see* Fig. 2.19) is relatively more common. One or more nails may be affected (polydactylous Bowen disease). Involvement of the nail folds presents as persistent periungual erythema with scales, crusts, fissures, or erosions that look like chronic eczema or paronychia. On the other hand, hyperkeratotic verrucous nodules of Bowen disease in this area may be erroneously diagnosed and treated as verruca vulgaris. Subungual (nail bed) lesions may lead to onycholysis and nail destruction. Sometimes Bowen disease presents as melanonychia striata simulating malignant melanoma of the nail.

Progression to invasive squamous cell carcinoma rarely occurs in Bowen disease and mostly after several months or even years. However, the metastasizing potential of the carcinoma arising in the setting of Bowen disease is usually high. Therefore, early diagnosis will prevent this risk. An indurated nodule more elevated than other parts of the plaque and sudden onset of foci of erosion or ulceration may be the signs of carcinomatous transformation (*see* Fig. 2.32). A biopsy should be performed, especially from the most indurated part of the plaque, to detect dermal invasion. Epithelial dysplasia is prominent in all layers of the epidermis. Multinucleated keratinocytes, loss of cell polarity and maturation toward the surface, individual keratinization, and numerous, sometimes atypical mitoses are the main features. Similar atypical cells and mitoses are also scattered throughout the follicle epithelium.

Management. Before deciding on the appropriate therapeutic modality, the clinician should be initially sure that the lesion is clear of any focus of invasive squamous cell carcinoma. If any doubt exists, the most suspected part of the lesion should be chosen for biopsy or total excision may be performed in order to yield histopathological evaluation.

Various therapeutic options are possible, but aggressive therapies do not have high priority because of the slow progressive course and low risk of carcinomatous transformation of Bowen disease. The number, size, and localization of the lesions are important when deciding on the treatment modality. Genital, perianal, and periungual Bowen disease is

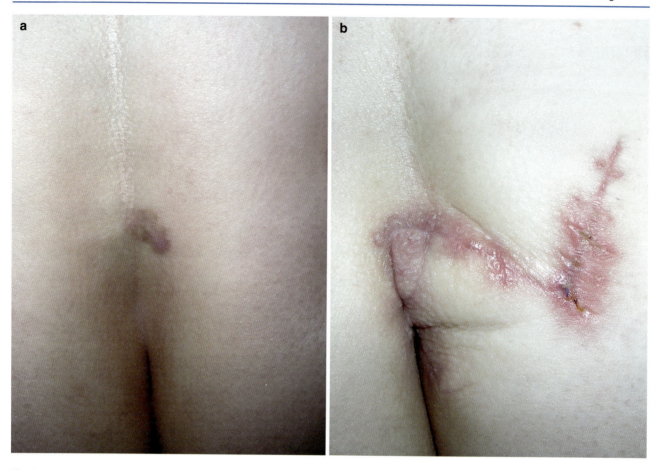

Fig. 2.33 (**a**) Solitary pigmented plaque of Bowen disease on the buttock. (**b**) Excision was performed because cosmetic concern could be disregarded on that site

technically more difficult to treat. Topical imiquimod, an immune response modifier, is effective in multiple small lesions and can also be used for larger lesions on the genitalia or on areas where cosmetic concern is higher. Topical 5-flourouracil is another medical option. The disadvantage of the topical therapies is that they are not very effective in the presence of deep follicular involvement and are associated with recurrence (*see* Fig. 2.29b and c).

Destructive methods such as cryotherapy, laser ablation, and photodynamic therapy are other alternatives. However, there is a high risk of recurrence after these therapies, especially because of the deep follicular involvement. Therefore close follow-up is mandatory after these treatment modalities. Radiotherapy is another option. Above all, excision with tumor-free margins will be curative when surgery is feasible (*see* Fig. 2.33a and b).

2.3 Erythroplasia of Queyrat

Erythroplasia of Queyrat is a premalignant lesion of the penis sharing major clinicopathologic features with Bowen disease. High-risk types of HPV are suggested to be major etiologic factors. It is more common in the older population, and most patients are uncircumcised or late circumcised males. Lesions tend to be located on the glans penis, prepuce, urethral meatus, corona, and frenulum. The shaft of the penis may rarely be involved.

The typical lesion is a solitary sharply demarcated, slightly raised, red, soft plaque measuring 1 to 3 cm in diameter (*see* Fig. 2.34). The surface of the lesion may be velvety or smooth. Erosion, crusting, and even bleeding may occur. It may sometimes be pruritic or tender. Lesions around the urethra may extend to the urethral meatus. Invasive squamous cell carcinoma occurring in the setting of this precancerous lesion shows highly aggressive behavior and early metastasizing potential. Development of carcinoma should be considered in the presence of indurated or ulcerated plaques or nodules.

Psoriasis vulgaris, lichen planus, pemphigus vulgaris, Zoon's plasma cell balanitis, and balanitis xerotica obliterans are the main differential diagnoses. The first three conditions may also cause similar lesions on other regions, which may simplify the diagnosis. Histologically, full-thickness epithelial dysplasia is diagnostic of erythroplasia of Queyrat.

Management. Because of the location of the lesion, conservative treatment may be initially preferred. Topical 5-fluorouracil and imiquimod are effective options that are also helpful in conserving the underlying tissue. Contrary

2.4 Leukoplakia

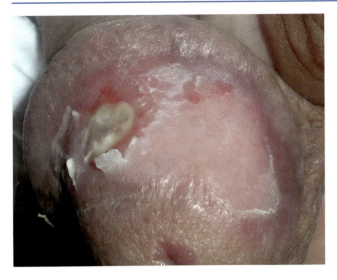

Fig. 2.34 Erythroplasia of Queyrat presenting as a flat plaque on the glans penis. The tumor can be observed exceptionally in a circumcised man as seen in this figure

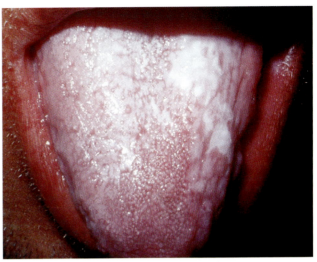

Fig. 2.35 Leukoplakia on the tongue as a manifestation of dyskeratosis congenita. The risk of development of squamous cell carcinoma is high in these patients

to Bowen disease, the recurrence rate of erythroplasia of Queyrat is low because follicular involvement is absent in this area. Surgical excision can be performed when lesions are unresponsive to topical therapies. On the other hand, lesions involving the distal part of the glans penis, together with invasion of the urethral meatus, may require Mohs microsurgery.

2.4 Leukoplakia

Leukoplakia is a potentially malignant lesion of the oral mucosa presenting as persistent whitish patches or plaques showing varying degrees of epithelial dysplasia. By contrast, there are similar mucosal lesions that only show nonspecific histopathologic changes. Accordingly, leukoplakia may also be accepted only as a clinical term encompassing any whitish mucosal lesion after exclusion of all possible diseases causing similar lesions. The white color is the result of the hydration of keratin.

Leukoplakia is usually seen in adults in their sixties and seventies. Tobacco smoking, use of smokeless tobacco, alcohol, and betel-areca quid (nut) are the only known risk factors of leukoplakia. On the other hand, some genodermatoses can present with leukoplakia as a major manifestation. In patients with dyskeratosis congenita (see Fig. 2.35), Howel-Evans syndrome (see Fig. 2.36), pachyonychia congenita (see Fig. 2.37), and Kindler syndrome (see Fig. 2.38) severe leukoplakia may develop in the first two decades of life.

Leukoplakia may appear anywhere on the oral mucosa as an isolated or as multiple lesions. The vermilion border of the lips (see Fig. 2.36), ventral and lateral surfaces of the tongue (see Figs. 2.39 and 2.40), floor of the mouth (see Figs. 2.41 and 2.42), buccal mucosa (see Fig. 2.43), gingivae (see Fig. 2.44), and soft palate (see Fig. 2.45) are

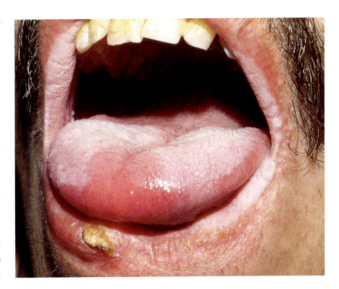

Fig. 2.36 Diffuse oral leukoplakia as a manifestation of Howel-Evans syndrome. Occasionally cutaneous horn may arise on leukoplakia as seen on the vermilion border of the lower lip

the commonly involved sites. In some patients, more than one area is affected (see Fig. 2.46). The size of the lesions is highly variable. As the disease is mostly asymptomatic, intraoral lesions in particular may not be noticed by the patient until they grow to 2 to 3 cm in size. The lesions may be incidentally detected during dental examination. Slightly raised, well-defined white lesions are adherent to the mucosa and cannot be removed. Lesions may be homogenous or may show a speckled pattern. Homogeneous lesions are usually smooth and flat (see Fig. 2.47). However, some lesions may be more elevated, thicker, and have a rough, wrinkled, or verrucous surface (see Fig. 2.48). Sometimes white and eroded red areas may

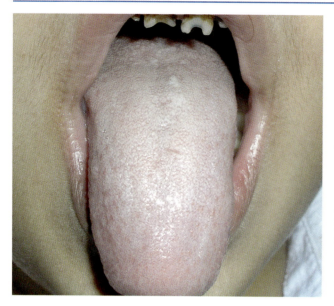

Fig. 2.37 Leukoplakia on the tongue of a child as a manifestation of pachyonychia congenita. Syndrome-associated leukoplakia may occur at young age

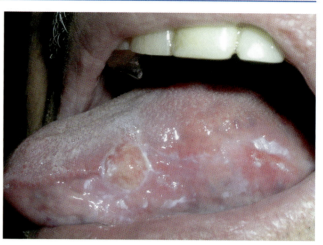

Fig. 2.40 Leukoplakia on the lateral surface of the tongue (*white patches*). Note also the eroded nodule representing early squamous cell carcinoma

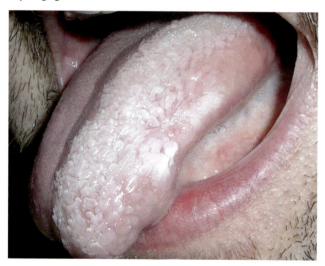

Fig. 2.38 Leukoplakia on the tongue as a manifestation of Kindler syndrome

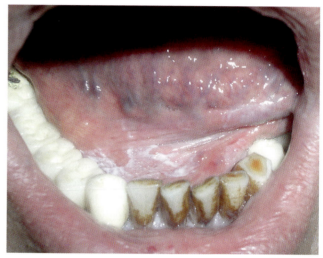

Fig. 2.41 Leukoplakia on the floor of the mouth; this is a high risk location for malignant degeneration

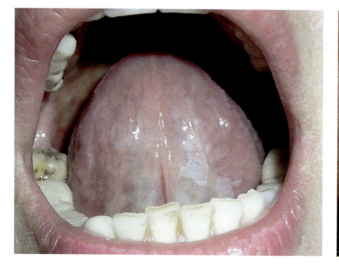

Fig. 2.39 Leukoplakia on the ventral surface of the tongue. Note the minimally raised white plaque

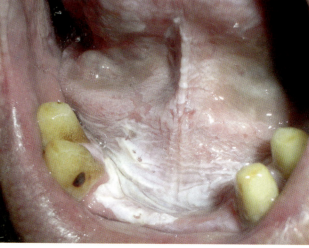

Fig. 2.42 Extensive leukoplakia involving the gingiva, floor of the mouth, and ventral surface of the tongue

2.4 Leukoplakia

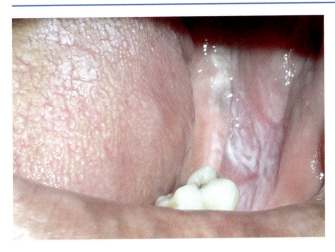

Fig. 2.43 Leukoplakia on the buccal mucosa. It may be clinically confused as lichen planus but lesions of leukoplakia rather show a homogenous pattern in contrast to the common reticular pattern of lichen planus

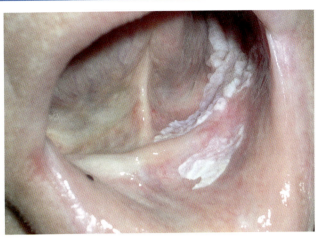

Fig. 2.46 Leukoplakia involving more than one area. Note that the white plaque on the floor of the mouth is thicker than the lesion on the lower lip

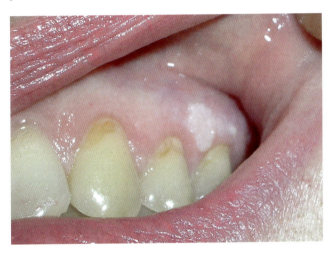

Fig. 2.44 Leukoplakia on the gingivae

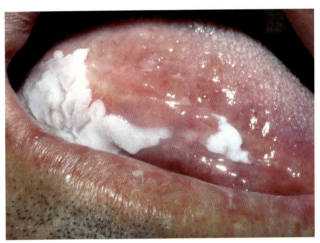

Fig. 2.47 Leukoplakia on the tongue causing homogenous flat white lesions

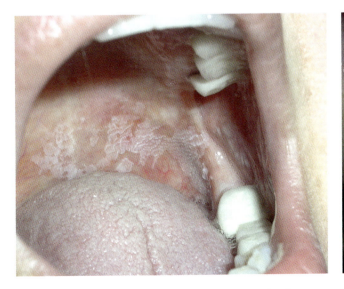

Fig. 2.45 Leukoplakia on the soft palate as a thin irregular plaque

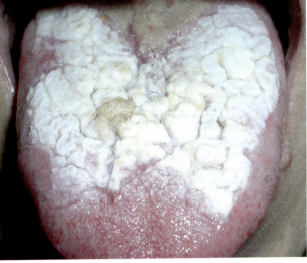

Fig. 2.48 Thick plaque of leukoplakia with a verrucous surface extending widely over the dorsum of the tongue

appear in a mixed pattern (erythroleukoplakia). The lesions tend to extend slowly to the periphery, and neglected plaques may become very large. Furthermore, the clinical appearance of the lesions may change over time.

Proliferative verrucous leukoplakia is a rare clinical variant of leukoplakia, usually presenting as multifocal lesions in older nonsmoking women. It shows a high risk of malignant transformation, an aggressive course, resistance to therapy, and a high recurrence rate.

A number of traumatic, infectious, inflammatory, and neoplastic diseases may also cause white lesions on the oral mucosa, posing a challenge in the differential diagnosis.

Although not very often, invasive squamous cell carcinoma and verrucous carcinoma of the oral mucosa may present as white nodules, plaques, or tumors. As these tumors have metastatic potential, misinterpretation with leukoplakia must be avoided. In a patient with leukoplakia, development of ulceration, induration and nodularity are clinical clues suggestive of a carcinoma (see Fig. 11.101). Oral lichen planus is a common inflammatory disease of the oral mucosa causing white, persistent, asymptomatic patches as well as erosive or ulcerative lesions. In patients lacking the typical papular skin lesions and classic reticular pattern of mucosal keratotic lesions, the differentiation from leukoplakia may only be possible with a biopsy. In discoid lupus erythematosus sharply demarcated white patches usually occur on the lips and sometimes on the other areas of the oral mucosa. Frictional keratosis (morsicatio buccarum) is another cause of localized white keratotic lesions on the oral mucosa. Furthermore, white sponge nevus (see Fig. 1.136) and hereditary benign intraepithelial dyskeratosis are associated with diffuse white, persistent plaques of the oral mucosa beginning at an early age. A biopsy is helpful in order to differentiate these lesions from genodermatoses causing diffuse leukoplakia. Oral hairy leukoplakia is an infectious disease of the tongue caused by Epstein-Barr virus seen mostly during the course of human immunodeficiency viral infection. Poorly demarcated lesions with white papillary projections bilaterally located on the sides of the tongue are typical of this condition. Actinic cheilitis causes irregular whiteness on the lower lip intermingled with erosions and crusts (see Fig. 2.52). Secondary syphilis and acute pseudomembranous candidiasis may also manifest with white oral lesions, but they develop acutely (sometimes as widespread plaques) and may be easily differentiated by laboratory investigation. In addition, mucosal candidal plaque is not adherent to the underlying area.

Any oral lesion about which there is doubt that resembles leukoplakia warrants a biopsy. The most elevated or indurated part of the lesion or the area with a suspicion of erythroleukoplakia is the preferred site for biopsy. The histopathologic appearance is heterogeneous. Epithelial dysplasia, the pathognomonic sign of leukoplakia, may be severe in most cases but may also be mild or even absent. The term carcinoma in situ is mostly used for cases with severe dysplasia and without maturation. However, dysplastic lesions do not have a specific clinical appearance, and a single biopsy specimen is not always sufficient for the exclusion of dysplasia. Hyperkeratosis or epidermal atrophy may be the sole histopathologic features in some cases. Biopsies can be repeatedly performed in the close follow-up of these patients. Epithelial dysplasia may be more prominent on the areas of erythroleukoplakia. If invasion of the subepithelial area is observed, invasive carcinoma is the appropriate diagnosis.

The main complication of leukoplakia is the development of squamous cell carcinoma (see Fig. 11.101). Leukoplakia is known to be the most common precancerous lesion of oral squamous cell carcinoma. However, the development of squamous cell carcinoma is seen in approximately 15 percent of the cases. The floor of the mouth and the ventral surface of the tongue are considered the high risk areas, but malignant degeneration may also occur at other sites. In patients with larger lesions and a nonhomogeneous clinical appearance, the risk of malignant transformation is increased. Speckled, verrucous, eroded, ulcerated, or indurated lesions or lesions intermingled with reddish areas should be flags for squamous cell carcinoma. Malignant degeneration may develop quickly or very slowly. Patients with progressive verrucous leukoplakia have a high risk of developing squamous cell carcinoma and verrucous carcinoma. In patients with dyskeratosis congenita and Howel-Evans syndrome, malignant degeneration of leukoplakia may occur at an earlier age.

Management. The main goal in the management of patients with leukoplakia is to prevent malignant degeneration or at least achieve an early diagnosis of invasive squamous cell carcinoma. Use of tobacco and alcohol should be avoided in all patients. Spontaneous clearance of the lesions upon stopping of smoking is reported anecdotally but a "wait and see" policy may be risky. The above described risk factors for malignant transformation are not absolute predictors for the development of carcinoma.

The appropriate therapy of leukoplakia should be tailored to its histopathologic features, clinical presentation, size, and site of the lesions. If a white plaque is confirmed to be leukoplakia showing moderate or severe grades of epithelial dysplasia, it should be treated aggressively. Verrucous plaques, nonhomogeneous lesions, or erythroleukoplakia are high-risk lesions that should be managed accordingly. Management of patients with white homogeneous patches or plaques showing only nonspecific histopathologic features in repeat examinations and who lack the association with other conditions causing similar lesions are rather challenging as there is no consensus regarding therapy or follow-up. On the other hand, it has also been suggested that lesions on the high-risk sites, even without epithelial dysplasia, should be treated immediately.

Surgical excision seems to be an ideal choice for leukoplakia but may be difficult, especially for large lesions and on some locations like the gingivae. The possibility of tissue destruction resulting in deformities limits the use of surgery. Carbon dioxide laser ablation and cryotherapy are alternatives that preserve the underlying tissue. It should be noted, however, that the recurrence rate is not low, even with all these surgical or ablative methods. Oral retinoids at high doses have been used in some high-risk patients to prevent malignant degeneration with variable efficacy.

If all the above treatment modalities cannot be applied and the patient has no risk factors, regular monitoring at short intervals is sometimes the only solution, but biopsy should be performed from the lesions with recent development of suspicious areas such as those with erosion and nodules. Close follow-up is also mandatory after the therapeutic interventions highlighted above.

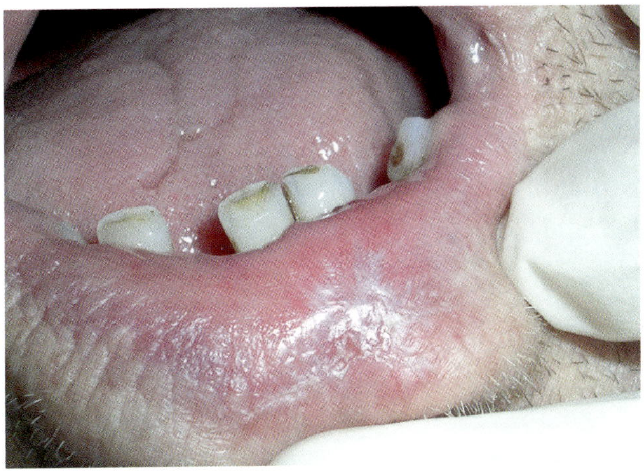

2.5 Actinic Cheilitis

Actinic cheilitis is a precancerous condition of the lower lip with a chronic course. It is more common in fair-skinned individuals. Cumulative sun damage is the main etiologic factor; therefore it is primarily seen in patients over 50 years of age. Men are more commonly affected. The clinical picture is variable; it may be localized as a poorly demarcated lesion on the lower lip or may diffusely involve the lower lip. The lower lip may be dry, atrophic, or slightly hyperkeratotic (*see* Fig. 2.49). Nonhomogeneous whiteness may be observed in a scattered pattern in this area (*see* Fig. 2.50). Erosions (*see* Fig. 2.51), scales, crusts (see Fig. 2.52) or fissures may be seen on the lesions. The margin between the vermilion border and the skin can appear indistinct (*see* Fig. 2.53). Cutaneous horn may rarely develop overlying actinic cheilitis. Regional induration, elevation (*see* Fig. 11.100), and ulceration may be the signs of malignant degeneration and warrant further urgent examination.

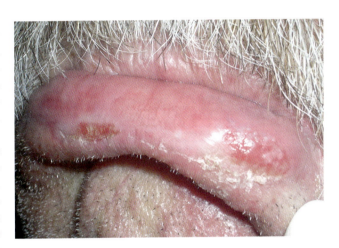

Fig. 2.50 Actinic cheilitis on the lower lip. A nonhomogeneous white area is noticeable

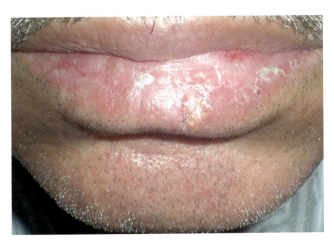

Fig. 2.49 Actinic cheilitis typically located on the lower lip of a man causing slight hyperkeratosis and crusting

Fig. 2.51 Actinic cheilitis on the lower lip. Small eroded areas and hyperkeratosis are seen

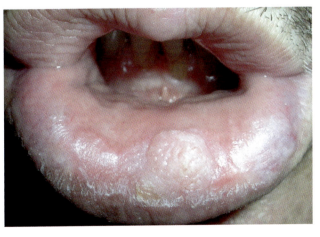

Fig. 2.52 Actinic cheilitis causing hyperkeratosis and crusts on the lower lip

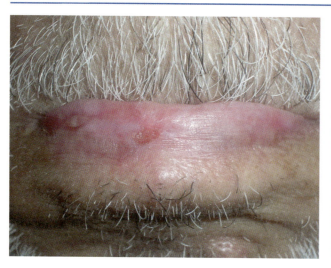

Fig. 2.53 A case of actinic cheilitis with indistinctive vermilion border of the lip. This was a relapsing lesion after vermilionectomy operation

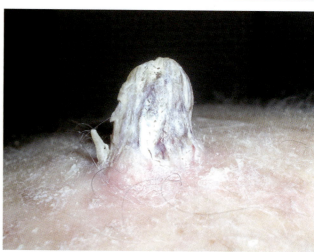

Fig. 2.54 Cutaneous horn overlying actinic keratosis on the scalp. The underlying lesion should always be investigated

Discoid lupus erythematosus, leukoplakia, and factitious lip crusting are the main differential diagnoses of actinic cheilitis. The diagnosis should be confirmed by histopathologic examination, but sometimes only one biopsy may not be sufficient. In addition to nonspecific changes such as acanthosis and hyperkeratosis, varying degrees of epithelial dysplasia may be observed.

Management. Because actinic cheilitis is a precancerous lesion, it should be treated accordingly. Most cases have widespread involvement of the lower lip. 5-fluorouracil and imiquimod may be used topically. Cryotherapy, carbon dioxide laser ablation, and photodynamic therapy are other alternatives. Vermilionectomy is a radical choice. Patients should be followed up regularly for possible recurrences. Sun protection measures should be used on a constant and long-term basis.

2.6 Cutaneous Horn (Cornu Cutaneum)

Cutaneous horn is morphologically a keratinous outgrowth of skin resembling the horn of an animal. It is caused by cohesion of keratin on a localized area. This harmless lesion shows abnormal keratinization of the epidermis overlying various cutaneous lesions which may be benign, precancerous, or malignant. The pathogenesis causing an increase in keratin cohesion is not understood. It occurs more commonly in the elderly patients but may appear at any age. Horns may appear anywhere on the body, but sun-exposed areas such as the face, the dorsum of the hands, and the scalp are more commonly involved. Ears, nose, and eyelids are the most involved parts of the face. Lesions may also be found on the penis. Underlying conditions include a variety of tumors producing keratin. Actinic keratosis is a well-known cause of cutaneous horn, especially on the face and scalp of elder men (*see* Fig. 2.54). Cutaneous horns may overlie filiform warts

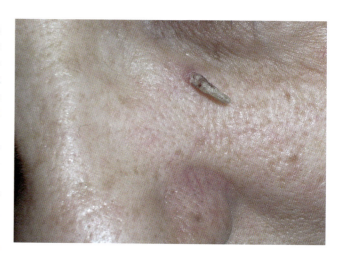

Fig. 2.55 A cone-shaped thin cutaneous horn on the basis of verruca filiformis

(*see* Figs. 2.55 and 2.56) at any age, including the children. Seborrheic keratosis (*see* Fig. 1.35), Bowen disease, keratoacanthoma (*see* Fig. 2.67), trichilemmoma, molluscum contagiosum, and angiokeratoma are other lesions that may be present on the base of a cutaneous horn. Among these conditions, cutaneous malignancies like squamous cell carcinoma (*see* Fig. 11.137) and verrucous carcinoma (*see* Fig. 11.152) are of greatest importance.

A typical lesion is a cone- (*see* Fig. 2.55) or pyramid-shaped (*see* Fig. 2.57), hard, dry, white to dark yellow, sometimes skin-colored, asymptomatic projection that is firmly adherent to its base. It may be thin or thick, with size usually smaller than 1 cm when diagnosed. However, in neglected cases, lesions may be 2 to 3 cm long and may be angulated or curved (*see* Fig. 2.58). Sometimes the tip of the lesion may be split into a few parts perpendicularly. The base of the lesion may be flat or elevated, depending on the underlying disease. It is usually asymptomatic unless it is traumatized,

2.6 Cutaneous Horn (Cornu Cutaneum)

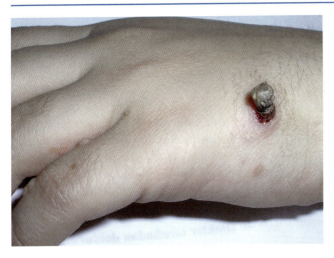

Fig. 2.56 Cutaneous horn overlying verruca filiformis on the dorsum of the hand

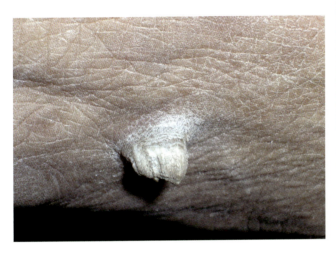

Fig. 2.57 Pyramid-shaped cutaneous horn

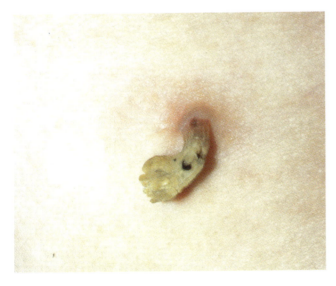

Fig. 2.58 Long, angulated cutaneous horn

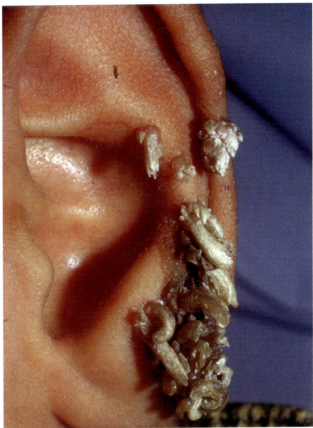

Fig. 2.59 Multiple cutaneous horns associated with verrucae on the ear

which may cause inflammation and pain. In cases with an underlying tumor, cutaneous horn is usually a solitary lesion, but more than one can appear in patients with multiple warts (*see* Fig. 2.59). Cutaneous horn overlying warts are usually thinner, but the ones overlying seborrheic keratosis tend to be larger and to have a verrucous surface (*see* Fig. 1.35). Although rare, a cutaneous horn may be seen on the lips overlying actinic cheilitis or leukoplakia (*see* Fig. 2.36).

Clinical diagnosis of a cutaneous horn is not difficult. However, in order to clarify the underlying pathology, an adequate biopsy including the base is usually necessary. An abnormally thick keratin layer formed by orthokeratotic hyperkeratosis, sometimes admixed with parakeratosis, is the main histopathologic feature of cutaneous horn. The histopathologic features of the base depend on the type of the underlying lesion.

Management. The initial consideration must be made according to the lesion type on the base. Total excision including the base is therapeutic and also yields histopathologic confirmation. When the possibility of an underlying malignancy is excluded with incisional biopsy, destructive methods such as electrocautery and cryotherapy may be used for the cutaneous horn. If the underlying lesion is compatible with a precancerous or malignant condition, then it should be treated accordingly.

2.7 Arsenical Keratosis

Arsenical keratosis is a rare precancerous lesion occurring in individuals with chronic arsenism. Patients usually have a history of previous arsenic exposure of 10 to 50 years. Causative factors may be contamination of the water supply with arsenic or medicinal exposure.

Lesions typically appear on the palmoplantar area, but other areas of the extremities (*see* Fig. 2.60), trunk, and face may also be involved. Tens to hundreds of yellowish, hard hyperkeratotic papules 2 to 10 mm in diameter are prone to occur on sites of pressure and friction. Cutaneous horn may overlie some lesions. Papules may coalesce into verrucous plaques. Hereditary punctate palmoplantar keratoderma may cause similar symmetric lesions, but it arises at a younger age. Verruca plantaris and Darier disease are other differential diagnoses. Histologically epithelial dysplasia seen in arsenical keratosis is similar to actinic keratosis. Progression to squamous cell carcinoma is the main risk of these lesions. Mees lines on the nails and mottled hyperpigmentation associated with hypopigmented macules over the body are other dermatologic features of chronic arsenism. Multiple lesions of Bowen disease and superficial basal cell carcinoma may also occur in these patients; therefore a full body examination is necessary. Cancers of the lung and urinary bladder owing to arsenic exposure may be associated in some of the cases.

Management. Destructive methods like cryotherapy, electrocautery, and carbon dioxide laser may be helpful. Surgery may be used for individual lesions, especially those showing rapid change. However the presence of numerous lesions is a limiting condition in therapy. Follow-up of the patient is mandatory because of the risk of development of squamous cell carcinoma.

2.8 Chronic Radiodermatitis

Chronic radiodermatitis is a localized chronic skin condition appearing months to years after x-ray exposure on irradiated fields. It is a precancerous lesion with a very long latent period of carcinogenesis. Overdose of radiotherapy is a risk factor for skin damage. Moreover, overexposure of hands to x-rays may be occupational, as may be seen in physicians. Fluoroscopic devices used in the past had caused chronic radiodermatitis on the hands of physicians years later (*see* Fig. 2.61). At present fluoroscopy is frequently used in cardiology (i.e., percutaneous transluminal coronary angioplasty); this may also be the cause of radiodermatitis in these patients, especially on the upper trunk.

The previously irradiated skin sites overlying a visceral malignant tumor are the most common locations of chronic radiodermatitis (*see* Fig. 2.62). A typical lesion is a geometric or angulated-shaped, well-defined, shiny plaque with a yellow hue and comprises depigmentation, hyperpigmentation, atrophic areas, multiple telangiectases, induration caused by fibrosis, and hair loss (*see* Figs. 2.62 and 2.63). The lesion is dry and may be pruritic. Sometimes chronic ulcerations and extensive fibrosis may develop.

Chronic radiation keratoses as discrete keratoses or hyperkeratotic plaques may overlie the poikilodermatous plaques of chronic radiodermatitis (*see* Fig. 2.62). Basal cell carcinoma (*see* Figs. 11.15, 11.16 and 11.17) and squamous cell carcinoma (*see* Fig. 11.106) may develop after a latency period of 20 to 40 years in the setting of chronic radiodermatitis or at areas that have been previously treated with radiotherapy but lack typical skin changes. Other malignancies such as sarcomas may also rarely develop. Cutaneous malignancies usually occur on the border of chronic radiodermatitis delineating normal skin (*see* Fig. 11.15).

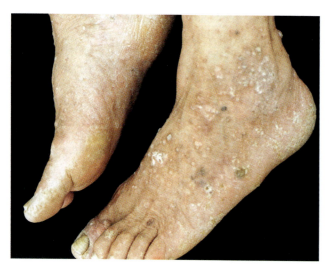

Fig. 2.60 Arsenical keratoses on the feet. Note the hyperkeratotic papules

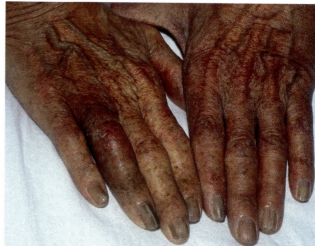

Fig. 2.61 Chronic radiodermatitis on the dorsum of the hands of an elderly. This patient was a physician who had worked with fluoroscopy devices in the past

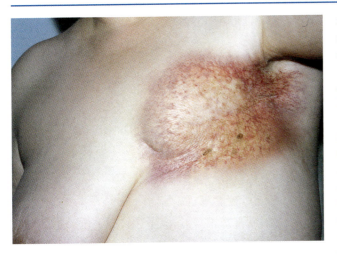

Fig. 2.62 Chronic radiodermatitis on the mastectomy site due to postoperative radiotherapy. Note the associated radiation keratoses in form of hyperkeratotic plaques overlying a poikilodermatous area

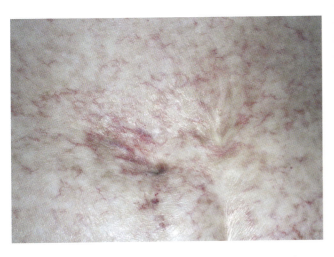

Fig. 2.63 Atrophy, hypopigmentation, and telangiectases on a circumscribed area associated with local sclerosis; typical presentation of chronic radiodermatitis

Morphea may be considered in the differential diagnosis of chronic radiodermatitis but lacks poikilodermatous appearance. Clinical features supported by the history of the patient enable the diagnosis. Histopathologic examination of chronic radiodermatitis reveals epidermal atrophy, sclerotic collagen bundles in the dermis, giant fibroblasts, loss of skin appendages, and dilated capillaries. Chronic radiation keratoses show epithelial dysplasia similar to that seen in actinic keratosis.

Management. There is no effective therapy for chronic radiodermatitis. Emollient creams may be used symptomatically. Lesions with persistent ulcers or causing functional impairment due to sclerosis may be excised with aggressive reconstructive surgery. However, this is not a routine procedure. Many patients are just followed because of the risk of development of basal cell carcinoma and squamous cell carcinoma. Chronic radiation keratoses may be treated with destructive methods and excision. Occurrence of a new nodule and ulceration on or around the sites of chronic radiodermatitis may be signs of cutaneous malignancies and should be biopsied.

2.9 Keratoacanthoma

Keratoacanthoma is a rapidly growing epithelial neoplasm of the skin and mucous membranes with a tendency to spontaneous involution. Tumors with typical umbilicated centers most often localize on sun-exposed areas such as the face, neck, forearms, and dorsum of the hands. It has been suggested that keratoacanthomas originate from hair follicles, but lesions may be seen also on hairless areas such as oral mucosa, nail beds, palms, and soles of the feet. Keratoacanthoma is mostly seen in patients over the age 40. Chronic sun damage may be a risk factor, as may immunosuppressive treatment after transplantation. Use of vemurafenib in melanoma therapy can be associated with the development of cutaneous neoplasms including keratoacanthoma. Keratoacanthomas may also arise during sorafenib therapy, another antineoplastic agent.

Although this tumor can be considered to show benign biological behavior without invading the tissue below the level of the eccrine sweat glands and undergo spontaneous regression, it has an unpredictable course that can occasionally show local destruction and may even cause metastasis. Therefore, classification of this tumor as benign or malignant is controversial. There are different views about its relationship to squamous cell carcinoma. One view is that keratoacanthoma is a well-differentiated squamous cell carcinoma; the opposing view is that it is a separate entity but may rarely progress to invasive squamous cell carcinoma. Both tumors have some overlapping histopathologic features, and a reliable method of differentiation has not yet been established.

There are many clinical types of keratoacanthoma, most of them occurring sporadically, but some are genetically inherited or occur in the setting of various syndromes. The classic solitary type of the tumor has a natural evolution period, an average time of 6 months, including proliferation, maturation, and regression. The lesion starts as a small pinkish or skin-colored, dome-shaped, smooth papule. It grows rapidly for several weeks, evolving into a scaly hemispheric nodule (*see* Fig. 2.64) and then remains stable. In the following maturation period an adherent keratin plug develops on the center, which forms a crater (*see* Figs. 2.65 and 2.66). The round or oval, pale red to reddish violet, well-defined nodule is 1 to 2 cm in size with a height less than 1 cm (*see* Fig. 2.67). Telangiectases may be prominent on the surface. Cutaneous horn may sometimes develop on the center of the tumor (*see* Fig. 2.68). Mature keratoacanthoma is firm but not fixed to deep structures. Solitary keratoacanthomas usually remain superficial and are asymptomatic. During the

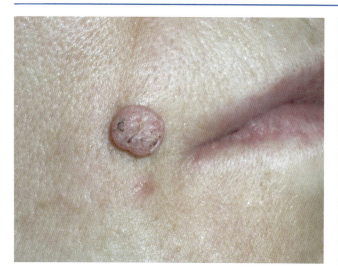

Fig. 2.64 Early lesion of keratoacanthoma; a scaly hemispheric nodule is seen

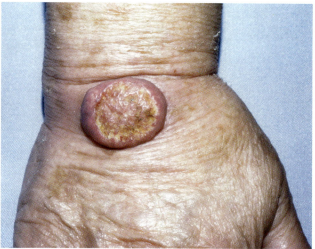

Fig. 2.67 Oval-shaped keratoacanthoma measuring more than 1 cm

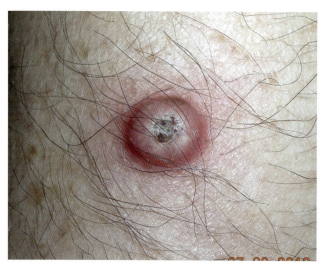

Fig. 2.65 Mature keratoacanthoma; a round, red nodule with keratin plug on the center is seen

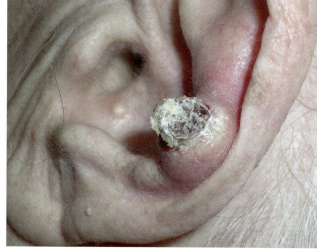

Fig. 2.68 Keratoacanthoma on the ear. Note the cutaneous horn protruding from the center of the lesion

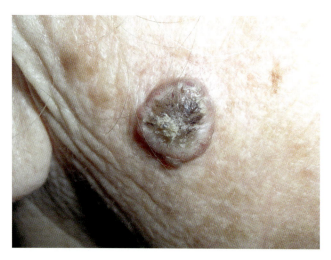

Fig. 2.66 Keratoacanthoma with a large central crater

involution period between 2 and 6 months the tumor shrinks, and the keratin plug may be expelled. At the end of this period, keratoacanthoma regresses, usually leaving an irregular atrophic hypopigmented scar.

A solitary keratoacanthoma may mimic squamous cell carcinoma showing central ulceration (*see* Fig. 11.115) but the latter one usually grows slower. However, invasive squamous cell carcinoma may sometimes grow more rapidly than expected, leading to confusion with keratoacanthoma. Giant molluscum contagiosum may be mistaken for a keratoacanthoma, but the core of this viral lesion can easily be evacuated. The nodular type of cutaneous metastasis (*see* Fig. 16.5) is another differential diagnosis, but these nodules are typically indurated to underlying deep tissue.

Other clinical types of keratoacanthoma are rare, and some are associated with increased morbidity. A keratoacanthoma

2.9 Keratoacanthoma

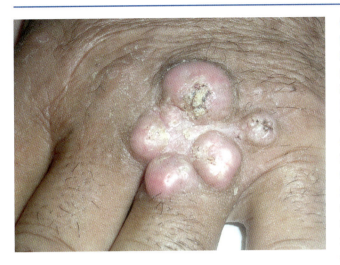

Fig. 2.69 Multinodular keratoacanthoma with a bunch of round nodules around a central atrophic area; a rare clinical type

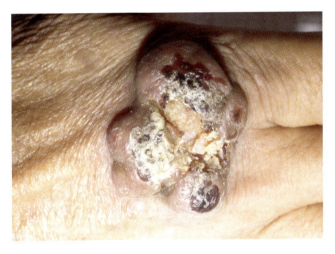

Fig. 2.70 Multinodular keratoacanthoma; multiple confluent nodular lesions compose a large mass

that grows larger than 3 cm in diameter is called a giant keratoacanthoma. The size may even reach 8 to 10 cm, with a height up to 2 to 3 cm. It may be locally invasive but has a tendency to spontaneous healing, similar to smaller solitary keratoacanthomas. Another rare type presenting with a large lesion is keratoacanthoma centrifigum marginatum. This variant manifests with a flat annular plaque showing central clearing and scarring as it continues to grow and move peripherally up to 20 cm. Lesions are typically seen on the dorsum of the hands and legs. The tumor has an elevated peripheral wall and may clinically resemble granuloma annulare. This type of keratoacanthoma is unlikely to show spontaneous regression. Multiple keratoacanthomas localized around a central atrophic area that show a tendency to expand are called multinodular keratoacanthomas (see Figs. 2.69 and 2.70). Keratoacanthoma may rarely show a verrucous surface without central umbilication and keratin plug. This presentation is called verrucous keratoacanthoma and is more common in multiple keratoacanthoma syndromes. If hyperkeratosis is massive, it may resemble cutaneous horn. Keratoacanthoma on the nose (see Fig. 2.71a and b), lips, ears, and eyelids can cause destruction of the normal tissue, including the underlying cartilage.

Keratoacanthoma may rarely be derived from the nail bed and nail folds. The subungual type of keratoacanthoma may affect the thumb, index, or middle fingers, causing rapidly growing local swelling that usually lacks the typical shape and keratin plug of the tumor. It may cause onycholysis related to nail bed deformity (see Fig. 2.72), bone destruction (osteolysis) on the distal phalanx, and be very painful. Keratoacanthoma may also involve the mucous membranes, including the lips, palate, nasal mucosa, conjunctiva, and anus. Subungual keratoacanthomas and mucosal keratoacanthomas are unlikely to undergo spontaneous regression.

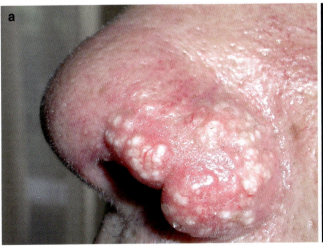 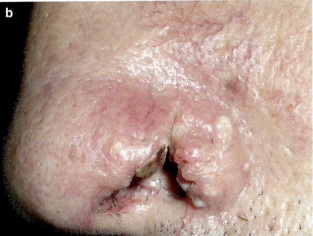

Fig. 2.71 (a) Keratoacanthoma on the nose: an ill-defined nodule with irregular surface. (b) Destruction of the deep tissue by the tumor

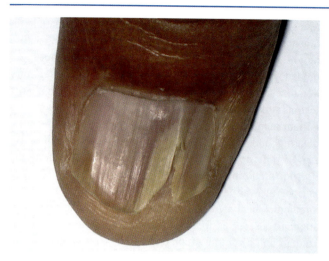

Fig. 2.72 Subungual keratoacanthoma causing onycholysis and longitudinal splitting of the nail. The diagnosis was established with radiologic examination followed by biopsy

Keratoacanthoma may rarely present as multiple lesions occurring anywhere on the body in different periods of life (multiple keratoacanthoma syndromes). In the non-hereditary variant called "multiple persistent keratoacanthomas," tumors occur simultaneously, have a tendency to heal slowly, and outbreaks of new lesions are possible. "Ferguson-Smith type multiple keratoacanthomas" is the familial presentation of these syndromes with onset at a young age. Various medium- to large-sized lesions in tens to hundreds are found. They have a tendency to slow spontaneous regression. Disfiguring scar formation, especially on the face, is observed after periodic recurrences over many years.

In "Grzybowski type generalized eruptive keratoacanthomas," the number of small tumors measuring 1 to 5 mm reaches thousands. This unusual variant shows no familial pattern of inheritance, and the patients are middle aged or older. Keratoacanthomas may occur anywhere on the skin, but facial involvement is prominent. The papules have a tendency to coalesce. They may be pruritic or painful. Lesions clinically mimic molluscum contagiosum and verrucae. In this variant, the involvement of oropharyngeal and laryngeal mucosal surfaces may cause serious complications.

Keratoacanthoma may occur in the setting of some genodermatoses. Patients with xeroderma pigmentosum may develop keratoacanthomas in addition to other ultraviolet-induced benign and malignant cutaneous neoplasia that begin in early childhood (see Fig. 2.73a and b). In Muir-Torre syndrome, solitary or multiple keratoacanthomas may accompany sebaceous skin tumors and visceral malignancies. Keratoacanthoma, particularly in subungual locations, may rarely occur in patients with incontinentia pigmenti as a late manifestation of the disease.

The clinical features of keratoacanthoma are usually sufficient for the diagnosis. However, a histopathologic confirmation is obligatory. Punch biopsy, shave biopsy, and a small incisional biopsy do not provide adequate specimens for histopathologic examination. This kind of material can support the clinical diagnosis but will not be completely adequate for exclusion of squamous cell carcinoma. As the general architecture of keratoacanthoma is distinctive, complete excision is necessary. A cup-shaped tumor with exophytic and endophytic architecture associated with a central keratin-filled invagination lined by proliferating atypical squamous epithelium are the main histologic features. Keratinocytes have a ground-glass cytoplasm, and there is a sharp outline between the tumor and stroma. Intraepidermal neutrophilic abscesses are common. Eosinophils may also be numerous both intraepithelially and in the surrounding dermis. If suspicion of squamous cell carcinoma cannot be eliminated histopathologically, a metastasis screening should also be performed.

Management. Although keratoacanthoma mostly shows spontaneous regression (see Fig. 2.73a and b), the possibility of progression is unpredictable. Therefore, treatment of this tumor is recommended. Clinical type, size, and location of the tumor play a role in determining the therapeutic modality, which includes surgery, radiotherapy, and medical therapy. Complete excision as early as possible is the therapy of choice in a classic small solitary lesion if the tumor is not located on sites like the eyelids, where surgery can be destructive. Advantages of surgery include rapid solution, definite histopathologic examination, exclusion of the possibility of invasive squamous cell carcinoma, relieving the anxiety of the patient, and providing mostly better cosmetic results than spontaneous healing. If the clinical presentation is typical but surgery is technically difficult or contraindicated, the patient can be monitored for 3 to 4 months while awaiting spontaneous resolution. However, if regression does not occur within this period, an aggressive treatment should be performed. The prognosis of most keratoacanthomas is good after standard surgery. The therapeutic approach for multiple and destructive keratoacanthomas may be different. Mohs surgery facilitates optimal margin control and can be chosen for larger lesions or for facial and subungual localization. The recurrence rate of keratoacanthomas after surgery is not high. Surgery may also be used for recurrent tumors. Amputation of the phalanx may sometimes be required for persistent subungual keratoacanthoma.

Destructive methods like electrocautery and cryotherapy are not preferred for keratoacanthoma because the recurrence rate is high and scar formation after therapy is more prominent when compared to postsurgical scars. Radiotherapy may be an effective option in older individuals, for large lesions and in certain locations such as the face. This method may also be used for recurrent lesions after surgery.

The most commonly used option for multiple lesions of keratoacanthoma is medical therapy. Various

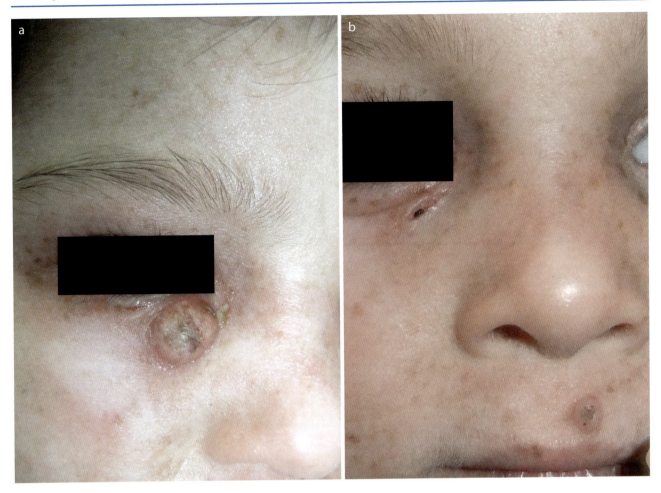

Fig. 2.73 (**a**) Keratoacanthoma on the periorbital area of a child with xeroderma pigmentosum. (**b**) Spontaneous regression of the periorbital tumor is seen. Note also the occurrence of a second lesion on the philtrum of the upper lip

alternatives exist that can be used systemically or intralesionally. Chemotherapeutic agents such as methotrexate, 5-fluorouracil, and oral retinoids (isotretinoin, acitretin) are used for very large and numerous lesions or for large facial lesions involving the eyelids, lips, and nose. Methotrexate, which inhibits dihydrofolate reductase may be used in patients with multiple lesions, for keratoacanthoma centrifugum marginatum, and for subungual keratoacanthoma.

Intralesional therapeutic agents such as methotrexate, 5-fluorouracil, and bleomycin have been used to treat keratoacanthomas with variable success. They are preferred for large lesions and for those in difficult locations that are not amenable to excision. Cosmetic outcome with intralesional methotrexate is mostly good. Topical imiquimod has also been used in some cases.

Sometimes even histopathologic examination does not permit a clear distinction between keratoacanthoma and squamous cell carcinoma, and there is a risk of relapse after any therapeutic intervention (*see* Fig. 2.74); thus follow-up of patients is mandatory, especially in the early postoperative period.

2.10 Paget Disease of the Breast

Paget disease of the breast (Paget disease of the nipple or mammary Paget disease) is an intraepithelial adenocarcinoma of the nipple and areola. In most if not all cases of mammary Paget disease (85 to 95 percent) an in situ or invasive ductal carcinoma of the underlying breast tissue is found. Accordingly, the prevailing view is that mammary Paget disease represents the intraepidermal spread of this tumor. But this theory fails to explain the origin of the intraepidermal neoplastic cells in cases where a breast neoplasm cannot be found. The breast tumor is generally centrally located and close to the nipple and areola. Patients having a palpable breast mass likely have an invasive tumor, whereas in mammary Paget disease with no palpable mass, ductal carcinoma in situ is likely to be found. Paget disease may also develop on ectopic breast tissue. It is seen predominantly in adult women but may very rarely be seen in males. It is most common in the sixth decade.

Lesions begin as a small erythematous scaly or crusted patch on one nipple (*see* Fig. 2.75) that subsequently extends

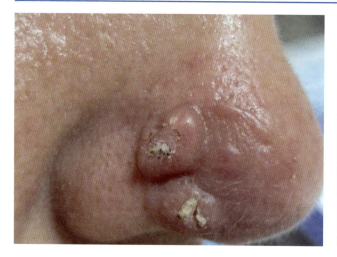

Fig. 2.74 Recurrent keratoacanthoma; a nodular lesion is remarkable on the left side of the scar

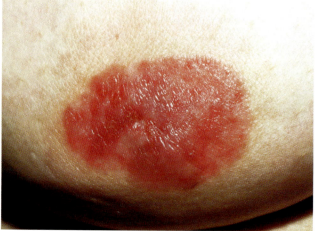

Fig. 2.76 Paget disease destroying the nipple and involving the areola as a sharply demarcated, reddish, eczema-like plaque. The unilateral lesion is a differentiating feature from contact dermatitis that typically presents with bilateral lesions

The suspicion of Paget disease always warrants a biopsy. Histologically, large epithelioid cells with abundant pale basophilic cytoplasm reflecting mucin content and large vesicular nuclei are distributed in an acanthotic epidermis. In pigmented cases the number of melanocytes is increased.

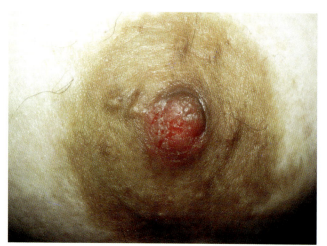

Fig. 2.75 Early lesion of Paget disease restricted to the nipple, unilaterally

to the areola as a result of the migration of malignant cells in the epidermis, forming a moist, well-defined eczematized plaque (*see* Fig. 2.76). Lesions may cause itching, burning, or even pain. Because of the draining serous fluid, it may be confused with eczema of the nipple, which is seen mostly in atopic individuals, but nipple dermatitis is nearly always bilateral and responds well to topical corticosteroids. In contrast, Paget disease is persistent, may be more infiltrated, and may have an eroded surface. Many patients with Paget disease have a history of an unsuccessful therapeutic intervention with topical corticosteroids. Erosive adenomatosis of the nipple (*see* Fig. 5.37) may also be a diagnostic challenge in this area. Clinically, the plaques may also resemble Bowen disease, but the breast location is typical for Paget disease. In neglected cases the skin surrounding the areola (*see* Fig. 2.77) may also be involved, and ulcerations may occur. Plaques of Paget disease may sometimes be hyperpigmented (*see* Fig. 2.78).

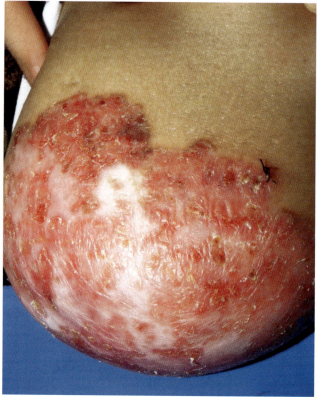

Fig. 2.77 Paget disease presenting as a large plaque extending over the margins of areola

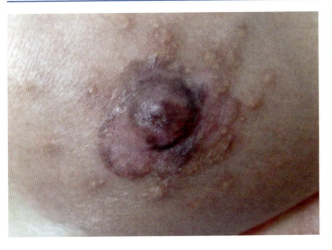

Fig. 2.78 Pigmented Paget disease, a rare clinical presentation

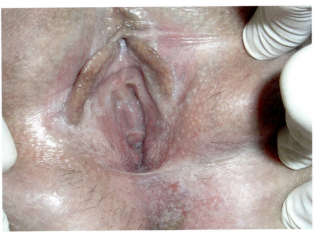

Fig. 2.79 Extramammary Paget disease causing scattered erosions around vulva and perineum

Management. Upon confirmation of the diagnosis, patients should be referred to surgeons and oncologists. A detailed examination of both breasts and the axillary lymph nodes should be carried out to search for an underlying mammary carcinoma and metastases. After the determination of the stage of the breast cancer, therapy can be planned. If modified radical mastectomy is used, there is certainly no need for therapy directed to the skin lesion. On the other hand, a mammary carcinoma may be clinically and radiologically (including by mammography) undetectable. In these cases, conservative surgery combined with radiotherapy may be an alternative therapeutic method. However, strict follow-up is essential.

2.11 Extramammary Paget Disease

Extramammary Paget disease is a rare localized cutaneous intraepidermal carcinoma seen in apocrine gland–bearing areas. The proportion of patients with extramammary Paget disease in which there is an associated in situ or invasive tumor of cutaneous adnexal structures (usually apocrine adenocarcinoma) or of contiguous gastrointestinal or genitourinary organs is much smaller than those with mammary Paget disease associated with breast cancer. Association with a malignancy is found in approximately 25 percent of cases, but this rate depends on the tumor location. According to the current view extramammary Paget disease represents a primary intraepidermal neoplasm of probable apocrine duct origin or of pluripotent keratinocyte stem cells. In perianal extramammary Paget disease an underlying anal or colorectal adenocarcinoma is found in 70 to 80 percent of the cases, whereas in vulvar disease an underlying contiguous organ neoplasm is less frequently found. Lesions with different etiopathogenesis have common clinical features. They are most commonly seen in the vulvar area of middle-aged or

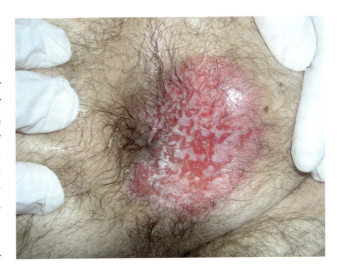

Fig. 2.80 Extramammary Paget disease manifesting as a sharply demarcated, eroded, flat plaque on the perianal area

elderly women (*see* Fig. 2.79) but may also be seen on the scrotum and penis of males. Perianal skin is another major site in both sexes (*see* Fig. 2.80). Rarely, axillae, umbilicus, cheeks, eyelids, and the external ear canal may be involved. The typical lesion is a unifocal, moist, oozing, well-defined, reddish flat plaque measuring 1 to 2 cm in diameter with scattered erosions and scales on the surface (*see* Fig. 2.79). It may sometimes be verrucous. Multifocal lesions may also be encountered. Lesions may be asymptomatic or pruritic, or may cause a burning sensation.

Inflammatory diseases such as lichen simplex chronicus, dermatophyte infections, lichen sclerosus et atrophicus, and intertriginous dermatitis may be the initial clinical diagnosis in different locations. The lesion of extramammary Paget disease expands slowly to involve larger areas, especially in patients with delayed diagnosis. Ulceration may occur. The main histopathologic features are similar to those of Paget disease of the breast. Large pale cells distributed throughout the epidermis may be single or clustered. Immunohistochemical stains (cytokeratin 7, cytokeratin 20) may be helpful in differentiating primary (intraepidermal extramammary Paget disease in which an underlying tumor cannot be identified) or secondary types (associated with underlying neoplasms) of the disease. Some lesions extend beyond the epidermis, invading the dermis (invasive extramammary Paget disease), and thus have the potential to metastasize.

Management. It should be kept in mind that extramammary Paget disease may be a marker of a systemic adenocarcinoma. Therefore, a cancer screening, including radiologic and endoscopic examinations of the gastrointestinal and genitourinary tracts, is mandatory. The sites of Paget disease give some clues as to the underlying carcinoma. For instance, in lesions of the perianal region the possibility of adenocarcinoma of the anal canal and rectum is higher. However, an underlying malignancy may not be found in all cases.

The therapeutic approach to extramammary Paget disease itself and the underlying malignancy differs. If a systemic carcinoma is detected, it should be treated accordingly. However, as this operation does not always include the area of extramammary Paget disease, further surgery is indicated for skin lesions. Wide local excision or Mohs microsurgery may be used for extramammary Paget disease. Sometimes even radical vulvectomy or scrotectomy can be performed. Postoperative radiotherapy and chemotherapy may be additionally indicated in some cases. Topical imiquimod can be used if surgery is technically not feasible. Photodynamic therapy may be an alternative. Topical 5-fluorouracil is not very effective for extramammary Paget disease but may be helpful to determine the surgical margins.

Suggested Reading

Amagasa T, Yamashiro M, Uzawa N. Oral premalignant lesions: from a clinical perspective. Int J Clin Oncol. 2011;16:5–14.

Aubut N, Alain J, Claveas J. Intralesional methotrexate treatment for keratoacanthoma tumors: a retrospective case series. J Cutan Med Surg. 2012;16:212–7.

Baykal C, Kavak A, Buyukbabani N, Gulcan P. Dyskeratosis congenita associated with three malignancies. J Eur Acad Derm Venereol. 2003;17:261–8.

Baykal C, Savcı N, Kavak A, Kurul S. Palmoplantar keratoderma and oral leucoplakia with cutaneous horn of the lips. Br J Dermatol. 2002;146:680–3.

Berman B, Cohen DE, Amini S. What is the role of field directed therapy in the treatment of actinic keratosis? Part 2: commonly used field-directed and lesion directed therapies. Cutis. 2012;89:294–301.

Burgdorf WHC, Plewig G, Wolff HH, Landthaler M. Braun-Falco's dermatology, edn 3. Italy: Springer-Verlag; 2009.

Caputo R, Tadini G. Atlas of Genodermatoses. Spain: Taylor and Francis; 2006.

Garcia Reitböck J, Feldmann R, Rühringer K, et al. Chronic radiodermatitis following percutaneous transluminal coronary angioplasty. J Dtsch Dermatol Ges. 2013;11:265–6.

James WD, Berger T, Elston D. Andrew's Diseases of the Skin: Clinical Dermatology, edn 11. China: Saunders Elsevier; 2011.

Kanitakis J. Mammary and extramammary Paget's disease. J Eur Acad Dermatol Venereol. 2007;21:581–90.

Ko CJ. Keratoacanthoma: facts and controversies. Clin Dermatol. 2010;28:254–61.

Koch A, Schönlebe J, Kötler E, Wollina U. Polydacytlous Bowen's disease. J Eur Acad Dermatol Venereol. 2003;17:213–5.

Kong HH, Cowen EW, Azad NS. Keratoacanthomas associated with sorafenib therapy. J Am Acad Dermatol. 2007;56:171–2.

Lloyd J, Flanagan AM. Mammary and extramammary Paget's disease. J Clin Pathol. 2000;53:742–9.

Lycka BA. Bowen's disease and internal malignancy. A meta-analysis. Int J Dermatol. 1989;28:531–3.

Napier SS, Speight PM. Natural history of potentially malignant oral lesions and conditions: an overview of the literature. J Oral Pathol Med. 2008;37:1–10.

Rigel DS, Robinson JK, Ross M, Friedman RJ, Corkerell CJ, Lim HW, et al. Cancer of the skin, edn 2. China: Saunders Elsevier; 2011.

Schimizu I, Cruz A, Chong KH, Dufrense RG. Treatment of squamous cell carcinoma in situ: a review. Dermatol Surg. 2011;37:1394–411.

Schwartz RA. Skin Cancer: Recognition and Management, edn 2. Singapore: Blackwell Publishing; 2008.

Sharma A, Shah SR, Illum H, Dowel J. Vemurafenib: targeted inhibition of mutated BRAF for treatment of advanced melanoma and its potential in other malignancies. Drugs. 2012;72:2207–22.

Siller G, Gebauer K, Welburn P, et al. PEP005 (ingenol mebutate) gel, a novel agent for the treatment of actinic keratosis: results of a randomized, double-blind vehicle-controlled, multicentre, phase IIa study. Australas J Dermatol. 2009;50:16–22.

Szeimies RM, Bichel J, Ortonne JP, et al. A phase II dose-ranging study of topical resiquimod to treat actinic keratosis. Br J Dermatol. 2008;159:205–10.

Taliaferro SJ, Cohen GF. Bowen's disease of the penis treated with topical imiquimod 5% cream. J Drugs Dermatol. 2008;7:483–5.

Vandergriff T, Nakamura K, High WA. Generalized eruptive keratoacanthomas of Gryzbowski treated with isotretinoin. J Drugs Dermatol. 2008;7:1069–71.

Yarosh D, Klein J, O'Connor A, et al. Effect of topically applied T4 endonuclease V in liposomes on skin cancer in xeroderma pigmentosum: a randomised study. Xeroderma Pigmentosum Study Group. Lancet. 2001;357:926–9.

Nevomelanocytic Benign Tumors

Nevomelanocytic benign tumors are commonly encountered skin problems. The proliferation of melanocytes or the presence of nevus cells (nevocytes) is the cause of these benign tumors. Melanocytes are elements of the basal layer of the epidermis. Their increase in the epidermis causes epidermal melanocytic tumors. These lesions also may be markers of some syndromes. Normally there are no melanocytes in the dermis. However, the presence of dendritic melanocytes in the dermis causes dermal melanocytic tumors. Melanocytic nevi (nevus cell nevi) are characterized by nevus cells that form nests in the epidermis and dermis. Different clinicopathologic variants of these nevi, either congenital or acquired, have been described. A large number of tumors of melanocytes or nevus cells and the related syndromes are the main topics of this chapter. On the other hand, lesions like ephelides only show an increase in melanin pigment (melanotic lesions) but are clinically similar to the nevomelanocytic tumors because of their brownish color. Although these lesions cannot be defined as real tumors because of the lack of proliferation of melanocytes or nevocytes, they are additionally discussed in this chapter for their overlapping clinical features and differential diagnostic importance.

3.1 Melanotic Lesions

3.1.1 Ephelides (Freckles)

Ephelides are common causes of hyperpigmentation on the facial skin. They are more frequent in fair-skinned people with blue or green eyes and blond or red hair. They may be familial in origin and tend to occur more commonly in females. Lesions appear in early childhood and are typically scattered symmetrically on the face, arms, and upper back. The cheeks and nose are most commonly involved (see Fig. 3.1). Lesions may be found on the lips but not on the intraoral mucosa. Asymptomatic, reddish or light brown irregularly-shaped macules measuring 1 to 3 mm in diameter are typical (see Figs. 3.1, 3.2 and 3.3). The lesions are usually discrete and in varying numbers, but some patients have profuse lesions showing a tendency to confluence. The

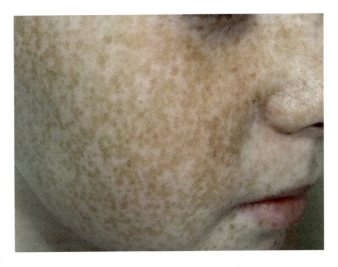

Fig. 3.1 Ephelides on the cheek, the most typical location

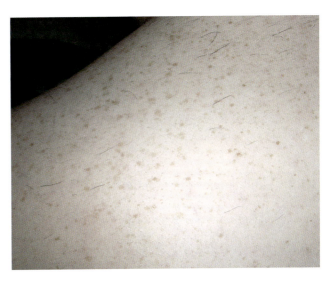

Fig. 3.2 Ephelides on the upper back. Note the small light brown macules

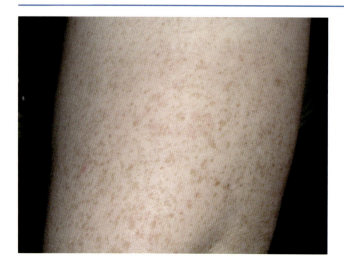

Fig. 3.3 Ephelides on the sun-exposed areas of the upper arm

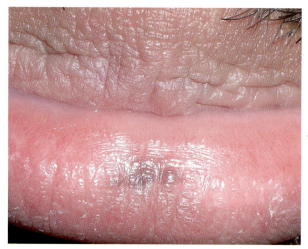

Fig. 3.4 Labial melanotic macule on the midline of the vermilion border of lower lip. This benign lesion has typically uniform brownish color

lesions may darken with sun exposure. Therefore, ephelides are relatively darker in summer and lighter in winter.

Xeroderma pigmentosum (see Figs. 3.27 and 11.20) and several other syndromes manifesting with multiple small pigmented lesions (e.g., lentigines) are the main clinical differential diagnostic challenges. But unlike ephelides, lentigines are stable and relatively darker. Additionally, photosensitivity is a differentiating feature of xeroderma pigmentosum. In neurofibromatosis, small café-au-lait macules grouped in the axillae or inguinal folds are called "axillary freckling" (see Fig. 3.38), but these are not real freckles since they have a persistent course and histologically show melanocytic hyperplasia. Ephelides are nearly always diagnosed clinically. Histologically, there is an increase in epidermal melanin without associated melanocytic proliferation.

Management. Ephelides are benign lesions. Sun protection, including the use of sunscreens, is essential to prevent the occurrence of new ephelides and darkening of lesions in summer. Patients with ephelides are more prone to solar damage, so may develop skin changes related with solar damage including skin tumors. Hence the importance of sun protection is increased in these individuals. Most patients do not seek any therapy. Cosmetic camouflage may be useful. Ephelides decrease or fade spontaneously later in life but usually do not vanish completely.

3.1.2 Labial Melanotic Macule

Labial melanotic macule is an acquired small hyperpigmented macule of the oral mucosa. It is usually seen on the lower lip of middle-aged women. The lesion is typically solitary and is located on the midline of the vermilion border (see Fig. 3.4) but may also be located on one side of the lip (see Fig. 3.5). An oval-shaped macule measuring 2 to 10 mm is flat or slightly raised and brownish to black-colored.

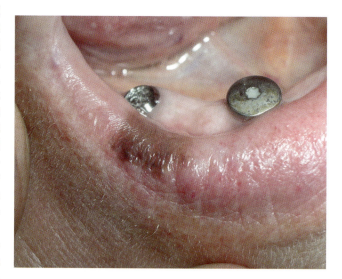

Fig. 3.5 A solitary small well-defined hyperpigmented macule on one side of the lower lip; labial melanotic macule

Rarely, more than one lesion may occur. Lesions do not show a tendency to enlarge. The predilection for the lower lip suggests solar etiology. However, the upper lip, buccal mucosa, gingivae, and palate are rarely involved. Despite its rare occurrence on these locations, the lesion is also called "oral melanotic macule."

An early lesion of mucosal melanoma is the main differential diagnostic challenge, especially in patients who lack a history of long duration of pigmentation. Other conditions in the differential diagnosis include acquired melanocytic nevi, blue nevus, ephelides, and lentigines. Melanocytic nevi and blue nevus are relatively elevated. Ephelides and lentigines located on the lips usually present with multiple lesions. The histologic features of a labial melanotic macule are similar to those of ephelides, with an increase of melanin and the absence of melanocytic hyperplasia. Additionally, there may be accompanying mild acanthosis and dermal melanophages.

Management. There is no risk of malignant degeneration of labial melanotic macules. Therefore, therapy is not mandatory. On the other hand, if there is any doubt of malignancy, the dark mucosal lesions should be excised for histopathologic examination. Cryotherapy and lasers are effective, but destructive methods can only be used for lesions in which malignant melanoma has been ruled out. Lesions evaluated as benign can be followed up for a period of time, and if they are stable they can be ignored.

3.1.3 Penile Melanotic Macule

This lesion is clinically and histopathologically similar to labial melanotic macule except for its localization. It is an acquired hyperpigmented small macule usually seen on the glans penis or prepuce of young adult men. Penile melanotic macule must primarily be distinguished from genital malignant melanoma.

Management. The lesion carries no risk of malignant transformation and therefore there is no need for therapy.

3.1.4 Vulvar Melanosis

This is a benign hyperpigmented condition seen in the female genitalia, either as a solitary lesion or as multiple scattered lesions. Brown to black, irregularly-shaped macules 5 to 15 mm in diameter are seen on the vulva (*see* Fig. 3.6), mostly on the labia minora, vagina and sometimes on the cervix. Since the lesions are asymptomatic, they may incidentally be detected during a gynecologic examination. When noticed, however, especially in diffuse lesions, they may cause concern. Irregularly-shaped, dark lesions should be differentiated from malignant melanoma. If any doubt exists, a biopsy should be performed. Vulvar lentigines seen in Carney syndrome may also show a similar picture (*see* Fig. 3.14). Vulvar melanosis is histologically characterized by an increase of epidermal melanin and dermal melanophages. Melanocyte hyperplasia and nest formation do not exist.

Management. There is no effective treatment. Total excision can be performed in small and solitary lesions.

3.2 Epidermal Melanocytic Tumors

3.2.1 Lentigo Simplex

Lentigo simplex is a pigmented macule showing melanocytic hyperplasia and may occur sporadically or in the setting of some syndromes. It may be seen in all races.

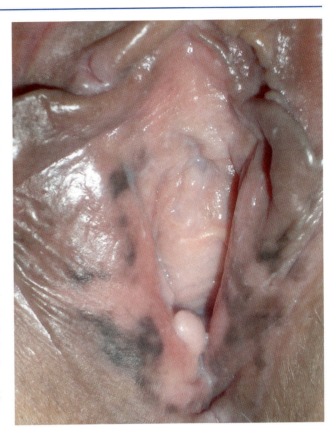

Fig. 3.6 Vulvar melanosis causing multiple irregularly distributed hyperpigmented macules on the vulva

Although it has been suggested as a precursor of junctional nevi, this transformation has not been observed, especially during the follow-up of several syndromes manifesting with lentigines.

Lentigines usually appear in childhood and may increase in number with age. They may rarely be congenital. A typical lesion is light brown or brownish-black, sharply demarcated, homogeneous, round or oval macule measuring 3 to 5 mm in diameter (*see* Fig. 3.7). Lentigo simplex has no connection with intense or cumulative sun exposure. Lesions may be seen anywhere on the body, and they are not restricted to sun-exposed areas. They may also be localized on mucocutaneous junctions and conjunctivae. Lentigo simplex is among the causes of melanonychia striata. In contrast to ephelides, which only show an increase of epidermal melanin, lentigines are characterized by an increase in melanocytes along the dermoepidermal junction, leading to overproduction of melanin.

On rare occasions genital lentigines may be superimposed on lichen sclerosus et atrophicus, causing a challenge in diagnosis (*see* Fig. 3.8).

Numerous lentigines distributed all over the body without the presence of any exogenous triggering factor is called lentigo profusa (*see* Figs. 3.9 and 3.10). There are some rare genodermatoses such as LEOPARD syndrome, Peutz-Jeghers syndrome, and Carney syndrome associated with

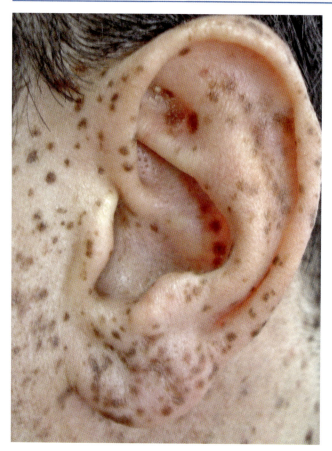

Fig. 3.7 Lentigo simplex presenting as multiple small hyperpigmented macules on the auricle

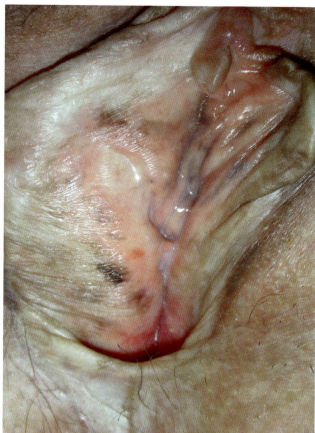

Fig. 3.8 Lentigo arising on white plaques of lichen sclerosis et atrophicus on the vulva

lentigo profusa. Apart from lentigines, these syndromes have other distinctive dermatologic features or systemic manifestations.

LEOPARD syndrome is a rare autosomal dominantly inherited disease. The term LEOPARD is an acronym reflecting **l**entigines, **e**lectrocardiographic conduction defects, **o**cular hypertelorism, **p**ulmonary stenosis, **a**bnormalities of the genitalia, **r**etardation of growth, and sensorineural **d**eafness. Not all systemic findings are present in the same patient. Delayed puberty is seen in both sexes. Arrhythmia is the main complication of the disease. Disseminated lentigines are present at birth or begin to occur in early childhood, localizing anywhere on the body but more commonly on the neck and upper trunk. The oral mucosa is usually not involved. There may be large, pigmented macules intermingled with small lentigines. The number of pigmented lesions increases with age. These patients need appropriate referral to the cardiology, endocrinology, ophthalmology, and ear-nose-throat departments.

Peutz-Jeghers syndrome is characterized by intestinal polyposis associated with mucocutaneous lentigines. It is an autosomal dominant syndrome related to a mutation in the *STK11/LKB1* gene. Lentigines (see Figs. 3.11 and 3.12) are present at birth or appear in childhood. The involvement of lips (mostly the lower lip), buccal mucosa, hard palate, and

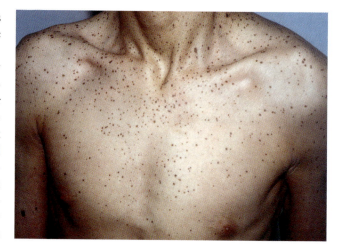

Fig. 3.9 Innumerable lesions of lentigo simplex called as lentigo profusa

perioral area is typical. The conjunctivae, periorbital and perinasal area, and genitalia are other main locations of lentigines. Small, brown or dark blue macules may be found on the face and may be accompanied by melanonychia striata and multiple lentigines on the fingertips (see Fig. 3.13) or palmoplantar area. Cutaneous lentigines may fade after puberty, but

3.2 Epidermal Melanocytic Tumors

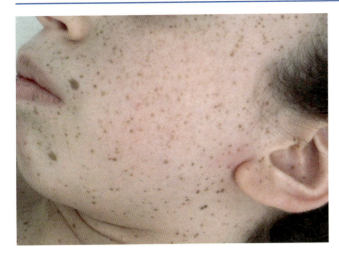

Fig. 3.10 Lentigo profusa on the face. This clinical picture should be alarming for some genodermatoses including LEOPARD syndrome

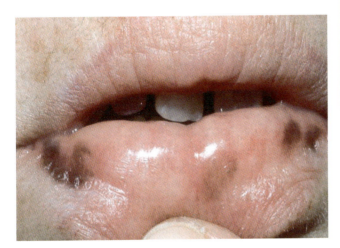

Fig. 3.11 Lentigines on the vermilion border of the lower lip in a patient with Peutz-Jeghers syndrome

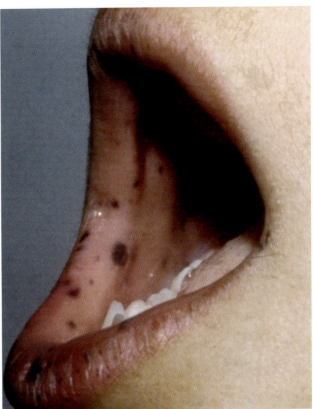

Fig. 3.12 Lentigines on the lip and buccal mucosa; the typical clinical clue of Peutz-Jeghers syndrome

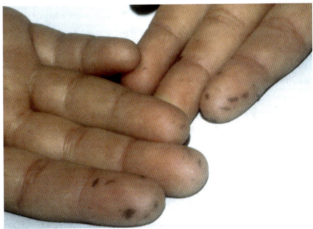

Fig. 3.13 Multiple lentigines on the volar aspect of the fingers; a dermatologic feature of Peutz-Jeghers syndrome

tend to persist in oral mucosa. Polyps are more commonly seen in the small intestine but may occur at any part of the gastrointestinal tract such as the stomach, colon, and rectum. They may cause intussusception resulting in bleeding and abdominal pain. Malignant change of these hamartomatous polyps is not clear. On the other hand, gastrointestinal malignancies (esophageal, gastric, small intestinal, colorectal, and pancreatic adenocarcinoma) are the most common neoplasms in this syndrome. The incidence of solid neoplasms of other visceral organs such as the breast, cervix, uterus, over and lung is also increased. In patients with mucocutaneous lentigines on typical locations, endoscopic and colonoscopic investigation for intestinal polyps should be done. Patients should also be screened and followed for life for the occurrence of malignancies. The dermatologic features of Peutz-Jeghers syndrome may resemble those of Laugier-Hunziker syndrome, which presents with lentigines of the lips, buccal mucosa, and hard palate associated with melanonychia striata of multiple fingers or toes. However, this rare syndrome is not associated with any systemic manifestations.

Carney syndrome and two other acronyms including LAMB (**l**entigines, **a**trial **m**yxomas, and **b**lue nevi) and NAME (**n**evi, **a**trial myxomas, **m**yxoid neurofibromas, **e**phelides or **e**ndocrine overreactivity) are accepted as the same disease. The autosomal dominant syndrome is related to mutations in the *PRKAR1A* gene. The major clinical sign of

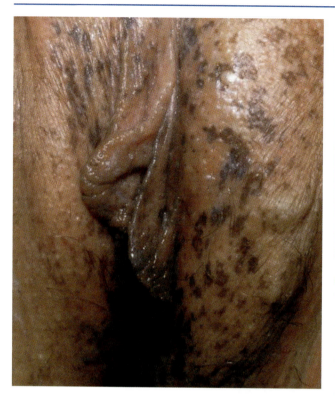

Fig. 3.14 Multiple lentigines on the vulva; a distinctive manifestation of Carney syndrome

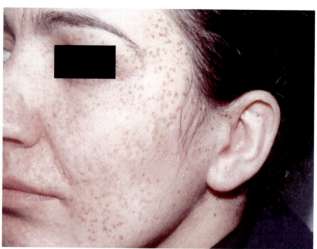

Fig. 3.15 Segmental lentiginosis; lentigines in a segmental distribution on one side of the face are seen

this syndrome is diffuse facial lentigines that are present at birth. Lentigines may also be found on the lips, genitalia (*see* Fig. 3.14), and conjunctivae. Multiple blue nevi may be seen on various locations. Cutaneous myxoma manifesting as an asymptomatic, skin-colored dermal papule or nodule is more commonly located on the eyelid, external ear canal and nipple. The coexistence of some of these skin findings are suggestive of the diagnosis. Echocardiography can be performed to detect myxomas of cardiac muscle. Pituitary adenomas, primary pigmented nodular adrenocortical hyperplasia, and testicular tumors (Sertoli cell tumors) are the endocrinologic manifestations. Psammomatous melanotic schwannoma, a rare nerve sheath tumor, may be also seen. Complications of atrial myxomas such as congestive heart failure, pulmonary edema, and embolization to different organs including the brain increase the morbidity of the syndrome.

Management. Lentigo simplex is a benign lesion without any risk of malignant degeneration. A periodic dermatologic follow-up is not mandatory. However, investigation of the associated syndromes is essential in patients with multiple lesions.

3.2.2 Segmental Lentiginosis

Segmental lentiginosis, also known as partial unilateral lentiginosis, is a circumscribed cluster of lentigines typically located on one side of the body (*see* Fig. 3.15). It may be segmental or dermatomal and sometimes may involve a large area of the body. The etiology of segmental lentiginosis is not understood. It is usually diagnosed in children but may even be present at birth. The individual lesions are sharply demarcated brown macules that are 2 to 10 mm in diameter. The patient does not have lentigines on other parts of the body. It is often diagnosed clinically. It may be confused with the segmental variant of nevus spilus, but segmental lentiginosis lacks diffuse pigmented macule on the background and overlying raised papules. The histopathologic features of an individual lesion are the same as those of lentigo simplex.

Management. Segmental lentiginosis is a benign condition. Association with any systemic disease is not known. Hence, further examination and therapeutic intervention are not necessary.

3.2.3 Actinic Lentigo (Lentigo Senilis)

Actinic lentigo is an irregular, flat, benign hyperpigmented lesion seen mostly on sun-exposed areas. There is no intimate association with skin type. Both cumulative and intermittent sun exposure play a role in the etiopathogenesis. Since sunburn in childhood is a risk factor for actinic lentigo, lesions may also occur at a young age. Therefore, the term lentigo senilis does not reflect the characteristic of the disease. In young individuals, lesions are more prevalent on the upper back (*see* Fig. 3.16), shoulders (*see* Fig. 3.17), and décolleté, while in older patients the face, dorsum of the hands (*see* Figs. 3.18 and 3.19), and forearms are more commonly involved in a symmetrical pattern. Typical lesions are approximately 6 to 10 mm, round or oval, light to dark brown discrete macules or slightly raised papules with irregular borders (*see* Figs. 3.20 and 3.21). The number of lesions varies from a few to hundreds. Lesions may increase in number

3.2 Epidermal Melanocytic Tumors

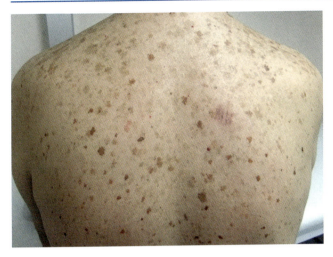

Fig. 3.16 Actinic lentigo typically located on the upper back of a young adult

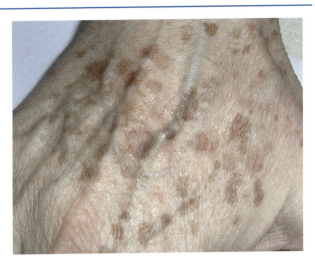

Fig. 3.19 Multiple lesions of actinic lentigo on the dorsum of the hand. In addition to flat lesions, a slightly raised lesion is also seen

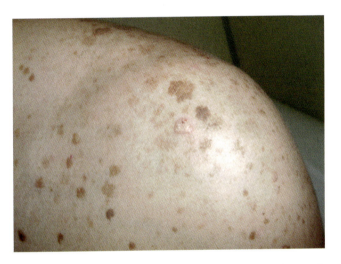

Fig. 3.17 Actinic lentigo on the shoulders. Most patients have typically multiple lesions as seen on the figure

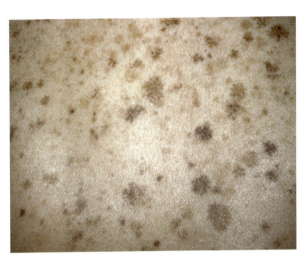

Fig. 3.20 Early lesions of actinic lentigo on the upper back. Brownish colored irregular lesions are just palpable

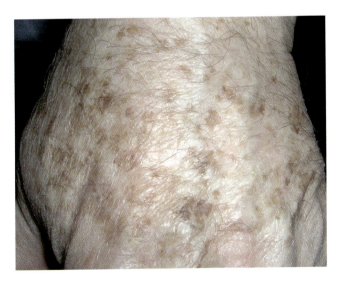

Fig. 3.18 Actinic lentigo on the dorsum of the hand. Lesions on this sun-exposed area are commonly seen in the elderly and they may be ill-defined

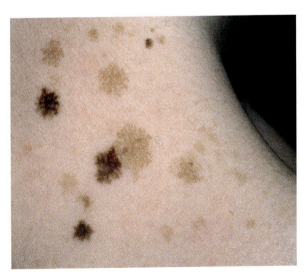

Fig. 3.21 Light- and dark-brown lesions of actinic lentigo are seen concomitantly in the figure

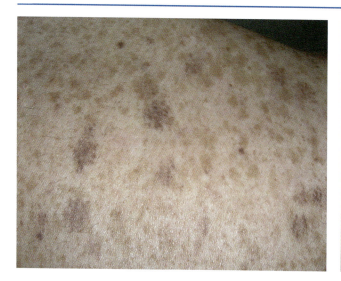

Fig. 3.22 Multiple actinic lentigines on the upper back. Lesions are typically discrete but some show tendency to confluence

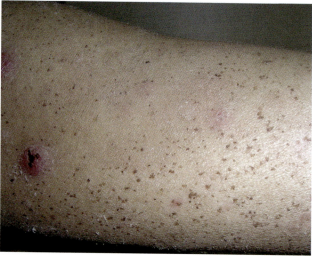

Fig. 3.23 PUVA lentigines on the arm of a patient with mycosis fungoides. This patient had a long-term treatment of phototherapy

in older patients. Lesions of various sizes may be observed concomitantly. Sometimes the lesions show a tendency to confluence (*see* Fig. 3.22). Patients, even those with multiple lesions, are asymptomatic.

Actinic lentigo is considered early flat seborrheic keratosis (*see* Fig. 1.43). Lesions may elevate later causing typical appearance of classical seborrheic keratosis. Unlike in lentigo simplex (*see* Fig. 3.9), lesions are restricted to sun-exposed areas of the skin and are relatively larger and irregular. Lentigo maligna (*see* Fig. 12.8) is the major differential diagnostic challenge on the face but presents as a solitary lesion, usually with a non-homogeneous appearance showing more variegated pigmentation than actinic lentigo, darker foci, and irregular borders. Dermoscopy may be helpful in the differentiation of these tumors. Histologically, an increase of melanocytes along the basement membrane, elongated ridges, and solar elastosis are the main features of actinic lentigo. Nest formation is not observed.

Actinic lentigines may also be seen in the setting of xeroderma pigmentosum at a very young age. But these patients are predisposed to other features of dermatoheliosis, including epidermal atrophy, telangiectases, and patchy hyper- or hypopigmentation.

Management. Transformation to malignant melanoma is not expected in actinic lentigo. Therefore therapy is not mandatory. Skin bleaching agents do not have any permanent effect. Because the lesions are usually multiple, destructive methods are not easy to use. Laser therapy (e.g., Q-switched Ruby laser, erbium Er:YAG laser) and cryotherapy are the main alternatives for aesthetic improvement. Cryotherapy carries the risk of postinflammatory dyspigmentation, especially in dark-skinned people. Patients should be instructed about lifelong sun protection.

3.2.3.1 PUVA Lentigines

PUVA (psoralen + ultraviolet A) therapy is used in dermatologic practice for various indications such as, mycosis fungoides, psoriasis and vitiligo. In patients treated for a long time or with high cumulative doses, the side effects of UVA are more frequently seen and are relatively common in fair-skinned people. PUVA lentigines are a special type of actinic lentigo occurring after 5 to 7 years of whole body irradiation. They are common on the trunk and proximal extremities (*see* Fig. 3.23), areas that are normally protected from the sun. The thighs, which are mostly preserved in patients with actinic lentigo, may also be involved. Skin folds and the palmoplantar area are usually spared. Lesions are also not usually found on genitalia, since this site is protected during PUVA therapy. The number of lesions is variable. Patients who have undergone long-term photochemotherapy may have numerous lesions (*see* Fig. 3.24). An individual lesion is 2 to 6 mm in size (*see* Fig. 3.25) and may be darker than that of lentigo simplex or actinic lentigo. It may have a stellate-like appearance. The diagnosis is always based on clinical examination, along with the presence of a history of photochemotherapy.

Management. These lentigines persist for years after discontinuation of PUVA therapy. They do not show malignant degeneration, but it should be kept in mind that these patients also have an increased risk of developing other cutaneous lesions caused by ultraviolet radiation, including precancerous lesions such as actinic keratosis or Bowen disease (*see* Fig. 3.26) and malignant tumors. Therefore, these patients should be followed indefinitely.

3.2.3.2 Xeroderma Pigmentosum

Xeroderma pigmentosum is an autosomal recessive genodermatosis characterized by sun damage–induced skin lesions

3.2 Epidermal Melanocytic Tumors

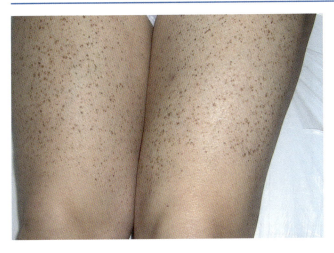

Fig. 3.24 PUVA lentigines presenting as symmetrically located profuse lesions on the leg. Note that the location is different than that of actinic lentigo

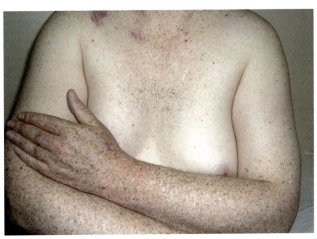

Fig. 3.27 Freckles and lentigines densely located on the sun-exposed areas in xeroderma pigmentosum

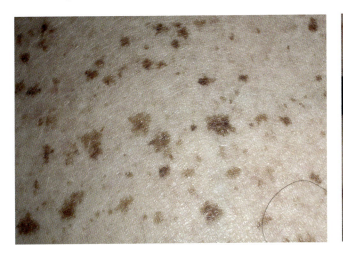

Fig. 3.25 Multiple dark-colored, stellate-like, small lesions of PUVA lentigines

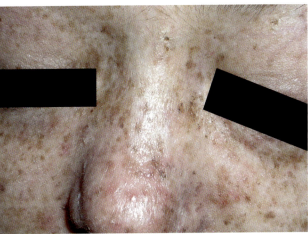

Fig. 3.28 Freckles, lentigines and skin atrophy on the face of a child with xeroderma pigmentosum

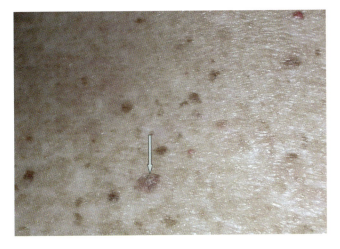

Fig. 3.26 PUVA lentigines associated with Bowen disease (erythematous papule), and skin atrophy related with chronic ultraviolet damage

and systemic involvement. Damage caused by ultraviolet exposure cannot be repaired adequately in these patients. Cutaneous and mucosal manifestations begin in early childhood with ultraviolet exposure. Marked photosensitivity of the child may be observed by the parents.

Early manifestations are freckles and lentigines. Atrophy, dyspigmentation, and telangiectases are also seen, especially on the face, neck, forearms, and dorsum of the hands (*see* Figs. 3.27, 3.28 and 3.29). The patients have an increased risk of developing precancerous lesions such as actinic keratosis and skin cancers, including basal cell carcinoma (*see* Fig. 11.21), squamous cell carcinoma (*see* Figs. 11.102 and 11.103), and malignant melanoma (*see* Fig. 12.15). It may be hard to diagnose early lesions of lentigo maligna melanoma (*see* Fig. 3.30) among freckles and lentigines.

Eye findings, neurologic involvement, ataxia, and microcephaly are systemic manifestations of the disease.

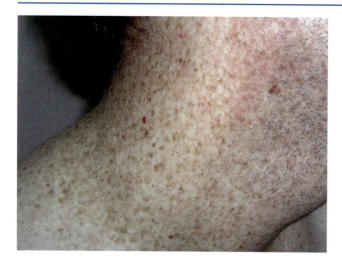

Fig. 3.29 Profuse lentigines on the neck of an adult patient with xeroderma pigmentosum

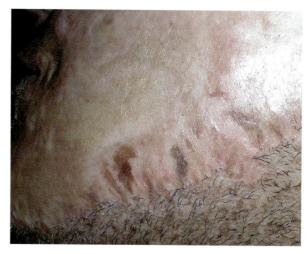

Fig. 3.31 Lentigines arising on surgical scar in a patient with xeroderma pigmentosum. Note the pigmented streaks on the scar

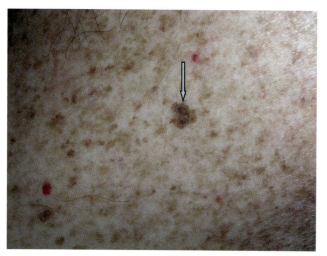

Fig. 3.30 Freckles and lentigines in a patient with xeroderma pigmentosum. Note the relatively larger and more irregular, hyperpigmented lesion of lentigo maligna (*arrow*) among the small lesions of lentigines

Management. Strict photoprotection from early childhood on is mandatory. Dermatologic surveillance is critical to diagnose precancerous lesions and skin cancers early. Precancerous and cancerous lesions can be treated with destructive techniques, topical medications, or surgery. Lentigines may occur on surgical scars as irregular hyperpigmentation (*see* Fig. 3.31) and should be differentiated from malignant melanoma.

3.2.4 Café-au-lait Macules

Café-au-lait macules are brown persistent patches that can be part of several syndromes. The name is derived from French and means "coffee with milk," reflecting the typical light brown color of these macules. Solitary lesions are common in all races but relatively more frequent in African Americans. Multiple lesions are mostly associated with neurofibromatosis, but they may also appear in other systemic diseases such as McCune-Albright syndrome, Fanconi anemia, Silver Russell syndrome, LEOPARD syndrome, and Westerhof syndrome. They are usually the first sign of neurofibromatosis type 1 (von Recklinghausen disease). Six or more café-au-lait macules larger than 5 mm in prepubertal or 15 mm in postpubertal individuals are among the diagnostic criteria of this type of neurofibromatosis. However, they may also be seen in neurofibromatosis type 2.

Café-au-lait macules are usually present at birth or appear in early infancy as faint patches. The macules may enlarge in size, darken in color, and become visible as the child grows. In cases associated with syndromes, the number of lesions may increase in years.

Café-au-lait macules are located mostly on the trunk, extremities, and face. Involvement of the palmoplantar area and genitalia is unusual. Mucosal surfaces are always spared. A typical lesion is a hairless, uniformly pigmented, pale brown macule with round, oval, or irregular shape and usually larger than 0.5 cm (*see* Figs. 3.32 and 3.33). However, lesions larger than 10 cm (*see* Fig. 3.34) or smaller than 0.5 mm are also possible. A patient with neurofibromatosis type 1 can have multiple lesions in different sizes (*see* Figs. 3.35 and 3.36). On the other hand, café-au-lait macules of McCune Albright syndrome are usually observed as unilateral large macules with irregular borders and are likely to follow the lines of Blaschko (*see* Fig. 3.37).

Multiple café-au-lait macules of a few millimeters localized in a symmetric fashion on the axillary region are called "axillary freckling" or "Crowe sign" (*see* Figs. 3.38 and 3.39). These tiny lesions are among the diagnostic criteria of neurofibromatosis type 1. They mostly occur in puberty and

3.2 Epidermal Melanocytic Tumors

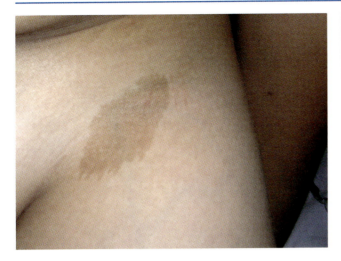

Fig. 3.32 Solitary, irregular café-au-lait macule in an otherwise healthy child

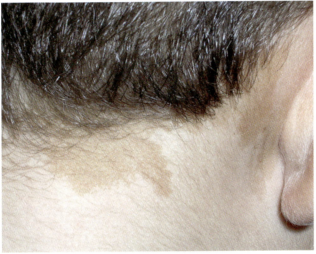

Fig. 3.33 Café-au-lait macules presenting as pale brown patches with irregular borders on the nape and retroauricular area

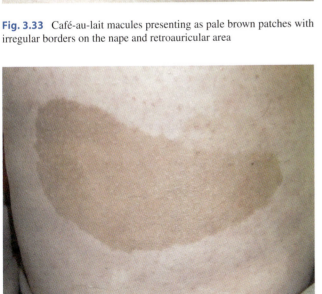

Fig. 3.34 A large café-au-lait macule on the trunk. Its even color is distinctive

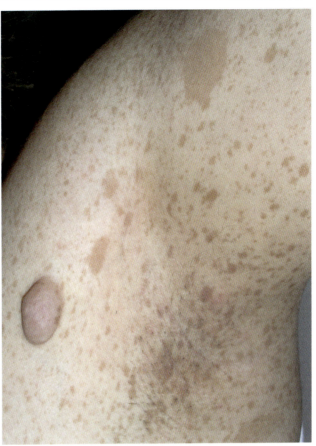

Fig. 3.35 Multiple café-au-lait macules of various sizes associated with neurofibromas in a neurofibromatosis patient

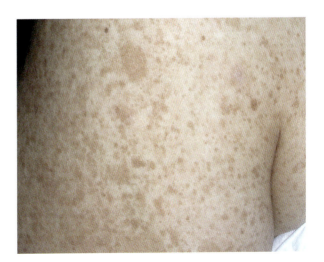

Fig. 3.36 Innumerable café-au-lait macules in an adult patient with neurofibromatosis

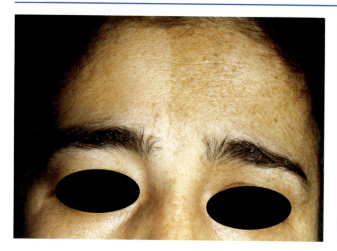

Fig. 3.37 Unilateral café-au-lait macules (*right*) in McCune Albright syndrome

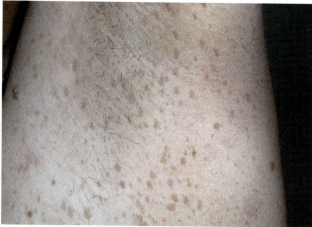

Fig. 3.39 Axillary freckling presenting as multiple brownish macules measuring a few millimeters. These lesions are typically bilateral in neurofibromatosis patients and may also be seen on other body folds

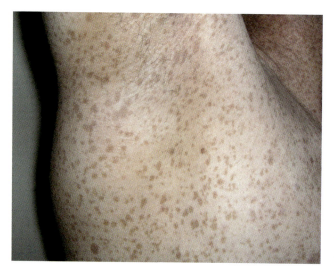

Fig. 3.38 Axillary freckling (Crowe sign); multiple small café-au-lait macules restricted to axilla in neurofibromatosis

do not show a tendency to enlarge. Similar lesions may also be seen in the inguinal folds.

Café-au-lait macules are usually persistent but sometimes they may fade or disappear spontaneously in adulthood. They are diagnosed clinically. Postinflammatory hyperpigmentation, the initial stage of nevus spilus, and Becker nevus (*see* Fig. 1.129) are among the differential diagnostic conditions. Histologic features include increased basal melanin content and a very subtle increase in melanocytes. Macromelanosomes may sometimes be seen.

Management. There is no need to search for any accompanying dermatoses in patients with one or two café-au-lait macules. However, if multiple lesions are present, an association with a genodermatose should be suspected. Café-au-lait macules are asymptomatic and do not cause any complications. Treatment can be sought for cosmetic purposes. Cosmetic camouflage may be advised for some lesions.

Hydroquinone and other bleaching agents are ineffective for café-au-lait macules. Various laser alternatives can be applied, but results of therapy are variable and include risks of irregular pigmentation, slight scarring, and recurrence.

3.3 Dermal Melanocytic Tumors

Mongolian spot, nevus of Ota, nevus of Ito, dermal melanocytosis, and blue nevus are congenital or acquired hamartomatous tumors presenting as cutaneous and/or mucosal macules, papules, or plaques. Most lesions occur separately, whereas some may be seen concomitantly. A common theory in the pathogenesis of all these tumors is that some embryonic melanocytes migrating from the neural crest were arrested in the dermis and failed to reach their normal location in the epidermis. All of these tumors have a bluish-gray color owing to dermal melanin produced by melanocytes. The dermal pigmentation scatters the shorter wavelength light, causing a bluish-gray color of the lesion which is called as Tyndall effect. Age of onset, anatomic location, and predominant type of elementary lesion are helpful clinical clues in differentiating these nevi from one another. Histopathologic differences are subtle or absent.

3.3.1 Mongolian Spot

Mongolian spot is a congenital hyperpigmented patch with a tendency to spontaneous healing. It is one of the most common cutaneous changes in newborns. It shares common clinicopathologic features with some other dermal melanocytic tumors but is not permanent, unlike these lesions. It is extremely prevalent among East Asians as the name suggests. African Americans and Native Americans are

3.3 Dermal Melanocytic Tumors

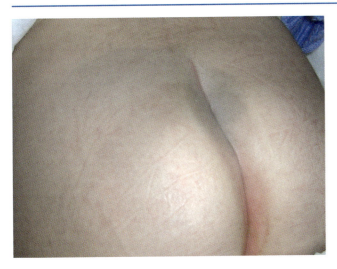

Fig. 3.40 Mongolian spot presenting as an ill-defined, bluish gray, small patch on the inner aspect of the buttocks of a child

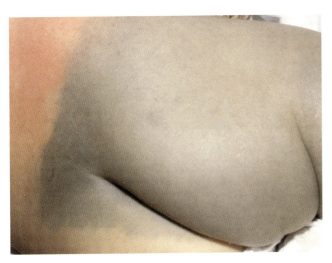

Fig. 3.41 A large Mongolian spot on the buttocks of a child

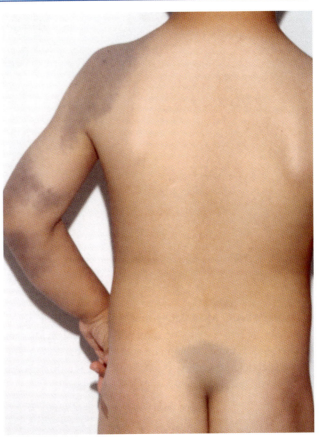

Fig. 3.42 Mongolian spot on the typical sacral location. There are also similar lesions on the shoulder and arm (ectopic Mongolian spots)

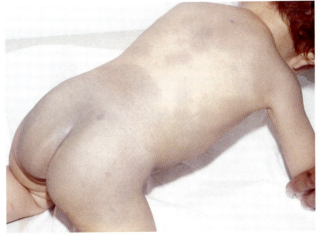

Fig. 3.43 Extensive ectopic Mongolian spots on the trunk of a child

also frequently targeted. A relatively rare appearance in Caucasians also reveals the prominent racial differences.

Lesions are apparent at birth or develop within the first weeks of life as multiple small coalescing spots or as one large patch. The blue, bluish-gray and bluish-black asymptomatic patches are round, oval, or irregularly shaped and have indistinct borders (see Fig. 3.40). Most lesions are a few centimeters in size but may sometimes be extensive (see Fig. 3.41). Large lesions may be sharply demarcated. Mongolian spot is generally located on the lumbosacral area, on the inner aspect of the buttocks and flanks. Sometimes lesions may be observed at other locations such as the shoulders or the dorsal aspect of the hands and feet, and these are called ectopic Mongolian spots (see Figs. 3.42 and 3.43).

Mongolian spot is usually not associated with systemic diseases. The typical location and color are indicative of the clinical diagnosis, and biopsy or further systemic examination is not necessary. Histologically, sparse dendritic melanocytes that contain melanin are present in the lower half of the dermis.

Phakomatosis pigmentovascularis is a rare disease associated with ectopic Mongolian spots in addition to other types of dermal melanocytic tumors and nevus flammeus (see Fig. 3.44).

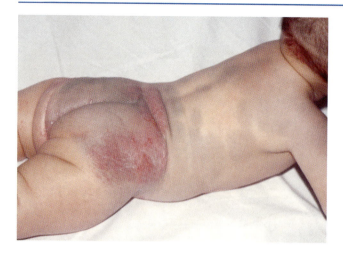

Fig. 3.44 Phacomatosis pigmentovascularis presenting with irregularly scattered ectopic Mongolian spots and a port-wine stain on buttocks

Management. Most Mongolian spots disappear spontaneously in 3 to 5 years or sometimes by puberty. Larger lesions and ectopic Mongolian spots may be permanent. A therapeutic intervention is not indicated for this benign melanocytic lesion.

3.3.2 Nevus of Ota

Nevus of Ota is a dermal melanocytic tumor of the skin and mucosal surfaces that are supplied by the first (ophthalmic) and second (maxillary) branches of the trigeminal nerve. It is also called nevus fuscoceruleus ophthalmomaxillaris. This nevus is more common in the Asian population and uncommon in Caucasians. It generally occurs sporadically. Females are more commonly affected than males. Tumors may be present at birth or develop in the first year of life or in early adolescence, appearing as a slight pigmented patch of variable size that gradually darkens and becomes more prominent. The face is usually unilaterally involved (*see* Fig. 3.45). However, oropharyngeal mucosa, nasal mucosa, tympanic membrane, and eye may also be affected on the same side as the skin lesions. Typical presentation of the nevus is blue, bluish-brown or bluish-grey, ill-defined, speckled or mottled pigmentation of the eyelids, forehead, temple, cheeks, nasal root, and alae nasi without extending to the other parts of the face (*see* Figs. 3.45 and 3.46). The pinna and retroauricular area may rarely be affected (*see* Fig. 3.47). Bluish-grey pigmentation of the conjuctivae and sclera may be prominent in some patients (*see* Figs. 3.48 and 3.49). Bilateral involvement of the skin and eyes may rarely be seen (*see* Fig. 3.50). Glaucoma may be associated in some cases.

Nevus of Ota is usually asymptomatic but may rarely be associated with sensory changes of the involved skin. It usually presents as a separate entity but sometimes may be accompanied by nevus of Ito or persistent ectopic Mongolian spots. It may also be a component of phakomatosis pigmentovascularis (*see* Fig. 3.51). We observed bilateral involvement of nevus of Ota on the palate in a patient with phakomatosis pigmentovascularis (*see* Fig. 3.52). Blue nevi may sometimes be found as small papules or nodules overlying the patches of nevus of Ota or on adjacent normal skin.

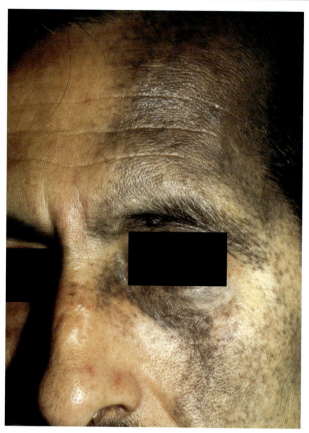

Fig. 3.45 Nevus of Ota showing typical unilateral involvement of the upper part of the face. This pigmentation is persistent

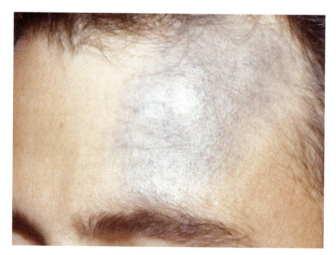

Fig. 3.46 Unilateral bluish patch on the forehead; a classic presentation of nevus of Ota

3.3 Dermal Melanocytic Tumors

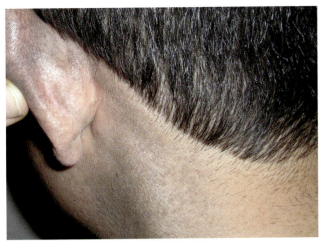

Fig. 3.47 Hyperpigmentation on the pinna in a patient with nevus of Ota. Any area supplied by the ophthalmic and maxillary branches of trigeminal nerve may be involved in this type of dermal melanocytic tumor

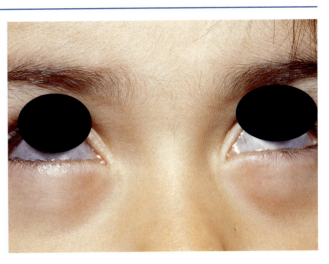

Fig. 3.50 Bilateral scleral involvement; a rare presentation of nevus of Ota

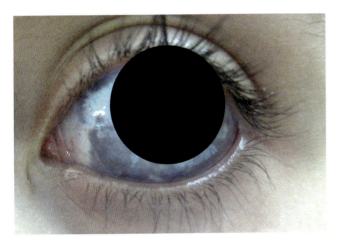

Fig. 3.48 Unilateral bluish grey pigmentation of the sclera; a distinctive clinical feature of nevus of Ota

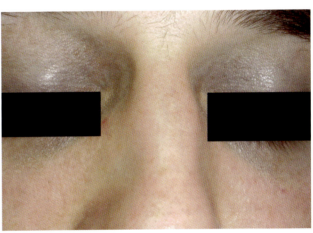

Fig. 3.51 Bilateral eyelid involvement of nevus of Ota in a patient with phacomatosis pigmentovascularis

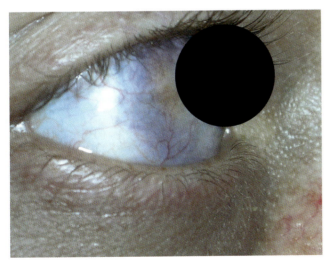

Fig. 3.49 Unilateral bluish grey pigmentation of the sclera. Association with ipsilateral periorbital hyperpigmentation is typical

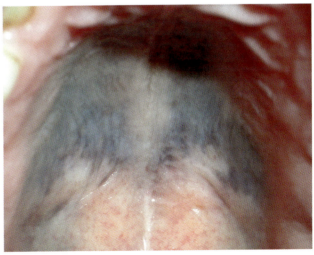

Fig. 3.52 Bilateral bluish pigmentation on the hard palate representing nevus of Ota in a patient with phacomatosis pigmentovascularis

Typical location and color of the lesions with coexisting skin, eye, and other mucosal surface involvement enable the clinical diagnosis of nevus of Ota. A biopsy is rarely performed. Histologically, dermal dendritic melanocytes are associated with surrounding fibrosis and dispersed melanophages.

Management. Most lesions remain unchanged. Although very rare, malignant melanoma can arise on the macular mucocutaneous patches or ocular lesions. Therefore, patients must be followed up both by a dermatologist and an ophthalmologist. Papules or subcutaneous nodules occurring on macular lesions and showing tendency to enlarge may be alarming signs of malignant degeneration. Nevus of Ota poses a serious cosmetic problem, eventually causing demand for therapy. Q-switched lasers may be helpful to reduce skin pigmentation, resulting in good cosmetic appearance. However, it is not certain whether this therapy can prevent malignant transformation. Cosmetic camouflage can also be advised. Eye lesions are generally not treated.

3.3.3 Nevus of Ito

Nevus of Ito is a dermal melanocytic tumor sharing the same clinicopathologic findings with skin lesions of nevus of Ota, but it has a different location. It is less common than nevus of Ota and is very rare in white individuals. Concomitant occurrence of both nevi may either be sporadic or be seen in the setting of phacomatosis pigmentovascularis. Nevus of Ito is located on the shoulder girdle (*see* Figs. 3.53 and 3.54), base of the neck (*see* Fig. 3.55), and upper arm, which are supplied by the posterior supraclavicular and lateral cutaneous brachial nerves. It is also called nevus fuscoceruleus acromiodeltoideus. Clinically, bluish-gray or brownish, uniform or speckled large unilateral patches are observed (*see* Fig. 3.55). These lesions are permanent. Nevus of Ito is usually diagnosed clinically. Inflammatory diseases causing dermal pigmentation such as fixed drug eruption and erythema dyschromicum perstans differ from nevus of Ito by their irregularly distributed small patches. The Mongolian spot has a typical anatomic location with a tendency to spontaneous regression. However,

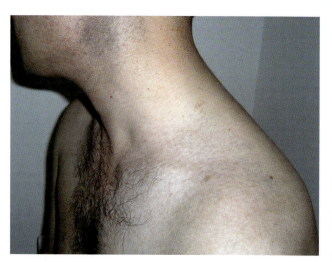

Fig. 3.53 Nevus of Ito typically located on the shoulder girdle unilaterally

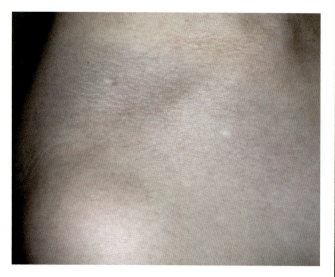

Fig. 3.54 Nevus of Ito causing bluish gray, ill-defined pigmentation on the shoulder

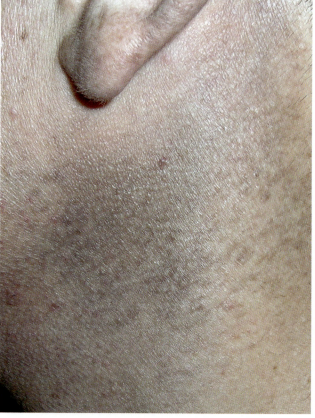

Fig. 3.55 Speckled pigmentation on the neck due to nevus of Ito

3.3 Dermal Melanocytic Tumors

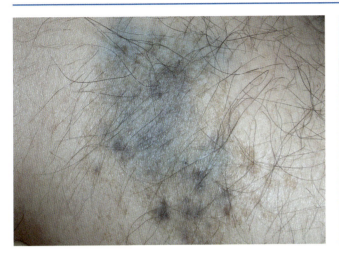

Fig. 3.56 Congenital dermal melanocytosis presenting as a speckled bluish patch measuring 4 cm size on the upper arm

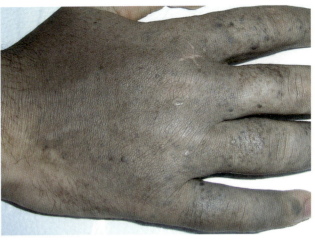

Fig. 3.57 Congenital dermal melanocytosis; scattered bluish macules are seen on the dorsum of the hand. This case showed unilateral involvement

atypically located (ectopic) Mongolian spots (*see* Fig. 3.42) may be challenging in the differential diagnosis. The amount of dermal melanocytes in this nevus is denser than seen in Mongolian spots histologically.

Management. Malignant transformation of nevus of Ito is extremely rare, and a routine follow-up is not mandatory. Cosmetic camouflage may be efficient. Q-switched lasers can also be used.

3.3.4 Congenital Dermal Melanocytosis (Dermal Melanocytic Hamartoma)

A subset of dermal melanocytic tumors cannot be classified under the above-mentioned main types. These cases can be described under the term "congenital dermal melanocytosis." The lesion is usually present at birth and may look like nevus of Ota or nevus of Ito clinically and histopathologically, but it is located on other regions such as the extremities or lower trunk. It may be seen as an isolated uneven small patch in varying sizes (*see* Fig. 3.56). Occasionally a dermatomal distribution can be observed. Small, well-demarcated grayish-blue macules coalesce to form a large patch (*see* Figs. 3.57 and 3.58). Darker areas or papules similar to blue nevus may be dispersed on the patches (*see* Fig. 3.59). These papules may arise later and have histopathologic features common with those of blue nevus. Lesions are persistent, but there is no known risk of malignant degeneration.

Apart from the isolated lesions of congenital dermal melanocytosis, "generalized dermal melanocytosis" is described as a rare condition with scattered pigmented patches resembling ectopic Mongolian spots distributed widely over the body (*see* Fig. 3.43). Unusual presentations of congenital dermal melanocytosis may also be seen in cases of phakomatosis pigmentovascularis (see Fig. 6.125).

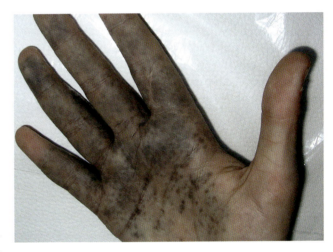

Fig. 3.58 Congenital dermal melanocytosis covering the great majority of the palm as grayish blue patches

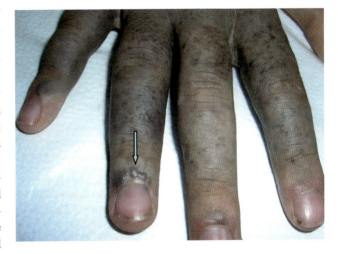

Fig. 3.59 Congenital dermal melanocytosis on the fingers. Note a papular component (*arrow*) overlying the irregular bluish patches

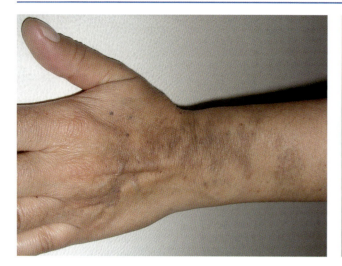

Fig. 3.60 Acquired dermal melanocytosis. Grey-colored patchy lesions on the back of the hand and forearm occurred in childhood in this patient

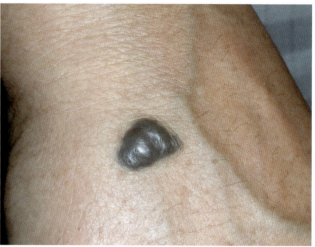

Fig. 3.61 Blue nevus presenting as a bluish black nodule on the dorsum of the hand

Furthermore, dermal melanocytosis may also be acquired (acquired dermal melanocytosis) and be located on various parts of the body (*see* Fig. 3.60).

Management. The approach to this benign condition is similar to that for nevus of Ito.

3.3.5 Blue Nevus

Blue nevus is a common benign tumor of the skin and mucous membranes, presenting mostly as a firm papule or nodule resulting from dermal collection of melanocytes. The bluish color of the tumor is the reflection of deep dermal melanin. Contrary to other dermal melanocytic tumors, blue nevus is usually elevated.

Most blue nevi occur in the second decade of life, but lesions may develop at any age and rarely may be congenital. The great majority of patients have solitary lesions. The dorsum of the hands and feet (*see* Fig. 3.61), the head (*see* Figs. 3.62 and 3.63), the neck and presacral area are the main locations. However, the nevus may be found on arms (*see* Fig. 3.64), legs (*see* Fig. 3.65), and the trunk. Blue nevus may rarely be located on mucosal surfaces like conjunctiva (*see* Fig. 3.66), oral mucosa (*see* Fig. 3.67), nasal mucosa (*see* Fig. 3.68), and vagina. A typical lesion is a well-circumscribed, blue (*see* Fig. 3.69), gray-blue (*see* Fig. 3.70), or bluish-black (*see* Figs. 3.71 and 3.72), slightly elevated, dome-shaped, round, usually firm papule or nodule measuring 0.5 to 1 cm in size. The surface of the tumor is smooth and symmetric but sometimes slightly raised areas may cause an irregular appearance (*see* Fig. 3.73).

Multiple clinical presentations of blue nevi other than the classic type have also been described. Some lesions may be slate gray or grayish-brown (hypochromic variant) (*see* Figs. 3.74 and 3.75). Macular (*see* Fig. 3.76) and plaque-like lesions (*see* Fig. 3.77) or rarely targetoid, and

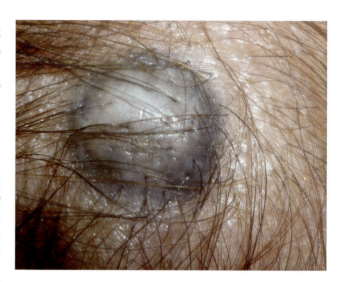

Fig. 3.62 A dome-shaped blue nevus on the scalp. Lesions are not uncommon on the head

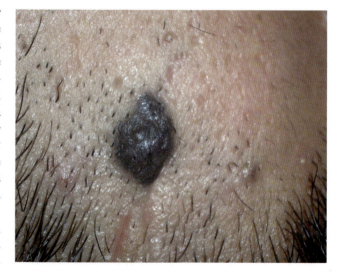

Fig. 3.63 Blue nevus on the face. Most patients have a solitary tumor uniform in shape and pigmentation

3.3 Dermal Melanocytic Tumors

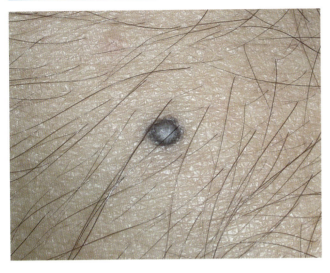

Fig. 3.64 Blue nevus on the arm. The papulonodular lesion has typically a smooth surface

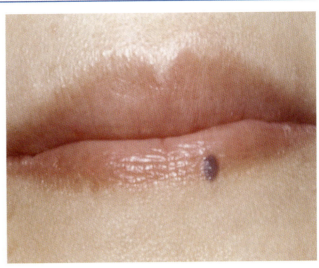

Fig. 3.67 Blue nevus on the lip. Intraoral mucosa may also be involved

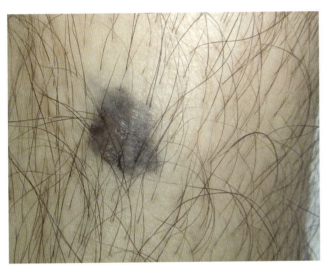

Fig. 3.65 Blue nevus on the leg

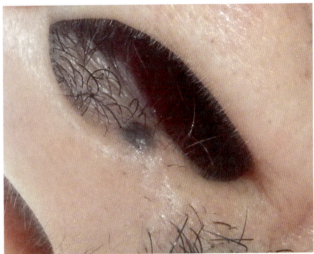

Fig. 3.68 Blue nevus on the nasal vestibule

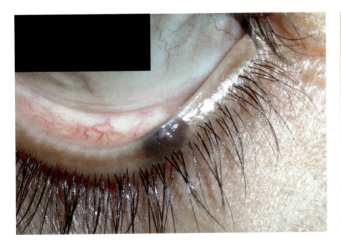

Fig. 3.66 Blue nevus on the conjunctiva

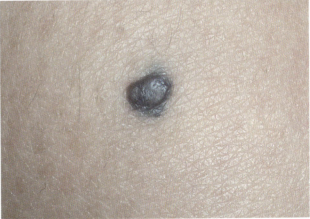

Fig. 3.69 Classic presentation of blue nevus as a well-circumscribed, round bluish papule less than 1 cm in size

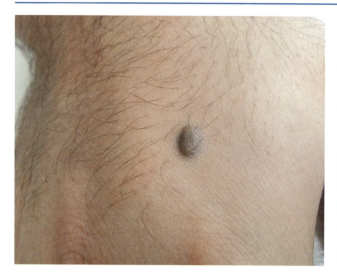

Fig. 3.70 Grayish blue-colored, slightly raised nodule on the dorsum of the hand representing blue nevus. The lesion is firm on palpation

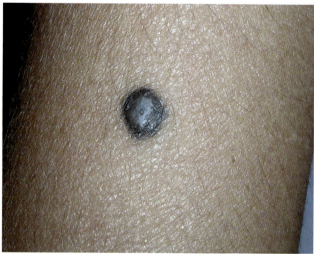

Fig. 3.72 Bluish black nodule that can be easily misdiagnosed as nodular melanoma. The diagnosis of blue nevus was confirmed by histopathological interpretation in this case

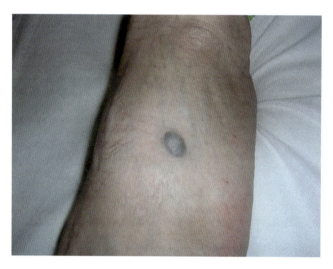

Fig. 3.71 Blue nevus on the dorsum of the foot, a typical location

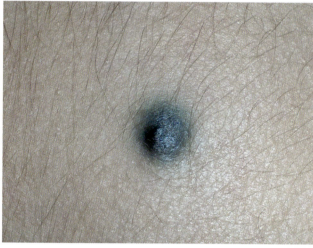

Fig. 3.73 A slightly raised second component is seen on blue nevus. The surface of blue nevi is not uniform in all cases

agminated (*see* Fig. 3.78) clinical subtypes of blue nevi may also be seen. Cellular blue nevus is a clinicopathologic type typically located on the buttocks and scalp as elevated nodules and plaques measuring 1 to 3 cm in diameter (*see* Fig. 3.79). The surface of these lesions may be relatively irregular. Blue nevus may also be seen in the setting of Carney syndrome.

Blue nevus usually has typical clinical features. Uniform color and symmetric appearance of a stable lesion is helpful in the differentiation from malignant melanoma (*see* Fig. 12.43). However, a recently developing blue nevus may be hard to distinguish from nodular melanoma. Dermoscopy is helpful to exclude Reed nevus (*see* Fig. 3.223) and angiomatous lesions like angiokeratoma (*see* Fig. 6.152) and venous lake (*see* Fig. 6.183). Hypochromic lesions may mimic dermatofibroma (*see* Fig. 8.4) and intradermal melanocytic nevus (*see* Fig. 3.114). It should be remembered that benign skin appendage tumors such as trichoblastoma (*see* Fig. 5.43) and poroma (*see* Fig. 5.17) may also appear as pigmented nodules mimicking blue nevus.

An excisional biopsy is indicated in cases in which the diagnosis of malignant melanoma cannot be excluded. The histopathologic appearance of blue nevus is different from most types of nevomelanocytic tumors but is similar to the histology of other dermal melanocytic tumors. Thus, clinicopathologic correlation is important in the diagnosis of blue nevus. Elongated, finely pigmented dendritic melanocytes forming groups among interwoven thickened collagen

3.3 Dermal Melanocytic Tumors

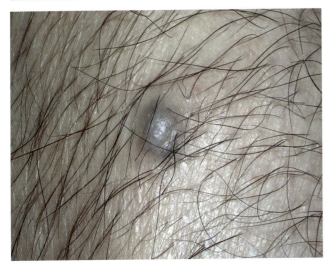

Fig. 3.74 Hypochromic variant of blue nevus. This slate gray lesion was diagnosed upon histopathological examination

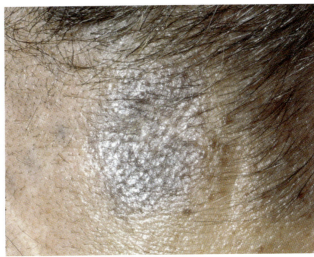

Fig. 3.77 Plaque-like lesion of blue nevus. This is a rare presentation

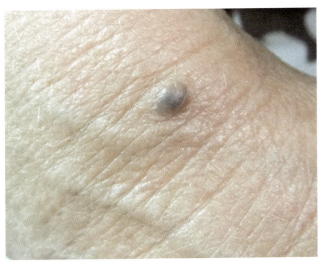

Fig. 3.75 Hypochromic variant of blue nevus on the dorsum of the hand. The location was helpful in the diagnosis of this tumor

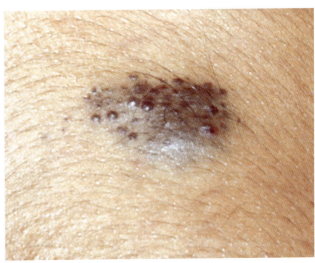

Fig. 3.78 Agminated blue nevus. Note the grouped papular lesions forming a plaque

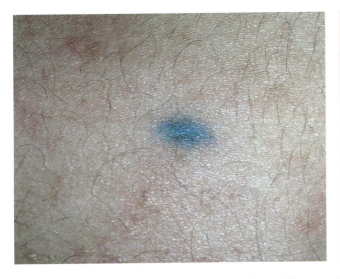

Fig. 3.76 Blue nevus presenting as a bluish macule. Some lesions are not elevated at all

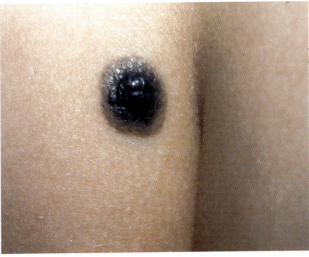

Fig. 3.79 A cellular blue nevus larger than 1 cm on the gluteal region, a typical location. This clinical appearance as a target-like nodule is not very common

bundles in the upper and middle dermis are the main features of the classic type of blue nevus. Scattered melanin-laden melanophages are also present. The overlying epidermis is normal. In cellular blue nevus, cellular density is clearly higher. In addition to dendritic melanocytes, nests of spindle-shaped melanocytes with pale cytoplasm are present. Subcutaneous fat tissue involvement is the rule.

Management. Most of the classic blue nevi remain unchanged, and a strict follow-up procedure is not indicated. Although very rare, malignant degeneration may occur, especially in the cellular type. A sudden increase in size and ulceration may herald a malignant process.

A simple excision can be performed for cosmetic concerns in classic blue nevi. Furthermore, cellular blue nevi may be excised for prophylactic purposes or in the presence of any secondary changes.

3.4 Melanocytic Nevi (Nevus Cell Nevi)

Melanocytic nevi (moles) are among the most common dermatologic problems. They are benign proliferations of melanocytes or so-called "nevus cells (nevocytes)." Therefore, they are also named "nevus cell nevi." These cells are slightly altered melanoblasts that migrate from the neural crest to the epidermis. Nevus cells tend to cluster, forming nests. The natural evolution of melanocytic nevi is not fully understood. As related to the Unna's "Abtropfung" hypothesis, nevus cells subsequently migrate into the dermis. There are many types of melanocytic nevi occurring in different periods of life. Melanocytic nevi found at birth (congenital nevi) constitute only a small proportion of all nevi. On the other hand, the acquired nevi start to appear in childhood and increase in number gradually in years. Young adults have the greatest number of acquired melanocytic nevi. Although new melanocytic nevi may continue to occur, the total number of nevi decreases progressively after adulthood, and most lesions completely vanish in the ninth decade.

Melanocytic nevi may be located on the skin, nails, and mucosae. Racial differences and environmental factors play a role in the etiology. Common acquired nevi and dysplastic nevi are more prevalent in Caucasians. On the other hand, acquired melanocytic nevi on the palmoplantar area and nails are common in Asians and African Americans. Although the familial trait of congenital and common acquired melanocytic nevi is unknown, dysplastic nevi may be familial. Intermittent sunlight exposure is considered a triggering factor for the development of acquired nevi. The role of hormonal factors cannot be denied because proliferation of melanocytic nevi can be observed during puberty or pregnancy. Other etiologic factors are poorly understood.

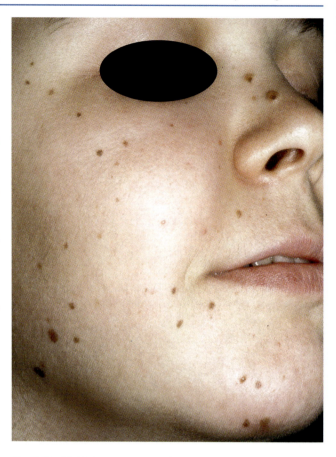

Fig. 3.80 Multiple common acquired melanocytic nevi in a patient with Turner syndrome

3.4.1 Common Acquired Melanocytic Nevus

The majority of melanocytic nevi are acquired. They are seen in all races and in general, they are not associated with systemic diseases. However, in a few rare diseases such as Turner syndrome (*see* Fig. 3.80), the number of melanocytic nevi is increased. They may be found anywhere on the body. Some patients have only a few lesions, but others have numerous nevi. In contrast to congenital melanocytic nevi, they are nearly always less than 1.5 cm in diameter. Collection of nevocytes may be in the lower part of the epidermis (junctional), dermis (intradermal), or both (compound). This histopathologic difference also contributes to the clinical features.

Common acquired melanocytic nevi are small and do not have a tendency to grow; most lesions do not require cosmetic treatment. Moreover, they are benign lesions with a very low potency toward malignant degeneration. However, the increased total number of melanocytic nevi is a well-known general risk factor for malignant melanoma.

Junctional nevi are usually seen in childhood. Nevus cells are usually restricted to the lower part of the epidermis at this age. Typical lesions are hairless macules or round to oval papules that are 2 to 7 mm in diameter (*see* Fig. 3.81). The

3.4 Melanocytic Nevi (Nevus Cell Nevi)

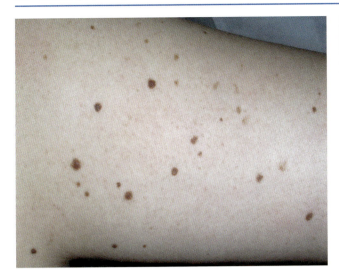

Fig. 3.81 Multiple junctional nevi on the arm. These lesions typically appear in childhood

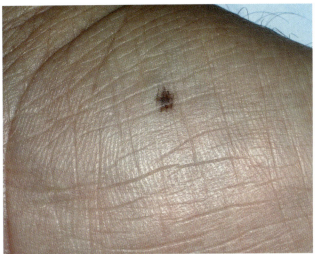

Fig. 3.83 Junctional nevus on the palm, a common location

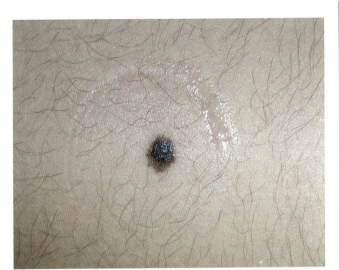

Fig. 3.82 Junctional nevus on the trunk. Note the symmetric appearance of the small black flat lesion

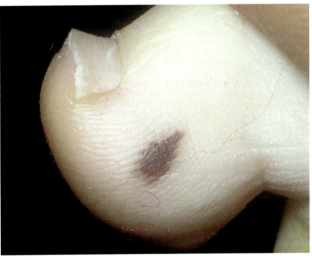

Fig. 3.84 Junctional nevus on the volar aspect of the toe. The lesion is typically small, and skin markings are accentuated

appearance of the nevus is symmetric, with regular borders and homogeneous color and may be in all shades of brown or black (*see* Fig. 3.82). Skin markings are accentuated. Lentigo simplex (*see* Fig. 3.7) is the main clinical differential diagnostic challenge.

Junctional nevi may be located anywhere on the body, but the palms or soles are the most typical locations (*see* Figs. 3.83 and 3.84). Palmoplantar lesions are usually small (*see* Fig. 3.85) and regular in shape (*see* Fig. 3.86). Compound nevi and congenital melanocytic nevi may rarely be located on the palmoplantar area, but they are usually raised and larger. A junctional nevus in this location should primarily be distinguished from early lesions of acral lentiginous melanoma (*see* Fig. 12.29). Lesions showing rapid enlargement, color variegation, and asymmetric appearance should always raise the suspicion

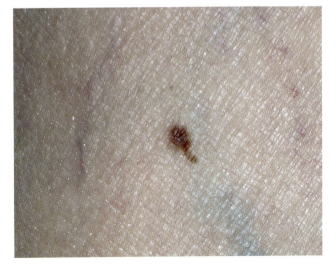

Fig. 3.85 Junctional nevus causing a quite flat small lesion with irregular shape

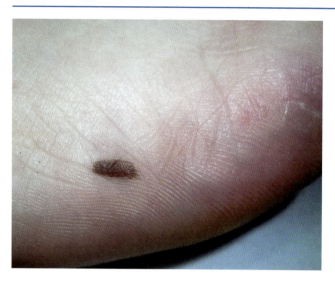

Fig. 3.86 Junctional nevus on the foot presenting as a slightly raised, regular lesion

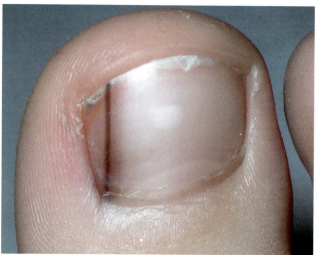

Fig. 3.88 Melanonychia striata due to junctional nevus; a typical thin pigmented longitudinal band is seen

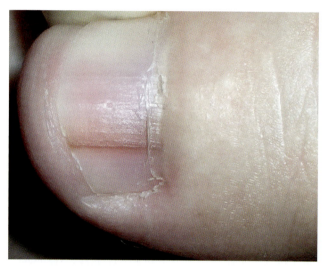

Fig. 3.87 Melanonychia striata due to a junctional nevus in a child. Nearly always only one nail is involved

of malignant melanoma. Moreover, according to the current view, melanoma is not expected to occur as a result of malignant degeneration of melanocytic nevi in the palmoplantar area; thus lesions evaluated as benign do not deserve special attention.

Junctional nevus may also appear as a subungual or ungual tumor. Nail nevi may involve any part of the nail, but mostly the nail matrix. Nail bed and lateral nail folds may also be affected. Junctional melanocytic nevus of the matrix presents as melanonychia striata, which is a persistent pigmented longitudinal band of the nail plate (see Figs. 3.87 and 3.88). Since there are various underlying causes of melanonychia striata, the clinical features are important in the differential diagnosis. Junctional nevus usually occurs in childhood and affects only one nail. The longitudinal band is thin and homogeneous, with brown or black monochromic color. It has definite borders and does not involve the cuticle or supramatrical skin (see Fig. 3.89). This pigmented band is stable and does not darken or enlarge over the years. Acral lentiginous melanoma may also appear as a monodactylic melanonychia striata, but its onset is mostly during adulthood. The band of malignant melanoma is usually wide and heterogeneous with different shades of brown and black (see Fig. 12.40a). This lesion has a tendency to darken in time and enlarge to periungual tissue, which is called the Hutchinson sign. However, melanonychia striata due to a heavily pigmented benign nevus may cause a pseudo-Hutchinson sign that appears as perionychial pigmentation seen through the translucent cuticle. Matrix biopsy is not indicated for the confirmation of the diagnosis, unless there is a suspicion of malignancy. On the other hand, melanonychia striata involving multiple nails (see Figs. 3.90 and 3.91) is mostly associated with systemic triggering factors such as drug eruption or PUVA therapy.

Compound nevi and intradermal (dermal) nevi are more elevated than junctional nevi, and they cannot always be differentiated from each other clinically. Compound nevi may present with variable clinical features. They may occur anywhere on the skin, including the palmoplantar and interdigital areas (see Figs. 3.92 and 3.93). They are always round or oval, well-demarcated, elevated tumors mostly 0.5 to 1.5 cm in diameter (see Fig. 3.94). Two different types of color can be seen in one nevus. Brown to black and pink are the most common colors. Some lesions have two components, especially an elevated part located in the center (see Fig. 3.95) or asymmetrically (see Fig. 3.96). The surface of the lesion is smooth, and skin creases are discernible (see Fig. 3.94). Most lesions are hairless, but one or a few long hairs may sometimes be seen on compound nevi (see Fig. 3.97). The surface of a compound nevus may rarely be hyperkeratotic

3.4 Melanocytic Nevi (Nevus Cell Nevi)

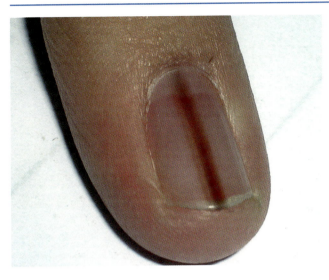

Fig. 3.89 Melanonychia striata due to junctional nevus without the involvement of the cuticle. This feature is helpful in differentiating this benign lesion from malignant melanoma

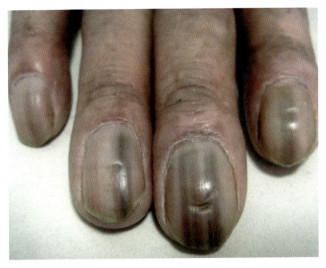

Fig. 3.91 Melanonychia striata presenting as large pigmented longitudinal bands on multiple fingers caused by PUVA therapy in a vitiligo patient

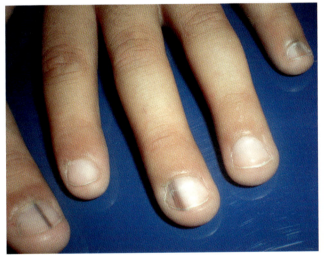

Fig. 3.90 Melanonychia striata involving multiple nails that occurred as a result of chemotherapy

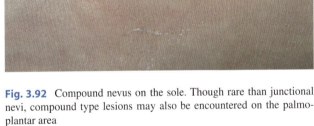

Fig. 3.92 Compound nevus on the sole. Though rare than junctional nevi, compound type lesions may also be encountered on the palmoplantar area

(*see* Fig. 3.98) or crusted, and the center may be lighter in color (*see* Fig. 3.97) or depressed (*see* Fig. 3.99). A ring-shaped lesion with peripheral pigmentation is called "nevus en cocarde" (*see* Figs. 3.100 and 3.101), which is more commonly seen on the scalp.

A compound nevus may sometimes present as a lesion with two components: a flat base and overlying polypoid or pendulous papules. Both components may be in different colors (*see* Figs. 3.102 and 3.103). An extreme presentation of compound nevus is two different papules attached together; one of these papules may show a papillomatous surface (see Fig. 3.104 and 3.105). We propose the term "non-identical attached nevus" for those lesions.

Intradermal nevi are more common after middle age, especially in women (*see* Fig. 3.106) but may also be seen in men (*see* Fig. 3.107). This type of nevus, also called the Miescher nevus, is frequently observed on the face (*see* Figs. 3.107 and 3.108) and scalp (*see* Figs. 3.109 and 3.110). Facial nevi are more commonly seen on nasolabial folds and around the mouth (*see* Fig. 3.111) but may also be found on eyelids (*see* Fig. 3.112) and ears. Palmoplantar involvement is rare (*see* Fig. 3.113). The typical lesion is a 0.5 to 1 cm, light brown or flesh-colored and dome-shaped nodular lesion with a broad base and smooth surface (*see* Figs. 3.114, 3.115 and 3.116). On the surface, darker dots (*see* Fig. 3.117), cyst-like structures (see Figs. 3.118 and 3.119), telangiectasia, and a few protruding hairs (*see* Figs. 3.111) may be noticed. Nevus cells located in deep dermis are small cells producing little melanin. Additionally, nevus cells on the dermoepidermal junction are absent in this type of nevus and lesions are usually lighter in color (*see* Figs. 3.109 and 3.115) compared

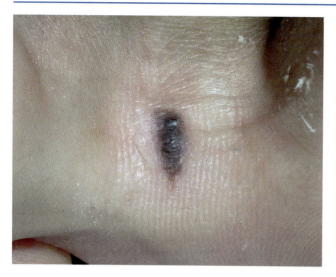

Fig. 3.93 Compound nevus on the interdigital area

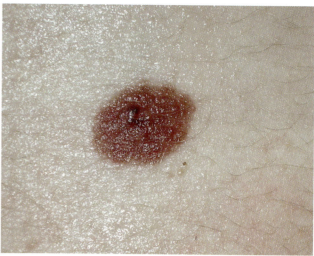

Fig. 3.96 Compound nevus with two components. In this case, the elevated part of the lesion is asymmetrically located

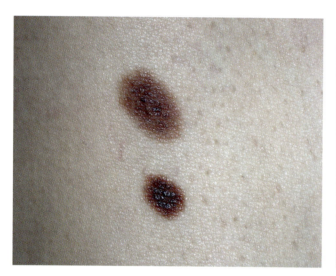

Fig. 3.94 Two, well-demarcated, round lesions of compound nevi with discernable skin creases

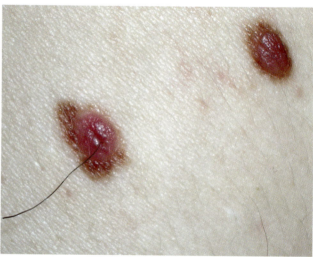

Fig. 3.97 Compound nevi with typical central and peripheral difference. Central part is lighter colored in these two lesions, and a long terminal hair is protruding from the lesion on the left

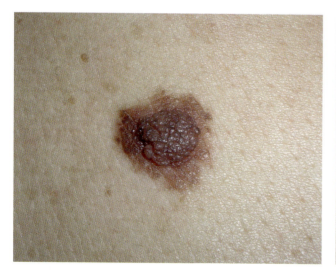

Fig. 3.95 Compound nevus with two components. Note the lesion has an elevated part in the center and a flat component on the periphery

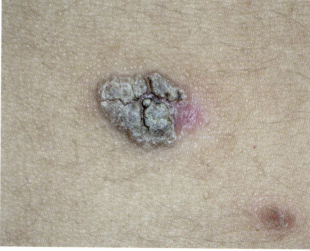

Fig. 3.98 A compound nevus with hyperkeratotic surface. Note the resemblance to seborrheic keratosis

3.4 Melanocytic Nevi (Nevus Cell Nevi)

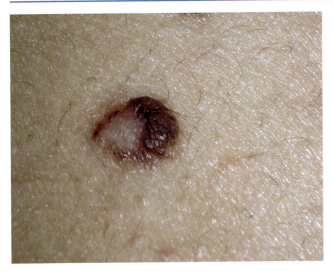

Fig. 3.99 A compound nevus with depressed center. This patient had a history of trauma on the lesion

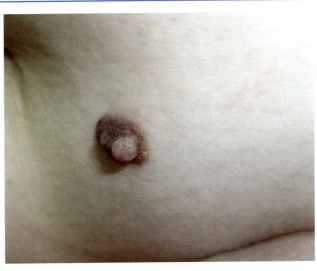

Fig. 3.102 A compound nevus composed of a flat component and overlying polypoid papules in different colors

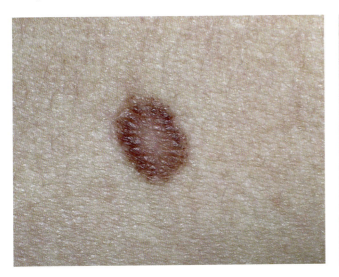

Fig. 3.100 A ring-shaped compound nevus with peripheral pigmentation called nevus en cocarde

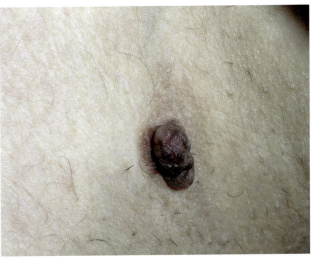

Fig. 3.103 A compound nevus exhibiting two components; flat base and overlying polypoid nodule

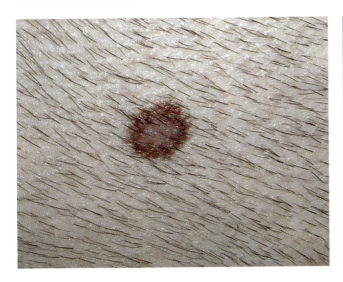

Fig. 3.101 Nevus en cocarde on the scalp, the most common location

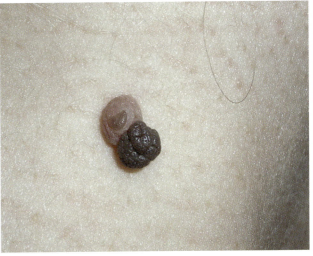

Fig. 3.104 A compound nevus composed of two unlike (non-identical) papules attached together; both components have different colors and different surface characteristics

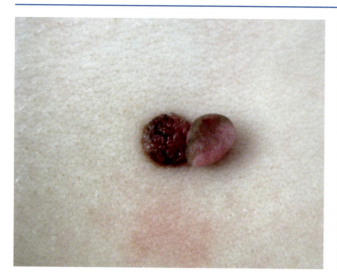

Fig. 3.105 A compound nevus composed of two completely different papules attached together. Note the nodule on the base has a papillomatous surface and the one on the top has a smooth surface

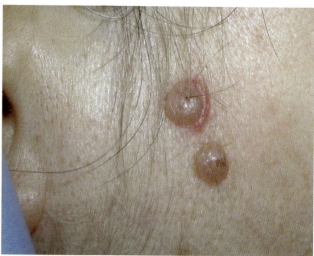

Fig. 3.108 Intradermal nevi on the face of an adult woman. These lesions occur typically after middle age

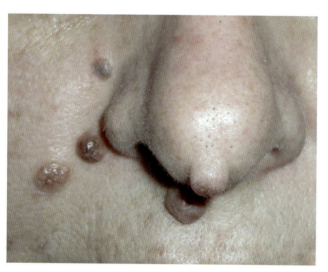

Fig. 3.106 Multiple lesions of intradermal nevus (Miescher nevus) on the face of a woman

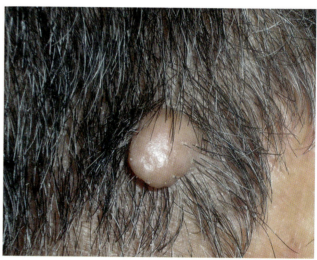

Fig. 3.109 Intradermal nevus presenting as a skin-colored raised nodule on the scalp. This is one of the most common locations of this nevi

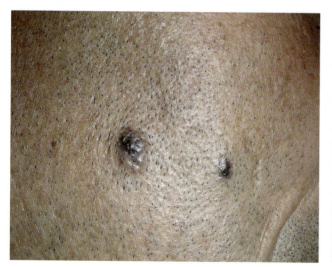

Fig. 3.107 Two intradermal nevi on the face of a man

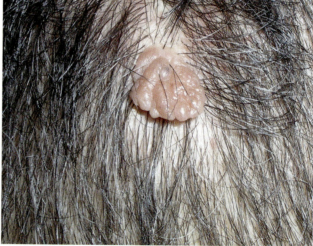

Fig. 3.110 Intradermal nevus on the scalp. The skin-colored nodule is polypoid in shape

3.4 Melanocytic Nevi (Nevus Cell Nevi)

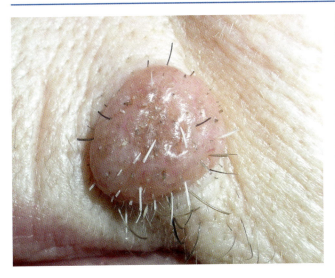

Fig. 3.111 Intradermal nevus above the upper lip. Multiple hairs are protruding from the lesion

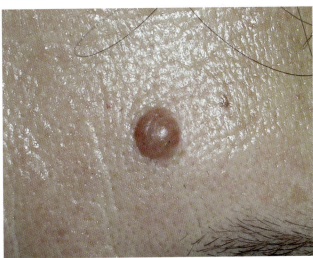

Fig. 3.114 Dome-shaped, smooth-surfaced, light brown-colored intradermal nevus on the forehead

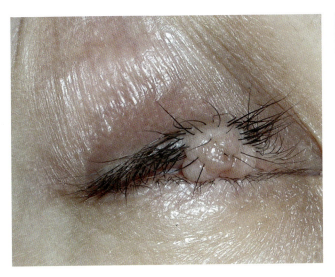

Fig. 3.112 Intradermal nevus on the eyelid

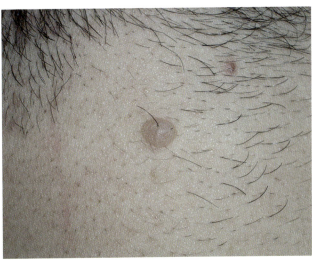

Fig. 3.115 Skin-colored dome-shaped intradermal nevus on the neck. The lesion is softish on palpation

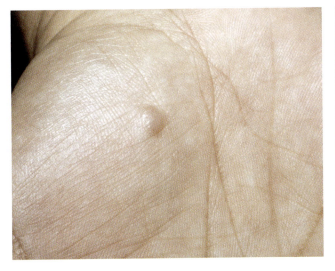

Fig. 3.113 Palmar intradermal nevus. In contrast to brownish-colored flat lesions of junctional nevi, palmoplantar lesions of intradermal nevi are mostly skin-colored and dome-shaped

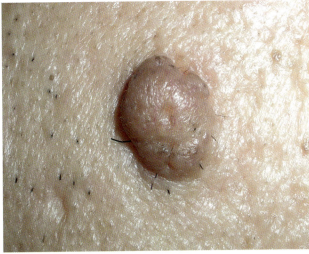

Fig. 3.116 Light brown-colored, well-defined facial nodule with a broad base; a typical presentation of intradermal nevus

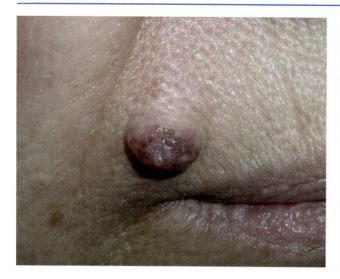

Fig. 3.117 Intradermal nevus on the face. Note the brown dots on the surface

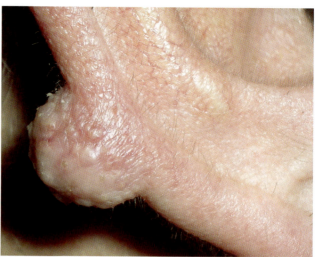

Fig. 3.119 Intradermal nevus with tiny cysts on the surface

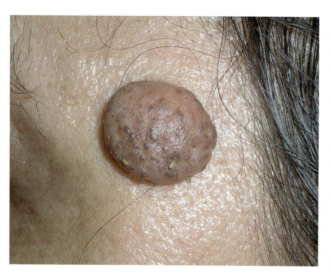

Fig. 3.118 Intradermal nevus with dark brown dots and tiny cysts on the surface

to junctional nevus. However, some intradermal nevi may be relatively dark-colored (*see* Figs. 3.120 and 3.121). The lesion may sometimes be confused with early nonulcerated basal cell carcinoma, but intradermal nevus is softer than this malignant tumor. There may be slight umbilicated areas (*see* Fig. 3.122) and foldings (*see* Fig. 3.123) on the surface of the tumor. Some lesions are pedunculated. Trichoepithelioma (*see* Fig. 5.38), neurofibroma (*see* Fig. 7.2), dermatofibroma (*see* Fig. 8.6) and fibrous papule of the nose (*see* Fig. 8.16) are the benign tumors considered in the differential diagnosis.

Intradermal nevi do not change for years and may only cause a cosmetic problem. They may be ulcerated or hemorrhagic as a result of trauma (*see* Fig. 3.124) but heal spontaneously in a short time. Sometimes cystic dilatation or secondary bacterial infection of follicles may cause acute local inflammation and erythema or swelling on the nevus (*see* Fig. 3.125). This may initially arouse a suspicion of malignant melanoma but symptoms resolve with therapy. On the other hand, if there is no clinical improvement, a biopsy may be performed.

Papillomatous nevus (Unna nevus) is another presentation of intradermal or compound nevi. Histologically this nevus shows epidermal changes like hyperkeratosis, acanthosis, and papillomatosis. It is mostly acquired but sometimes congenital nevi (even the large one) may also have a papillomatous surface (*see* Fig. 3.159). The exophytic tumor is mostly located on the trunk, arms, and neck. The homogeneous papillomatous surface resembling a mulberry (*see* Figs. 3.126 and 3.127) is distinctive. This soft tumor has pink (*see* Fig. 3.126) or light to dark brown color (*see* Fig. 3.128). Intradermal papillomatous nevi are typically lighter (*see* Fig. 3.129). Some lesions have a verrucous surface and may rarely be polypoid. As most papillomatous nevi are histologically compound type tumors, clinically two components may be noticed: a raised papillomatous lesion and a surrounding flat area (*see* Fig. 3.130). Due to common surface features, especially in the presence of hyperkeratosis (*see* Fig. 3.131) and minute cysts (*see* Fig. 3.132), papillomatous nevus may mimic seborrheic keratosis (*see* Fig. 1.32). Irritation by trauma or clothes occurs easily on the elevated tumors. Therefore lesions may show inflammation or may bleed, but these changes resolve spontaneously.

Multiple pigmented nevi of the same kind forming a group or cluster on a localized area are called agminated nevus (*see* Fig. 3.133). The clinical features are variable depending on the type of the nevi. This condition is different from nevus spilus (*see* Fig. 3.227) in that it lacks the underlying pigmented macule (*see* Fig. 3.134).

The above-mentioned clinical features mostly enable the diagnosis of acquired melanocytic nevi. Dermoscopy is a useful tool in the differentiation of common acquired melanocytic nevi from malignant melanoma and nonmelanocytic tumors.

3.4 Melanocytic Nevi (Nevus Cell Nevi)

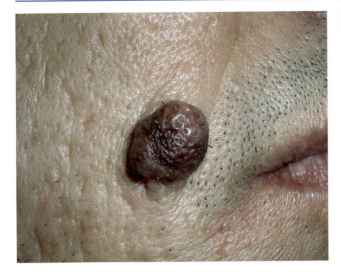

Fig. 3.120 Dark-colored intradermal nevus. The dark lesions are not as common as the light ones

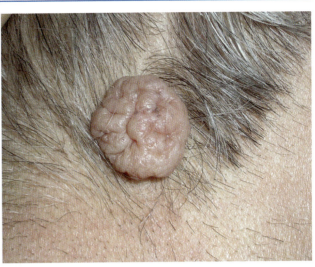

Fig. 3.123 Pedunculated intradermal nevus with a folded flabby surface

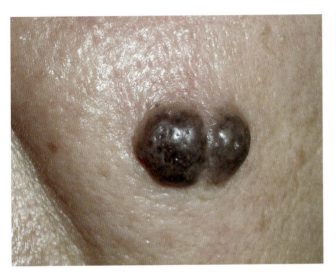

Fig. 3.121 Two dark-colored nevi adjacent to each other representing intradermal nevi

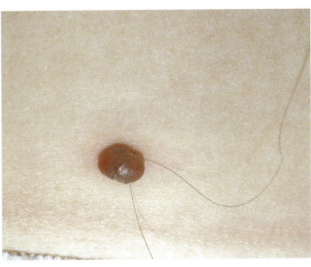

Fig. 3.124 Intradermal nevus showing hemorrhage due to trauma (strangulation of a hair surrounding the lesion)

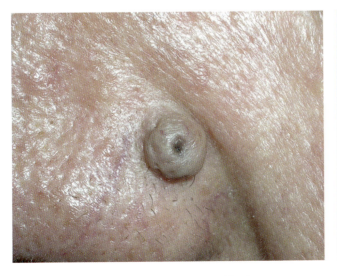

Fig. 3.122 Intradermal nevus with central umbilication

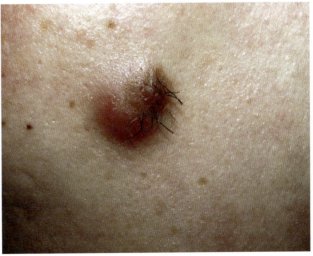

Fig. 3.125 Intradermal nevus showing acute local inflammation. This sudden change should not be confused with malignant degeneration

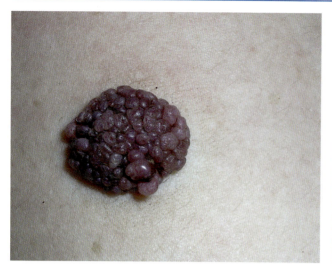

Fig. 3.126 Papillomatous nevus (Unna nevus) on the trunk resembling to mulberry. The pinkish lesion has a symmetric surface

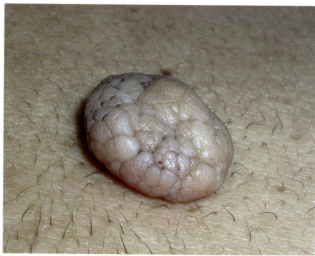

Fig. 3.129 A polypoid, skin-colored papillomatous nevus. This lesion represented an intradermal nevus histologically

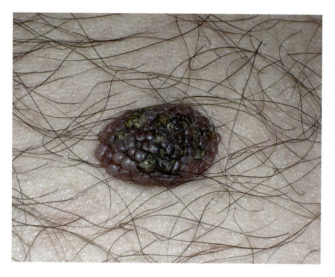

Fig. 3.127 A sessile papillomatous nevus on the leg

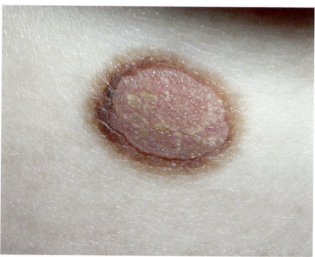

Fig. 3.130 A raised, light-colored papillomatous nevus surrounded by a darker thin flat rim. This lesion represented a compound nevus histologically

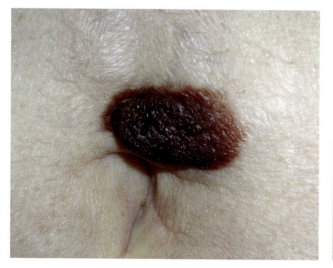

Fig. 3.128 A dark brown papillomatous nevus above umbilicus

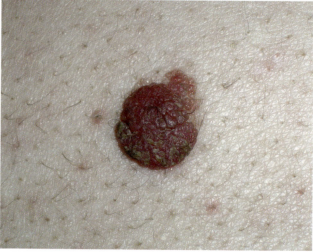

Fig. 3.131 Papillomatous nevus with partial hyperkeratotic areas that resemble those of seborrheic keratosis

3.4 Melanocytic Nevi (Nevus Cell Nevi)

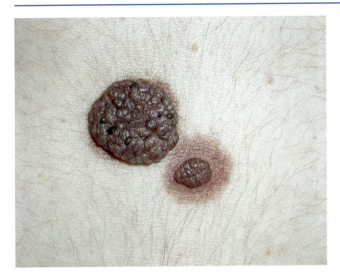

Fig. 3.132 Papillomatous nevus (*left*) and compound nevus (*right*) are seen concomitantly. Note the black-colored tiny cysts on the surface of the papillomatous nevus mimicking seborrheic keratosis

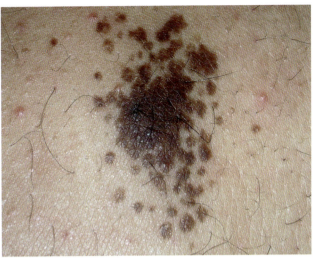

Fig. 3.134 Agminated nevus. There is no hyperpigmented patch on the base of multiple small melanocytic nevi in contrast to nevus spilus

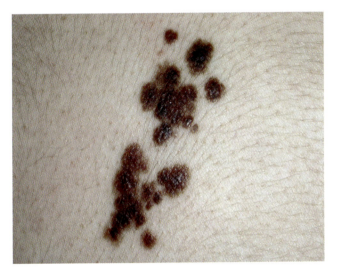

Fig. 3.133 Agminated nevus; a cluster of melanocytic nevi describes this lesion

Management. In general, common acquired melanocytic nevi are benign lesions, and any therapeutic intervention and routine follow-up are not mandatory. On the other hand, some patients may be worried about malignant transformation, and therefore reassurance may be required. Prophylactic excision of these lesions is not indicated. However, as malignant melanoma is also an acquired pigmented tumor, it needs to be excluded when an acquired pigmented lesion with atypical features is found. Skin lesions with any suspicion of malignancy, especially those fulfilling the criteria of melanoma when assessed by ABCDE rule, can be excised for histopathologic examination. Cosmetic concern may be another indication for therapy. Incisional biopsy for diagnostic purposes is not a preferred option but may be used in large lesions and in difficult locations. Total excision is the best modality for the removal of the nevus. Destruction with laser, cryotherapy and electrocautery are not favored as it eliminates the chance of histopathologic examination if

needed and is associated with the possibility of recurrence leading to pseudomelanoma. Moreover, these methods may sometimes cause an unsightly cosmetic appearance.

Though nail nevi are not high risk lesions, a special approach is needed. The major concern in the management of melanonychia striata is to rule out malignant melanoma. Although biopsy of the nail matrix is advised for the confirmation of the diagnosis, it is a technically difficult procedure and may not always reveal the diagnosis. Furthermore, biopsy may cause permanent nail dystrophy. Therefore in lesions without clinical criteria of malignant melanoma, unnecessary biopsy should be avoided. Benign lesions that are determined by clinical and dermoscopic findings do not need treatment. If there is a need for excision, then complete removal of the lesion must be performed. Melanonychia striata, which is clinically accepted as junctional nevus, can be followed up for a period of time, and if the bands show no enlargement, lesions do not need to be closely observed thereafter as there is no increased risk of malignant degeneration.

3.4.2 Mucosal Melanocytic Nevi

Although less commonly observed than on the skin, nevomelanocytic benign tumors may also be found on mucous membranes such as intraoral, ocular, intranasal, and genital mucosae. Blue nevus and melanocytic nevi of different types, predominantly acquired melanocytic nevus, may be located in the oral mucosa. The most common histopathologic type of melanocytic nevi in the oral mucosa is intramucosal nevus, which is the counterpart of intradermal nevus of the skin. Junctional and compound nevi are rare. Oral melanocytic nevi are usually small, round or oval, brown, bluish or black, slightly raised papules with smooth or rarely irregular surfaces (*see* Fig. 3.135). Since these lesions are mostly asymptomatic, they are usually first noticed during physical examination. Lesions may be

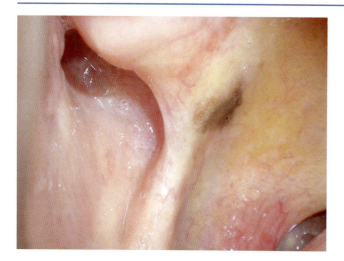

Fig. 3.135 A melanocytic nevus on the oral mucosa. Mucosal nevi may be congenital or acquired

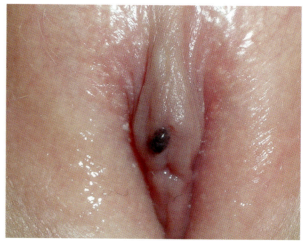

Fig. 3.136 Melanocytic nevus on the vulva. This acquired lesion revealed a compound nevus on histopathological examination

found anywhere in the mouth but are most commonly seen on the hard palate, followed by the buccal mucosa. A labial melanocytic macule (*see* Fig. 3.4) may be confused with oral melanocytic nevus, but the typical location of a labial melanocytic macule, especially on the lower lip, is helpful in diagnosis. Vascular tumors may also be misdiagnosed as melanocytic nevi, but melanocytic nevi do not blanch on compression, unlike vascular lesions. Oral mucosal malignant melanoma is the most important diagnostic consideration in the differential diagnosis. Malignant melanoma is usually an irregular dark lesion that can be variable in color and has a tendency to rapid growth and ulceration (*see* Fig. 12.52).

Congenital and acquired melanocytic nevi are not among the common pigmented lesions of the anogenital region. On the other hand, common acquired melanocytic nevi are relatively more frequent. Initial detection of an anogenital nevus is usually during physical examination. The vulva (labia majora, labia minora, and clitoris) is the main location (*see* Fig. 3.136) in women, but lesions on the perineum and mons pubis can also be seen. Penile melanocytic macule, vulvar melanosis (*see* Fig. 3.6) and malignant melanoma (*see* Fig. 12.53) are the main differential diagnostic considerations. Among the melanocytic nevi, a special variant is determined as "atypical genital melanocytic nevus," which deserves special attention because of its similarity to malignant melanoma. It is more frequent among young women, but lesions may also appear in childhood. A personal or family history of dysplastic nevus or melanoma elsewhere is not uncommon. Usually, this nevus appears as a dark-colored, atypical lesion that may mimic malignant melanoma clinically and histopathologically. However, the lesion has a benign course. Total excision of the lesion is required for histopathologic confirmation. Histology reveals a symmetric sharply demarcated melanocytic proliferation. However, slight cytologic atypia of the melanocytes, architectural disorder, focal pagetoid spread, and superficial dermal fibrosis may be found, causing suspicion of malignant melanoma.

Ocular nevomelanocytic tumors are not uncommon. They may be detected during ophthalmologic examination, but many of them are already visible. Benign epithelial melanosis, nevus of Ota (*see* Figs. 3.48 and 3.49), melanocytic nevi, and primary acquired melanosis are among the examples of benign nevomelanocytic tumors of the ocular surface. Benign epithelial melanosis is observed as the pigmentation of perilimbal and interpalpebral bulbar conjunctivae, which is mobile with conjunctival movement. It may be congenital or acquired. Chronic irritation of the conjunctiva, irradiation, Addison disease, pregnancy, and arsenic poisoning are among the etiologic factors. On the other hand, the presence of this lesion in dark-skinned people may also reflect racial melanosis. The lesion is usually bilateral, flat, and brown-colored. Histologically pigmentation is observed at the basal layer of the conjunctiva with no nest formation. Nevus of Ota, a dermal melanocytic tumor, is observed as episcleral pigmentation. Unlike benign epithelial melanosis, it does not move with the conjunctiva. It may also be accompanied by orbital and uveal pigmentation. Proliferation of melanocytes can be seen histologically. Follow-up of these patients is essential because the risk of development of malignant melanoma is slightly increased.

Melanocytic nevi of the conjunctivae are mostly located in the bulbar area. The limbus, caruncle, and palpebral area are other sites of involvement (*see* Figs. 3.137, 3.138 and 3.139). They may be localized at the epithelial-subepithelial junction (junctional nevus) and/or subepithelium (compound or intradermal nevus). Among these types, compound nevus is more common. Subepithelial (localized in the substantia propria) lesions move with the conjunctiva. Most ocular nevi are acquired, but congenital ones may also be seen. Lesions may become apparent at puberty or during pregnancy as a result of increase of pigmentation and may enlarge. Most lesions

3.4 Melanocytic Nevi (Nevus Cell Nevi)

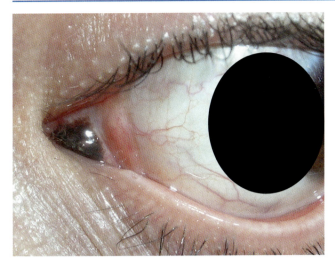

Fig. 3.137 Melanocytic nevus on the caruncle of the eye

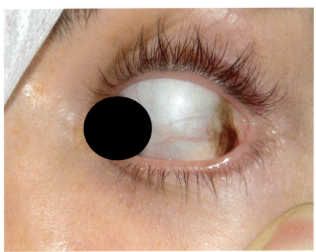

Fig. 3.139 Melanocytic nevus on the bulbar conjunctiva

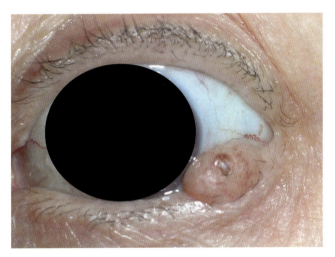

Fig. 3.138 Melanocytic nevus on the palpebral conjunctiva

are pigmented. But amelanotic lesions may also be found. Histologically, nests of nevus cells are seen. Conjunctival nevi are usually benign and must be differentiated from malignant melanoma and primary acquired melanosis.

Primary acquired melanosis is an acquired melanocytic lesion of the conjunctiva that has the potential to evolve into malignant melanoma. It is usually unilateral and more commonly seen in adulthood and in Caucasians. Clinically it has flat, brown-colored pigmentation. Conjunctival lesions are more common, but corneal and caruncle lesions may also be seen. Although the extent of primary acquired melanosis is variable, most lesions are small. Racial melanosis and melanocytic nevus are among the differential diagnoses. A bilateral and symmetric appearance favors racial melanosis. Primary acquired melanosis may show enlargement during follow-up. Large lesions are thought to be more prone to develop into malignant melanoma. Histologically these lesions may or may not be associated with atypia. Primary acquired melanosis with atypia, which is also considered a kind of intraepithelial malignant melanoma, has a higher risk of malignant degeneration than primary acquired melanosis without atypia.

Management. Most types of mucosal melanocytic nevi do not have different biological behavior than melanocytic nevi of the skin. Accordingly, an aggressive approach is not indicated. The correct diagnosis of atypical genital melanocytic nevus will prevent unnecessary aggressive surgery resulting from suspicion of malignant melanoma. Treatment indications for conjunctival melanocytic nevi include suspicion of malignancy with recent change of the nevi and cosmetic concerns.

3.4.3 Congenital Melanocytic Nevus

Congenital melanocytic nevus is a benign nevus that is present at birth or appears in the first weeks or months of life and persists throughout life. In contrast to the acquired variant, congenital melanocytic nevus is seen only in a small subset of the individuals (1 to 6%). The occurrence is almost always sporadic, and familial inheritance is not known. Even monozygotic twins do not have similar congenital nevi (*see* Fig. 3.140). Divided nevus of the eyelid, which refers to congenital melanocytic nevus on the opposing margins of the lower and upper eyelids of the eye (*see* Fig. 3.141) is accepted as an indicator that congenital nevi occur in utero during early embryogenesis, namely before the separation of the eyelids.

In contrast to the acquired melanocytic nevi, congenital ones may be very large. However, lesions of a few millimeters are also possible. Since clinical features and especially prognosis are different depending on the size, congenital melanocytic nevi are classified as small, medium, and large (giant). A small congenital nevus is less than 1.5 cm, medium type is between 1.5 to 19.9 cm, and the large one is over

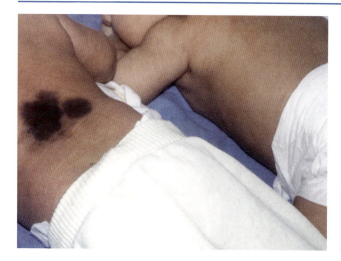

Fig. 3.140 Congenital melanocytic nevus is seen in only one of the monozygotic twins supporting sporadic occurrence

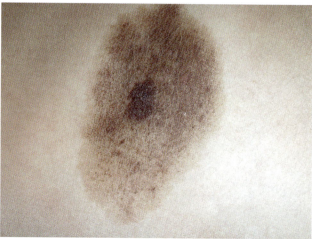

Fig. 3.142 A hairless congenital melanocytic nevus on the trunk

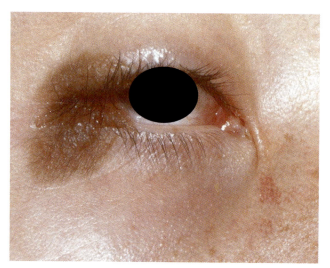

Fig. 3.141 Divided nevus. This picture further suggests the development of congenital melanocytic nevus in the early period of embryogenesis

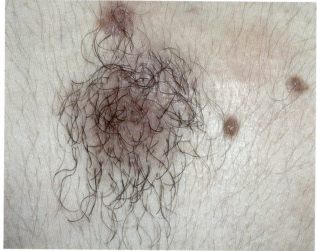

Fig. 3.143 Congenital melanocytic nevus with overlying long terminal hairs

20 cm in diameter. This classification is based on clinical observation and depends on the size that the nevi are predicted to attain in adulthood. Certainly, a few millimeters of difference in size will not have an influence on the prognosis, but this classification is useful for making a rough estimate about the prognosis and is helpful in designing the appropriate management modality. In addition, various definitions concerning the size of the lesions are present.

Most congenital nevi are stable and grow only in proportion to the child's growth, but some may grow slightly in the first year of life. Pale lesions that are not apparent at birth may be noticed later in infancy. Furthermore, flat lesions at birth may become raised later. While some lesions may be hairless (*see* Fig. 3.142) or contain a few long terminal hairs, some nevi are covered with dense terminal hairs (*see* Fig. 3.143). On rare occasions, scalp lesions may be alopecic (*see* Fig. 3.144). The great majority of congenital nevi, even the very large ones, are asymptomatic, but sometimes pruritus or tenderness is present and the overlying skin may be xerotic.

Small congenital melanocytic nevus is the most common subtype of these nevi. It may be located anywhere on the body (see Fig. 3.145), including the genitalia (*see* Fig. 3.146). Most patients have a solitary nevus (see Fig. 3.145) or a few small nevi (*see* Fig. 3.147). On the other hand, an individual with a large congenital melanocytic nevus may have additionally multiple small- or medium-sized nevi that are called satellites (*see* Fig. 3.148). The typical small congenital melanocytic nevus is usually a regular, round or oval, brown or heavily pigmented, flat (*see* Fig. 3.149) or raised lesion (*see* Fig. 3.150). Sometimes the borders may be irregular and

3.4 Melanocytic Nevi (Nevus Cell Nevi)

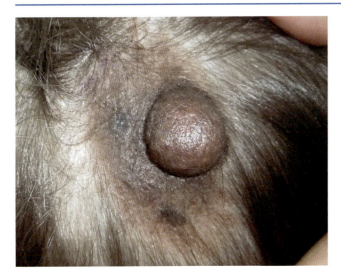

Fig. 3.144 Congenital melanocytic nevus causing alopecia on the scalp. The dome-shaped nodule overlying the flat plaque was histologically diagnosed as a hamartoma of neural origin

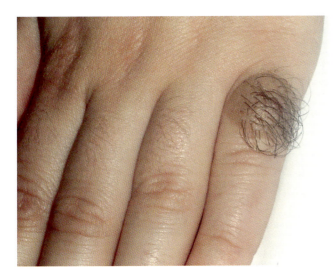

Fig. 3.145 Solitary congenital melanocytic nevus on the dorsum of the finger. Hand is not a common location as trunk, leg and arm

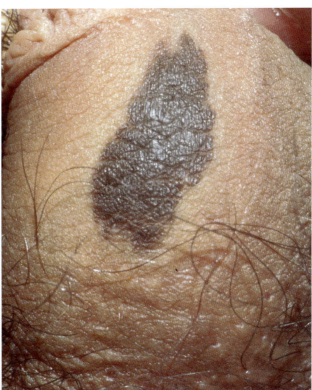

Fig. 3.146 Congenital melanocytic nevus on the male genitalia, a rare location

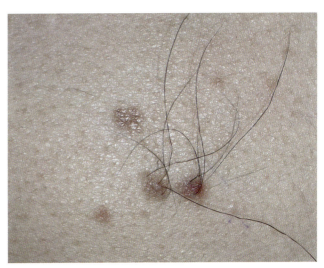

Fig. 3.147 Two small congenital melanocytic nevi with a few protruding hairs

notched (*see* Fig. 3.151). The surface of the tumor may be smooth or pebbly (mamillary), and skin markings may be accentuated. Overlying long hairs are mostly localized on the nevus but sometimes may also be seen on the normal skin at the periphery of the lesion (*see* Fig. 3.152). Lesions smaller than 0.5 cm are clinically difficult to differentiate from acquired compound nevi.

Medium-sized congenital melanocytic nevi may be seen anywhere but are more common on the trunk (*see* Fig. 3.153). They generally have clinical features similar to those of small nevi. However, they may be more heterogeneous, with irregular surface and nonuniform pigmentation (*see* Figs. 3.154, 3.155, 3.156 and 3.157). Some lesions have a papillomatous surface (*see* Figs. 3.158, 3.159 and 3.160). Darker or lighter colored papules or nodules that mimic the invasive stage of malignant melanoma may be found on the tumor (*see* Figs. 3.161, 3.162, 3.163 and 3.164). On the contrary of malignant melanoma, patients usually have a history of a stable lesion. Furthermore, congenital melanocytic nevi may be covered with diffuse terminal hairs (*see* Fig. 3.153), a characteristic feature that is not observed in malignant melanoma. Association of satellite lesions are unusual for

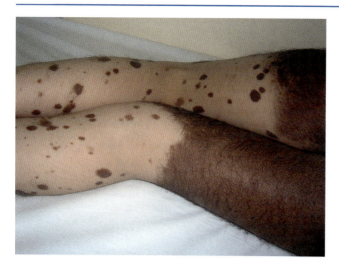

Fig. 3.148 A giant congenital melanocytic nevus and accompanying multiple small- and medium-sized nevi (satellite nevi)

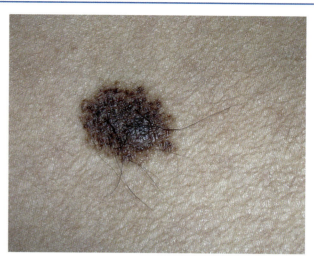

Fig. 3.151 Small congenital melanocytic nevus with irregular notched borders

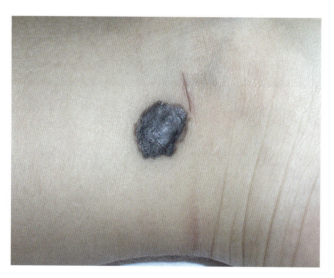

Fig. 3.149 Small congenital melanocytic nevus presenting as a black-colored, hairless, flat lesion

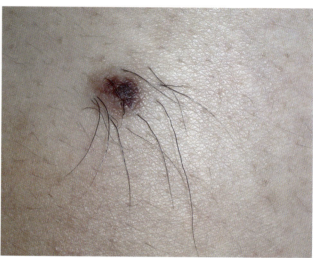

Fig. 3.152 A small congenital melanocytic nevus with protruding coarse dark hairs. Note that long hairs exceed the mass of the nevus

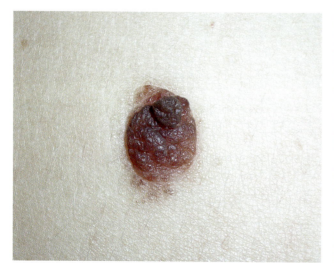

Fig. 3.150 Small congenital melanocytic nevus presenting as a round, brownish, raised nodule

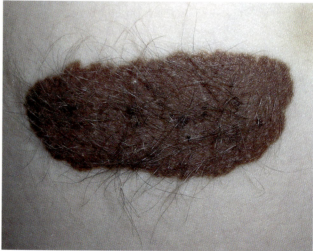

Fig. 3.153 Medium-sized congenital melanocytic nevus with uniform surface and long hairs located on the trunk

3.4 Melanocytic Nevi (Nevus Cell Nevi)

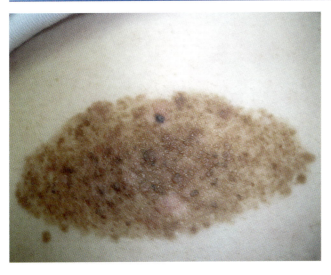

Fig. 3.154 Medium-sized congenital melanocytic nevus with heterogeneous surface. Note the multiple irregularly distributed papules overlying the mass of the nevus

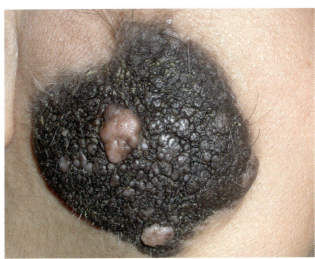

Fig. 3.157 Dark-colored, medium-sized congenital melanocytic nevus with partially papillomatous surface and overlying light-colored papules

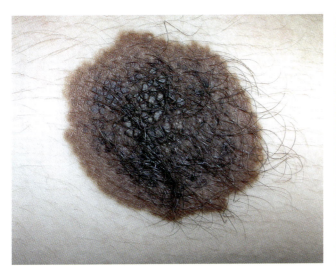

Fig. 3.155 Medium-sized congenital melanocytic nevus exhibiting a pebbled, nonhomogeneous surface

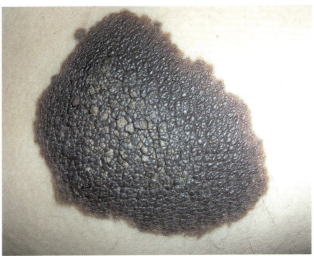

Fig. 3.158 Medium-sized congenital melanocytic nevus with homogenous papillomatous surface

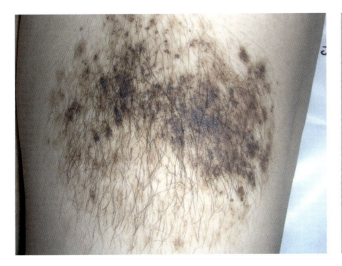

Fig. 3.156 Hairy medium-sized congenital melanocytic nevus. Note that some parts of the lesion is more elevated

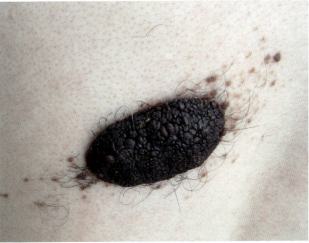

Fig. 3.159 Medium-sized congenital melanocytic nevus with papillomatous surface showing multiple small papules (satellites) in the near vicinity; an unusual presentation

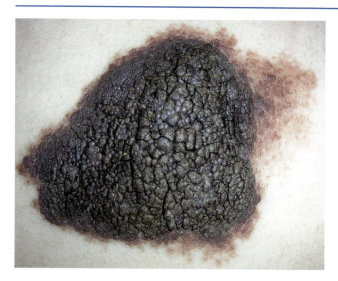

Fig. 3.160 Medium-sized congenital melanocytic nevus presenting with two components; a raised darker-colored plaque with papillomatous surface and a flat lighter-colored part (*upper right*)

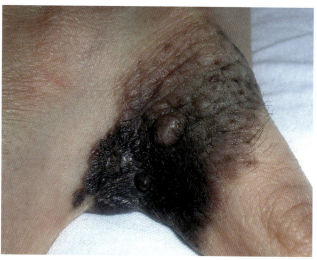

Fig. 3.162 Medium-sized congenital melanocytic nevus on the finger, a rare location

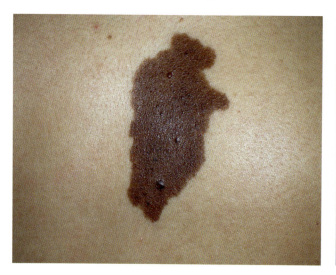

Fig. 3.161 Irregularly scattered small papules overlying a flat, medium-sized congenital melanocytic nevus. Different from the invasive stage of malignant melanoma, overlying papules or nodules are not ulcerated

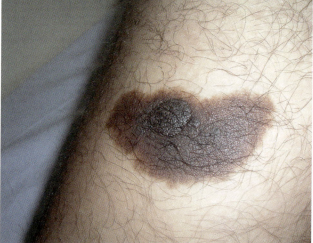

Fig. 3.163 A nodule overlying a flat medium-sized congenital melanocytic nevus

medium-sized congenital nevi (see Fig. 3.159). Congenital follicular melanocytic nevus is a special variant of congenital nevi composed of clustered follicular papules (see Fig. 3.165) showing histologically periadnexial localization of nevus cells.

Large congenital melanocytic nevus shows marked variability of clinical features. Some lesions are 20 to 30 cm in diameter (see Figs. 3.166 and 3.167), but others are larger (see Figs. 3.168 and 3.169) and may even exceed 50 cm and occupy completely one or more body sites or most of the integument (see Fig. 3.170). The most typical pattern is the involvement of the lower part of the trunk together with the upper part of the thighs, thus giving rise to the term "bathing trunk nevus" (see Figs. 3.171 and 3.172). However, involvement of the face, nape (see Fig. 3.173), scalp (see Fig. 3.174), and arms (see Fig. 3.175) is not rare. Lesions located on the hands and feet (see Fig. 3.176) are relatively rare. Generally an individual has only one large nevus that is usually accompanied by multiple satellite congenital nevi as small- or medium-sized lesions (see Figs. 3.148 and 3.177). These satellites may be near the vicinity of the main lesion (see Fig. 3.169) or distant from it, locating anywhere on the body (see Fig. 3.177). Some patients have profuse satellites.

Large congenital melanocytic nevi may have irregular configurations with variable surface features. Coloring may be uniform (see Fig. 3.176), irregular, or speckled (see Fig. 3.154). Hypopigmented or depressed foci may also be found (see Fig. 3.178). The surface may be homogeneous

3.4 Melanocytic Nevi (Nevus Cell Nevi)

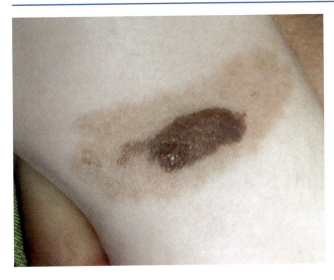

Fig. 3.164 A medium-sized congenital melanocytic nevus composed of two components; a large light brown patch and a central darker-colored plaque

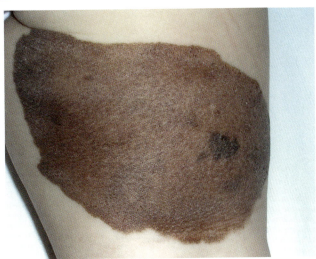

Fig. 3.166 Large congenital melanocytic nevus on the leg of a child. This subtype of congenital nevi have a projected adult size larger than 20 cm

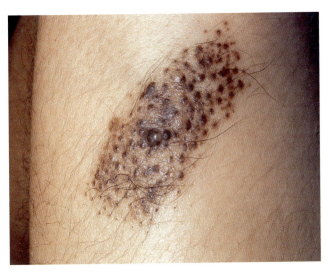

Fig. 3.165 Congenital follicular melanocytic nevus manifesting as a group of brownish or black follicular papules. This is a rare subtype of congenital melanocytic nevi with diagnostic histopathologic features

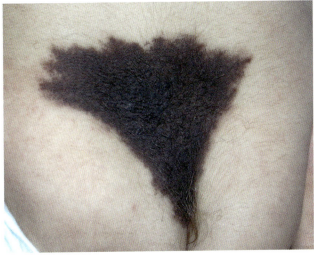

Fig. 3.167 A large congenital melanocytic nevus measuring nearly 20 cm on the sacral area with overlying hypertrichosis as dark terminal hairs. There are no associated satellite nevi in this case

(*see* Fig. 3.169) or heterogeneous (*see* Fig. 3.173). Lesions with papillomatous (*see* Fig. 3.179), lobular, verrucous, rugous (wrinkled) (*see* Fig. 3.180) and cerebriform (*see* Fig. 3.181) surface may be observed. Besides more raised papules, nodules, and plaques (*see* Figs. 3.173 and 3.182), plexiform or pendulous overgrowths may develop (*see* Figs. 3.180 and 3.183). Some lesions on the scalp may cause a cutis verticis gyrata-like appearance (*see* Fig. 3.181). Extensive lesions of the arms and legs involving sometimes the whole extremity may be associated with soft tissue atrophy, causing underdevelopment of the extremity (*see* Figs. 3.175 and 3.184).

Large congenital melanocytic nevi do not enlarge after the first year of life but may get darker in color, raise a little, and become more heterogeneous over time. Excessive growth of the terminal hairs (*see* Fig. 3.167), especially on the facial and extremity lesions, redoubles the cosmetic concerns. A few new small satellites may continue to occur in the early period. On the other hand, the color of the lesion may become lighter in adulthood.

Congenital melanocytic nevi including the giant lesions are generally not linked to any syndromes. However, in patients with neurofibromatosis large congenital melanocytic nevi are more commonly seen than in healthy individuals (see Fig. 3.185).

Congenital melanocytic nevi can be easily diagnosed on clinical examination. Differential diagnoses include mainly other types of melanocytic nevi. Since common acquired melanocytic nevi and dysplastic nevi are usually smaller

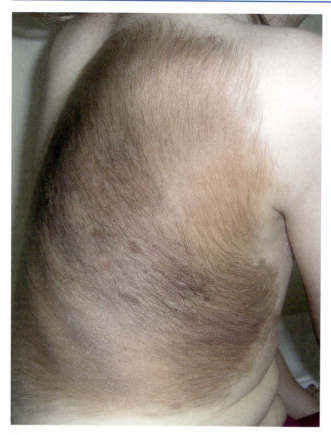

Fig. 3.168 Large congenital melanocytic nevus measuring approximately 40 cm on one side of the trunk. The relatively thinner lesion is light brown in color

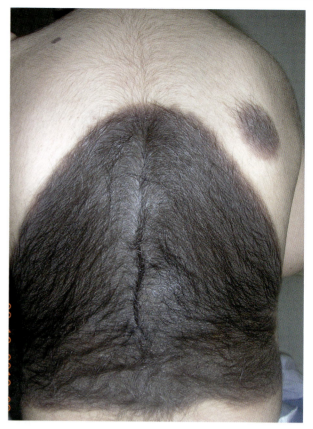

Fig. 3.169 Large congenital melanocytic nevus on the trunk. The surface of the hairy lesion is homogenous in this case. A satellite nevus near the main lesion is also seen

than 1.5 cm, they may be clinically confused with small congenital nevi. A history of onset since birth is in favor of small congenital melanocytic nevus, but adults may not always remember the time of onset of the nevus. At birth, small or medium-sized pale congenital nevi may look like café-au-lait macules. Medium or large congenital melanocytic nevi may also be confused with other types of tumoral lesions or pigmentation disorders such as nevus spilus, Becker nevus, congenital smooth muscle hamartoma, segmental lentiginosis, and café-au-lait macules. Nevus spilus (*see* Fig. 3.229) may present as a large heterogeneous lesion, but there is a hyperpigmented macule on the base. Becker nevus (*see* Fig. 1.131) is a hairy pigmented large lesion but is mostly acquired and not raised. Congenital smooth muscle hamartoma is also covered with hairs, but these are thin vellus hairs. Segmental lentiginosis (*see* Fig. 3.15) may involve a large area, but the lesion is flat and hairless with a nonhomogeneous appearance and typical distribution pattern. Finally, it is important to differentiate malignant melanoma from congenital melanocytic nevi. Malignant melanoma occurring on normal skin is hairless, is mostly seen in adults, and is usually associated with a typical history of recent change.

Histopathologic confirmation is rarely needed for congenital melanocytic nevi. They share main histopathologic features with acquired melanocytic nevi of compound or intradermal types and absolute specific findings do not exist. However, nevus cells usually invade deeper parts of the reticular dermis and subcutis. Large lesions typically tend to invade deeper tissue, along neurovascular bundles and adnexal structures, mostly hair follicles. Maturation of the nevus cells is also observed in these lesions.

Congenital melanocytic nevus is one of the most problematic nevi. Complications mainly correlate with the size of the tumor. In addition to giant lesions, nevi located on the face and genitalia, and lesions diffusely covered with hairs may cause major psychological problems for patients and parents. Moreover, affected patients are at risk for the development of malignant melanoma or soft tissue sarcoma and neurocutaneous melanosis. Cosmetic disfigurement and scar formation after excision may be another cause of concern. Therefore, an individualized approach is needed to determine the best management plan.

Xerosis and pruritus seen in large nevi may be disturbing. Folliculitis (*see* Fig. 3.186) and abscess formation are rare problems of hairy nevi and may easily be treated with antibiotics.

3.4 Melanocytic Nevi (Nevus Cell Nevi)

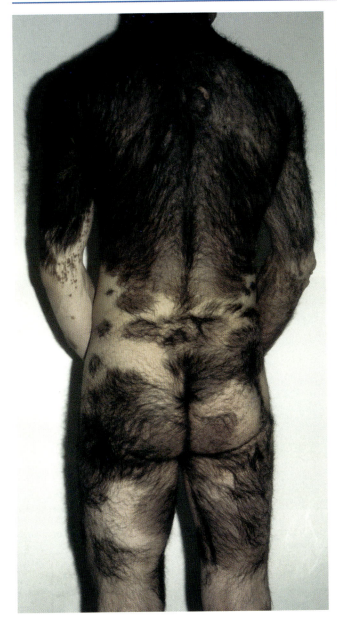

Fig. 3.170 Large congenital melanocytic nevus covering an extensive area of the integument

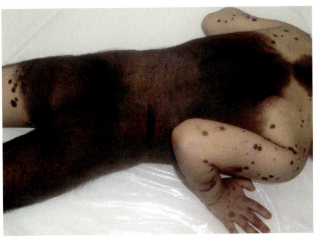

Fig. 3.171 Bathing trunk nevus; a common pattern of large congenital melanocytic nevus involving lower part of the trunk and upper part of the thighs circumferentially

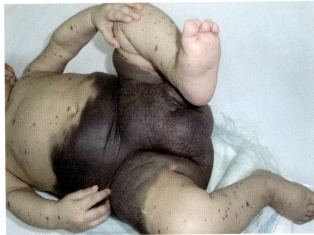

Fig. 3.172 Bathing trunk nevus. Genitalia may also be involved

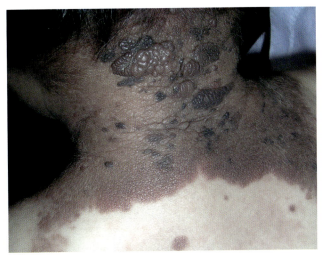

Fig. 3.173 Large congenital melanocytic nevus with heterogeneous surface extending from scalp to the upper back. Note the darker colored, raised papules and nodules on the neck

The risk of malignant transformation developing within small- and medium-sized congenital nevi is reported in varying rates (0 to 6%). Malignant melanoma may develop sometimes before but mostly after puberty. It develops usually within the dermoepidermal junction and may be detected early as a papular or nodular lesion on the surface of the nevus (see Fig. 3.187). In our clinical practice, we rarely observe melanoma developing within these nevi.

The lifetime risk of malignant melanoma's developing within a large congenital melanocytic nevus is approximately 5 to 10 percent. Lesions larger than 50 cm have a relatively increased risk for the development of malignant melanoma.

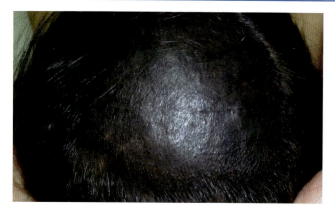

Fig. 3.174 Large congenital melanocytic nevus causing alopecia

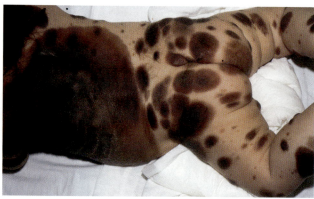

Fig. 3.177 Large congenital melanocytic nevus associated with widely distributed small- and medium-sized melanocytic nevi, namely satellites

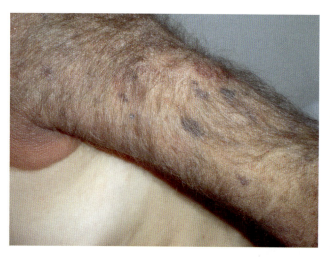

Fig. 3.175 Large congenital melanocytic nevus involving the upper arm circumferentially. The whole arm or leg may be covered unilaterally

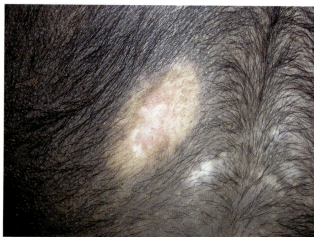

Fig. 3.178 A hairless, slightly atrophic, well-defined area on a large congenital melanocytic nevus

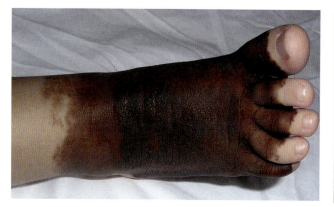

Fig. 3.176 A large congenital melanocytic nevus on the dorsum of the foot. Involvement of fingers and toes is relatively rare

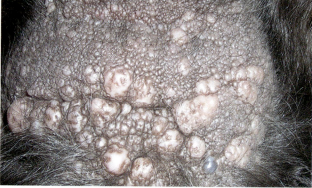

Fig. 3.179 Large congenital melanocytic nevus with papillomatous surface associated with alopecia

3.4 Melanocytic Nevi (Nevus Cell Nevi)

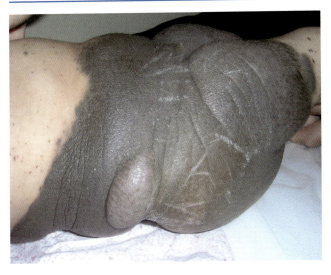

Fig. 3.180 Large congenital melanocytic nevus exhibiting a rugose surface. There is also a plexiform overgrowth on the flank

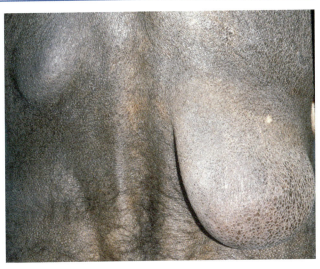

Fig. 3.183 Multiple subcutaneous masses due to soft tissue hamartomas on a large congenital melanocytic nevus. Note that one of these overgrowths is very large and pendulous (*right*)

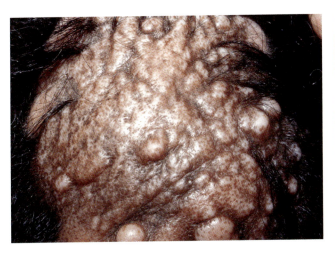

Fig. 3.181 Large congenital melanocytic nevus with a cerebriform surface causing alopecia and cutis verticis gyrate-like appearance

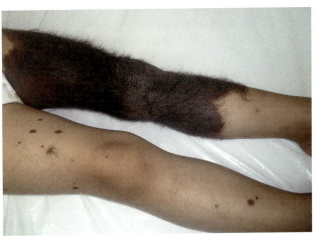

Fig. 3.184 Circumferential large congenital melanocytic nevus on one leg. Atrophy or hypertrophy of the underlying soft tissue may be associated with large nevi of the limbs

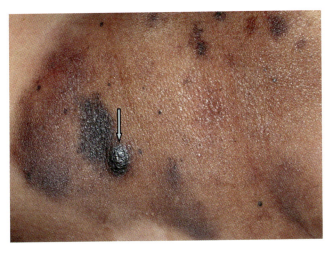

Fig. 3.182 Heavily pigmented small nodule within a large congenital melanocytic nevus (*arrow*). It was diagnosed as a proliferative nodule histopathologically

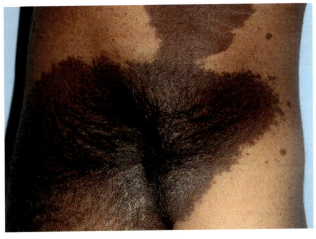

Fig. 3.185 Large congenital melanocytic nevus associated with multiple café-au-lait macules in a patient with neurofibromatosis

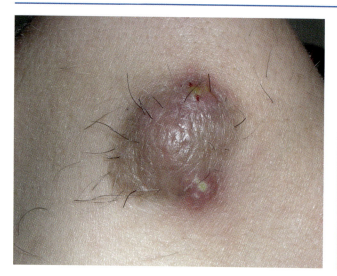

Fig. 3.186 Secondarily infected congenital melanocytic nevus

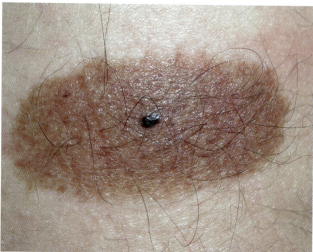

Fig. 3.187 Malignant melanoma arising on a medium-sized congenital melanocytic nevus. Note the dark papule on the brownish plaque, which was diagnosed as in-situ melanoma histologically

Malignant degeneration may occur at any age, but more than half of the melanomas are diagnosed in patients under the age of 10. The most common cause of melanomas in infancy is large congenital melanocytic nevus. Axial large nevi have the greatest risk for malignant transformation. Different from what occurs in small- and medium-sized ones, malignant melanoma develops from the deep part (deeper than the dermoepidermal junction) of the large congenital melanocytic nevus and usually cannot be detected early. The sudden appearance of a pigmented superficial or subcutaneous nodule, new foci of hyperpigmentation, persistent erosion, nonhealing ulceration, spontaneous bleeding, and extension of the lesion into previously unaffected normal skin are the possible signs of malignant degeneration. Although they have been suggested to pose a general risk for the development of malignant melanoma, satellite nevi usually do not undergo malignant degeneration in patients with large congenital melanocytic nevi.

Not all papulonodular lesions developing within the giant nevi are signs of malignant melanoma. Benign small (<1 cm) or large (>1 cm) dermal nodules or plaques may arise within these nevi. Small nodules, which are more frequent, may be present at birth or develop later in life, especially in childhood. They may be lighter or darker in color when compared to the other flat parts of the nevus (see Fig. 3.173). The surface of these nodules is smooth, and ulceration is uncommon. On the other hand, large nodules are rare. They are usually deeply pigmented showing rapid growth and occasionally may be ulcerated. A small nodule (see Fig. 3.182) usually corresponds to a proliferative nodule histopathologically, showing high cellularity of atypical melanocytes. These benign nodules may become smaller and softer or completely regress in time. Apart from these, dermal or subcutaneous nodules corresponding to hamartomatous lesions containing various cell types like muscle cells, nerve cells, adipose cells or cartilage may also arise within congenital melanocytic nevi (see Fig. 3.146), especially within the giant subtype. These may sometimes present as large pendulous masses (see Fig. 3.183).

Neurocutaneous (leptomeningeal) melanocytosis is another serious complication of congenital melanocytic nevi. It is more common in men and is mostly seen in individuals with giant nevi localized on the posterior axis (midline of the back, head, and neck) that is associated with multiple satellites. Uncontrolled leptomeningeal proliferation of melanocytes may lead to impaired cerebrospinal fluid circulation and cisternal blockage, causing neurologic symptoms such as hydrocephaly and seizures. The prognosis of leptomeningeal melanocytosis is poor after the occurrence of neurologic symptoms. Magnetic resonance imaging may enable the diagnosis. However, not every patient with positive findings in imaging studies will develop clinical symptoms. Another complication of neurocutaneous melanocytosis is leptomeningeal melanoma, which usually has high metastatic potential.

Management. Approach to the patients with congenital melanocytic nevi depends on the size, localization, and number of the lesions. Solar protection is essential for all individuals with these nevi. Neurologic examination is mandatory for patients with dorsal midline congenital melanocytic nevi, especially in the presence of large ones.

Treatment of congenital nevi depends on two factors: reducing the risk of developing cutaneous malignant melanoma and improving the cosmesis. There is no urgency to remove a small congenital nevus in childhood as the risk of malignant transformation is not high. Malignant melanoma generally arises from the junctional area in this subtype, allowing a relatively earlier detection. Excision can be

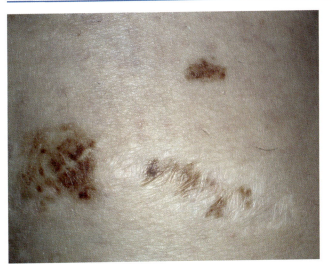

Fig. 3.188 Irregular hyperpigmentation developed on the excision scar of a medium-sized congenital melanocytic nevus

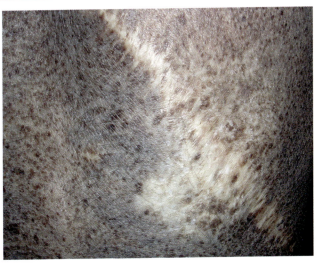

Fig. 3.189 Irregular hyperpigmentation developed along the partial excision scar of a large congenital melanocytic nevus. This is not a sign of malignant transformation

performed at any age for prophylactic or cosmetic purposes if technically easy. On the other hand, routine prophylactic removal of medium-sized nevi is controversial. Excision eliminates the risk of malignant melanoma but cosmetic disfigurement after surgery may be worrisome.

Management of large congenital melanocytic nevi is more complicated. The risk of malignant melanoma development is increased and begins in the early period of life. Malignant melanoma originates from deeper parts of the skin in these giant lesions with a low possibility of early detection. Parents or patients can be extremely worried about the development of malignant melanoma when informed about the risk of the nevus. Moreover, serious cosmetic disturbance of the nevus affects the psychology of the individual starting from childhood. Therefore, large congenital melanocytic nevi should primarily be evaluated for excision. Unfortunately, definite prevention from malignant melanoma is not possible. Surgery is technically difficult in these patients because it usually requires general anesthesia and deep resection, sometimes extending to the fasciae for the removal of nevus cells that invade deep tissue. Furthermore, postsurgical scars are usually troublesome and may be associated with pruritus and fragility of skin. If the whole nevus cannot be removed, scars will be hyperpigmented afterward (see Figs. 3.188 and 3.189) and cosmetic appearance may be worsened.

Multistaged full-thickness surgical excision is the main option of surgery to reduce the risk of malignant melanoma, but the above-mentioned difficulties of surgery limit the use of this option. Tissue expanders may be applied to facilitate large excisions. They are useful in reconstruction of large congenital melanocytic nevi and provide satisfactory cosmesis. Methods especially preferred for cosmetic improvement, such as dermabrasion, curettage, partial thickness excision or laser therapy that are performed in different periods of life are relatively easier and safer to use and scars might be less than excision. However, as these procedures only destruct melanocytes or nevus cells in the epidermis and dermis, the risk of malignant melanoma development from residual nevus cells in deeper tissue still remains. In addition, after the application of these methods, early clinical detection of malignant melanoma may not be easy on the treated sites.

On the other hand, some congenital melanocytic nevi are extremely large, and any therapeutic intervention is difficult; in these cases observation may be the only alternative. Covered areas such as the scalp, perianal area, and genitalia are difficult to follow up. Baseline photographs are helpful for monitoring all patients. Patients or parents should also be taught about self-examination like following the changes of the nevus in color, size, shape, and surface features.

3.4.4 Dysplastic Nevus (Atypical Nevus)

Dysplastic nevus is a special type of acquired melanocytic nevus with distinct clinicopathologic features. Congenital lesions with features of dysplastic nevus are rare. Dysplastic nevus is accepted as a marker of increased risk for malignant melanoma, but the lesions infrequently transform into malignant melanoma (see Fig. 12.1). Genetic and environmental factors, especially intense sun exposure, are suggested to play a role in the etiopathogenesis. The onset of the nevus is usually around the end of the first decade.

The presence of multiple dysplastic nevi associated with a personal or family history of malignant melanoma is referred to "dysplastic nevus syndrome" or "atypical mole syndrome." These people have a significantly higher risk of developing malignant melanoma, but melanomas usually

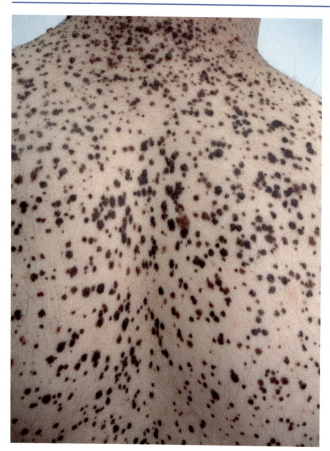

Fig. 3.190 Numerous dysplastic nevi in a patient with dysplastic nevus syndrome. These type of nevi are most common on the back

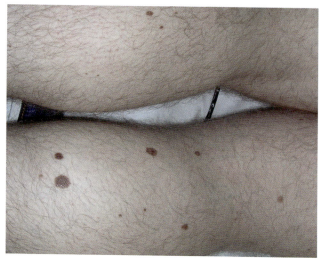

Fig. 3.191 Multiple dysplastic nevi on the legs. Lesions are mostly smaller than 1 cm as in this case

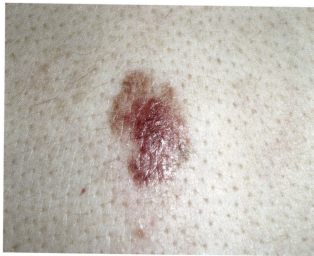

Fig. 3.192 A relatively large dysplastic nevus measuring 13 to 15 mm in size. Note the irregular borders of the lesion simulating melanoma

arise on normal skin. The number of nevi correlates with the increased risk of malignant melanoma. Some individuals have innumerable lesions (*see* Fig. 3.190). New nevi continue to develop in these patients in adulthood.

Dysplastic nevi may also develop in individuals lacking a personal or familial history of similar nevi and melanoma. There may be a solitary nevus or multiple nevi. In people with multiple nevi, dysplastic nevi and common (ordinary) acquired melanocytic nevi are usually found concomitantly. The trunk is the typical location of dysplastic nevus. However, the buttocks, limbs (*see* Fig. 3.191), scalp, face, and genitalia may also be involved. Lesions are usually larger than 5 mm and smaller than 15 mm (*see* Figs. 3.191 and 3.192). In particular patients with "dysplastic nevus syndrome" have relatively larger nevi (*see* Fig. 3.193). In general, a dysplastic nevus is a minimally elevated, hairless, small lesion, usually with an irregular shape (*see* Figs. 3.194, 3.195, and 3.196). Pigmentation of the nevus is variable but shades of tan, brown (*see* Fig. 3.197), or pink color (see Fig. 3.193) predominate. The center or the periphery (Fig. 3.197) of the nevus may be relatively darker, and some parts may be slightly elevated (*see* Figs. 3.193 and 3.198). The outline border is usually irregular and partially indistinct, sometimes with asymmetric notching (*see* Figs. 3.192 and 3.199). Lesions with atypical features and irregularity may even fulfill the ABCD rule of melanoma criteria. The number of dysplastic nevi may increase during adolescence, pregnancy, a state of immunosuppression, or after intense sun exposure. They do not follow the typical evolutionary pattern of common acquired nevi.

Small and flat dysplastic nevi may not be easily distinguished from lentigo simplex (*see* Fig. 3.9) or common junctional nevi (*see* Fig. 3.82). On the other hand, large lesions may be confused with early lesions of superficial spreading melanoma (*see* Fig. 12.16) or early lesions of pigmented superficial basal cell carcinoma (*see* Fig. 11.58). The diagnosis of dysplastic nevus is based on clinical examination together with dermoscopy supporting the diagnosis. However, biopsy must be performed for lesions suspicious for malignant melanoma. As the nevus is not usually large,

3.4 Melanocytic Nevi (Nevus Cell Nevi)

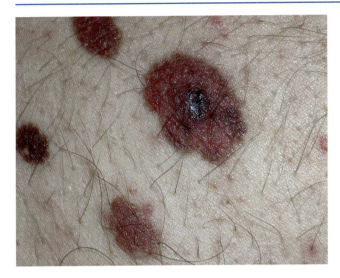

Fig. 3.193 A few pinkish brown-colored dysplastic nevi in a patient with dysplastic nevus syndrome. Note one of them (*right*) is larger and shows a central slightly elevated black area

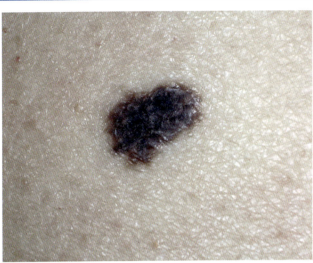

Fig. 3.196 Dysplastic nevus with irregular outline. This lesion mimics in-situ superficial spreading melanoma

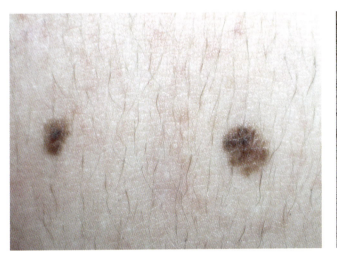

Fig. 3.194 Two dysplastic nevi on the trunk. Note that they are minimally elevated and ill-defined

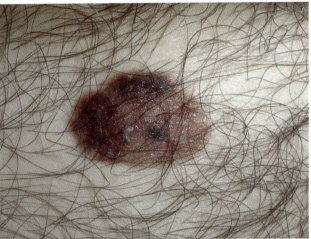

Fig. 3.197 A large dysplastic nevus with non-homogeneous surface; multifocal areas of brown and black colors are seen

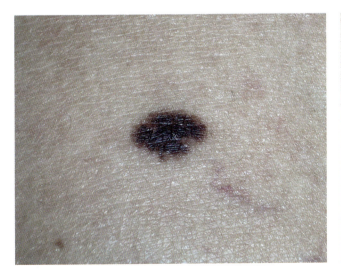

Fig. 3.195 Dysplastic nevus presenting as a small, oval-shaped, brownish, flat lesion

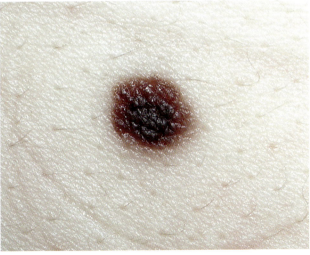

Fig. 3.198 Dysplastic nevus with a relatively darker center

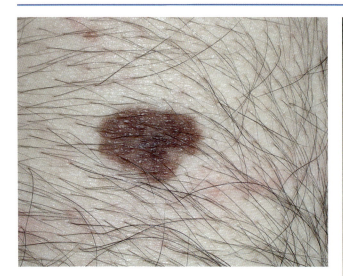

Fig. 3.199 Dysplastic nevus presenting as a flat hyperpigmented lesion showing asymmetric notching

complete excision is preferred. Dysplastic nevi show irregular, bridging nests forming a junctional or compound nevus. Melanocytes show variable atypia, from slight to severe. Lentiginous elongation of rete ridges, patchy lymphocytic infiltration, and lamellar and concentric fibroplasia in the papillary dermis are other histopathologic features of this nevus.

Management. The initial step in evaluating a patient with dysplastic nevus is to rule out malignant melanoma. Whole body dermatologic examination should be performed. Additionally, an ophthalmologic examination is also useful in dysplastic nevus syndrome because of the increased risk of conjunctival and intraocular melanoma. Prophylactic excision of dysplastic nevus is not indicated unless there is a suspicion of malignant melanoma. Patients with dysplastic nevi must be followed regularly for life. Photographic and dermoscopic documentation are essential for regular controls. Digital dermoscopy enables comparison of sequential images. Self-examination of the skin can be advised and taught to patients, since it may allow earlier detection of malignant melanoma.

Some patients with dysplastic nevus syndrome develop more than one malignant melanoma during their lifetimes. Any new appearing lesion or major change in the morphology of a preexisting nevus detected during examination should be considered for malignant melanoma. If the suspicion of malignant melanoma cannot be eliminated, total excision followed by histopathologic examination is obligatory. Many patients with multiple dysplastic nevi have small scars due to removal of the lesions (*see* Fig. 3.200). Risky lesions are inevitably removed but unnecessary excisions should be avoided. Lifelong sun protection should be advised to the patients. The family of the patients must also be meticulously screened for the presence of dysplastic nevi and malignant melanoma.

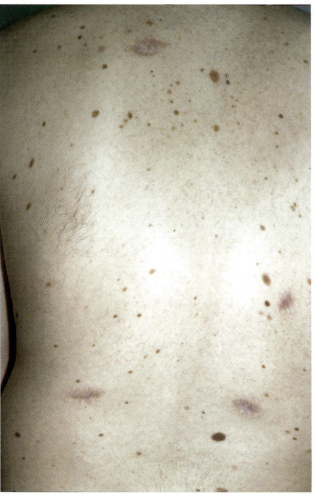

Fig. 3.200 A patient with multiple dysplastic nevi on the back. Note the multiple scars due to previous surgical excisions performed to exclude malignant melanoma

3.4.5 Halo Nevus (Sutton Nevus)

Halo nevus is a benign lesion with two different components, namely, a central melanocytic nevus surrounded by a white (depigmented or hypopigmented) halo. An autoimmune mechanism triggered by nevus cells has been suggested as an etiopathogenetic factor for hypopigmentation. It develops mostly in adolescence but sometimes appears either earlier or later in adulthood. The preferred site is the trunk (*see* Fig. 3.201), especially the upper back, but it may be seen nearly anywhere on the skin, including the face and scalp (*see* Fig. 3.202). Patients usually have more than one lesion (*see* Fig. 3.201) and have a history of sudden onset.

The center of melanocytic nevus is mostly a pink to dark brown, homogeneous, 3 to 6 mm-sized (*see* Fig. 3.203), relatively flat (*see* Fig. 3.204), or sometimes raised (*see* Fig. 3.205) papule. The surface of some lesions may be mildly crusted (*see* Fig. 3.206). The well-defined halo is approximately 0.5 to 1.5 cm in size with a round or oval shape and homogeneous color (*see* Figs. 3.207 and 3.208).

3.4 Melanocytic Nevi (Nevus Cell Nevi)

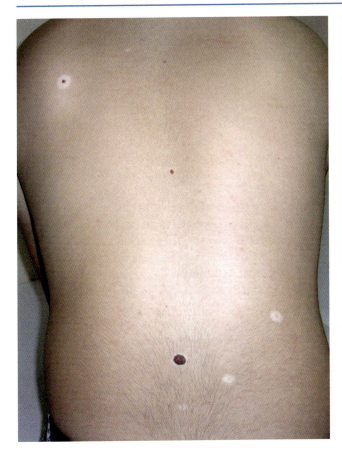

Fig. 3.201 Multiple halo nevi irregularly scattered on the back, a common location

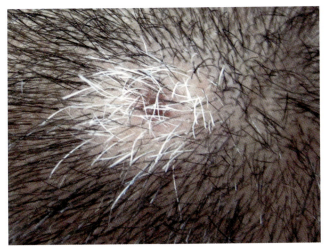

Fig. 3.202 Halo nevus may rarely be located on the scalp. Note the associated leukotrichia restricted to the lesion site

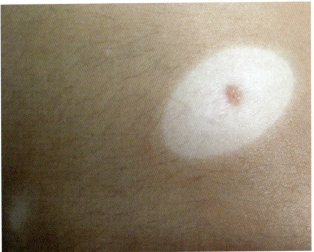

Fig. 3.203 Oval, symmetrical, well-demarcated hypopigmented rim around a central small acquired melanocytic nevus; halo nevus

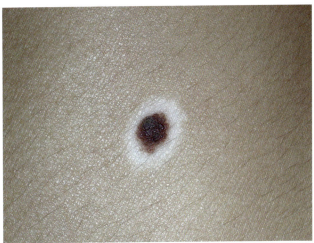

Fig. 3.204 A flat hyperpigmented melanocytic nevus surrounded with a round-shaped, white, narrow halo; a typical halo nevus

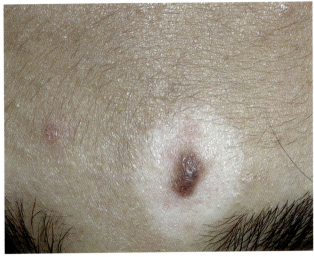

Fig. 3.205 Halo nevus on the face with a raised, uniformly colored papule in the center of the lesion

On dark skin, the halo can be more striking. Sometimes, leukotrichia may overlie the hypopigmented area. This is especially remarkable on scalp lesions (*see* Fig. 3.202).

The frequency of melanocytic nevi, including halo nevus, is increased in individuals with Turner syndrome. Halo nevi are relatively common in patients with vitiligo (*see* Fig. 3.209).

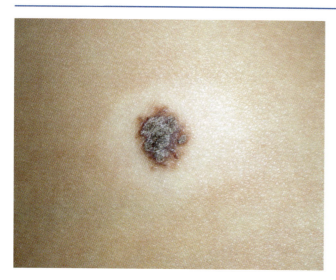

Fig. 3.206 Halo nevus showing mild crusting on the central nevus

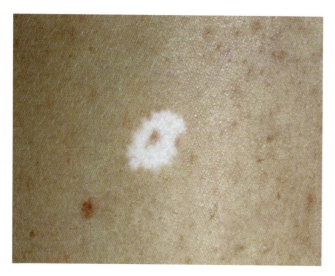

Fig. 3.207 Halo nevus with a fading central papule and an irregularly-shaped halo

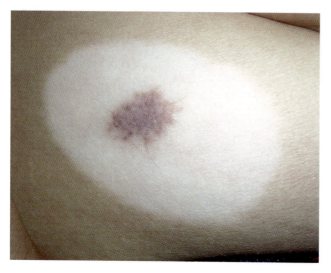

Fig. 3.208 Halo nevus with a flat small central nevus and a relatively large, oval-shaped rim

The hypopigmented component of the nevus is similar to that of vitiligo macules except for its specific localization around a tumor. Halo nevus has a typical evolution period. Perilesional depigmentation develops around an acquired nevus over a period of several months. After persistence for months to years, the central nevus may undergo involution (*see* Fig. 3.210) and may disappear. The remaining halo may also gradually disappear, sometimes with complete repigmentation after months or years. However, not all lesions follow the same pathway. Lesions at various stages of involution may be seen in one patient (*see* Fig. 3.211).

Sometimes the central nevus is of papillomatous type (*see* Fig. 3.212), a congenital melanocytic nevus, or a dysplastic nevus. The presence of large and relatively irregular central lesions is more indicative of congenital nevi (*see* Fig. 3.213). On the other hand, an acquired pigmented lesion with a white halo can be a sign of a regressing melanoma and confusion with a halo nevus causes diagnostic delay. Malignant melanoma with a halo is solitary, can be located anywhere on the skin, and depigmentation mostly occurs in adulthood. In addition to the atypical clinical features of the central lesion, the halo is also asymmetric with an irregular shape and border. Nevi protected with sunscreens and tapes during sunbathing or phototherapy may have transient light-colored pseudohalos. Although rare, a white halo may also be observed around nonmelanocytic tumors such as dermatofibroma and seborrheic keratosis.

Halo nevus is usually diagnosed clinically. Dermoscopic examination can also be helpful. In lesions with atypical clinical features a biopsy should be performed from the central nevus to rule out malignant melanoma. A compound or intradermal nevus is usually found. A dense inflammatory infiltration of predominantly lymphocytes in the dermis is the major finding of halo nevus. The surrounding halo is characterized by the absence of melanocytes and melanin.

Management. Halo nevus is a benign melanocytic lesion. However, exclusion of a regressing malignant melanoma is the first step of an approach. Sometimes removal of the lesion may be necessary for histopathologic examination allowing a definite diagnosis. Patients with halo nevi should also be examined for vitiligo. The malignant transformation of this type of nevus is unusual, and a prophylactic excision or destructive therapies that may cause undesirable scars (*see* Fig. 3.214) are not indicated. Reassuring the patients about the natural course of the nevus is enough. Cosmetic camouflage can be recommended for facial lesions. In patients with multiple lesions, sun-protection must be advised.

3.4.6 Spitz Nevus

Spitz nevus is an uncommon type of benign acquired melanocytic nevi which most commonly appears during childhood and rarely in adulthood. Because of its histopathologic

3.4 Melanocytic Nevi (Nevus Cell Nevi)

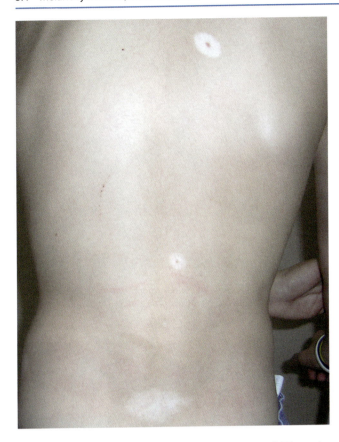

Fig. 3.209 Halo nevus associated with vitiligo that is visible on the lower part of the figure

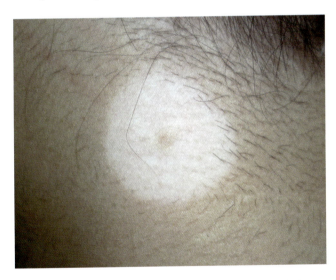

Fig. 3.210 Spontaneous involution of halo nevus. Only slight hyperpigmentation can be noticed on the center

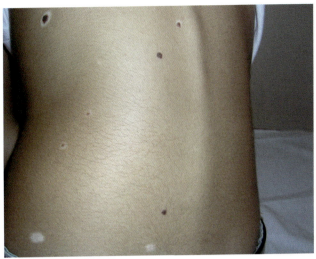

Fig. 3.211 Multiple lesions of halo nevus on the trunk showing different stages of involution. Note that some white round patches lack the central papule due to fading of the nevus

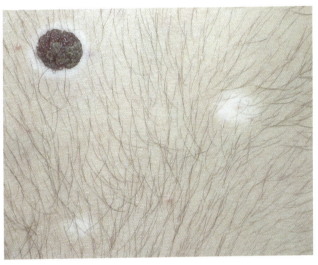

Fig. 3.212 Halo nevus with a central large papillomatous nevus (*upper left*)

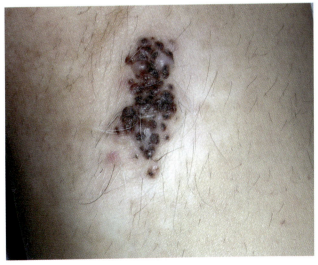

Fig. 3.213 A congenital nevus with halo phenomenon. White halo is irregular in this case and leukotrichia is remarkable

resemblance to malignant melanoma, the term "juvenile melanoma" has historically been used. It appears suddenly, then grows progressively within a few months and remains unchanged thereafter. Many patients have a history of a recently developing lesion that may cause suspicion of a malignant lesion. Face, neck, and lower extremities are the preferred sites. The typical presentation is a solitary, dome-shaped, hairless, firm papule or nodule approximately

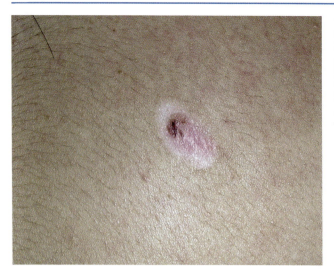

Fig. 3.214 Recurrence of a nevus as irregular hyperpigmentation on the scar tissue surrounded by hypopigmentation. This is a site of previously mistreated halo nevus with a destructive method

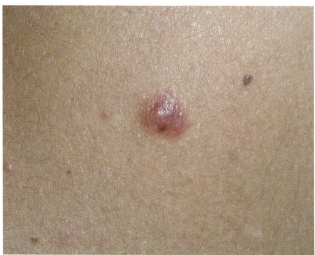

Fig. 3.216 A solitary pink-colored, smooth-surfaced nodule measuring 8–9 mm in size; distinctive appearance of Spitz nevus

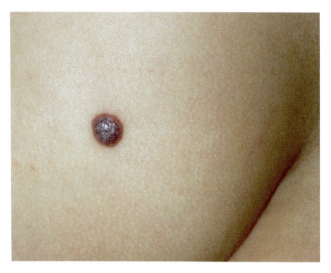

Fig. 3.215 Spitz nevus presenting as a solitary dome-shaped, hyperpigmented nodule on the gluteal area of a child

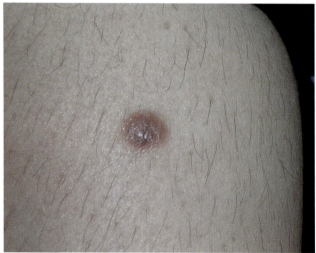

Fig. 3.217 Spitz nevus shown as a dome-shaped, brownish hairless nodule with smooth-surface

1 cm in diameter (*see* Figs. 3.215 and 3.216). The color of the lesions is variable; brown (*see* Figs. 3.215 and 3.217), flesh or pink to red-colored (*see* Figs. 3.216 and 3.218) nevi can be seen. The reddish color occurs as a result of increased dermal vascularity, a histopathologic feature that is unusual for other melanocytic nevi. Lesions localized on the lower extremities may be more pigmented. Telangiectasia on the surface and bleeding after trauma are rare findings. The surface is mostly smooth but may sometimes be rough due to hyperkeratosis.

Multiple lesions are rarely encountered. Multiple lesions restricted to one site of the body or in a segmental pattern are called agminated Spitz nevi. Rarely, disseminated eruptive Spitz nevi are observed. A desmoplastic (sclerotic) variant of Spitz nevus has also been described. This lesion is more commonly seen in young adults as a red or reddish brown smooth, firm papule, nodule, or plaque (*see* Fig. 3.219), mostly localized on the trunk or extremities.

Clinical diagnosis of Spitz nevus is harder than diagnoses of other melanocytic nevi. Rapidly growing tumors of Spitz nevus usually have a symmetric appearance with well-defined margins, contrary to the irregular lesions of malignant melanoma. Reddish tumors occurring in childhood may also be confused with nonmelanocytic tumors such as pyogenic granuloma (*see* Fig. 6.56), angiolymphoid hyperplasia with eosinophilia (*see* Fig. 6.81), pseudolymphoma (*see* Fig. 14.194), isolated mastocytoma (*see* Fig. 9.19), and juvenile xanthogranuloma (*see* Fig. 15.21). Pyogenic granuloma grows more rapidly, is typically pedunculated, and bleeds easily. Darker lesions may resemble other acquired melanocytic

3.4 Melanocytic Nevi (Nevus Cell Nevi)

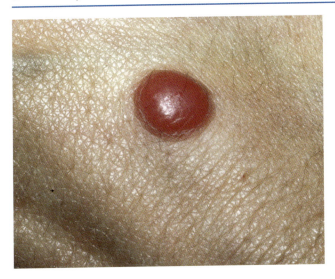

Fig. 3.218 Spitz nevus may appear as a red nodule as seen in the figure. This presentation is unusual for other melanocytic nevi

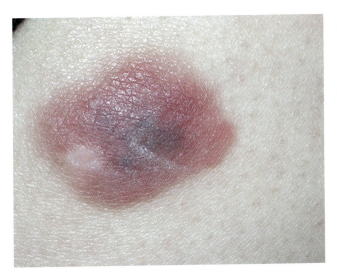

Fig. 3.219 Desmoplastic Spitz nevus presenting as a reddish plaque

nevi, especially the intradermal type (*see* Fig. 3.120) and dermatofibroma (*see* Fig. 8.10). Desmoplastic variant of Spitz nevus may also mimic dermatofibroma. Hyperkeratotic lesions must be differentiated from viral warts. If there is any diagnostic difficulty from the clinical point of view, lesions must be removed for histopathologic examination. However, as some histologic features may overlap with those of malignant melanoma, clinicopathologic correlation is crucial for the diagnosis. Spitz nevus is mainly a compound nevus composed of large spindle and epithelioid cells usually forming nests and bundles. Thin-walled dilated capillaries in the dermis are correlated with the reddish color of the tumor. Symmetric appearance, maturation in the deeper part of the lesion, scattered lymphocytic infiltration, multinucleated giant cells, and Kamino bodies on the dermoepidermal junction are other histopathologic features of this nevus. In the desmoplastic variant, nevus cells are distributed in abundant fibrotic dermal stroma of thickened collagen bundles.

The relation between Spitz nevus and spitzoid malignant melanoma is a matter of debate. It is suggested that benign (classical) Spitz nevus, atypical spitzoid melanocytic neoplasm and spitzoid malignant melanoma form a spectrum. Moreover, the potential of benign lesions to progress towards the malignant end of this spectrum is unclear.

Management. Spitz nevus is accepted as a benign tumor with a very low risk of malignant degeneration. Some lesions may even involute spontaneously in a few years. Routine removal of childhood lesions without atypical features is not mandatory. Monitoring the lesions for at least 1 to 3 years may be efficient. On the other hand, Spitz nevus in adults is more difficult to diagnose both clinically and histopathologically; as a result lesions in adulthood are usually excised to rule out malignant melanoma.

Apart from the above-mentioned approach, there is another opinion that holds that all tumors suggestive of Spitz nevus noticed at any age should be removed. The entire lesion can be excised with a narrow margin in order to perform an accurate histopathologic examination. If Spitz nevus is not completely excised, the recurrent lesion may mimic malignant melanoma histopathologically, leading to confusion.

The therapeutic approach to atypical spitzoid melanocytic neoplasm is rather complicated. This tumor is better treated as it were spitzoid malignant melanoma.

3.4.7 Reed Nevus (Pigmented Spindle Cell Nevus)

Reed nevus is a rare benign acquired melanocytic nevus regarded as a distinct entity or a variant of Spitz nevus. It is usually seen in young adults or children. It is more common on the extremities but may occur anywhere. Patients have almost always a solitary, homogeneous heavily pigmented lesion (*see* Fig. 3.220).

A typical lesion is a sharply circumscribed, smooth-surfaced, hairless, blue-black, relatively flat (*see* Fig. 3.221) or raised (*see* Figs. 3.222 and 3.223) papule or nodule varying in size from 0.3 to 0.8 mm. Because this darkly pigmented lesion appears suddenly, patients usually come to physicians within a short time with concern of a malignancy. In general, the homogeneous pigmentation and symmetric appearance are different from that of malignant melanoma. Blue nevus (*see* Fig. 3.61) and pigmented basal cell carcinoma (*see* Fig. 11.71) are other differential diagnostic challenges. Dermoscopy is usually helpful in the diagnosis of Reed nevus. Histologically it is a junctional or compound nevus composed of nests of uniform spindle-shaped cells that form interconnecting fascicles. Dense melanin content of the nevus cells and many melanophages in the papillary

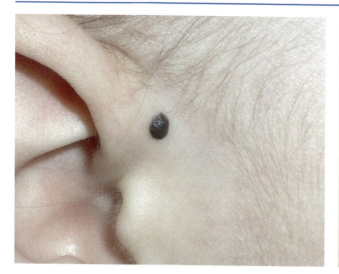

Fig. 3.220 Reed nevus causes a heavily pigmented solitary lesion as shown in the figure. Different from malignant melanoma this lesion has a homogenous appearance

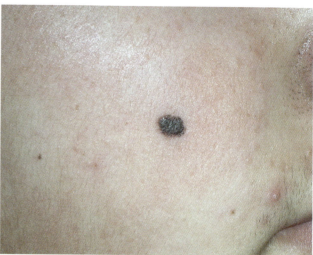

Fig. 3.222 Reed nevus on the cheek of a child. It is nearly always less than 1 cm

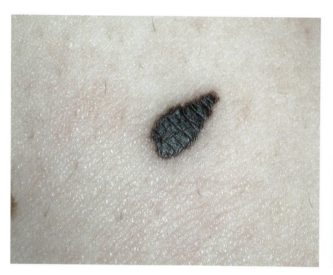

Fig. 3.221 A darkly pigmented, flat, oval lesion exhibiting symmetry; typical Reed nevus

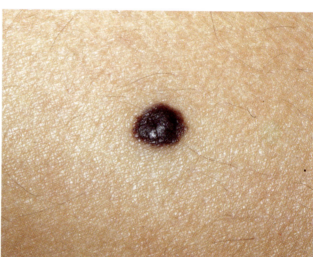

Fig. 3.223 A dome-shaped, bluish-black solitary nodule with acute onset is a typical presentation of Reed nevus at admission. Heavy pigmentation may cause some concern but the lesion is benign

dermis are the cause of the darkness of the tumor. Nevus cells show maturation like other benign melanocytic nevi.

Management. Although Reed nevus follows a benign clinical course, it is usually excised with a clear margin to exclude malignant melanoma. Since the lesion is small, a wide excision is not necessary, so fine cosmetic outcome is expected after surgery. Unless the lesion is completely excised, the histopathologic features of recurring lesion will be particularly difficult to distinguish from malignant melanoma.

3.4.8 Deep Penetrating Nevus

Deep penetrating nevus is a rare benign acquired tumor showing a rich spectrum of histopathologic features causing controversies in classification. It is suggested to be a distinct type of melanocytic nevus but also shares some similar features with several other types of nevi. It may be seen at any age but mostly appears in young adults. It is usually found on the face and neck but may also be found on other body sites, including the trunk and limbs. The typical lesion is a heavily pigmented, pink to black, dome-shaped, 2 to 10 mm papule or nodule (*see* Fig. 3.224).

The clinical diagnosis is challenging because the nevus can easily be mistaken for a malignant melanoma. Blue nevus, Reed nevus and Spitz nevus are other challenging points in the differential diagnosis. In fact, whereas some have suggested that it could be a type of blue nevus, others have considered it to be a type of plexiform Spitz nevus. Deep

3.4 Melanocytic Nevi (Nevus Cell Nevi)

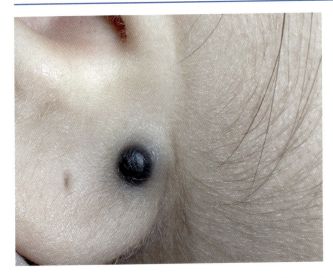

Fig. 3.224 Deep penetrating nevus on the ear. This heavily pigmented lesion may not be easily distinguished from blue nevus or pigmented Spitz nevus

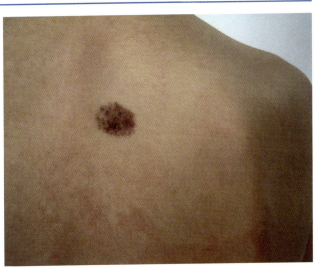

Fig. 3.225 Nevus spilus associated with nevus anemicus in a patient with phacomatosis pigmentovascularis

penetrating nevus may have clinicopathologic overlapping features with both of these lesions. In addition, histopathologically, deep penetrating nevus may be associated with common acquired melanocytic nevi, most commonly compound nevus. Furthermore, a nevus with a focal atypical epithelioid component (clonal nevus) is suggested to be the superficial variant of deep penetrating nevus. Histologically, deep penetrating nevus is sharply demarcated and has a wedge shape, with the apex pointing toward subcutaneous fat. Cells form nests or fascicles located in the reticular dermis or extending to the subcutis. Plump fusiform to spindle cells compose the fascicles. Some may have an epithelioid cell component. The lesion is rich in melanin.

Management. Differentiation from malignant melanoma is essential. Complete excision is almost always needed for histopathologic confirmation. The correct diagnosis will prevent the patient from the unnecessary troublesome surgery of melanoma. The lesion has no metastatic potential and is not expected to recur after removal with a narrow margin.

3.4.9 Nevus Spilus (Speckled Lentiginous Nevus)

Nevus spilus is a melanocytic nevus characterized by two components causing a speckled pattern. The occurrence is mostly sporadic, but it may sometimes be associated with nevus flammeus and/or nevus anemicus, indicating phacomatosis pigmentovascularis (*see* Fig. 3.225); or it may be associated with nevus sebaceus, indicating phacomatosis pigmentokeratotica (*see* Figs. 1.108 and 3.226).

Nevus spilus usually develops in childhood but may also be present at birth or appear in adulthood. The most

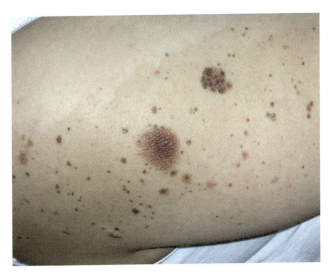

Fig. 3.226 An extensive nevus spilus in a patient with phacomatosis pigmentokeratotica

common locations are the trunk (*see* Fig. 3.227) and proximal extremities. The size is variable. Typical lesions range from 1 to 4 cm (*see* Figs. 3.227 and 3.228), but very large lesions in a segmental or zosteriform pattern (e.g., involving one extremity) may also be observed (see Fig. 3.226). There is an oval or irregularly shaped, sharply demarcated, light brown patch on the background resembling a café-au-lait macule (*see* Fig. 3.229). Overlying this macule, dark brown or black, tiny (1 to 4 mm) macules or slightly elevated papules (papular type) are irregularly distributed without exceeding the background, giving rise to a speckled appearance (*see* Figs. 3.229 and 3.230). Some patients describe occurrence of the second component months or years after the first one. The large lesions are seen especially in patients

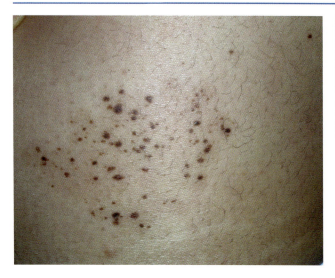

Fig. 3.227 A typical nevus spilus on the trunk; dark brown macules and papules irregularly scattered throughout a light brown patch measuring 3–4 cm in size

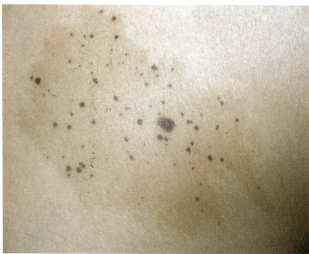

Fig. 3.229 Nevus spilus on the trunk. Darker macules as well as papules do not exceed the border of the café-au-lait-like macule on the background

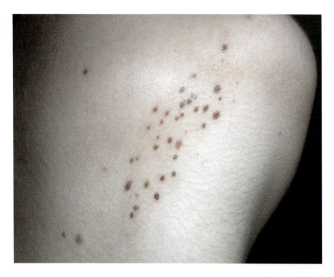

Fig. 3.228 Nevus spilus on the neck. Only darker areas contain nevus cells

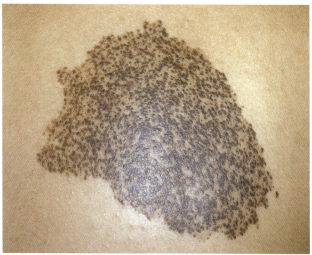

Fig. 3.230 Pigmented patch covered with numerous papules. Congenital melanocytic nevus showing speckled pattern cannot be easily differentiated from nevus spilus in this case, that possibly reflects an overlap between the two types of melanocytic nevi

with phakomatosis pigmentovascularis and phakomatosis pigmentokeratotica (*see* Fig. 3.226). In the latter disease, the papular type of nevus spilus is mostly present.

The diagnosis of nevus spilus depends on clinical examination. It may be confused with medium-sized or large congenital melanocytic nevi, which may also show a speckled pattern, but the background of congenital nevus is typically irregular and infiltrated (see Fig. 3.182) contrary to the preserved skin markings in nevus spilus. Becker nevus is another diagnostic challenge but unlike Becker nevus (*see* Fig. 1.125), nevus spilus shows nonhomogeneous pigmentation and is hairless. A small biopsy from nevus spilus may not be diagnostic as it would not involve the two components of the nevus, which have separate histologic features. Hyperpigmentation on the background shows an increased number of melanocytes as in lentigo simplex or café-au-lait macules. The overlying darker spots or papules are usually junctional nevi or sometimes compound nevi. Dysplastic nevus, Spitz nevus, and blue nevus rarely occur on the background of nevus spilus.

Management. Although rare, there are reports of malignant melanoma arising on nevus spilus. However, it is not accepted as a melanocytic nevus associated with increased risk of malignant transformation. Therefore, routine removal of nevus spilus is not necessary. Moreover, removal of large lesions may require grafting and result in scarring. Regular follow-up is the most adequate method of approach.

3.4 Melanocytic Nevi (Nevus Cell Nevi)

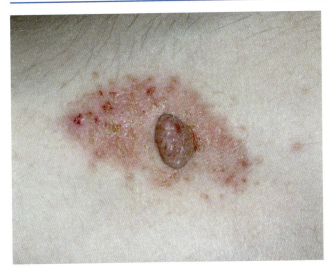

Fig. 3.231 Eczematous halo developing about a classical acquired melanocytic nevus acutely. This phenomenon is called Meyerson nevus

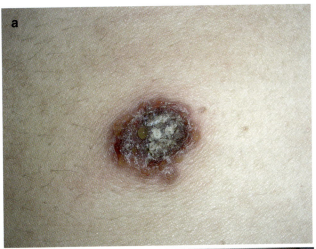

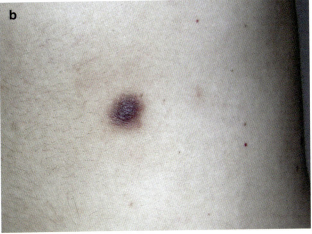

Fig. 3.233 (**a**) Meyerson nevus before therapy. (**b**) The healing of eczematous reaction after a short term topical corticosteroid therapy

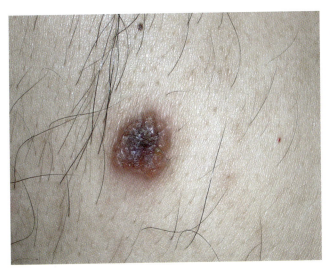

Fig. 3.232 Eczematous reaction surrounding a melanocytic nevus. The underlying cause of Meyerson nevus is mostly unknown

3.4.10 Meyerson Nevus (Meyerson Phenomenon)

The term "Meyerson nevus" implies a benign melanocytic nevus surrounded by a transient halo of eczema. The pathogenesis of this rare condition is not understood. It occurs mostly in young adults and more commonly on the trunk and proximal extremities. A peripheral halo of erythema and scaling (*see* Fig. 3.231) develops suddenly around one or more melanocytic nevi at various locations. The surface of the nevus also shows eczematization (*see* Fig. 3.232). Similar circumscribed eczematous lesions may also develop simultaneously elsewhere without nevi. Some lesions may be slightly pruritic.

This phenomenon is almost always diagnosed clinically. Central nevus may either be a junctional or compound type. The eczematous halo reveals spongiotic dermatitis and mononuclear cell infiltration predominantly in perivascular distribution in the dermis. Atypical features of the nevus component are not expected.

Management. Eczematous halo clears spontaneously within several weeks to months without leaving postinflammatory changes. Therapy with topical corticosteroids may induce rapid healing (*see* Fig. 3.233a and b). The central melanocytic nevus remains unchanged after the resolution of eczema.

3.4.11 Epidermolysis Bullosa Nevus

Epidermolysis bullosa nevus is a benign acquired melanocytic lesion developing mainly in epidermolysis bullosa patients. It is predominantly seen in dystrophic and junctional forms of epidermolysis bullosa but may also develop

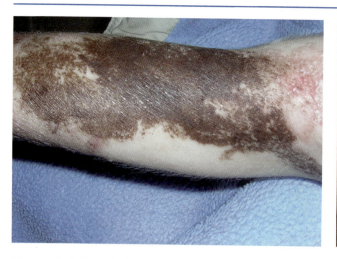

Fig. 3.234 Epidermolysis bullosa nevus presenting as a very large, heavily pigmented, irregular, flat lesion. The nevus had spread radially in months in this child with epidermolysis bullosa

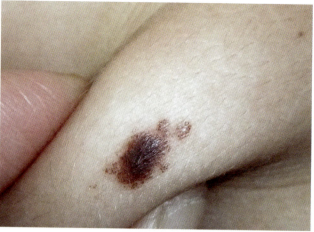

Fig. 3.236 Epidermolysis bullosa nevus depicted here has developed after healing of Stevens-Johnson syndrome

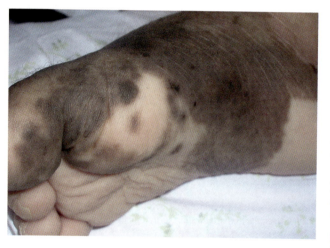

Fig. 3.235 Epidermolysis bullosa nevus covering a large area on the foot. Especially smaller lesions of this nevus variant is not uncommon in epidermolysis bullosa patients

in other forms (see Figs. 3.234 and 3.235). It tends to appear suddenly and grow rapidly. It usually occurs in childhood and is more common in areas subject to exogenous trauma where recurrent bullae are common. Etiopathogenesis is not fully understood and several theories have been proposed. According to one theory, it is postulated that a bullous reaction could cause spread of melanocytes and also induce proliferation of the same cells that are already present in the skin. Similar nevi are also described in Stevens-Johnson syndrome following improvement of the bullous skin lesions (see Fig. 3.236) or after severe burns. Epidermolysis bullosa nevus presents as an asymmetric flat or slightly raised patch or plaque with irregular shape, color variety including very dark and light areas, and regression foci (see Figs. 3.234 and 3.235). The pigmentation may be stippled. The lesion may be persistent or may lose partial or complete pigmentation in time and become lighter. The surface features may also change, such as becoming papillomatous. The lesion may

be large as 10 to 15 cm, which is unusual for any benign acquired nevomelanocytic tumor. There may also be satellite lesions. Both clinical and dermoscopic features may resemble malignant melanoma. Therefore in addition to the history of the associated disease, a biopsy is crucial for the diagnosis. Histologically the lesion may reveal a compound congenital nevus pattern or a junctional lentiginous melanocytic proliferation, which has been referred to as the "persistent nevus/pseudomelanoma" pattern.

Management. Awareness of clinicians and dermatopathologists of epidermolysis bullosa nevus phenomenon can avoid a diagnostic error like malignant melanoma. This may also prevent unnecessary troublesome surgical procedures. In the beginning of the follow-up period the lesion may enlarge, but this condition has no prognostic significance. Malignant degeneration of epidermolysis bullosa nevus is not expected. Reassurance of the patients or parents is important.

3.4.12 Pseudomelanoma (Recurrent Melanocytic Nevus)

Pseudomelanoma is a distinct clinicopathologic appearance of melanocytic nevus recurring at sites of any incompletely excised melanocytic nevus. The name of the disease implies common features with malignant melanoma, but pseudomelanoma has a completely benign biological behavior. Shave removal of a melanocytic nevus is the most common cause of pseudomelanoma (see Fig. 3.237). Destruction of a melanocytic nevus with methods like laser therapy or electrocautery (see Fig. 3.238) may also be a reason. If the nevi that are incidentally found on surgical incision sites are not completely excised, pseudomelanoma may develop around the operation scar (see Fig. 3.239). The great majority of the lesions occur within six months after the initial procedure.

Suggested Reading

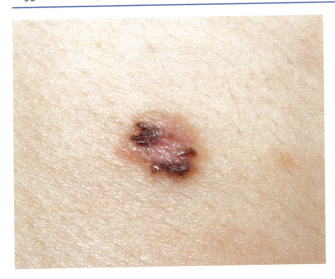

Fig. 3.237 Pseudomelanoma occurred after shave excision of a melanocytic nevus. Note that the mottled brownish pigmentation is restricted to the surgical scar

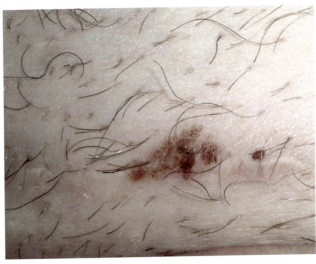

Fig. 3.239 Pseudomelanoma on the scar site of an abdominal operation. Coincidentally a nevus on the excision site has been partially removed during the operation but recurred in a short time causing irregular pigmentation

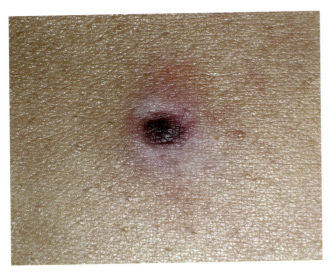

Fig. 3.238 Recurrence of a melanocytic nevus on the scar site of electrocautery; pseudomelanoma. This lesion was biopsied to exclude malignant melanoma

Proliferation of residual melanocytes in the epidermis is the pathogenetic factor.

Pseudomelanoma is more commonly seen in young adults. The trunk is the most common site of involvement. Brown or black mottled, irregular hyperpigmentation occurs within white areas of scars (*see* Fig. 3.237). The lesion is usually smaller than 1 cm and has an asymmetric appearance with irregular borders.

The clinical appearance of pseudomelanoma may look like a superficial spreading melanoma showing foci of regression. The main differential diagnostic challenges are recurrent malignant melanoma and benign lentiginous proliferation on melanoma scars. Recurrent melanoma (*see* Figs. 12.75 and 12.76) may occur any time after the operation, and the pigmentation may show extension beyond the surgical scar contrary to pseudomelanoma. Dermoscopy is not useful to exclude recurrent malignant melanoma. The histology of pseudomelanoma is characterized by abundant melanin-laden melanocytes that show minimal cytologic atypia distributed in all levels of epidermis overlying dermal scar tissue. Residual nevus cells may be seen beneath scar tissue, but there is no lateral spread of melanocytes. The history of the previous surgical procedure can sometimes be more helpful for diagnosis. In these cases, if available, the initial biopsy material must be reevaluated in order to verify the residual benign melanocytic nevus and exclude a recurrent malignant melanoma. In cases with recurrent Spitz nevus, Reed nevus, or blue nevus, histopathologic differentiation between malignant melanoma and pseudomelanoma can even be more difficult, necessitating the reevaluation of the initial biopsy.

Management. Pseudomelanoma is a persistent lesion but is not associated with an increased risk of malignant melanoma. Therefore if there is no doubt about the diagnosis of the initially excised tumor, a reexcision is not indicated. However, if a recurrent melanoma cannot be ruled out, complete excision must be performed.

Suggested Reading

Abecassis S, Spatz A, Cazeneuve C, et al. Melanoma within naevus spilus: 5 cases. Ann Dermatol Venereol. 2006;133:323–8.

Alikhan A, Ibrahimi OA, Eisen DB. Congenital melanocytic nevi: where are we now? Part I. Clinical presentation, epidemiology, pathogenesis, histology, malignant transformation, and neurocutaneous melanosis. J Am Acad Dermatol. 2012;67:495.e1–17.

Alkatan HM, Al-Arfaj KM, Maktabi A. Conjunctival nevi: Clinical and histopathologic features in a Saudi population. Ann Saudi Med. 2010;30:306–12.

Aouthmany M, Weinstein M, Zirwas MJ, Brodell RT. The natural history of halo nevi: a retrospective case series. J Am Acad Dermatol. 2012;67:582–6.

Argenziano G, Agozzino M, Bonifazi E, et al. Natural evolution of Spitz nevi. Dermatology. 2011;222:256–60.

Barnhill RL. The spitzoid lesion: rethinking Spitz tumors, atypical variants, 'spitzoid melanoma' and risk assessment. Mod Pathol. 2006;19 (Suppl 2):S21–33.

Barnhill RL, Fitzpatrick TB, Fandrey K, Kenet RO, Mihm MC, Sober AJ. Color atlas and synopsis of pigmented lesions. USA: McGraw-Hill; 1995.

Bauer JW, Schaeppi H, Kaserer C, et al. Large melanocytic nevi in hereditary epidermolysis bullosa. J Am Acad Dermatol. 2001;44:577–84.

Baykal C, Kurul S. Large congenital melanocytic naevi: clinical considerations based on 27 patients. J Eur Acad Dermatol Venereol. 2003;17:241–4.

Beggs AD, Latchford AR, Vasen HF, et al. Peutz-Jeghers syndrome: a systematic review and recommendations for management. Gut. 2010;59:975–86.

Bogart MM, Bivens MM, Patterson JW, Russell MA. Blue nevi: a case report and review of the literature. Cutis. 2007;80:42–4.

Burgdorf WHC, Plewig G, Wolff HH, Landthaler M. Braun-Falco's dermatology, edn 3. Italy: Springer-Verlag; 2009.

Caputo R, Tadini G. Atlas of Genodermatoses. Spain: Taylor and Francis; 2006.

Cotrim CP, Simone FT, Lima RB, et al. Epidermolysis bullosa nevus: case report and literature review. An Bras Dermatol. 2011;86:767–71.

Gleason BC, Hirsch MS, Nucci MR, et al. Atypical genital nevi. A clinicopathologic analysis of 56 cases. Am J Surg Pathol. 2008; 32:51–7.

High WA, Alanen KW, Golitz LE. Is melanocytic nevus with focal atypical epithelioid components (clonal nevus) a superficial variant of deep penetrating nevus? J Am Acad Dermatol. 2006;55:460–6.

Ibrahimi OA, Alikhan A, Eisen DB. Congenital melanocytic nevi: where are we now? Part II. Treatment options and approach to treatment. J Am Acad Dermatol. 2012;67:515. e1-13.

James WD, Berger T, Elston D. Andrew's Diseases of the Skin: Clinical Dermatology, edn 11. China: Saunders Elsevier; 2011.

Kanzler MH, Mraz-Gernhard S. Primary cutaneous melanoma and its precursor lesions. J Am Acad Dermatol. 2001;45:260–76.

Karam SL, Jackson SM. Malignant melanoma arising within nevus spilus. Skinmed. 2012;10:100–2.

Krengel S, Marghoob AA. Current management approaches for congenital melanocytic nevi. Dermatol Clin. 2012;30:377–87.

Krengel S. New aspects of congenital melanocytic nevi. Hautarzt. 2012;63:82–8.

Lee S, Kim DH, Lee G, et al. An unusual case of congenital dermal melanocytosis. Ann Dermatol. 2010;22:460–2.

Leech SN, Bell H, Leonard N, et al. Neonatal giant congenital nevi with proliferative nodules: a clinicopathologic study and literature review of neonatal melanoma. Arch Dermatol. 2004;140:83–8.

Manganoni AM, Pavoni L, Farisoglio C, et al. Report of 27 cases of naevus spilus in 2134 patients with melanoma: is naevus spilus a risk marker of cutaneous melanoma? J Eur Acad Dermatol Venereol. 2012;26:129–30.

Othman IS. Ocular surface tumors. Oman J Ophthalmol. 2009;2:3–14.

Ribé A. Melanocytic lesions of the genital area with attention given to atypical genital nevi. J Cutan Pathol. 2008;35(Suppl 2): 24–7.

Rigel DS, Robinson JK, Ross M, Friedman RJ, Corkerell CJ, Lim HW, et al. Cancer of the Skin, edn 2. China: Saunders Elsevier; 2011.

Robson A, Morley-Quante M, Hempel H, et al. Deep penetrating naevus: clinicopathological study of 31 cases with further delineation of histological features allowing distinction from other pigmented benign melanocytic lesions and melanoma. Histopathology. 2003;43:529–37.

Sahin S, Levin L, Kopf AW, et al. Risk of melanoma in medium-sized congenital melanocytic nevi: a follow-up study. J Am Acad Dermatol. 1998;39:428–33.

Salopek TG. The dilemna of dysplastic nevus. Dermatol Clin. 2002;20:617–28.

Schwartz RA. Skin cancer: recognition and management, edn 2. Singapore: Blackwell Publishing; 2008.

Shah KR, Boland CR, Patel M, et al. Cutaneous manifestations of gastrointestinal disease: part I. J Am Acad Dermatol. 2013;68:189. e1–21.

Shields JA, Shields CL, Mashayekhi A, et al. Primary acquired melanosis of the conjunctiva: experience with 311 eyes. Trans Am Ophthalmol Soc. 2007;105:61–72.

Sinha S, Cohen PJ, Schwartz RA. Nevus of Ota in children. Cutis. 2008;82:25–9.

Soyer HP, Argenziano G, Hofmann-Welenhof R, Johr R. Color Atlas of Melanocytic Lesions of the Skin. Germany: Springer-Verlag; 2010.

Stratakis CA, Kirschner LS, Carney JA. Clinical and molecular features of the Carney complex: diagnostic recommendations for patient evaluation. J Clin Endocrinol Metab 2001;86:4041–6.

van Houten AH, van Dijk MC, Schuttelaar ML. Proliferative nodules in a giant congenital melanocytic nevus-case report and review of the literature. J Cutan Pathol. 2010;37:764–76.

Cutaneous Cysts

In addition to occurring in many visceral organs, cysts may also appear on the skin and mucous membranes. Various types of cutaneous cysts containing fluid or semi-solid material and showing variable histopathologic features and clinical significance have been defined. Some cysts are surrounded by an epithelial cell wall, which is either stratified squamous or nonstratified squamous epithelium. These are generally called true cysts. On the other hand, a subset of cysts, namely pseudocysts, is not lined by an epithelium but instead is surrounded by connective or granulation tissue. Generally, cutaneous cysts are round, dome-shaped, protruding, or deeply located dermal or subcutaneous papules or nodules seen at different locations. Confirmation of the diagnosis is mostly via histopathologic examination. However, some clinical features, including the location of the cyst, may serve as diagnostic clues leading to a presumptive diagnosis.

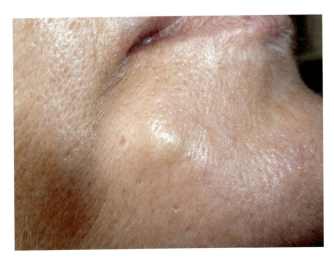

Fig. 4.1 Epidermoid cyst presenting as a solitary dermal nodule with a white-yellow hue on the chin

4.1 Epidermoid Cyst (Infundibular Cyst)

Epidermoid cyst is a common type of cutaneous cyst with an epidermis-like epithelial lining (wall). The lining of the cyst produces keratin. The term sebaceous cyst, which has formerly been used as a synonym for epidermoid cyst, is inappropriate because of the absence of sebaceous glands within the cyst lining. Lesions usually occur spontaneously. However, implantation of epithelium as a result of injury is considered an etiologic factor. Therefore, it may also be called epidermal inclusion cyst. Moreover, epidermoid cysts may also occur as a result of the obstruction of the follicular orifice as seen in patients with acne vulgaris.

Epidermoid cyst can occur at any age, but it is more frequent in adulthood. The face (see Fig. 4.1), neck, periauricular area (see Fig. 4.2), and upper trunk (see Fig. 4.3) are more commonly involved, but any part of the body including sites such as the nipple (see Fig. 4.4), genitalia, and palmoplantar area (see Fig. 4.5) may be involved. Lesions may be solitary (see Figs. 4.1 and 4.3) or multiple (see Figs. 4.2 and 4.6).

Multiple epidermoid cysts may be encountered as irregularly distributed lesions on the whole body or localized grouped lesions which is common on the retroauricular area (see Fig. 4.6). Most lesions are sporadic but familial inheritance is also possible, especially in individuals with multiple lesions. Gardner syndrome (familial adenomatous polyposis), Gorlin syndrome, and pachyonychia congenita (see Fig. 4.7) are among the rare diseases associated with multiple epidermoid cysts. Early-onset and atypical localization of epidermoid cysts such as limb involvement may be signs of Gardner syndrome, a disease associated with colorectal polyps that have high risk for the development of malignancy. Multiple epidermoid cysts on the trunk and extremities may also be seen in patients with Gorlin syndrome (see Figs. 4.8 and 4.9).

The typical epidermoid cyst is a well-demarcated, dome-shaped, skin-colored, yellowish or pinkish, mobile dermal nodule with a smooth surface (see Figs. 4.10, 4.11, 4.12, 4.13, and 4.14). Furthermore, a visible central blackhead-like punctum is common on the surface (see Figs. 4.15,

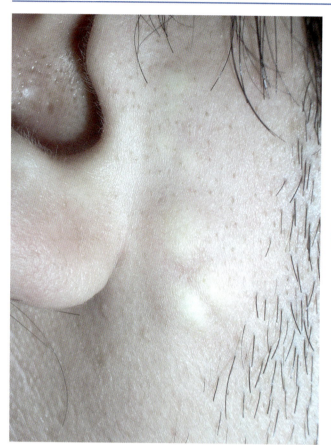

Fig. 4.2 A few small epidermoid cysts on the periauricular area. The distinctive comedo-like opening may not be visible on smaller lesions as in this case

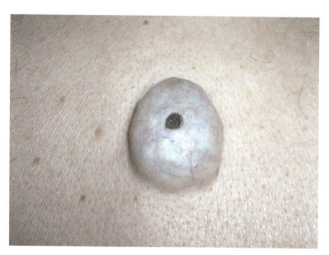

Fig. 4.3 Solitary epidermoid cyst on the trunk. Note the prominent blackhead-like punctum in the center of the large lesion

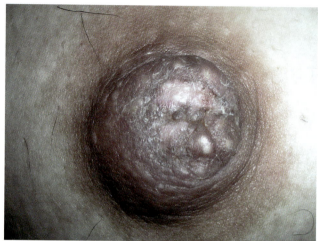

Fig. 4.4 Epidermoid cyst on the nipple, a rare location

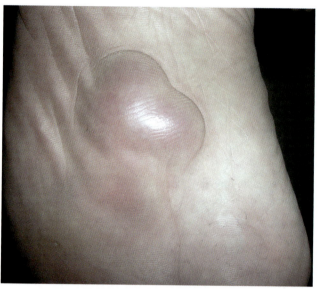

Fig. 4.5 A large epidermoid cyst on the sole

4.16, and 4.17). This punctum is the clinical sign indicating a connection between the cyst surface and the cyst lining. The central punctum is more prominent on large lesions (see Fig. 4.18). Rarely, more than one punctum may be noticed (see Fig. 4.19). Telangiectasia may also be seen on the surface of some lesions (see Fig. 4.17). Giant comedones with a black keratinous plug (see Figs. 4.20, 4.21, and 4.22) are also epidermoid cysts and are usually localized on the back.

An epidermoid cyst may be confused with other cutaneous tumors such as lipoma (see Fig. 10.2), cystic basal cell carcinoma (see Fig. 11.49), and other variants of cutaneous cysts. A single lesion of epidermoid cyst is more protruding and firm than lipoma. The cystic lesion of a basal cell carcinoma may also have telengiectases on the surface, but does not have a marked central punctum. Trichilemmal cyst is usually found on the scalp, is mildly alopecic and lacks a central punctum. Protrusion of cheese-like, malodorous material seen spontaneously (see Fig. 4.23) or by compression (see Fig. 4.24 a–c) is a helpful clue in the diagnosis of an

4.1 Epidermoid Cyst (Infundibular Cyst)

epidermoid cyst. A biopsy is rarely performed. Histologically, an epidermoid cyst is lined by an epithelial cell wall. This epithelium is stratified squamous epithelium resembling epidermis and includes a granular layer and keratin lamellae in the lumen. Additionally, epidermoid cysts in Gardner

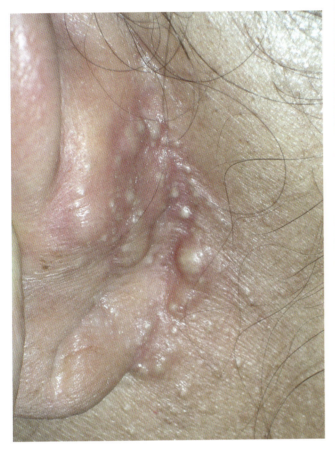

Fig. 4.6 Closely set milia and small epidermoid cysts on the retroauricular area

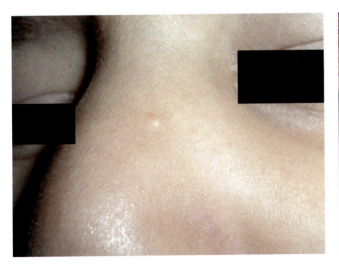

Fig. 4.7 A small epidermoid cyst on the nose of a patient with pachyonychia congenita

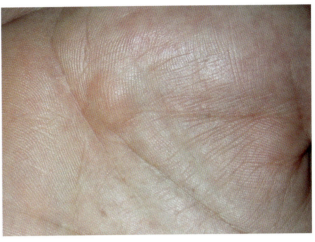

Fig. 4.8 Epidermoid cyst on the palm of a patient with Gorlin syndrome. Cysts may be more commonly seen on unusual locations in the setting of some syndromes

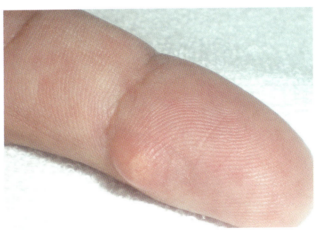

Fig. 4.9 Epidermoid cyst on the volar aspect of the finger in a patient with Gorlin syndrome. No punctum is present in this case

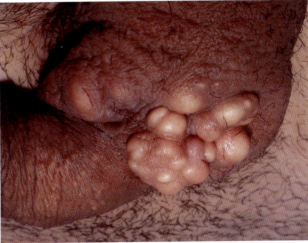

Fig. 4.10 Epidermoid cyst manifesting as multiple dome-shaped nodules with smooth surface on the male genitalia

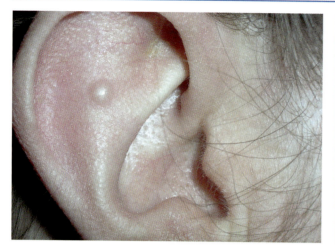

Fig. 4.11 Epidermoid cyst on the auricle. Note the solitary skin-colored small nodule

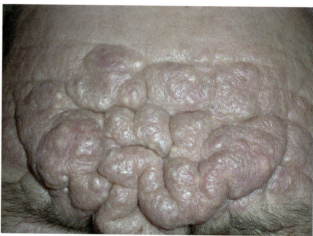

Fig. 4.14 Clustering of epidermoid cysts causing protuberance on the forehead. An unusual presentation

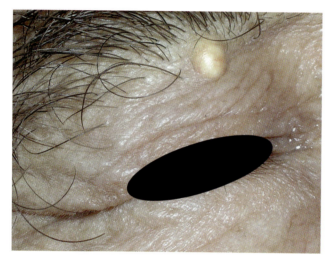

Fig. 4.12 Yellow-colored solitary nodule on the eyelid. Epidermoid cysts may exhibit various colors, such as yellow, and so may be considered in the differential diagnosis of xanthelasma on the periorbital area

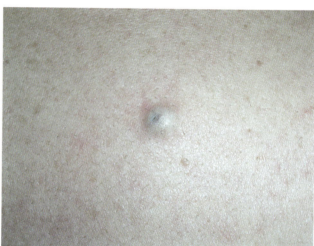

Fig. 4.15 Epidermoid cyst with a tiny blackhead-like punctum

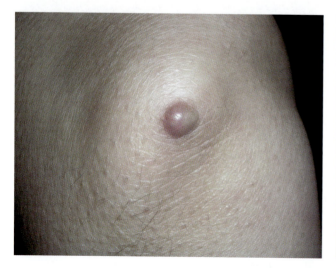

Fig. 4.13 Epidermoid cyst presenting as a pinkish dermal nodule on the elbow

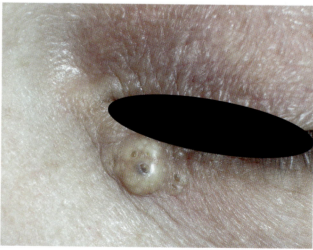

Fig. 4.16 Epidermoid cyst with a typical blackhead-like punctum

4.1 Epidermoid Cyst (Infundibular Cyst)

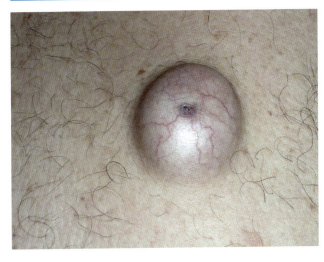

Fig. 4.17 Large epidermoid cyst with a central blackhead-like small punctum and telangiectases on the surface

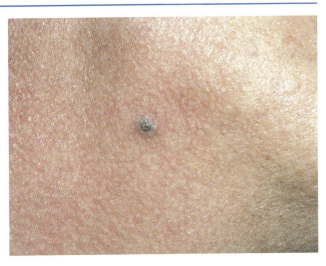

Fig. 4.20 Giant comedo. These black lesions look like an open comedo of acne but histologically they are true epidermoid cysts

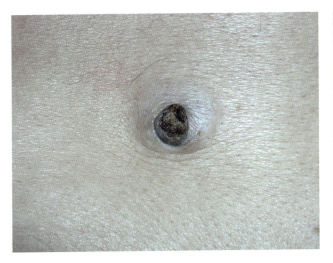

Fig. 4.18 Epidermoid cyst with a central blackhead-like broad punctum

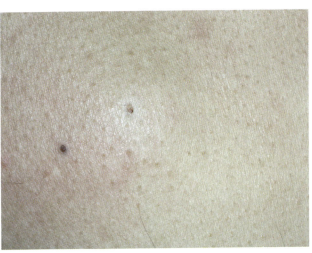

Fig. 4.21 Two giant comedones. The lesion on the right has become a small pit due to the discharge of the keratinous material

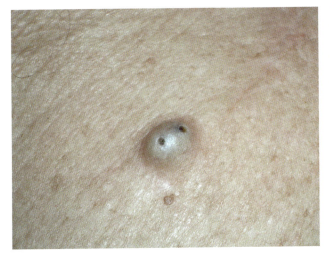

Fig. 4.19 Epidermoid cyst with two punctums. This presentation is not very common

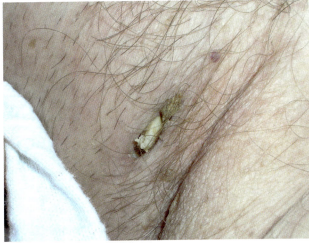

Fig. 4.22 A giant comedo on the groin

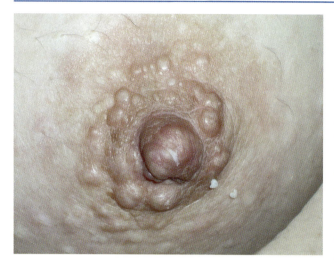

Fig. 4.23 Spontaneous protrusion of cheese-like material from an epidermoid cyst on the nipple. This material is typically foul-smelling

syndrome may show uncommon histologic features such as hybrid cysts or pilomatricoma-like changes.

Although epidermoid cysts usually remain asymptomatic, they may become inflamed as a result of the rupture of the cyst lining. Erythema (*see* Figs. 4.25 and 4.26), swelling (*see* Figs. 4.27 and 4.28), tenderness, pain, and fluctuation may occur suddenly, caused by inflammation. Inflamed cysts may be mistaken for a furuncle or carbuncle. Spontaneous (*see* Fig. 4.29) or surgical drainage will facilitate the healing process. Scrotal epidermoid cysts may be calcified, leading to calcinosis cutis.

Management. Epidermoid cysts are benign lesions. Treatment is indicated in recurrent inflammatory lesions and can also be done for cosmetic reasons. Excision with various surgical techniques can be performed. The whole cyst, including the cyst wall, must be removed, either intact or by enucleation through a small incision, extracting the parts of the cyst wall. Cosmetic results are usually satisfactory.

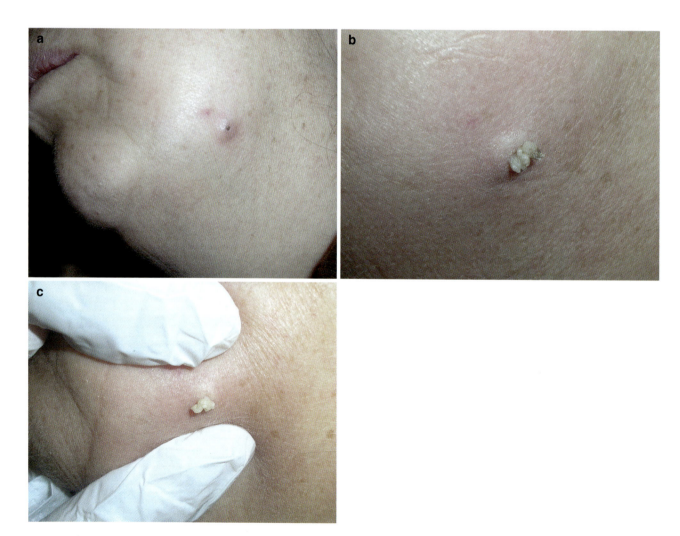

Fig. 4.24 (**a**) Epidermoid cyst with a blackhead-like punctum. (**b**) Protrusion of cheese-like material from the cyst after compression. (**c**) The mass of the cyst has declined after continuous compression

4.1 Epidermoid Cyst (Infundibular Cyst)

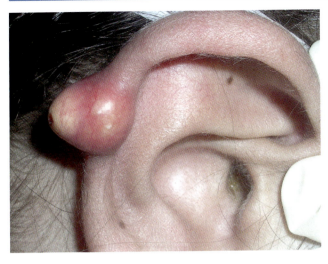

Fig. 4.25 Inflamed epidermoid cyst on the helix. Note the erythema on the lesion

Inflamed cysts may be treated with incision and drainage if possible through the orifice. Although it is usually not very effective, topical and systemic antibiotic treatment can be used for inflamed lesions. Intralesional injection of corticosteroids (triamcinolone acetonide) may reduce inflammation.

4.1.1 Milium

A milium is a minute epidermoid cyst occurring at all ages of life. This very common variant of cutaneous cyst may be idiopathic (so-called primary milia), or may occur on sites of trauma such as burns and in the course of some dermatoses (so-called secondary milia). Moreover, milia may appear as a feature of some genodermatoses.

Transient milia of the face is a very common problem, arising in approximately half of newborns (*see* Fig. 4.30).

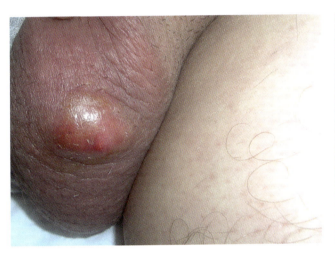

Fig. 4.26 Epidermoid cyst on the scrotum. Erythema has appeared suddenly due to inflammation

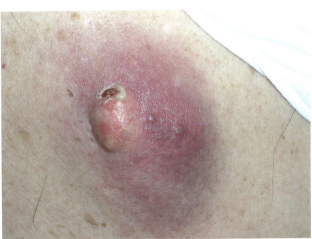

Fig. 4.28 Swelling and redness on and around the lesion due to inflammation of an epidermoid cyst. Protrusion of the cyst content is also remarkable

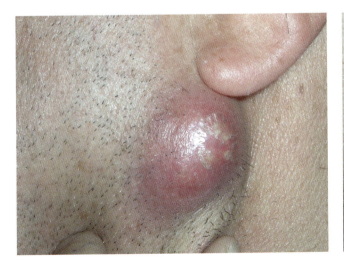

Fig. 4.27 Swelling due to intense inflammation of an epidermoid cyst. Such lesions may be misdiagnosed as pyoderma

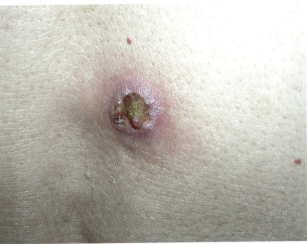

Fig. 4.29 An inflamed and ruptured epidermoid cyst that has declined after spontaneous drainage

Bullous dermatoses involving the dermoepidermal junction, such as variants of inherited epidermolysis bullosa (*see* Fig. 4.31), acquired epidermolysis bullosa, bullous pemphigoid, porphyria cutanea tarda, and sunburn may cause milia at different ages on sites of the healing bullae. Milia may also appear following cosmetic procedures such as dermabrasion or after cryotherapy of skin tumors. In some instances, milia may occur following treatment of cutaneous leishmaniasis and lupus vulgaris (*see* Fig. 4.32). Multiple milia appearing at a young age may be seen in the setting of Bazex-Dupré-Christol syndrome (*see* Fig. 11.96), Rombo syndrome, Gorlin syndrome (*see* Figs. 4.33 and 4.34), hereditary trichodysplasia (Maria-Unna hypotrichosis), oral facial digital syndrome type I, and Brooke-Spiegler syndrome.

A typical papule of milium is white or cream-colored, firm, asymptomatic, and 1 to 2 mm in size (*see* Fig. 4.35). Idiopathic lesions mostly occur on the face, especially on the cheeks,

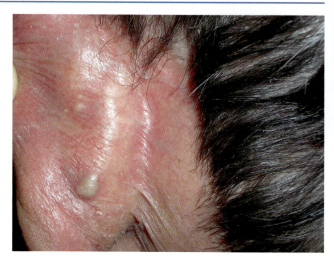

Fig. 4.32 Milia occurred after healing of lupus vulgaris

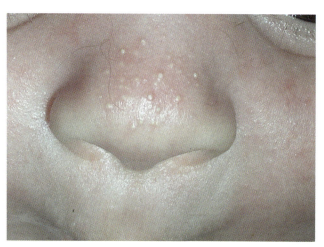

Fig. 4.30 Transient milia on the face of a newborn

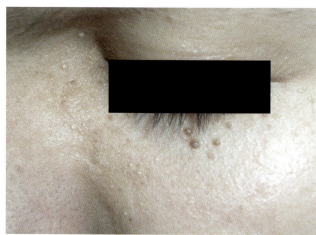

Fig. 4.33 White papules of milia (left) associated with darker papules (under eyelashes) representing early basal cell carcinomas in a child with Gorlin syndrome

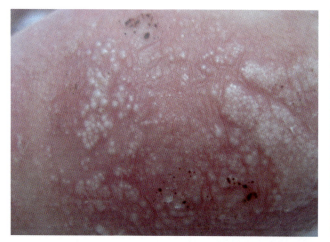

Fig. 4.31 Innumerable milia showing tendency to clustering associated with scars of recurrent bullae in a patient with epidermolysis bullosa

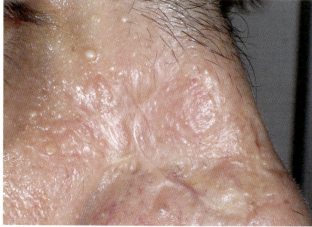

Fig. 4.34 Milia associated with surgical scars in an adult patient with Gorlin syndrome

nose, periorbital areas (see Fig. 4.36), and ears (*see* Figs. 4.37 and 4.38). They may sometimes be numerous. Lesions developing in association with dermatoses or as a result of skin injury may be seen at any site. Most lesions are discrete papules, but the secondary lesions may be grouped (*see* Fig. 4.31).

Multiple milia within an erythematous, edematous base are called milia en plaque (*see* Fig. 4.39). The etiology is not clear. Most patients are middle-aged women. These lesions are mostly located on the face, especially the retroauricular area. Multiple eruptive milia are defined as the sudden onset of numerous extensive milia.

Disorders presenting with multiple tiny papules on the face such as the comedones of acne, perifollicular fibroma (*see* Fig. 8.39), trichilemmoma (*see* Fig. 5.45), or syringoma (*see* Fig. 5.3) may be confused with milia. Milia-like papules may be observed on plaques of folliculotropic mycosis

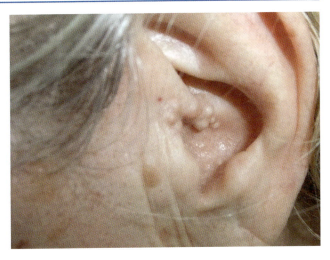

Fig. 4.37 Idiopathic milia on the concha of the ear

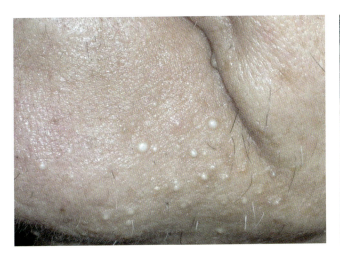

Fig. 4.35 Idiopathic milia shown as multiple cream-colored tiny papules on the face of an old woman

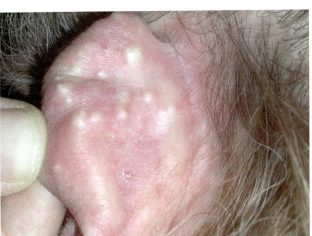

Fig. 4.38 Idiopathic milia on the retroauricular area

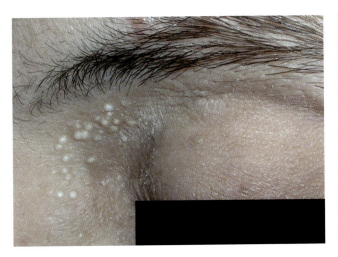

Fig. 4.36 Idiopathic milia on the periorbital area. These hard lesions may be persistent for a long time

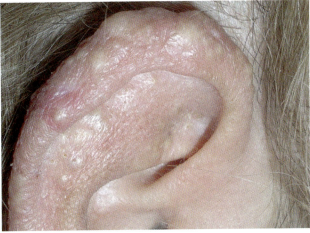

Fig. 4.39 Milia en plaque. Note grouped milia with slightly erythematous background

fungoides (see Fig. 14.53). Clinical features are mostly diagnostic of milium. The history of an associated disease or other triggering factors may also support the diagnosis. Histopathologic examination reveals small epidermoid cysts in the superficial dermis.

Management. The course of milia is unpredictable. Whereas some lesions heal spontaneously in several months, others are persistent. Multiple lesions in newborns generally resolve spontaneously in a few weeks without scar formation. Topical retinoids may be used for multiple facial lesions in adults or in patients with milia en plaque but have a limited effect. Incision of the overlying epidermis with a sterile needle or scalpel followed by manual compression and evacuation of the cyst content is an easy method for the removal of a milium. A small excision may be used for a relatively larger lesion. Electrocautery and laser ablation are also effective in management but may be complicated with minute scars.

4.2 Trichilemmal Cyst (Pilar Cyst)

Trichilemmal cyst deriving from the outer root sheath of the hair follicle is the second most common type of cutaneous cyst after epidermoid cyst/milium. It is located on sites with dense hair follicles; therefore most lesions are observed on the scalp (see Fig. 4.40). The face (see Fig. 4.41), neck, and other hairy regions of the body are rarely involved. The cyst may be sporadic or autosomal dominantly inherited. A positive family history is a frequent finding. Trichilemmal cyst does not show association with other types of cutaneous cysts or systemic diseases. It is more commonly seen in women than in men and is more common in middle age.

More than half of the cases have multiple cysts. Typical lesion is a round, large, mobile, firm intradermal nodule (see Fig. 4.42). The surface is smooth and a blackhead-like punctum is not present in contrast to an epidermoid cyst (see Fig. 4.3). Some lesions may be very large and protuberant. Unlike lipomas (see Fig. 10.2), these lesions are firm and may seem mildly alopecic due to thinning of the overlying hairs (see Fig. 4.43). A scalp cylindroma (see Fig. 5.22) may also be confused with a trichilemmal cyst. The former is softer and irregular in shape.

Trichilemmal cysts are asymptomatic unless secondarily infected. Inflamed or secondarily infected cysts may be erythematous, tender, or painful. A great majority of the trichilemmal cysts on the scalp are diagnosed clinically. However, since the clinical appearance of the lesions on trunk and limbs is not always diagnostic (see Figs. 4.44 and 4.45), histopathologic examination is crucial. An excisional biopsy

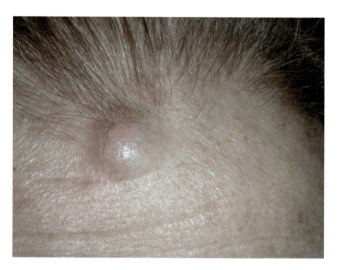

Fig. 4.41 Trichilemmal cyst on the forehead. Note the smooth surface of the round nodule

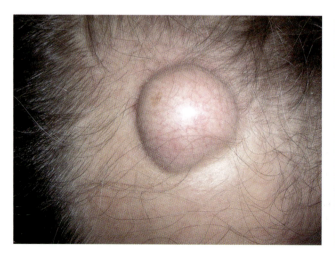

Fig. 4.40 Trichilemmal cyst located on the scalp, the classical location. There may be sometimes multiple lesions

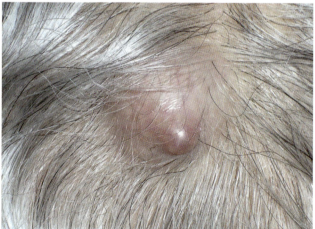

Fig. 4.42 Trichilemmal cyst on the scalp. Different from an epidermoid cyst, comedo-like punctum is not present on the surface of this raised round nodule

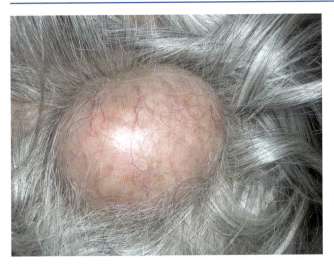

Fig. 4.43 Trichilemmal cyst presenting as a large mass with prominent telangiectases running on the surface. Localized alopecia of varying degree is a typical feature of this cyst

is preferred for confirmation of the diagnosis. Histologically the lining of the cyst is stratified squamous epithelium that closely mimics the outer root sheath of the hair follicle. The innermost layer is composed of large keratinocytes with pale cytoplasm. Trichilemmal keratinization with the absence of a granular layer is typical. The cyst contains homogeneous eosinophilic compact keratin and may show focal calcification. Metaplastic ossification is rarely observed.

Management. Most of these cysts remain benign and stable, but some have the potential to enlarge, causing a cosmetic problem. A trichilemmal cyst may rarely evolve into a proliferating trichilemmal cyst, which has tendency to enlarge more rapidly and may sometimes be locally invasive. Therefore, trichilemmal cyst is usually removed prophylactically. Removal of the entire tumor, especially in large lesions, may leave undesirable scars. Enucleation through a small incision with extraction of parts of the cyst wall is an alternative method providing better cosmetic results. Systemic antibiotics may be used for infected cysts.

4.3 Proliferating Trichilemmal Cyst

Proliferating trichilemmal cyst is a rare tumor with biological behavior that alternates between benign and malignant. Some patients have associated trichilemmal cysts. It is supposed that proliferating trichilemmal cyst originates from a preexisting trichilemmal cyst.

Most lesions are solitary, but rarely multiple tumors may also be seen. The lesion appears as a cystic nodule in the elderly patient and grows slowly. It is usually more inflammatory than classic trichilemmal cyst. Patients may present with an exophytic large mass that may be lobulated, ulcerated, and crusted (*see* Fig. 4.46). Lesions with a discharge may be malodorous. Lesions are mostly located on the scalp and nape but may also

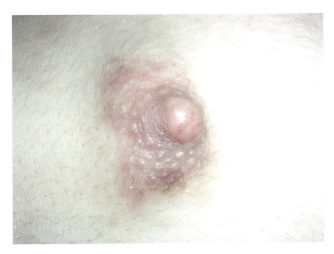

Fig. 4.44 A large trichilemmal cyst with lobulated structure on the trunk

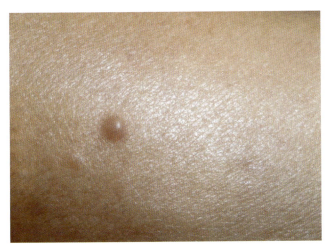

Fig. 4.45 A small trichilemmal cyst localized on the arm

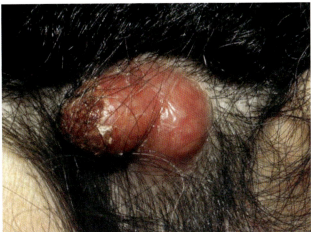

Fig. 4.46 Proliferating trichilemmal cyst on the scalp. Note the lobulated large lesion

be seen on the trunk and extremities. Local invasion of the underlying structures and distant metastasis may rarely occur.

Differential diagnoses in the advanced stage include malignant skin tumors such as squamous cell carcinoma (*see* Fig. 11.124) and basal cell carcinoma (*see* Fig. 11.13). Histopathologic examination reveals the diagnosis. It is a well-circumscribed tumor in the dermis and subcutis, composed of cellular aggregates showing trichilemmal differentiation and keratinization. A variable degree of cellular atypia and mitosis may be seen. When focal necrosis, squamous eddies, and individual cell keratinization are found, differentiation from squamous cell carcinoma may become difficult. The presence of an ordinary trichilemmal cyst in direct continuity with the lesion can sometimes be seen and indicates the origin of this unusual tumor.

Management. Because of the potential for local invasion, surgical excision is the therapy of choice. Although rare, local recurrence is possible.

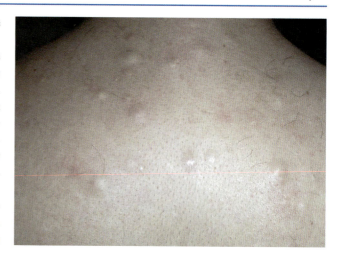

Fig. 4.47 Steatocystoma multiplex on the neck and upper back. Existence of multiple lesions are typical

4.4 Steatocystoma Multiplex

Steatocystoma multiplex is a rare type of cutaneous cysts that contains a cyst wall with sebaceous glands and presents with multiple lesions. It may occur sporadically or be familial with an autosomal dominant inheritance. The gene mutation of steatocystoma multiplex is localized on *keratin 17 (K17)*; the same mutation is found in pachyonychia congenita type 2, a rare type of palmoplantar keratoderma syndrome. In addition to the major findings of pachyonychia congenita type 1 like palmoplantar hyperkeratosis and thickening of the fingernails and toenails, patients with pachyonychia congenita type 2 may also have steatocystoma multiplex. However, not all familial cases of steatocystoma multiplex have other manifestations of pachyonychia congenita type 2. Steatocystoma multiplex may sometimes be associated with eruptive vellus hair cysts.

Cysts of steatocystoma multiplex are usually noticed in adolescence or early adulthood. They may increase gradually in number, and some patients may have numerous lesions (*see* Fig. 4.47). Lesions are dispersed especially in sebaceous gland–rich areas. They are typically located on the chest but involvement of the back (*see* Fig. 4.47), arms, axillae (*see* Fig. 4.48), neck, face (*see* Fig. 4.49), scalp, and genital area can also be frequently seen. Typical lesions are 3 to 10 mm, flesh-colored or yellowish, smooth-surfaced papules (*see* Figs. 4.50 and 4.51) or nodules (*see* Fig. 4.48). Occasionally larger lesions may be observed. Cysts show elastic to firm consistency on palpation. A punctum on the surface is not present, as opposed to the epidermoid cyst (*see* Fig. 4.15). Moreover, the content of steatocystoma multiplex is oily and odorless. These cysts are usually asymptomatic but may sometimes be tender due to the inflammation caused by the

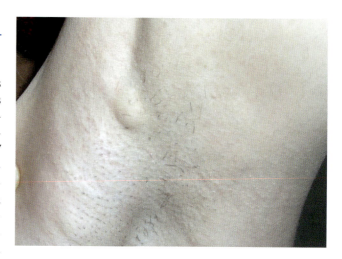

Fig. 4.48 Steatocystoma multiplex on the axilla. Note the skin-colored, raised nodule with smooth surface

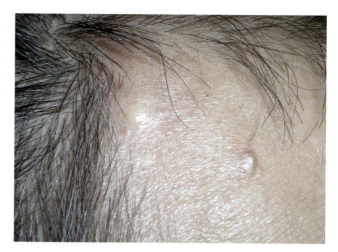

Fig. 4.49 Steatocystoma multiplex presenting as multiple yellowish papules on the forehead

rupture of the cyst wall. Inflamed erythematous lesions (*see* Fig. 4.52) should be differentiated from acne cysts. Multiple eruptive vellus hair cysts (*see* Fig. 4.53) which usually present as smaller lesions, are the biggest challenge in the clinical as well as in the histopathologic differential diagnosis. Histologically, the thin wall of steatocystoma multiplex is stratified squamous epithelium without a granular layer, and sebaceous glands are seen in the vicinity. Sometimes vellus hair follicles may be seen in the cyst wall and vellus hairs in the cavity. These are hybrid cysts with features of both a steatocyst and a vellus hair cyst.

Management. Steatocystoma multiplex is a benign lesion, but patients with widespread cysts mostly request therapy for cosmetic reasons. Medical interventions have been tried in these patients. Systemic isotretinoin, a retinoid mostly used for acne vulgaris, can be useful to decrease the sebum production and size of the sebaceous glands. It may be effective in some cases, but the results are controversial and the relief is temporary. Tetracycline may be useful for inflamed lesions. Although it is mostly not practical in patients with widespread cysts, surgical excision can be performed for individual lesions. A small incision with extraction of the parts of the cyst wall is also an alternative method.

4.5 Eruptive Vellus Hair Cyst

Eruptive vellus hair cyst, which is one of the rarest variants of cutaneous cysts, presents as multiple tiny lesions containing vellus hairs as a pathognomonic sign. It may be sporadic or autosomal dominantly inherited. It may be seen in association with steatocystoma multiplex. Some patients with pachyonychia congenita type 2 also have eruptive vellus hair cysts. Steatocystoma multiplex and eruptive vellus

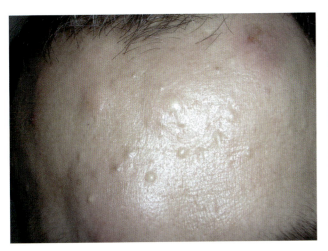

Fig. 4.50 Small, smooth-surfaced papules and nodules of steatocystoma multiplex are seen concomitantly on the forehead

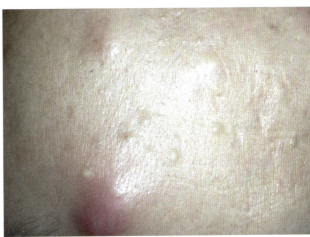

Fig. 4.52 Multiple lesions of steatocystoma multiplex on the forehead. Note some of them are erythematous and swollen due to inflammation

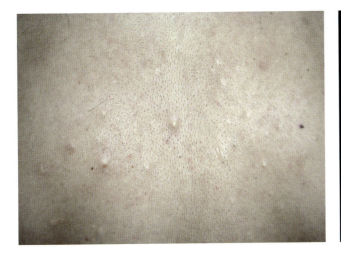

Fig. 4.51 Steatocystoma multiplex manifesting as multiple skin-colored small papules on the back

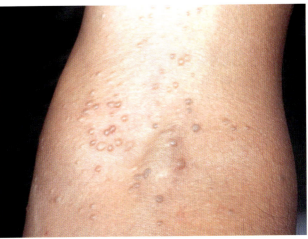

Fig. 4.53 Multiple lesions of eruptive vellus hair cyst on the antecubital fossa of the arm

hair cysts are considered to be related to each other and to represent clinicopathologic variants of the same entity, as they may show overlapping clinical and histologic features. Furthermore, association of vellus hair cysts with hidrotic and anhidrotic ectodermal dysplasia is possible.

In familial cases cysts are present at birth or appear in early childhood and gradually increase in number. Sporadic cysts may occur in eruptive form at a young age following the onset of puberty. There may be a few or sometimes more than hundreds of cysts. Solitary lesions are rare. The chest, abdomen, back, and extremities (*see* Fig. 4.53) are commonly involved, but lesions may also be seen on the eyelids, periorbital area, ears, or elsewhere. Typical lesions of eruptive vellus hair cyst are dome-shaped, smooth-surfaced, flesh to yellowish, grey, or bluish-colored papules that are 2 to 4 mm in diameter (*see* Figs. 4.54, 4.55, and 4.56). Lesions are relatively smaller than cysts of steatocystoma multiplex (*see* Fig. 4.47) and epidermoid cysts (*see* Fig. 4.3). They are softer than milia. Contrary to acne cysts, they are mostly noninflammatory and asymptomatic.

In most cases, the diagnosis of eruptive vellus hair cyst is confirmed by histopathologic examination. The cyst is lined with thin stratified squamous epithelium containing keratin and vellus hairs. A vellus hair follicle may be attached to the wall. Except for the hybrid form associated with steatocystoma multiplex, there is no sebaceous gland in the cyst wall.

Management. Some vellus hair cysts resolve spontaneously, possibly due to the transepidermal elimination of the cyst material. However, most are persistent. They are only a cosmetic problem. Since most patients have numerous lesions, surgical procedures are not easily used. Topical tretinoin, tazarotene, and keratolytic agents may be helpful in some cases. Evacuation of the cyst with a needle is an alternative. Destructive methods like the carbon dioxide laser and Er:YAG laser can also be effective. Complete traditional excision of the vellus hair cyst can cause undesirable scars and thus is not recommended.

4.6 Digital Mucous Cyst (Mucoid Cyst, Myxoid Cyst)

Digital mucous cyst is a pseudocyst of digits that contains mucinous fluid. There are two types of digital mucous cysts. The one that generally involves the proximal nail fold is smaller, its etiopathogenesis is not fully understood, and it is suggested that it occurs as a result of mucoid degeneration of connective tissue. Histopathology shows dermal accumulation of mucin and an increased number of fibroblasts in this area. Therefore, this type has been considered a variant of dermal mucinosis. A history of rheumatologic disease is usually not present in these patients.

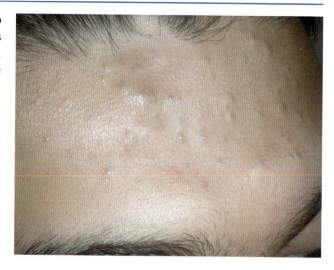

Fig. 4.54 Eruptive vellus hair cyst causing multiple papules on the forehead. The clinical differentiation from steatocystoma multiplex is not easy in this case

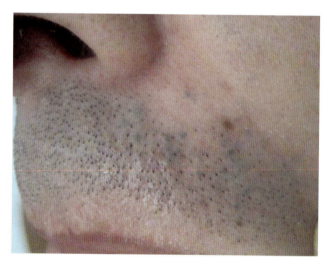

Fig. 4.55 Eruptive vellus hair cyst presenting as multiple bluish-colored tiny papules on the face

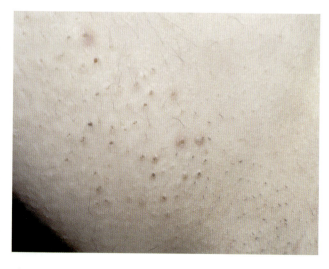

Fig. 4.56 Flesh-colored lesions of eruptive vellus hair cyst on the arm

4.6 Digital Mucous Cyst (Mucoid Cyst, Myxoid Cyst)

The second type of digital mucous cyst is the ganglionic type, generally seen in proximity to the distal interphalangeal joint (*see* Fig. 4.57) and also ankles (*see* Fig. 4.58). There may be communication between the cyst and the adjacent joint in some cases. According to this theory, the origin of the cyst content may be derived from the synovial fluid. A history of trauma or accompanying osteoarthritis of the adjacent joint may be present in these cases. Histopathology results show a dermal cyst with a fibrous wall of varying thickness.

Digital mucous cyst mostly occurs in middle age and in the elderly as a solitary lesion. Women are more commonly affected than men. Rarely, patients have more than one cyst. Typical lesions are located on the dorsum of the fingers between the proximal nail fold and the distal interphalangeal joint (*see* Fig. 4.59). Fingers (*see* Fig. 4.60) are more commonly involved than toes.

Most digital mucous cysts are 0.5 to 1 cm in size but larger lesions are possible. These cysts are round or oval, translucent, flesh- or bluish-colored, smooth-surfaced nodules (*see* Fig. 4.60). They may be firm or fluctuant on palpation. They are mostly asymptomatic, but large lesions may be painful because of the compression on adjacent nerve fibers and may rarely limit the function of digits.

Lesions over the proximal nail fold typically cause distortion of the nail plate, leading to the appearance of irregular longitudinal grooves (*see* Fig. 4.60). Sometimes lesions are located beneath the nail and appear only as a swelling with indistinct borders, causing increased transverse curvature accompanied by secondary nail changes such as discoloration of the lunula, distal or longitudinal splitting, or onycholysis (*see* Fig. 4.61). The fluid of the cyst, which is clear, viscous, thick and sticky, may drain spontaneously but refill in a short time. Digital mucous cysts are usually diagnosed clinically. Simple puncturing of the cyst to observe the discharge of the typical content is usually confirmatory for diagnosis

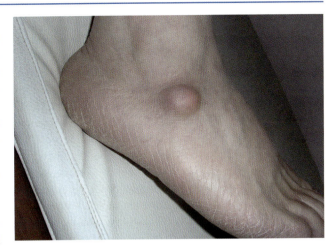

Fig. 4.58 Ganglion cyst on the ankle

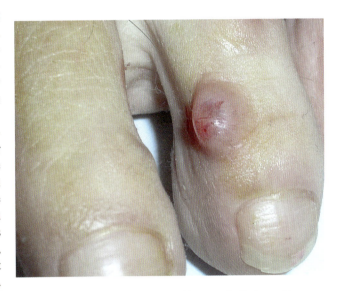

Fig. 4.59 Digital mucous cyst on the big toe typically located between the distal interphalangeal joint and the nail

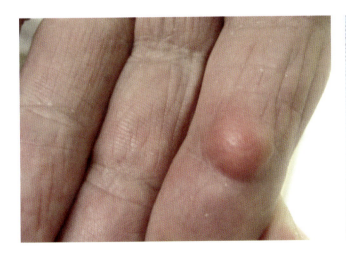

Fig. 4.57 Digital mucous cyst of ganglionic type on the volar aspect of the finger. Note that the solitary lesion with smooth-surface is located on the distal interphalangeal joint

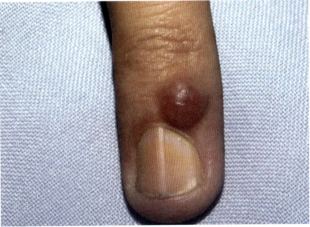

Fig. 4.60 Digital mucous cyst overlying the nail matrix of the finger. Note the prominent longitudinal groove on the nail aligned with the distal part of the cyst

without requiring a biopsy (*see* Fig. 4.62a and b). Rarely, more than one mucous cyst may be seen on the same area (*see* Fig. 4.63a and b).

Management. Digital mucous cysts are benign. Spontaneous resolution is possible. However, most lesions are persistent and may be unsightly, especially in cases with accompanying nail dystrophy. Therefore, most lesions are treated. Multiple factors should be taken into account for a therapeutic decision. Various therapeutic options exist. Total excision accompanied by cutting the communication between the cyst and the adjacent joint has a high cure rate and a low risk of recurrence. However, radical surgery may be associated with various complications, such as dysfunction of the joint and secondary infection. Therefore, conservative methods are mostly preferred. Repeated puncture of the cyst is a common and effective therapy when cysts are easily accessible. On the other hand, there is a risk of cutaneous or joint infection and a high rate of recurrence, which occurs mostly in a few months. Intralesional corticosteroid injection (triamcinolone acetonide) is an alternative therapy of choice. Sclerotherapy may be considered in the treatment, but escape of the chemical into the joint space is a troubling side effect. Cryotherapy and carbon dioxide laser may be effective in some cases. However, these destructive methods may be complicated by scarring.

4.7 Mucocele (Mucous Cyst of Oral Mucosa)

Mucocele is a pseudocyst of the oral mucosa containing mucinous material. It usually occurs as a result of trauma or injury to the minor salivary gland ducts, leading to the escape of mucus into adjacent connective tissue. This is followed by inflammation and surrounding granulation tissue formation. It has a sudden onset and is more common in the second decade of life. No dermatologic or systemic disease is known to be associated with mucocele. It appears as a translucent or bluish, dome-shaped, 5 to 10 mm tense solitary papule or nodule with an intact surface (*see* Figs. 4.64 and 4.65). Most lesions are located on the lower lip as a result of trauma from biting. The ventral surface of the tongue, floor of the mouth, and buccal mucosa are rarer locations. Mucocele has a fluctuant course. The size of the cyst may show variations; it sometimes enlarges suddenly and then shows spontaneous involution. The lesions are usually asymptomatic.

Apart from the classic presentation, two different clinical variants of mucocele are described. Superficial mucocele

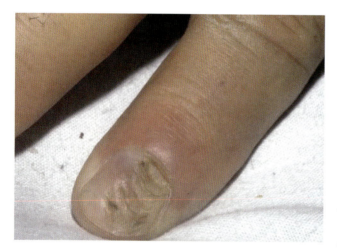

Fig. 4.61 Digital mucous cyst beneath the nail plate causing severe nail dystrophy. Note the multiple transverse grooves

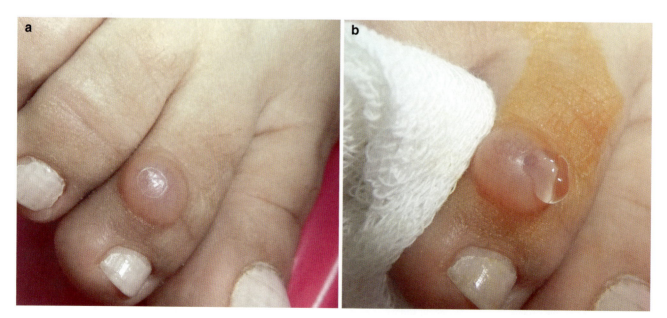

Fig. 4.62 (**a**) Digital mucous cyst on the second toe. (**b**) Discharge of thick cyst fluid after simple puncturing

4.7 Mucocele (Mucous Cyst of Oral Mucosa)

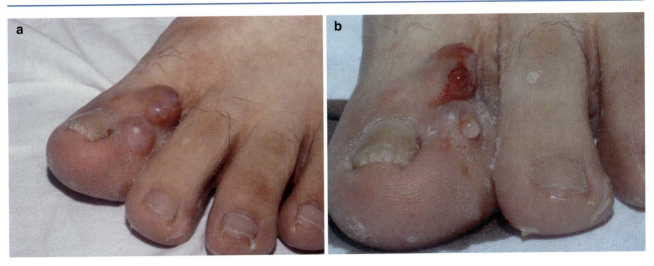

Fig. 4.63 (**a**) Two digital mucous cysts on the big toe. (**b**) Note the discharged fluid on both cysts after simple puncturing. One of the cysts' content is hemorrhagic

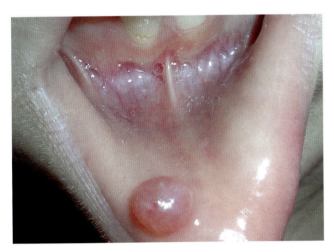

Fig. 4.64 Mucocele, typically presenting as a solitary painless nodule on the inner part of lower lip

presents as a tense, clear vesicle of a few millimeters on the soft palate, retromolar area, or posterior buccal mucosa. There may be multiple lesions. In these patients, the clinical appearance can initially be mistaken for autoimmune bullous dermatoses or herpes zoster.

A large mucocele, namely ranula, is typically located unilaterally on the floor of the mouth. The major salivary glands are more commonly involved than the minor ones.

Mucocele may sometimes be confused with pyogenic granuloma (*see* Fig. 6.43) when it appears reddish as a result of bleeding into the cyst. In contrast to venous lake (*see* Fig. 6.180), mucocele does not blanch with compression. Some lesions have a white keratotic surface secondary to sucking that may resemble oral fibroma (*see* Fig. 8.47).

Mucocele is usually diagnosed clinically. Histology reveals a cystic space with mucin deposition surrounded by granulation tissue in the submucosa. There may be an opening of ruptured salivary duct in the wall of the cyst.

Mucous retention cyst is clinically hard to distinguish from mucocele. It results from the obstruction of the salivary gland excretory duct leading to retention of the mucus and dilatation of the duct. In contrast to mucocele, mucous retention cyst is a true cyst with an epithelial lining, usually not associated with trauma, more common in the elderly, and mostly located on the floor of the mouth followed by the buccal mucosa. Moreover, it may enlarge slowly but does not show a fluctuant course.

Management. Mucocele is a benign lesion, not associated with serious complications and may spontaneously resolve. However, it may rarely affect mastication and swallowing which necessitate treatment. A conservative approach is usually preferred, especially for the lip lesions of children. Aspiration of the cyst's content is one of the therapeutic modalities. High-potency topical or intralesional corticosteroids may also be useful but recurrence

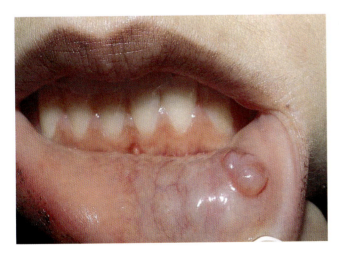

Fig. 4.65 Mucocele causing a translucent nodule with intact surface on the inner aspect of lower lip

is possible. Destructive methods like cryotherapy and laser ablation are among the possible therapeutic interventions with good results. However, the most effective method is the excision of the cyst along with adjacent minor salivary glands. While surgery is not routinely indicated for mucocele, ranula is mostly treated with surgery.

4.8 Auricular Pseudocyst

Auricular pseudocyst is a nodular ear lesion that does not have a cyst wall. Patients usually have a history of chronic trauma such as rubbing or pulling the ear, boxing, or wrestling. Therefore, it is also called wrestler's ear or boxer's ear. A minor auricular embryologic defect is suggested to be an underlying factor.

Auricular pseudocyst is usually seen unilaterally on the anterior or lateral part of the upper pinna, especially on the scaphoid or triangular fossa of middle-aged men. It is a painless, tense swelling within the auricular cartilage with an intact, smooth surface (*see* Fig. 4.66) containing a clear or bloody fluid composed of glycosaminoglycans. The cystic lesion enlarges within 2 to 3 months, reaching a size of 1 to 5 cm. It may be confused with an epidermoid cyst (*see* Fig. 4.25), which is a firm lesion in contrast to the fluctuant nature of auricular pseudocyst. Auricular pseudocyst is often diagnosed clinically. Histologically, there is an intracartilaginous cavity that is not lined by an epithelium. The surrounding cartilage includes areas of degeneration.

Management. In order to prevent a possible development of an ear deformity, early treatment is indicated. Aspiration or drainage of the cyst's content can be effective, and pressure dressings should be applied after these procedures in order to prevent recurrence. The aspiration fluid material is yellow or orange in color and of olive oil consistency. Intracystic injection of different drugs such as corticosteroids, fibrin sealant, or minocycline may also be helpful. However, perichondritis (inflammation of the cartilage and the surrounding vascular structures) is a possible complication of these interventions. Different surgical procedures have also been tried with variable success.

4.9 Preauricular Cyst (Preauricular Sinus)

Preauricular cyst or sinus is a congenital defect appearing as a solitary cystic nodule or as a small opening on the preauricular area. There is often a family history. It develops as a result of imperfect embryologic fusion of the primitive ear tubercles. It is typically located in the front or anterior crux of the helix, usually being unilateral and right-sided. It may be a small superficial pit (*see* Fig. 4.67) or a deep sinus that is located outside the temporal fasciae without involving the tympanic membrane or external auditory canal. The epithelium of the sinus may secondarily be infected, leading to erythema (*see* Fig. 4.68), tenderness, and purulent discharge with an unpleasant odor. Patients may initially seek medical advice at this stage. Diagnosis of preauricular cyst is based upon clinical findings.

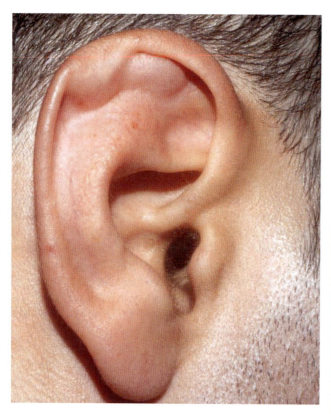

Fig. 4.66 Auricular pseudocyst on the upper pinna. It is a fluctuant, deep nodule with smooth surface. (With kind permission from Springer Science + Business Media: Baykal C, Yazganoğlu KD. *Dermatological diseases of the nose and ears*; 2010)

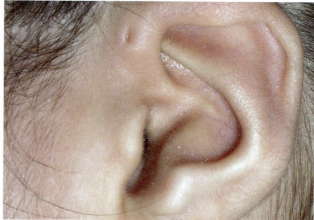

Fig. 4.67 Preauricular cyst typically manifesting as a solitary superficial pit on the anterior crux of the helix

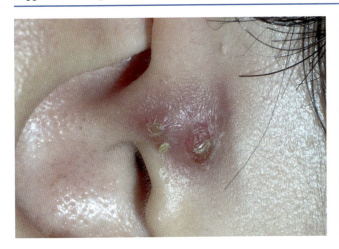

Fig. 4.68 Secondarily infected preauricular cyst. Erythema, swelling, and purulent discharge may be signs of infection

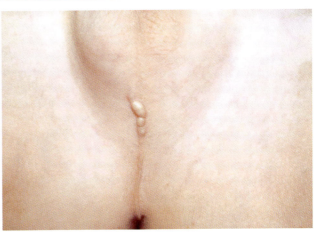

Fig. 4.69 Median raphe cyst. Note the midline cyst extending from perineum to scrotum

Most patients are otherwise healthy, although preauricular cysts may sometimes be associated with hearing loss and renal abnormalities, as in cases with branchio-oto-renal syndrome. Renal ultrasound examination and auditory testing can be useful in detecting accompanying congenital abnormalities. Preauricular cyst may also be seen in a number of other congenital conditions, such as Treacher-Collins syndrome, Waardenburg syndrome, and trisomy 22 mosaicism.

Management. In patients without associated abnormalities and who are asymptomatic, a further action is usually not taken. Systemic antibiotics are used in the presence of secondary bacterial infection. Incision and drainage of an abscess may sometimes be necessary. While complete excision is definitely indicated in the recurrent infected preauricular cysts, some authors also recommend excision of the asymptomatic ones.

4.10 Median Raphe Cyst

Median raphe cyst is a rare type of developmental anomaly presenting as a midline cyst that may be seen along a line extending from the anus via the perineum and scrotum (*see* Fig. 4.69) to the external urethral meatus. Though this asymptomatic lesion is present since birth, it may initially be detected in late childhood. It is more commonly found on the penis. Cystic lesions are usually less than 1 cm in diameter. Larger cysts located near the urethral meatus may cause urinary symptoms. It may be confused with epidermoid cyst and the pilonidal sinus. Histologically the cystic cavity is lined by a pseudostratified columnar or stratified epithelium. It has no connection with the overlying epidermis.

Management. Regular follow-up is sufficient in uncomplicated cases. Surgical excision can be performed in symptomatic lesions or for cosmetic purposes.

Suggested Reading

Bolognia JL, Jorizzo JL, Schaffer JV. Dermatology, edn 3. London: Mosby; 2012.
Burgdorf WHC, Plewig G, Wolff HH, Landthaler M. Braun-Falco's dermatology, edn 3. Italy: Springer-Verlag; 2009.
Choudhary S, Koley S, Salodkar A. A modified surgical technique for steatocystoma multiplex. J Cutan Aesthet Surg. 2010;3:25–8.
Giannokopoulus S, Makris NE, Kalaitzis C, et al. Two unusual cases of median raphe penile cyst. Eur J Dermatol. 2007;17:342–3.
Han A, Li LJ, Mirmirani P. Successful treatment of auricular pseudocyst using a surgical bolster: a case report and review of the literature. Cutis. 2006;77:102–4.
Juhn E, Khachemoune A. Gardner syndrome: skin manifestations, differential diagnosis and management. Am J Clin Dermatol. 2010; 11:117–22.
Li K, Barankin B. Digital mucous cysts. J Cutan Med Surg. 2010; 14:199–206.
MacKie RM. Skin cancer: an illustrated guide to aetiology, clinical features, pathology and management of benign and malignant cutaneous tumors, edn 2. England: Martin Dunitz; 1996.
Ogato K, Ikeda M, Miyoshi K, et al. Naevoid basal cell carcinoma syndrome with a palmar epidermoid cyst, milia and maxillary cysts. Br J Dermatol. 2001;145:508–9.
Park CO, Chun EY, Lee JH. Median raphe cyst on the scrotum and perineum. J Am Acad Dermatol. 2006;55(5 Suppl):141–5.
Satyaprakash AK, Sheehan DJ, Sanqüeaza OP. Proliferating trichilemmal tumors: a review of the literature. Dermatol Surg. 2007;33:1102–8.
Suliman MT. Excision of epidermoid (sebaceous) cyst: description of the operative technique. Plast Reconstr Surg. 2005;116:2042–3.
Takeshita T, Takeshita H, Irie K. Eruptive vellus hair cyst and epidermoid cyst in a patient with pachyonychia congenita. J Dermatol. 2000;67:655–7.
Tan T, Constantinides H, Mitchel TE. The preauricular sinus: a review of its aetiology, clinical presentation and management. Int J Pediatr Otorhinolaryngol. 2005;69:1469–74.
Torchia D, Vega J, Schachner LA. Eruptive vellus hair cysts: a systematic review. Am J Clin Dermatol. 2012;13:19–28.
Weedon D. Weedon's skin pathology, edn 3. China: Elsevier; 2010.
Zaharia D, Kanitakis J. Eruptive vellus hair cysts: report of a new case with immunohistochemical study and literature review. Dermatology. 2012;224:15–9.

Skin Appendage Tumors

Skin appendages located in the dermis but that are connected with the epidermis are the hair follicle, the sebaceous gland, the arrector pili muscle, and the sweat glands. The first three and the apocrine sweat glands form a complex called the pilosebaceous (folliculosebaceous-apocrine) unit. Eccrine sweat glands are localized separately. A great number of benign tumors may originate from these structures. Some of them have malignant counterparts, which will not be discussed in this chapter. Although some benign adnexal tumors show malignant degeneration, the great majority remain benign throughout life. But, some of these tumors are markers for syndromes associated with systemic findings or internal malignancies; therefore their diagnosis may be crucial in early detection or prevention of cancers. A number of these tumors do not have a typical clinical appearance or the clinician is not experienced enough to diagnose such very rare tumors, so they may first be diagnosed by dermatopathologists after removal. However, we assume that many skin appendage tumors have a few clinical clues before they are diagnosed histopathologically. This chapter concentrates on the relatively common benign skin appendage tumors. Tumors are classified mostly according to their adnexal origin. However, it should be kept in mind that some tumors may display more than one line of differentiation which are called composite tumors.

5.1 Sweat Gland Tumors

There are many types of sweat gland tumors that originate from eccrine or apocrine glands. In a substantial number of cases the eccrine or apocrine origin or differentiation is difficult to determine on histopathologic examination. Accordingly, the classification of some sweat gland tumors has been changed from eccrine to apocrine or vice-versa. Spiradenoma and poroma can be cited as examples of this situation.

5.1.1 Syringoma

Syringoma is one of most common benign sweat gland tumors of eccrine origin occuring as multiple small papules. It arises from the intradermal straight portion of the eccrine sweat gland. It may develop at any age but is predominantly seen in adults between 20 and 40 years. In most of the cases, lesions are multiple and are limited to the periocular area and the upper part of the cheeks in a symmetric distribution (*see* Figs. 5.1 and 5.2). However, the nose, forehead, chest, axillae, abdomen, and vulva or penis may also be involved. Facial lesions of syringoma are typically 1 to 3 mm in size and are flat, round, firm papules with smooth-surface (*see* Figs. 5.3 and 5.4). These lesions may be mistaken for eccrine hidrocystoma (*see* Fig. 5.14), verruca plana, xanthelasma, or milia (*see* Fig. 4.36). In contrast to eccrine hidrocystoma, syringoma is not translucent, and it is usually skin-colored or yellowish-white and may rarely be darker. Verruca plana usually appears at a younger age with irregularly distributed lesions. Eyelid syringomas are

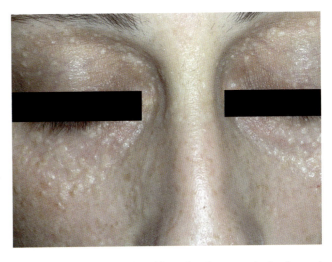

Fig. 5.1 Syringoma showing bilateral and symmetric involvement of the periocular areas. These lesions may cause a cosmetical problem

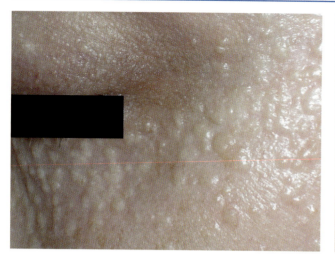

Fig. 5.2 Aggregation of numerous yellowish white lesions of syringoma on the periocular area and temple

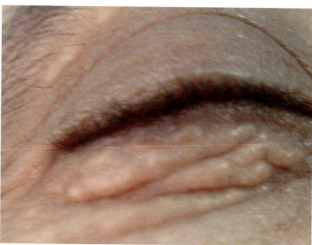

Fig. 5.5 Coalescing papules of syringoma forming a plaque on the eyelid

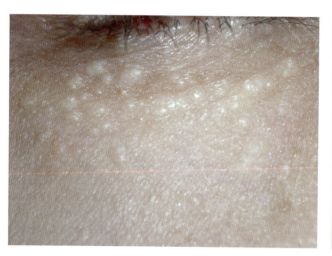

Fig. 5.3 Small, round facial papules of syringoma. They are asymptomatic

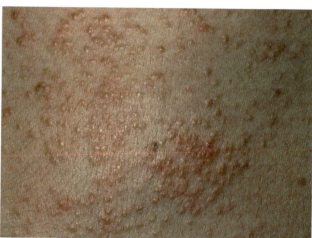

Fig. 5.6 Eruptive syringoma. Innumerable papular skin-colored lesions on the upper trunk have developed in an eruptive manner in this patient

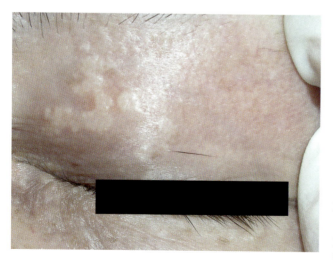

Fig. 5.4 Flat, yellowish papules of syringoma on the eyelid

usually smaller than xanthelasma. Rarely, eyelid lesions of syringoma may coalesce to form plaques (*see* Fig. 5.5). Scalp syringomas may cause alopecia.

Hundreds of papular lesions appearing simultaneously in a short period on the neck, chest, abdomen, arms, and sometimes genitalia are called "eruptive syringomas" (*see* Fig. 5.6). Lesions on the trunk (*see* Fig. 5.7) and limbs may be confused with eruptive vellus hair cysts (*see* Fig. 4.53) or non–Langerhans cell histiocytoses such as generalized eruptive histiocytosis (*see* Fig. 15.41) and benign cephalic histiocytosis. Penile lesions may even be misdiagnosed as ectopic sebaceous glands (*see* Fig. 5.68) or as venereal diseases such as verruca anogenitalis.

Syringomas are mostly asymptomatic but rarely may be pruritic. The clinical diagnosis of syringoma in a typical location is not difficult. Histologic examination reveals a proliferation of multiple cystic structures (ducts) lined by two rows of

5.1 Sweat Gland Tumors

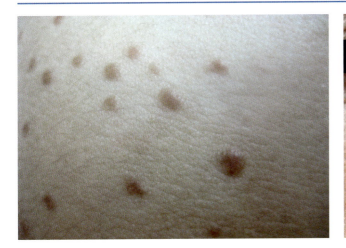

Fig. 5.7 Syringoma on the trunk. Note the irregularly scattered slightly brownish monomorphic papules

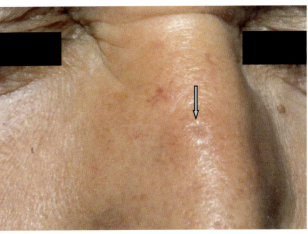

Fig. 5.8 Chondroid syringoma presenting as a solitary nonspecific nodule (*arrow*) on the nose

epithelial cells in a fibrous stroma. These ducts or epithelial chords sometimes form comma- or tadpole-shaped structures. There is no connection with the overlying epidermis.

Most patients with syringomas are otherwise healthy, but there are a few syndromes associated with syringomas. In Down syndrome, the frequency of syringomas is markedly high. Periorbital lesions are more commonly seen in this syndrome. Syringomas may also be encountered in Castello syndrome, which is considered a variant of Noonan syndrome. In Nicolau-Balus syndrome syringomas are associated with milia and atrofoderma vermiculata.

Management. Although syringomas are persistent, there are no complications or malignant degeneration of these tumors. Therapy is not necessary except for cosmetic purposes. A solitary syringoma can be excised. However, as lesions are almost always multiple, destructive methods such as gentle cautery, cryotherapy, and laser ablation may be preferred. On the other hand, these methods are neither very effective nor produce satisfactory cosmetic results. In addition to the risk of scarring, recurrence is also possible.

5.1.2 Chondroid Syringoma (Mixed Tumor of the Skin)

Chondroid syringoma is a rare benign adnexal tumor predominantly located in the head and neck region particularly on the nose, cheeks and upper lip. The tumor usually occurs in patients between 20 and 60 years of age as a solitary, slow-growing, painless, firm, intradermal or subcutaneous nodule (see Fig. 5.8). The area around the nose is a common location. The extremities and back may also be involved. The clinical presentation is nonspecific. The lesions are usually larger than those of syringoma. Thus, histopathologic diagnosis is usually required. Chondroid syringoma is accepted as a counterpart of salivary gland tumors (pleomorphic adenoma). It shows proliferation of epithelial cells in a myxoid and chondroid matrix. There are eccrine and apocrine variants of chondroid syringoma called eccrine mixed tumor and apocrine mixed tumor.

Chondroid syringoma generally has a benign course, but rarely lesions of long duration may show malignant transformation. Malignant chondroid syringoma is an uncommon tumor, usually not originating from the benign type but showing malignant features from the onset. In opposition to its benign counterpart, it is predominantly located on the trunk and extremities. It has a potential of widespread metastasis, including to regional lymph nodes, bones, and visceral organs.

Management. Complete surgical excision of the tumor is the best therapeutic option in order to avoid recurrences. Destructive methods are not preferred. When excision is not possible, close follow-up is recommended owing to the possibility of the development of malignant transformation.

5.1.3 Eccrine Hidrocystoma

Eccrine hidrocystoma is a benign cystic tumor occurring as a result of a blocked and secondarily dilated eccrine duct. It is more common in middle-aged women. The face, especially the eyelids, lateral canthus, nose, and malar areas (see Fig. 5.9) are typically involved. But lesions may also be seen on the chin (see Fig. 5.10), neck, trunk, and popliteal fossa. Most lesions are multiple and symmetrically distributed (see Fig. 5.11), but solitary lesions (see Fig. 5.12) may also occur. In patients with multiple lesions there are papules measuring 1 to 3 mm in size (see Fig. 5.13), but a solitary lesion may be relatively larger (see Fig. 5.12). Tense cystic papules have translucent appearance with a bluish tinge (see Fig. 5.14). Lesions are asymptomatic. The pathognomonic feature of this adnexal tumor is the seasonal variability in symptoms.

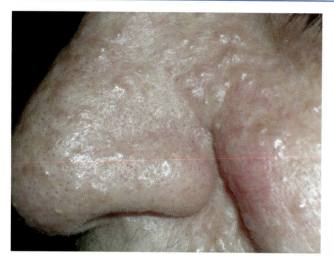

Fig. 5.9 Eccrine hidrocystoma presenting as multiple translucent papules on the nose and malar area

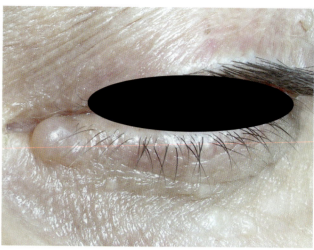

Fig. 5.12 Eccrine hidrocystoma presenting as a solitary nodule on the lateral canthus of the eye

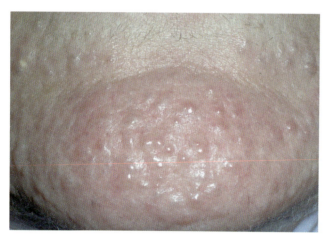

Fig. 5.10 Eccrine hidrocystoma involving the chin. The waxing and waning course of the lesions related to the seasons is distinctive

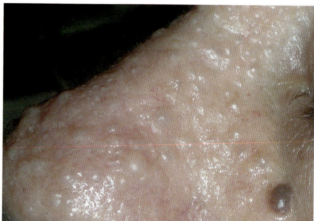

Fig. 5.13 Close-up view of small, transclucent, round papules of eccrine hidrocystoma located on the nose

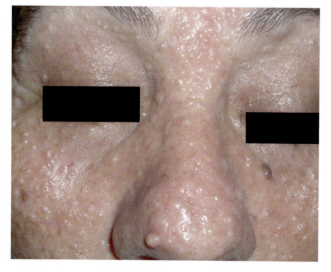

Fig. 5.11 The multiple symmetrically arranged papules of eccrine hidrocystoma in a middle-aged woman (With kind permission from Springer Science + Business Media: Baykal C, Yazganoğlu KD. *Dermatological diseases of the nose and ears*; 2010)

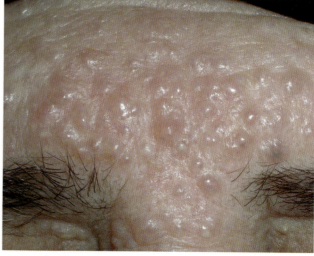

Fig. 5.14 Eccrine hidrocystoma on the forehead. Note the slight bluish tinge of the papules

Papules may enlarge and become prominent in hot weather and virtually become smaller in the winter.

Syringoma is the main diagnostic challenge, but small papules of syringomas are flat, mostly yellowish white (*see* Fig. 5.2), and do not show a prominent waxing and waning course. Eruptive vellus hair cyst may also arise on the face as multiple papular lesions, but usually there are accompanying cysts located on the trunk and extremities (*see* Fig. 4.53). Histopathologic examination is mostly performed on solitary lesions in order to exclude cystic basal cell carcinoma (*see* Fig. 11.49). A unilocular cyst in the dermis lined by two layers of cuboidal or a single layer of flattened epithelial cells is the main histopathologic feature of eccrine hydrocystoma.

Management. Since malignant degeneration is not expected, aggressive treatment is not necessary. However, multiple lesions on the face usually cause cosmetic disturbance. Symptomatic measures can be recommended, such as the avoidance of hot and humid weather and the use of air conditioning. A solitary lesion can be excised, but excision of multiple lesions is impractical and may lead to scarring. The results with the use of cautery and laser are also unsatisfactory. Therefore medical therapies are the main alternatives in management. Topical and systemic anticholinergic drugs such as atropine, scopolamine, and glycopyrrolate may be used in order to reduce sweat production. Adverse reactions such as blurred vision and photophobia limit the long-term use of these drugs. Same side effects may also be seen with the topical use of anticholinergic drugs because of their systemic absorption. On the other hand, the therapeutic effects of these drugs are transient and recurrences occur after cessation of therapy. In order to reduce hyperhidrosis intradermal botulinum toxin has been tried, which also leads to the regression of eccrine hydrocystoma.

5.1.4 Poroma (Eccrine Poroma)

Poroma is a benign adnexal neoplasm that was previously thought to originate solely from the eccrine gland. However, it can be of either eccrine or apocrine origin. The lesions initially appear in adulthood. The soles (*see* Fig. 5.15) and sides of the feet are well-known locations of this tumor. However, it may also arise on the hands, face, scalp, trunk, and other parts of the extremities. Periungual lesions (*see* Fig. 5.16) are rare. Poroma is among the secondary tumors that may develop on a nevus sebaceus. The typical clinical presentation is a solitary, soft, sessile, pink or reddish papule, nodule, or plaque that extrudes from a shallow depression (*see* Fig. 5.17). It may have a dry, hyperkeratotic and scaly or moist and eroded surface. The size of the tumor ranges from a few millimeters to a few centimeters.

A rare clinical presentation is "poromatosis," which is described as numerous, occasionally more than a hundred lesions that are mostly located on the palms and soles or uncommonly observed in a widespread distribution. In rare

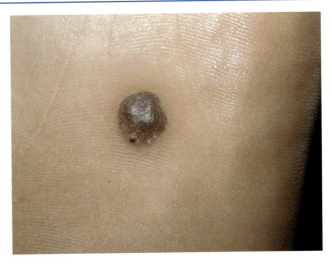

Fig. 5.15 Poroma typically presenting as a solitary nodule on the sole of foot. It should always be considered in the differential diagnosis of tumoral lesions of the plantar area

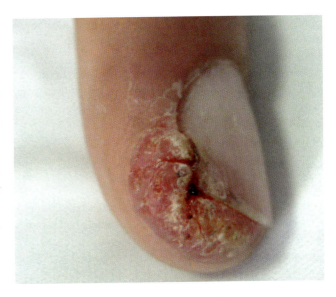

Fig. 5.16 Poroma located on the periungual area; not a common presentation

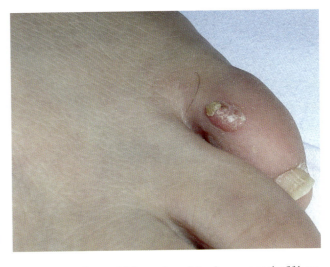

Fig. 5.17 A solitary reddish, sessile nodule of poroma on the fifth toe

instances, poroma may be hyperpigmented, resembling melanocytic nevi. Poroma with a thickened collar of epidermis may be confused with pyogenic granuloma (see Fig. 6.57), but growth of poroma is not as rapid as pyogenic granuloma. Because of the common location of poroma on the hands and feet, verruca vulgaris is another diagnostic challenge.

The diagnosis of this adnexal tumor may be considered clinically by an experienced dermatologist, but most lesions are diagnosed histologically. The tumor arises within the epidermis and extends into the dermis. Lobular growth of the monomorphic cuboidal small cells and dispersed duct-like structures are seen on histopathologic examination. There are some histologic variants of the tumor. Hidroacanthoma simplex may simply be described as an intraepidermal poroma. Poromas limited to the dermis consisting of tumor islands containing ductal lumina are called dermal duct tumors.

Most of the lesions stay unchanged during lifetime. However, rarely they can precede their malignant counterpart, namely, porocarcinoma. Rapid enlargement, ulceration, spontaneous bleeding and pain are the possible signs of malignant degeneration.

Management. Because of the risk of malignant transformation, complete excision is recommended with narrow margins of normal tissue. Reccurrence is possible if tumors are not adequately excised.

5.1.5 Poroid Hidradenoma

This rare tumor presents as a solitary lesion, usually in adults after middle age. A light red intradermal nodule measuring 1 to 2 cm may appear anywhere on the skin (see Fig. 5.18). Histopathology reveals a dermal tumor with solid and cystic components. The tumor is composed of neoplastic poroid cells and is not connected to the epidermis.

Management. The tumor may rarely show malignant transformation and therefore should be removed. In order to prevent recurrence, complete excision with deep margins should be performed. Ultrasonography may help to identify the limits of the tumor before surgery.

5.1.6 Tubulopapillary Hidradenoma (Papillary Tubular Adenoma)

Tubulopapillary hidradenoma is a rare benign sweat gland tumor that can either be of eccrine or apocrine differentiation. The term "papillary eccrine adenoma" is usually used for the former and "tubular apocrine adenoma" for the latter. These tumors resemble each other but show some slight differences, especially histologically.

Papillary eccrine adenoma usually appears as a solitary, firm, skin-colored or yellowish dermal nodule that is often smaller than 4 cm in diameter and is commonly located on the extremities and less commonly on the trunk or face. It may appear at almost any age, including childhood. It is more commonly seen in women.

Tubular apocrine adenoma also appears as a solitary dermal nodule, but it more commonly occurs on the scalp. It may also be seen on the anogenital area. It may be associated with syringocystadenoma papilliferum in some instances, especially on the background of a nevus sebaceus.

Clinical diagnosis of these benign tumors is difficult (see Figs. 5.19 and 5.20). They may be confused with various benign adnexal tumors, including cylindroma (see Fig. 5.21), spiradenoma (see Fig. 5.26), pilomatricoma (see Fig. 5.47) and trichoblastoma (see Fig. 5.43). They should also be differentiated from malignant adnexal neoplasms. Papillary eccrine adenoma should especially be distinguished from aggressive digital papillary adenoma or adenocarcinoma, and eccrine carcinomas.

Histopathologic examination of papillary eccrine adenoma reveals a well-circumscribed dermal nodule with dilated tubules that are lined by two layers of epithelial cells. An eosinophilic material is often present in the lumen of the tubules, and there are papillary projections extending into the lumina. The tubules are surrounded by a fibrous stroma. The tumor does not connect with the overlying epidermis. Papillary projections are fewer in tubular apocrine adenoma, and the distinguishing histologic feature is the presence of decapitation secretion of the luminal cells in many areas. These two tumors also have differences in enzyme biochemistry and electron microscopy findings.

Management. Malignant transformation of these tumors is extremely rare, but a complete excision is important in order to perform a detailed histopathologic examination, allowing differentiation from malignant adnexal neoplasms.

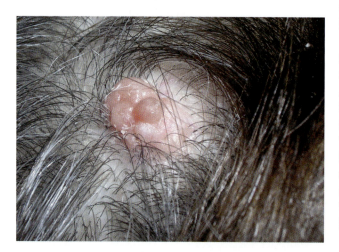

Fig. 5.18 Poroid hidradenoma presenting as a pinkish intradermal nodule with lobulated surface. The definite diagnosis is usually established upon biopsy

5.1 Sweat Gland Tumors

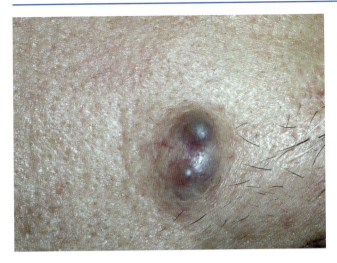

Fig. 5.19 Tubulopapillary hidradenoma on the face. The clinical presentation of the solitary nodule is nonspecific

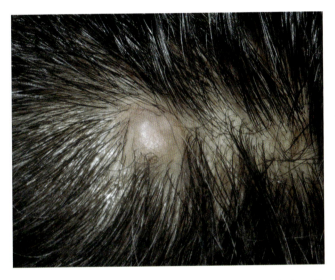

Fig. 5.20 A firm dermal nodule on the scalp representing tubulopapillary hidradenoma

Mohs micrographic surgery may allow a proper complete resection of the tumor, especially when the tumor margins are not well-defined.

5.1.7 Cylindroma

Cylindroma is an uncommon adnexal neoplasm that was formerly considered of apocrine origin but is now thought to originate from a pluripotent stem cell in the folliculo-sebaceous-apocrine unit. Lesions are typically located on the scalp (*see* Figs. 5.21 and 5.22) but may also be found on the face (*see* Fig. 5.23), ears (*see* Fig. 5.21), or trunk (*see* Fig. 5.24). It may occur as solitary (*see* Fig. 5.22) or multiple lesions (*see* Figs. 5.21, 5.23, and 5.24). It is an asymptomatic, slow-growing tumor measuring in size from a few milimeters to several centimeters. The typical presentation is a pinkish, dome-shaped, smooth nodule with prominent telangiectases (*see* Fig. 5.22). The tumor is firm or rubber-like on palpation.

Multiple cylindromas are usually familial. They can be seen in familial cylindromatosis and Brooke-Spiegler syndrome. Both syndromes are of autosomal dominant inheritance and considered within the same spectrum of diseases with numerous mutations of the *CYLD* tumor suppressor gene on chromosome 16q. Cylindromas commonly begin to occur in late childhood and adolescence, and increase with age. There may be disseminated lesions that can coalesce and cover the entire scalp and form a disfiguring mass. These cylindromas are called "turban tumors."

Brooke-Spiegler syndrome is characterized by various types of skin appendage tumors such as cylindroma, spiradenoma, and trichoepithelioma. All skin tumors may not be encountered in the same patient. Milia may also be found. Basal cell adenomas, basal cell adenocarcinomas and adenoid cystic carcinomas of the parotid and submandibular glands are also reported.

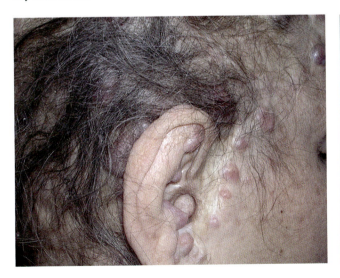

Fig. 5.21 Multiple cylindromas on the scalp and ears. In familial cases, patients may have numerous lesions (With kind permission from Springer Science + Business Media: Baykal C, Yazganoğlu KD. *Dermatological diseases of the nose and ears*; 2010)

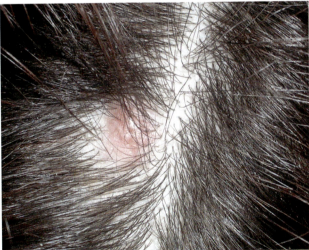

Fig. 5.22 A solitary cylindroma is seen on the scalp. This pinkish dermal nodule has a smooth surface

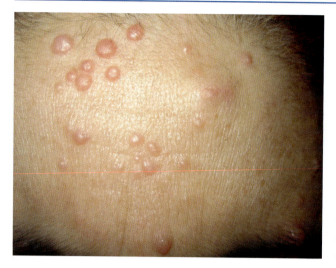

Fig. 5.23 Cylindromas manifesting as dome-shaped, pinkish papules and nodules on the forehead

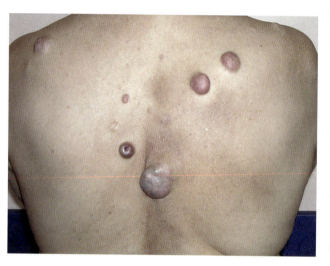

Fig. 5.24 Several large cylindromas on the back

Scalp cylindromas may resemble trichilemmal cysts (*see* Fig. 4.43), but rather soft consistency and irregularity may be a distinguishing feature of cylindromas. Cylindroma may also be mistaken for nonulcerated nodules of basal cell carcinoma (*see* Fig. 11.27). Patients with multiple lesions may be more easily diagnosed clinically, but biopsy is often required in the diagnosis of a solitary lesion. Histologically, cylindroma resembles spiradenoma with some differences. Cylindromas are well-demarcated dermal nodules consisting of variably sized lobules with two types of cells. In the center there are large, pale cells, and at the periphery there are small basaloid cells. These lobules are lined by a hyaline membrane and arranged in a characteristic "jigsaw puzzle" pattern.

Most cylindromas are benign. However, malignant cylindromas with metastatic potential have also rarely been described both in sporadic and familial cases. Ulceration, bleeding and rapid growth are among the clinical signs of malignant transformation.

Management. Patients with Brooke-Spiegler syndrome should be screened for salivary gland tumors. Treatment is considered due to the predisposition of cylindromas to malignant transformation and for cosmetic aspect, especially in the presence of a large lesion or turban tumor. Moreover, tumors on some locations may cause functional impairment (e.g., the ones on the concha and external auditory meatus may cause occlusion leading to conductive deafness). The number and location of the tumors should be also considered when deciding on the appropriate therapy. Treatment options include conventional excision, Mohs micrographic surgery, electrosurgery, and ablative laser surgery. Recurrence is possible since it is not always feasible to excise the tumor with wide surgical margins, especially in patients with numerous tumors. The cosmetic results of these procedures are not always satisfactory, especially in cases with large or multiple tumors of the scalp. Therefore, it is more convenient to remove the tumor before it enlarges.

Multiple scalp cylindromas, namely turban tumors, can be managed with total scalp excision or removal accompanied by split-thickness skin grafting. However, this is a high-risk procedure associated with various complications such as severe bleeding, hypotensive shock, and graft failure.

If excision is not feasible, patients should be monitored regarding the risk of malignant transformation. In addition to the patients, the family members of those with familial cylindromatosis and Brooke-Spiegler syndrome should be followed up for the development of skin tumors. Genetic testing may be considered in these families in order to detect *CYLD* mutation carriers. This will allow early recognition of skin tumors before their enlargement and malignant degeneration.

5.1.8 Spiradenoma

Spiradenoma, formerly called "eccrine spiradenoma," is a rare benign sweat gland tumor that is often tender or painful upon palpation. It may occur sporadically as a solitary lesion. On the other hand, multiple spiradenomas tend to be familial and are especially seen in Brooke-Spiegler syndrome.

Spiradenoma usually occurs in early adulthood. While it may occur anywhere on the body, most lesions appear on the trunk and proximal parts of the extremities. The tumor presents as a slowly growing, pinkish-, skin- or bluish-colored, smooth-surfaced, firm papule or nodule measuring 0.5 to 3 cm in size (*see* Figs. 5.25 and 5.26). Sometimes larger tumors are found, and in rare instances tumors may reach 10 cm. Rarely there may be grouped lesions arranged in a zosteriform or linear pattern. Lesions may be asymptomatic or tender or painful. Spiradenomas causing pain may be confused with other painful or tender cutaneous tumors such as angiolipoma, glomus tumor, angioleiomyoma, or schwannoma. The diagnosis is mostly based on histopathologic examination. which reveals one or more well-circumscribed intradermal nodules resembling a lymph node on scanning magnification. Two types of

5.1 Sweat Gland Tumors

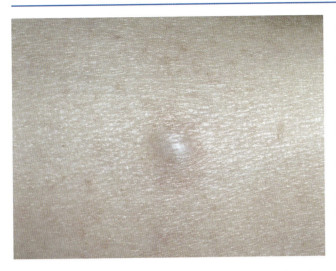

Fig. 5.25 A skin-colored subcutaneous nodule with smooth surface causing pain; typical presentation of a spiradenoma

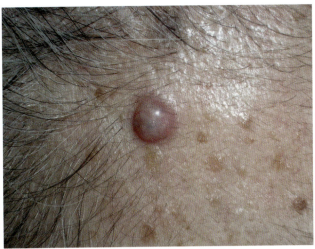

Fig. 5.27 Spiradenocylindroma. The illustrated dome-shaped nodule with overlying telangiectases has showed histologic features of spiradenoma and cylindroma concomitantly

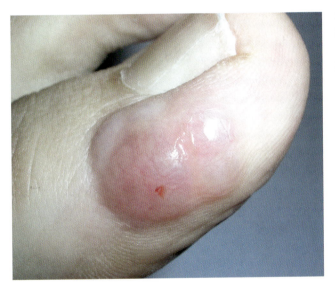

Fig. 5.26 Spiradenoma on the big toe. The solitary, smooth-surfaced nodule has a bluish tinge and is slightly telangiectatic

epithelial cells arranged in cords or clusters can be identified. Large cells with pale nuclei are seen in the center of the islands, while small basaloid cells with dark nuclei are observed at the periphery.

Spiradenomas may coexist with cylindromas and trichoepitheliomas, especially in the setting of Brooke-Spiegler syndrome. These tumors may occur separately in the same patient or histologic features of two or even three tumors within the same lesion may be observed. A hybrid tumor showing histologic features of both spiradenoma and cylindroma is called a spiradenocylindroma (*see* Fig. 5.27). Because of the close association of these tumors, it is suggested that they had a common cell of origin arising from pluripotent cells and that they represented tumors of the folliculosebaceous-apocrine unit. Therefore, today spiradenomas are not considered tumors of pure eccrine origin.

Malignant transformation, namely spiradenocarcinoma, is a rare complication of spiradenoma that may appear in long-standing tumors. Rapid growth, change in color, ulceration, and pain are alerting signs for malignant degeneration. On the other hand, spontaneous intralesional hemorrhage may cause transient enlargement of the tumor, mimicking a malignant transformation.

Management. Painful lesions are usually excised for the relief of pain. Because of the risk of malignant transformation, prophylactic excision of all tumors may be considered. Recurrence is uncommon.

5.1.9 Syringocystadenoma Papilliferum

Syringocystadenoma papilliferum is an uncommon benign tumor of the apocrine glands showing a variety of clinical presentations. It may occur primarily on normal skin or secondarily on nevus sebaceus (*see* Figs. 1.111, 1.112 and 5.28). Primary lesions may be present at birth or in most cases appear in childhood. However, syringocystadenoma papilliferum arising on nevus sebaceus is more common in young adults. The scalp (*see* Fig. 5.29) and face are the main locations, but tumors may also arise on the trunk, extremities, and genitalia. Skin-colored, grey, pink, red or brown, irregular-shaped tumors may have a smooth or hyperkeratotic surface (*see* Fig. 5.30). The size of the tumors ranges from 0.5 to 4 cm. The tumor may appear as a solitary papule, nodule, or plaque whereas in some cases multiple lesions in groups may be observed. Multiple papulonodular lesions may be arranged in a linear pattern (*see* Figs. 5.31 and 5.32). While some tumors are pedunculated (*see* Fig. 5.29), others are umbilicated resembling lesions of molluscum contagiosum. Some lesions may have an eroded

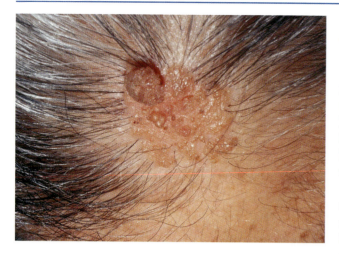

Fig. 5.28 Syringocystadenoma papilliferum manifesting as a polypoid nodule with hyperkeratotic surface overlying a flat yellowish verrucous plaque of nevus sebaceus

surface (*see* Fig. 5.33). Most lesions are asymptomatic, but due to the presence of pruritus in some cases, excoriations on the surface, superficial ulcerations, and bleeding can be seen.

A primary lesion of syringocystadenoma papilliferum is likely to be mistaken for irritated seborrheic keratosis (*see* Fig. 1.51), verruca vulgaris, or epidermal nevus (*see* Fig. 1.71). Moreover, it may be confused with basal cell carcinoma (*see* Fig. 1.119) when encountered secondarily on nevus sebaceus. Furthermore, both tumors may be observed concomitantly on nevus sebaceus in the same patient (*see* Fig. 5.33).

Although the typical lesions located on the scalp or linearly arranged on various locations are relatively easy to diagnose clinically, for other tumors the diagnosis is generally based on histopathologic examination. Numerous duct-like papillary projections invaginating from the surface epithelium into the dermis are distinctive. These may form cysts lined by two layers of cells. The outer layer is composed of cylindrical

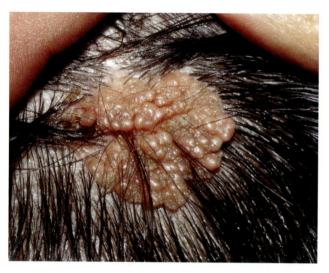

Fig. 5.29 Syringocystadenoma papilliferum on the scalp. The large pedunculated lesion has a papillomatous surface mimicking a papillomatous melanocytic nevus

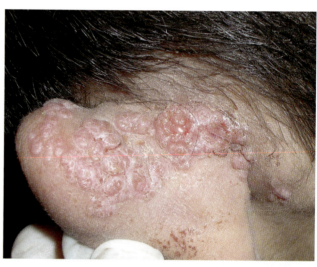

Fig. 5.31 Papulonodular lesions arranged in a linear pattern on the ear mimicking epidermal nevus. This is a rare but distinctive presentation of syringocystadenoma papilliferum

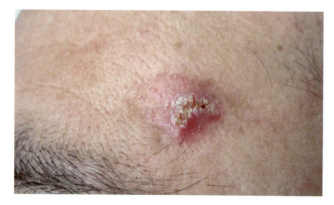

Fig. 5.30 Syringocystadenoma papilliferum on the face. Note that the lesion is partially hyperkeratotic

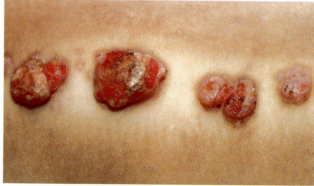

Fig. 5.32 Linear syringocystadenoma papilliferum on the trunk. Note that the large nodules have hyperkeratotic surface that cause clinical confusion with prurigo nodularis

5.1 Sweat Gland Tumors

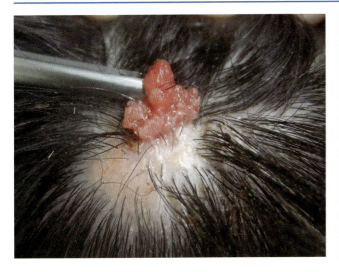

Fig. 5.33 A polypoid red tumor with eroded surface arising in nevus sebaceus on the scalp. Histopathological examination revealed features of both syringocystadenoma papilliferum and basal cell carcinoma in this lesion

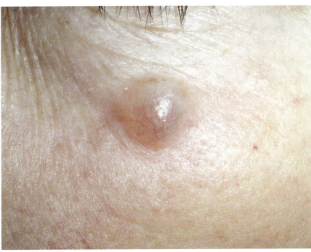

Fig. 5.34 Apocrine hidrocystoma presenting as a dome-shaped nodule on the face

cells with apical snouting, revealing apocrine differentiation. Numerous plasma cells are typically seen in the stroma.

In rare instances with long duration of lesions, malignant degeneration of the tumor, namely syringocystadenocarcinoma papilliferum develops. Verrucous carcinoma may rarely arise in the background of this appendageal tumor.

Management. Because of the risk of malignant degeneration, removal of lesions is recommended. Excision is the single best therapeutic choice.

5.1.10 Apocrine Hidrocystoma (Cystadenoma)

Apocrine hidrocystoma is an adnexal tumor arising from the apocrine secretory glands. Most lesions appear on the normal skin of middle-aged individuals and rarely on nevus sebaceus. They are more common on the face (*see* Fig. 5.34) but may also be seen on the trunk (*see* Fig. 5.35) and limbs. In contrast to eccrine hidrocystoma, the tumors are larger (3 to 15 mm), darker in color, and less likely to be periorbital (*see* Fig. 5.36). Bluish, dome-shaped nodules do not show a difference in size during hot weather. Telangiectases may be observed on the surface of the lesions, which can lead to confusion with cystic basal cell carcinoma (*see* Fig. 11.49). The histopathologic examination reveals a cyst lined by one to several layers of cuboidal to columnar epithelial cells with papillary projections and luminal decapitation secretions.

Schöpf-Schulz-Passarge syndrome is a rare inherited disorder associated with multiple late-onset apocrine hidrocytomas (especially on the eyelids), palmoplantar keratoderma, hypotrichosis, hypodontia, and onychodystrophy. There may be accompanying palmoplantar eccrine syringofibroadenomas.

Management. Since the tumor is asymptomatic and remains benign, therapy is not necessary. However, as the

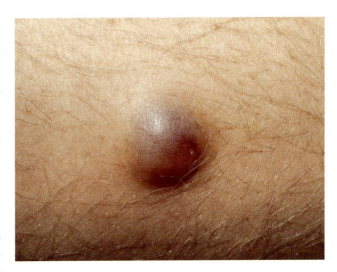

Fig. 5.35 Apocrine hidrocystoma on the trunk. Note the bluish, smooth-surfaced nodule

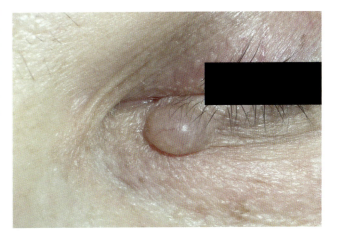

Fig. 5.36 Apocrine hidrocystoma on the eyelid. Different from eccrine hidrocystoma it does not wax and wane with temperature changes

clinical diagnosis is difficult in most cases, a definite diagnosis can be achieved with histopathologic examination after simple excision which will be therapeutic as well. Furthermore, some eyelid lesions may enhance vision and thus may require a special surgical approach.

5.1.11 Hidradenoma Papilliferum

Hidradenoma papilliferum is a benign sweat gland tumor of females mostly seen on the vulva and perianal area. It appears a solitary papule or nodule. Large masses with tendency to ulcerate is rare. Diagnosis is established upon biopsy. The dermal nodule without connection to the epidermis shows tubulopapillary structures lined by epithelial cells with apical secretion and myoepithelial cells.

Management. Large lesions can be removed.

5.1.12 Erosive Adenomatosis of the Nipple (Papillary Adenoma of the Nipple)

Erosive adenomatosis of the nipple is a benign proliferation of the lactiferous ducts on the nipple. It is an uncommon disease of middle-aged women in their fourth to fifth decades. Rarely, men or children may be affected. It may be asymptomatic or associated with various symptoms such as serous, bloody or serosanguineous discharge of the breast, tenderness, pain, and pruritus. It mostly involves one nipple; in rare cases two sides are affected. Clinically, it may appear as an eczematous lesion with inflammation, edema, erythema, erosions, and crusting (*see* Fig. 5.37). There may be a palpable nodule on the nipple. The nipple may become firm in later stages, and ulceration may be predominant. In the early period, from the clinical point of view the disease can be confused with Paget disease of the breast (*see* Fig. 2.75) and cutaneous metastasis of breast carcinoma. Although the disease is benign, some authors suggest performing mammography or ultrasound examination in order to exclude an underlying carcinoma.

Histologically, the disease must be differentiated from a carcinoma. There are two layers of cells surrounding the tubular structure. The outer layer demonstrates myoepithelial cuboidal cells, and the inner layer demonstrates columnar secretory cells. Keratin cysts are observed in the upper dermis. Immunohistochemical staining helps to distinguish the lesion from malignant tumors such as invasive carcinoma of the breast.

Management. The disease can be diagnosed with punch or wedge biopsy, but a complete excision of the tumor will be both curative and diagnostic. Unnecessary, aggressive surgery should be avoided. However, an incomplete excision will lead to recurrence. Resection of the tumor may involve the removal of the entire nipple, necessitating subsequent reconstruction, especially in women of child-bearing age. Mohs micrographic surgery is an effective alternative to classic complete excision of the tumor, allowing the preservation of the nipple unless the disease is extensive. Risk of recurrence is reduced by this method. Cryotherapy may also be useful in treating this tumor.

5.2 Hair Follicle Tumors

There are several benign tumors that are primarily classified according to their differentiation towards parts of the hair follicle such as germinative cells, matrix, outer root sheath, and infundibulum. Pilomatricoma is the commonest type of this rare tumor group.

5.2.1 Trichoepithelioma

Trichoepithelioma is a rare benign tumor with follicular germinative differentiation. Lesions are skin- or pink-colored, shiny, smooth, dome-shaped papules or small nodules predominantly located on the midface, especially around the nose and nasolabial folds (*see* Fig. 5.38). They can also occur on the scalp (*see* Fig. 5.39), ears, neck, or trunk. Trichoepitheliomas are asymptomatic lesions, 2 to 10 mm in size (*see* Fig. 5.40), and firm on palpation. Multiple tumors on the face are usually observed as symmetrically located discrete lesions that may sometimes be grouped (*see* Fig. 5.41).

A solitary trichoepithelioma is usually nonhereditary, but multiple lesions (*see* Fig. 5.41) may be part of "multiple familial trichoepithelioma" or Brooke-Spiegler syndrome. Multiple familial trichoepithelioma is within the same spectrum as Brooke-Spiegler syndrome and familial cylindromatosis. Multiple trichoepitheliomas usually appear in childhood or around puberty. Additionally spiradenomas, cylindromas and salivary gland tumors can be seen in Brooke-Spiegler syndrome. Trichoepithelioma may also be seen in Rombo syndrome. Basal cell carcinoma, atrophoderma vermiculata, milia, hypotrichosis and telangiectasia are other manifestations of this syndrome.

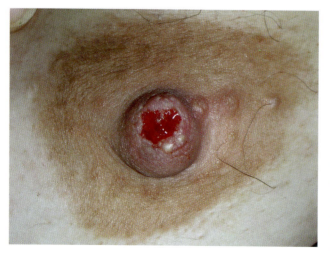

Fig. 5.37 Erosive adenomatosis of the nipple; an erythematous firm nodule located on the nipple showing a superficial ulceration

5.2 Hair Follicle Tumors

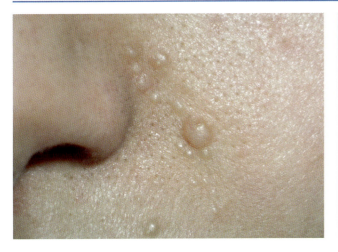

Fig. 5.38 Trichoepithelioma typically located on the midface. This patient does not have any other extrafacial lesions

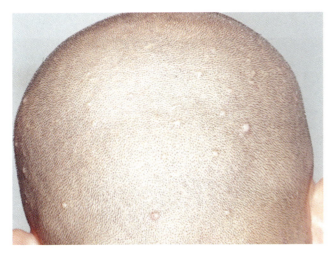

Fig. 5.39 Irregularly scattered papules of trichoepithelioma on the scalp

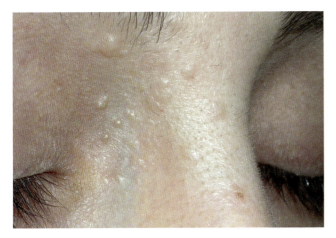

Fig. 5.40 Trichoepithelioma presenting as small, skin-colored firm papules on the face

Owing to the lack of distinctive features, a solitary trichoepithelioma is often difficult to diagnose clinically. It can be

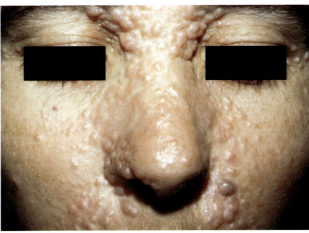

Fig. 5.41 Multiple trichoepitheliomas showing tendency to confluence. Other family members of the patient had also trichoepitheliomas (With kind permission from Springer Science + Business Media: Baykal C, Yazganoğlu KD. *Dermatological diseases of the nose and ears*; 2010)

confused with early lesions of basal cell carcinoma (*see* Fig. 11.23), fibrous papule of the nose (*see* Fig. 8.19), palisaded encapsulated neuroma (*see* Fig. 7.41), intradermal melanocytic nevus (*see* Fig. 3.114), or other benign adnexal tumors. Multiple tumors on the face may resemble multiple papules of syringoma (*see* Fig. 5.2), eccrine hydrocystoma (*see* Fig. 5.11), or angiofibroma (*see* Fig. 8.23). A simple distinction can be based on clinical features since syringomas are flat, angiofibromas are smaller, and hydrocystomas are translucent lesions. Yet, an exact diagnosis depends on the histopathologic examination. Histologically, trichoepitheliomas appear in nests or cribriform cords that are composed of basaloid cells and keratin cysts, and surrounded by fibroblastic stroma.

Management. Trichoepithelioma does not carry a risk of malignant transformation. While a solitary small lesion is not a cosmetic problem in most cases, multiple trichoepitheliomas appearing on the face may be disfiguring. Relatively larger trichoepitheliomas can be removed with conventional excision, but this method is not feasible for multiple lesions. Electrosurgery or ablative laser techniques such as carbon dioxide or erbium Er:YAG laser may be tried in these cases. However, recurrence is possible, and cosmetic results may not always be satisfactory. Trichoepitheliomas occluding the concha and external auditory meatus may be removed with loop cautery.

5.2.1.1 Desmoplastic Trichoepithelioma

A desmoplastic trichoepithelioma is a clinicopathologic variant of trichoepithelioma characterized by stromal sclerosis in the dermis (desmoplasia). It is more commonly seen in young to middle-aged females. The tumor is usually solitary and appears mostly on the cheeks, forehead, or chin as an asymptomatic, slowly growing, firm, skin- or yellow-colored annular plaque with a central depression. The tumor may be clinically confused with morpheic basal cell carcinoma (*see* Fig. 11.63) and microcystic adnexal carcinoma. Histologically, thin strands of basaloid cells along with desmoplastic stroma in the dermis are observed.

Management. Therapy is not indicated for this benign lesion, but it should be differentiated from sclerosing malignant cutaneous tumors and may be excised for histopathological examination.

5.2.2 Trichoblastoma

Trichoblastoma is a rare benign tumor with hair follicle differentiation that presents typically as a solitary nodule. Most lesions appear on the background of nevus sebaceus (*see* Fig. 5.42), but rarely the tumor may occur on normal skin. Trichoblastoma is the most common benign tumor developing on nevus sebaceus. It generally appears as an asymptomatic, skin-colored or grey, smooth-surfaced papule or nodule on the scalp or neck of adults. Some tumors may be as large as 1 to 2 cm. Since clinical features may not be helpful in the differentiation of trichoblastoma from most other benign cutaneous tumors, histologic examination is usually required. A nonulcerated nodular basal cell carcinoma is the main consideration both in the clinical and histopathologic differential diagnosis of trichoblastoma. Trichoblastomas overlying nevus sebaceus were formerly misdiagnosed as basal cell carcinomas. Trichoblastoma is a dermal tumor with islands of basaloid cells demonstrating peripheral palisading and a fibrocellular stroma. There is no connection with the epidermis. Occasionally, large tumors may extend into subcutaneous tissue. There are various histopathologic subtypes of this adnexal tumor including a pigmented form. Pigmented trichoblastoma (*see* Fig. 5.43) is one of the rarest forms and mimics pigmented basal cell carcinoma (*see* Fig. 11.71) and nodular malignant melanoma (*see* Fig. 12.42) clinically.

Rare cases of trichoblastoma exhibiting malignant degeneration or invasive growth have been described, called "trichoblastic carcinoma." However, these lesions are considered to represent basal cell carcinoma from the outset.

Management. Although not always necessary, excision of lesions on normal skin is the best approach for therapy and facilitates histopathologic analysis and the confirmation of the diagnosis. Similarly, lesions on nevus sebaceus are mostly evaluated histologically after excisional biopsy to exclude the diagnosis of basal cell carcinoma.

5.2.3 Trichofolliculoma

Trichofolliculoma is a rare hamartoma of the pilosebaceous unit and it features hairs. There may be a solitary lesion or multiple lesions. Most tumors occur on the face, scalp, or

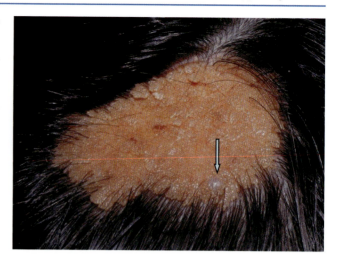

Fig. 5.42 A grey, dome-shaped, smooth small papule of trichoblastoma (*arrow*) on nevus sebaceus

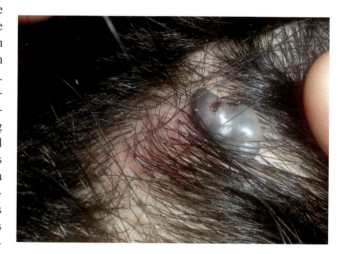

Fig. 5.43 Trichoblastoma as a pigmented nodule, a rare presentation

neck. A trichofolliculoma typically appears in adults as a flesh- or pink-colored, dome-shaped, small, centrally depressed papule or nodule. A tuft of immature hairs protrudes through a central pore. Lesions are asymptomatic. However, they may be inflamed when overlying hairs are pulled out. Intradermal or compound nevi with long hairs (*see* Fig. 3.111) are the main challenges in the differential diagnosis. However, hairs emerging from these melanocytic nevi are of the terminal type and are not tufted. Histologically, there are one or more dermal large cystic spaces or enlarged hair follicle (primary hair follicle). There are smaller secondary hair follicles radiating from the wall of the primary hair follicle. Some histologic variants of the tumor are described and sebaceous trichofolliculoma is one of them.

Management. The tumor poses only a cosmetic problem because of the hairs. Thus, excision may be performed for cosmetic improvement.

5.2.4 Trichilemmoma

Trichilemmoma is a rare tumor of the hair follicle showing differentiation toward the outer root sheath cells. It appears mostly in adulthood as solitary or multiple facial lesions. Solitary lesions occur sporadically as slow-growing, flesh- or yellowish-colored, flat-topped or hyperkeratotic (verrucous) papules or nodules (*see* Fig. 5.44). Trichilemmoma may also arise secondarily on nevus sebaceus.

Multiple lesions presenting as scattered, 1–3 mm papules (*see* Figs. 5.45 and 5.46) may be a sign of Cowden syndrome (multiple hamartoma syndrome), an autosomal dominant disease characterized by multiple dermatologic manifestations associated with internal malignancies. This syndrome is caused by mutations in *PTEN*, a tumor suppressor gene. Early diagnosis of the disease may reduce the morbidity and mortality. In more than 80 percent of patients with Cowden syndrome, trichilemmomas exist. Head and neck are the most commonly involved sites, especially the ears and the periorificial sites such as the perioral and perinasal regions. However, they may also be seen on unusual sites such as the genitalia. Therefore, numerous small persistent papules especially located on the face should always alert the clinician to the possibility of trichilemmoma, and a biopsy should be performed for histopathologic confirmation. Cobblestone appearance secondary to oral papillomas, acral keratotic papules on the dorsum of the hands, palmoplantar punctate keratoses, lipomas, hemangiomas, and scrotal tongue are other mucocutaneous signs of Cowden syndrome that may be seen in varying frequency. Macrocephaly may also be noticed. Moreover, there is a high risk of hamartomatous tumors of the breast, endometrium, thyroid, gastrointestinal tract, and brain. Malignancies of the breast, endometrium, and thyroid are the major concern. All patients should be investigated for the presence of solid cancers.

While a solitary trichilemmoma may be mistaken for verruca vulgaris, seborrheic keratosis, or basal cell carcinoma, multiple small papules of trichilemmoma may be confused with perifollicular fibromas (*see* Fig. 8.42), syringomas (*see* Fig. 5.1), comedones, or milia (*see* Fig. 4.36). Histology reveals a lobular tumor with peripheral palisading and thickened basement membrane that is connected to the epidermis and extending to the dermis. The cells are rich with glycogen and therefore look like clear cells. The overlying epidermis is hyperplastic and hyperkeratotic.

Management. Trichilemmomas are benign, and therapy is not indicated. Solitary lesions that are challenging for diagnosis can be excised for histopathologic examination. Multiple lesions may be treated with dermabrasion or carbon dioxide laser ablation for cosmetic reasons. Yet, occurrence of new lesions is inevitable. Patients diagnosed with Cowden syndrome should be followed periodically for the possible development of the associated internal malignancies. Family members should also be screened for these malignancies.

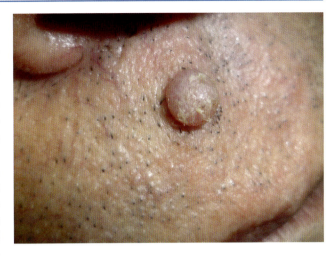

Fig. 5.44 Solitary trichilemmoma presenting as a skin-colored nodule with hyperkeratotic surface

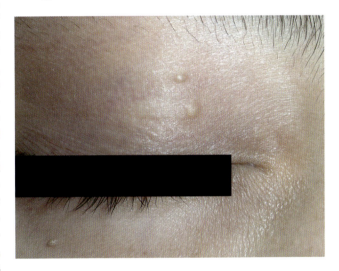

Fig. 5.45 Multiple trichilemmomas on the eyelid clinically mimicking milia. After the diagnosis is confirmed, patients should be evaluated about Cowden syndrome

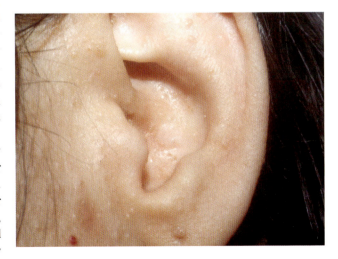

Fig. 5.46 Multiple trichilemmomas on the auricle of a patient with Cowden syndrome. Note the tiny papules (With kind permission from Springer Science + Business Media: Baykal C, Yazganoğlu KD. *Dermatological diseases of the nose and ears*; 2010)

5.2.5 Pilomatricoma (Calcifying Epithelioma of Malherbe)

Pilomatricoma is a relatively common, benign hamartoma of the hair follicle matrix and is one of the hardest lesions of the skin. It is more common in childhood and adolescence but may occur at any age. It may appear on any part of the skin involving hair follicles, but the face, neck, and upper limbs are more commonly affected. The periorbital area, cheeks (*see* Fig. 5.47), preauricular area and forehead are the major predilection sites on the face. Only palmoplantar area is spared. Typical solitary lesions are not usually associated with systemic diseases. However, multiple lesions may be seen, especially in myotonic dystrophy, a rare neuromuscular disease. The incidence of pilomatricoma is also increased in Rubinstein-Taybi syndrome and Turner syndrome. Epidermoid cysts in Gardner syndrome may reveal pilomatricoma-like changes histologically.

The clinical presentation of pilomatricoma is variable. The tumor may appear as a 0.5 to 3 cm, deep-seated nodule with overlying normal skin (*see* Figs. 5.48 and 5.49) or as a markedly raised nodule with a faint blue (*see* Fig. 5.50), slightly yellow (*see* Fig. 5.51), or reddish-blue (*see* Fig. 5.52) color. Some tumors may be lobulated. Occasionally giant tumors larger than 10 cm may be observed, especially on the trunk and extremities. The surface of the tumors is usually smooth (*see* Fig. 5.53). On the other hand, due to epidermal atrophy, the overlying skin may appear loose and folded, leading to an anetodermic appearance (*see* Fig. 5.52). The characteristic clinical feature of a pilomatricoma is the firm to hard consistency of the tumor upon palpation. Sometimes it may be as hard as a bone. This is related to the tendency of the tumor to calcification and osseous metaplasia. Lesions may sometimes be inflamed, and erythema may be seen. Ulceration is rare. Occasionally, rupture of the tumor may lead to the extrusion of the calcified material.

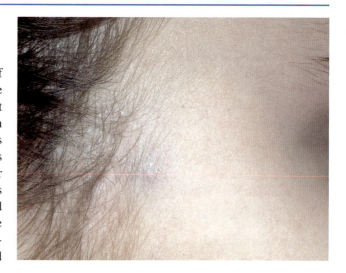

Fig. 5.48 Pilomatricoma presenting as a deep-seated solitary nodule on the temple of a child

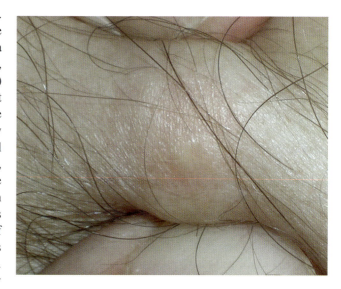

Fig. 5.49 A deep-seated, skin-colored nodule representing pilomatricoma. It is one of the hardest benign skin tumors and palpation is usually helpful in clinical diagnosis

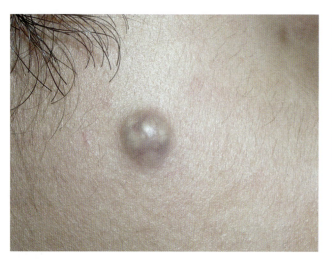

Fig. 5.47 Pilomatricoma on the cheek. A yellowish nodule is seen

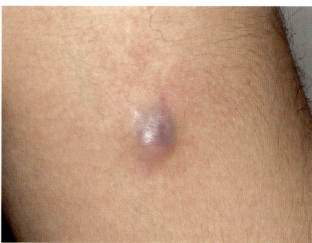

Fig. 5.50 A slightly raised, faint blue nodule of pilomatricoma located on the arm

5.2 Hair Follicle Tumors

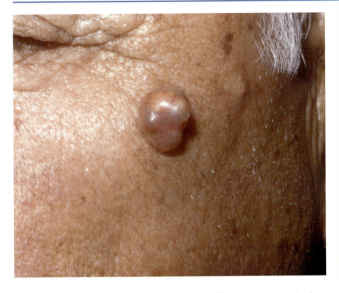

Fig. 5.51 An exophytic yellowish nodule of pilomatricoma on the face in an elder patient

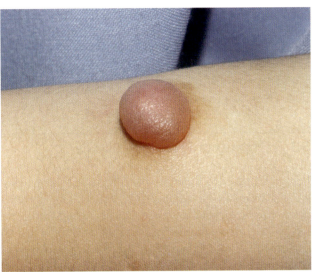

Fig. 5.53 A large smooth, cyst-like solitary nodule of pilomatricoma on the arm

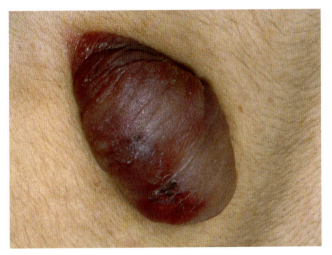

Fig. 5.52 Pilomatricoma occuring as a reddish blue, large nodule. Note the folded surface of the lesion causing anetodermic appearance

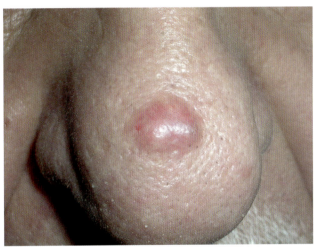

Fig. 5.54 Malignant pilomatricoma; a minute erosion is seen on the surface of the solitary tumor

Most pilomatricomas can be diagnosed clinically. An epidermoid cyst is the main diagnostic challenge, but it has a typical comedo-like central punctum (see Fig. 4.3). Nodules of cutaneous metastasis may also be hard, but indurated as well (see Fig. 16.24). Osteoma cutis, foreign body granuloma, and dermatofibroma are other differential diagnostic considerations. Some imaging procedures may be helpful in the diagnosis of pilomatricoma. Plain radiography may reveal cutaneous calcification. Ultrasonography is another noninvasive technique that helps to differentiate pilomatricoma from subcutaneous tumors. Incisional biopsy is not ideal for the diagnosis of this hair follicle tumor. Histopathologic examination of a completely excised lesion reveals an encapsulated tumor in the dermis and/or subcutis with two types of cells: areas of basophilic cells that evolve into eosinophilic "shadow" cells, which are cornified hair matrix cells. The type of the cells is related to the age of the lesion. Areas of calcification are commonly present. Even ossification may be seen.

Most tumors remain stable. Rarely, pilomatricomas may show malignant transformation. On the other hand, some tumors may initially start as malignant (see Fig. 5.54), which is referred to as malignant pilomatricoma (pilomatrix carcinoma). It is usually seen in the sixth to seventh decades occurring mostly on the head and neck, upper limbs and buttock. Histologically it shows asymmetrical growth pattern, significant nuclear atypia and tendency to invade the adjacent tissue. This malignant tumor is locally invasive, can metastasize to regional lymph nodes and visceral organs, and has a tendency to recur following excision.

Management. Patients with multiple lesions should be searched for accompanying diseases. Although pilomatricomas are asymptomatic, large lesions may be disfiguring. Excision of pilomatricomas is performed for cosmetic or prophylactic reasons. This will also allow a histopathologic confirmation of the diagnosis and help to exclude the possibility of a malignancy. Recurrence is possible after inadequate excision.

5.3 Tumors of Sebaceous Glands

Sebaceous gland is a part of the folliculosebaceous-apocrine unit and is located in hairy regions. On the other hand, ectopic location on other sites, including the mucosae, is also common as a result of minor developmental abnormality. Proliferation of sebaceous glands may be a component of a hamartomatous lesion such as nevus sebaceus, which is composed of different skin structures, or may cause an isolated hamartomatous tumor such as senile sebaceous hyperplasia and sebaceous neoplasms. The degree of differentiation and resemblance to normal sebaceous glands determine the type of the tumor. Senile sebaceous hyperplasia, which is the most common one in this group, is considered a hamartomatous lesion and is composed of nearly normal-looking sebaceous glands. Sebaceous adenoma, epithelioma (sebaceoma), and carcinoma form the spectrum of sebaceous neoplasms, and the degree of differentiation diminishes toward the sebaceous carcinoma end. All of these tumors are rare.

5.3.1 Senile Sebaceous Hyperplasia

Senile sebaceous hyperplasia is a common benign papular lesion caused by enlarged sebaceous glands around the follicular infundibulum. The etiology is not fully understood. Chronic sun damage is suggested to be a causative factor of this hamartoma. It is more common in transplant recipients treated with cyclosporine. It usually occurs after the fourth decade in otherwise healthy individuals and may gradually increase in number. Lesions are mostly located on the face, especially on the forehead (see Fig. 5.55), temples (see Fig. 5.56), cheeks (see Fig. 5.57), and nose (see Fig. 5.58). It is relatively rarely seen on the chin and ears (see Fig. 5.59). The neck and trunk may also be affected. Most patients have multiple but discrete lesions (see Fig. 5.60). The typical lesion is a flesh- or yellow-colored, glistening, soft, 2–5 mm dome-shaped papule mostly with central umbilication (see Figs. 5.55 and 5.60). Larger lesions are rare (see Fig. 5.57). Telangiectasia may be observed on the surface of some lesions (see Fig. 5.55), but ulceration does not occur. Asymptomatic small lesions pose only a minor cosmetic problem. Most lesions are diagnosed clinically. However, trichoepithelioma (see Fig. 5.38), intradermal nevus (see Fig. 3.122), and early lesion of basal cell carcinoma (see

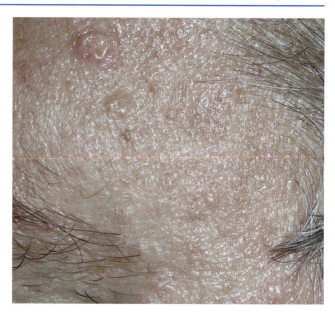

Fig. 5.55 Multiple lesions of senile sebaceous hyperplasia. Central umbilication and telangiectases on the surface are noticeable

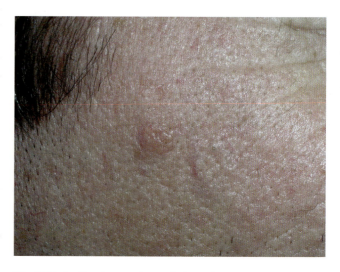

Fig. 5.56 Senile sebaceous hyperplasia on the temple. Yellowish papules are usually smaller than 5 mm

Fig. 11.24) may be confused with senile sebaceous hyperplasia. Histologically, large lobules of sebaceous glands with normal morphology are seen. These open to a central duct connected to the epidermis.

Apart from senile sebaceous hyperplasia, another type of sebaceous hyperplasia may be observed at a young age that gradually increases with time, leading to numerous lesions. This condition is called "premature sebaceous hyperplasia" (familial presenile sebaceous hyperplasia).

Management. The need for treatment of senile sebaceous hyperplasia arises only for cosmetic reasons. Light electrocautery, cryotherapy, shave excision, and laser therapy can be performed but may leave scars. In patients with

5.3 Tumors of Sebaceous Glands

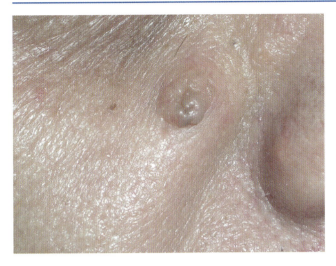

Fig. 5.57 A relatively larger papulonodular lesion of senile sebaceous hyperplasia. Even large lesions are soft in consistency

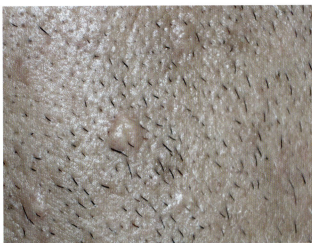

Fig. 5.60 Senile sebaceous hyperplasia on the cheek. Central umbilication is noticeable in this lesion

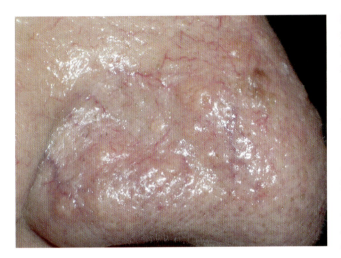

Fig. 5.58 Senile sebaceous hyperplasia presenting as several yellowish papules on the nose. Most patients have more than one lesion

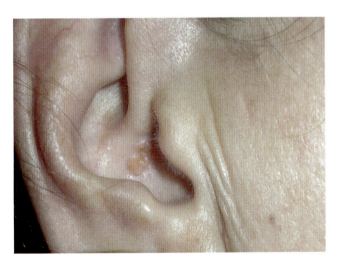

Fig. 5.59 Senile sebaceous hyperplasia on the concha of the ear. This is not a very common location

numerous lesions, low-dose systemic isotretinoin may be used; this causes a decrease in sebaceous gland size. However, discontinuation of the medication may cause recurrence of the lesions.

5.3.2 Sebaceous Adenoma and Sebaceous Epithelioma

Sebaceous adenoma is a rare benign tumor that may be a marker of a hereditary tumor syndrome. It may occur as a solitary sporadic tumor in the elderly. On the other hand, it is the most common sebaceous neoplasm, presenting as a solitary or multiple lesions in patients associated with Muir-Torre syndrome. The typical locations of the sporadic tumors are the head and neck, especially the eyelids and nose. In contrast, the trunk and extremities are more often involved than the head and neck in Muir-Torre syndrome. An individual lesion is a yellow papule or nodule less than 1 cm (*see* Fig. 5.61). The surface of the lesion may be intact and smooth, although it may sometimes be eroded, ulcerated, crusted, or verrucous (*see* Fig. 5.62). Contrary to umbilicated papular lesions of senile sebaceous hyperplasia (*see* Fig. 5.55), the lesions of sebaceous adenoma usually do not have a central dell. Sometimes sebaceous adenoma may be confused with an early lesion of basal cell carcinoma (*see* Fig. 11.24). The diagnosis is based upon histopathologic examination. Histopathology shows a well-circumscribed tumor with multiple sebaceous lobules consisting of mainly mature vacuolated sebocytes and also basaloid cells.

Sebaceous epithelioma (sebaceoma) is another benign sebaceous gland neoplasm (*see* Fig. 5.63) that is clinically difficult to differentiate from a sebaceous adenoma or basal cell carcinoma. The nomenclature of this tumor is controversial. Histologically basaloid cells are predominant but mature

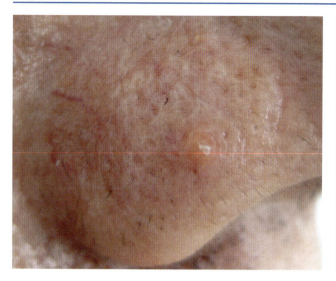

Fig. 5.61 A yellow, nonumbilicated papule on the nose histologically diagnosed as sebaceous adenoma in this patient with colon cancer

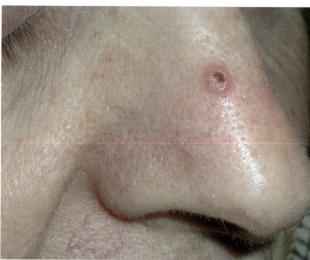

Fig. 5.63 Nonspesific eroded and crusted papule histologically diagnosed as sebaceous epithelioma

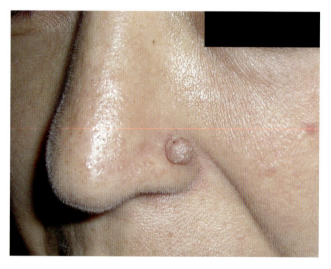

Fig. 5.62 Sebaceous adenoma presenting as a raised nodule with verrucous surface in an otherwise healthy woman

sebocytes may also be seen. Sebaceous epitheliomas may also be associated with Muir-Torre syndrome.

Muir-Torre syndrome is characterized by solitary or multiple, benign and malignant skin tumors of the sebaceous glands and visceral malignancies. It is accepted as a variant of hereditary non–polyposis colon cancer syndrome and is associated with *MSH2*, *MLH1* or *MSHG* gene mutations. Visceral malignancies may precede or follow the development of sebaceous gland tumors of the skin. All patients diagnosed with sebaceous adenoma, sebaceous epithelioma, and sebaceous carcinoma should be evaluated for Muir-Torre syndrome. Especially cystic histologic variants of these sebaceous lesions are suggested to be closely associated with Muir-Torre syndrome. Young age, multiple lesions and trunk involvement of sebaceous adenomas and epitheliomas should arouse suspicion for Muir-Torre syndrome. Occurrence of nonocular sebaceous carcinoma is another clue for this syndrome. Additionally single or multiple keratoacanthomas may be seen in approximately 20 percent of patients with this syndrome. Patients with Muir-Torre syndrome are at particularly high risk for the development of gastrointestinal and genitourinary cancers mostly in adulthood. Breast cancer and hematologic malignancies may also be observed. Some patients have more than one type of visceral cancer throughout their lives. Colonic polyps can also be seen, and colon cancer is the major concern in this syndrome. On the other hand, visceral malignancies in these patients are often relatively low-grade. Rarely, metastasis may occur.

Management. Sebaceous adenoma or sebaceous epithelioma does not have any malignant potential. Therefore therapy is only considered in patients with cosmetic concerns. However, excision may be performed in order to exclude other cutaneous tumors. Because of their close association with Muir-Torre syndrome, visceral malignancies should be screened in patients after the diagnosis of sebaceous adenoma or sebaceous epithelioma has been confirmed. Regular multidisciplinary follow-up is important. Family members of the patients must also be screened for visceral malignancies.

5.3.3 Fordyce Spots

Fordyce spots are ectopic sebaceous glands without activity localized on the oral mucosa. They are very common and accepted as a normal variant. Lesions are usually diagnosed after puberty. Tiny (1 to 2 mm), yellowish, slightly raised

5.4 Tumors of Smooth Muscles of Skin

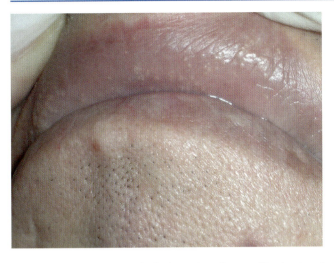

Fig. 5.64 Fordyce spots typically located on the vermilion border of upper lip. They are asymptomatic

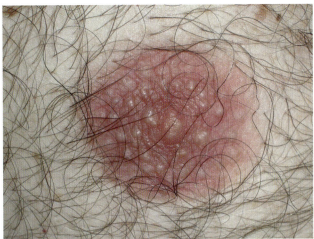

Fig. 5.67 Montgomery tubercules on the areola

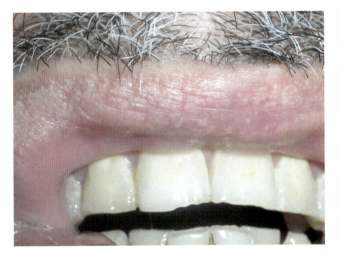

Fig. 5.65 Yellowish, tiny papules showing confluence on the lip; distinctive appearance of Fordyce spots

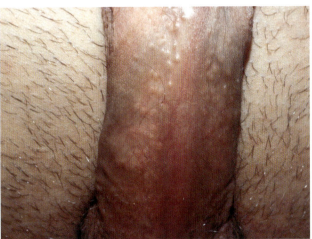

Fig. 5.68 Ectopic sebaceous glands on the corpus penis

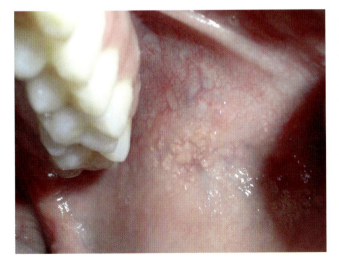

Fig. 5.66 Fordyce spots located on the retromolar area of the buccal mucosa. The lesions show tendency to confluence

papules showing a tendency to confluence are mostly localized on the vermilion border of the lips (*see* Figs. 5.64 and 5.65) and the buccal mucosa, especially on the retromolar area (*see* Fig. 5.66). Because they are asymptomatic, they may be initially diagnosed during physical examination. They are not associated with any systemic disease.

Ectopic sebaceous glands may also be seen on the areola (Montgomery tubercules) (*see* Fig. 5.67), penis (*see* Fig. 5.68), and vulva as similar yellowish papules.

Management. Therapeutic intervention is not necessary.

5.4 Tumors of Smooth Muscles of Skin

Leiomyoma, which is a real smooth muscle tumor, and congenital smooth muscle hamartoma may be seen on the skin.

5.4.1 Leiomyoma

Cutaneous leiomyoma is a rare benign tumor of smooth muscles located on various sites. It may be sporadic or familial. There are three subtypes classified regardless of location but according to the origin of the muscle. Piloleiomyoma arises from the arrector pili muscle, genital (dartoic) leiomyoma arises from the dartos muscles of the scrotum, labia majora, or erectile muscles of the nipple and areola, and angioleiomyoma arises from the muscles of veins.

Piloleiomyoma appears between the ages of 15 and 40 years and mostly on the upper trunk, neck, and extensor parts of the extremities. Multiple lesions (*see* Figs. 5.69 and 5.70) are more common than a solitary lesion. The lesions may be arranged in a linear, grouped (*see* Fig. 5.71), or

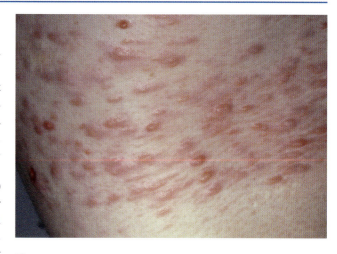

Fig. 5.71 Grouped papules of piloleiomyoma with tendency to confluence

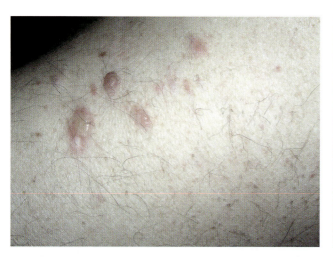

Fig. 5.69 Leiomyoma seen as multiple papular lesions on the trunk; these are piloleiomyomas

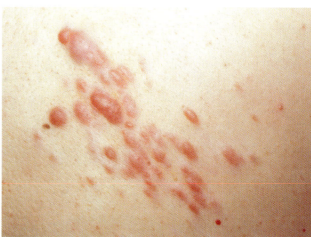

Fig. 5.72 Piloleiomyoma in a segmental pattern. History of associated pain that may be precipitated by trauma is helpful in diagnosis

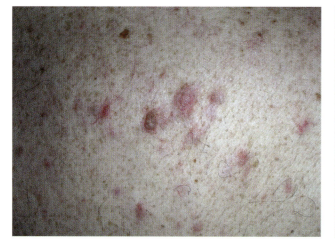

Fig. 5.70 Several discrete, light-brown colored, smooth-surfaced papules of piloleiomyoma is commonly restricted on one body site; lesions on upper trunk is depicted

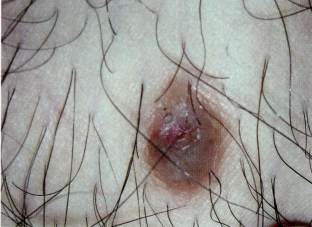

Fig. 5.73 A solitary brownish large nodule diagnosed histopathologically as piloleiomyoma

segmental pattern (*see* Fig. 5.72). Sometimes hundreds of lesions in more than one region of the body may be observed. Individual lesions are flesh, pink, or light brown, smooth-surfaced, firm, oval papules or nodules varying in size between 2 mm and 2 cm (*see* Fig. 5.73). Pain or paresthesia precipitated by trauma, pressure, cold exposure, emotion, or exercise are the main symptoms of piloleiomyomas. Pain occurs as a result of muscle contraction and sometimes may be paroxysmal.

Genital leiomyoma and angioleiomyoma are clinically different from piloleiomyoma. Genital leiomyoma appears on the vulva, scrotum, penis, nipple, and areola, usually as a solitary lesion smaller than 2 cm. It may occur at any age. Lesions may sometimes be pedunculated. Unlike piloleiomyomas, genital leiomyomas are usually asymptomatic.

Angioleiomyoma usually presents with a solitary, firm, large plaque located on the lower limbs, especially on the plantar area. It is more common in middle-aged women. The lesions of angioleiomyoma are painful.

Leiomyomas may sometimes be the sign of some syndromes. Multiple piloleiomyomas may be associated with uterine leiomyomas in Reed syndrome. Multiple cutaneous leiomyomas associated with uterine leiomyomas and renal cell carcinoma is observed in the syndrome "hereditary leiomyomatosis and renal cell cancer" (HLRCC). A germline mutation in the *fumarate hydratase* (FH) gene has been identified in this rare syndrome, which has an autosomal dominant inheritance. Uterine leiomyomas occur in a considerable number of women with HLRCC, especially at young ages. Most patients diagnosed are younger than 30 years of age and need early hysterectomy. Renal cell cancer develops in a small number of patients with HLRCC. This visceral cancer is more common in middle-aged patients but may also appear at young age. Because of its aggressive course, renal cell cancer is of a higher significance and concern in patients with HLRCC. When multiple piloleiomyomas are detected at a young age, patients should be considered for HLRCC, which can allow the early detection of renal cell carcinoma. Since renal cell carcinoma may also appear in children, it is suggested that children of HLRCC families with a pathogenic *FH* mutation could be considered for genetic testing. Appropriate screening measures directed to renal cell carcinoma are advised in children with *FH* mutations.

Genital leiomyoma in females may be seen in Alport syndrome, an X-linked condition of diffuse leiomyomatosis involving the digestive tract, especially the esophagus, tracheobronchial wall, and lower intestinal tract (perirectal area). Hematuric nephropathy, deafness, and ocular abnormalities are other features of this syndrome.

The clinical diagnosis of a solitary leiomyoma is more difficult than that of multiple lesions. Dermatofibroma (*see* Fig. 8.6), dermatofibrosarcoma protuberans (*see* Fig. 13.59), and cutaneous metastasis can be differentiated with a punch or incisional biopsy. Histology reveals broad interlacing fascicles of spindle-shaped smooth muscle cells in the dermis. Subtypes of cutaneous leiomyomas have some slightly different histologic features.

Management. There is no risk of malignant transformation in cutaneous leiomyomas. However, spontaneous regression does not occur, and pain may impact the quality of life. Therefore a therapeutic intervention is generally required. Solitary lesions may be excised. However, multiple lesions are more frequent, rendering surgical excision an inappropriate alternative. Moreover, some lesions are also difficult to excise owing to their size and location. Destructive methods are not preferred for this tumor. Overall, cosmetic results are usually not satisfactory, and recurrence is common. Thus, various medical therapies are used to relieve the pain of cutaneous leiomyomas, promoting smooth muscle relaxation. Amitriptilyn (antidepressant), nifedipine (calcium channel blocker), doxazosin (alfa-1 adrenoreceptor antagonist), phenoxybenzamine (alfa-adrenergic blocker), oral nitroglycerin, and gabapentin (antiepileptic) are among the medical alternatives with different mechanisms of action that are used with variable success. Intralesional botulinum toxin may also be an alternative for the resolution of the pain. Apart from these therapeutic modalities, it is important to avoid the triggering factors of pain.

5.4.2 Congenital Smooth Muscle Hamartoma

Congenital smooth muscle hamartoma is a rare congenital lesion characterized by proliferation of smooth muscles. It is more commonly seen on the trunk, especially on the lumbosacral region and extremities. The typical lesion is a flesh-colored or slightly hyperpigmented, irregularly shaped patch or plaque up to 8 to 10 cm in diameter. It is covered with hairs but these are thin vellus hairs in contrast to the thicker terminal hairs seen in congenital melanocytic nevi (*see* Fig. 3.153). The hyperpigmentation may increase and the hairs overlying may become more prominent with age. The lesion may typically show transient elevation and induration after rubbing, which is called the pseudo-Darier sign. This sign is helpful for diagnosis. Biopsy can be performed to confirm the diagnosis. Well-defined intersecting bundles of smooth muscle fibers in the dermis are the main histopathologic feature.

Management. Since congenital smooth muscle hamartoma does not show malignant transformation, any surgical intervention is not necessary. The correct diagnosis and differentiation from congenital melanocytic nevi avoid unnecessary prophylactic excision.

Suggested Reading

Ali SM, Sangueza OP. What is new in adnexal tumors of the skin. Adv Anat Pathol. 2013;20:334–46.

Alsaad KO, Obaidat NA, Ghazarian D. Skin adnexal neoplasms part 1: an approach to tumours of the pilosebaceous unit. J Clin Pathol. 2007;60:129–44.

Badeloe S, Frank J. Clinical and molecular genetic aspects of hereditary and multiple cutaneous leiomyomatosis. Eur J Dermatol. 2009;19:545–51.

Baykal C, Yazganoglu KD, Buyukbabani N, Erbudak E. Pigmente trikoblastom: olgu sunumu. Turk J Dermatol. 2011;5:107–9.

Blake PW, Toro JR. Update of cylindromatosis gene (CYLD) mutations in Brooke-Spiegler syndrome: novel insights into the role of deubiquitination in cell signaling. Hum Mutat. 2009;30:1025–36.

Bolognia JL, Jorizzo JL, Schaffer JV. Dermatology, edn 3. London: Mosby; 2012.

Bumgardner AC, Hsu S, Nunez-Gussman JK, Schwartz MR. Trichoepitheliomas and eccrine spiradenomas with spiradenoma/cylindroma overlap. Int J Dermatol. 2005;44:415–7.

Burgdorf WHC, Plewig G, Wolff HH, Landthaler M. Braun-Falco's dermatology, edn 3. Italy: Springer-Verlag; 2009.

Cosechen MS, Wojcik AS, Piva FM, Erosive adenomatosis of the nipple. Ann Bras Dermatol. 2011;86(4 Suppl 1):S17–20.

Eisen DB, Michael DJ. Sebaceous lesions and their associated syndromes: part I. J Am Acad Dermatol. 2009;61:549–60.

Eisen DB, Michael DJ. Sebaceous lesions and their associated syndromes: part II. J Am Acad Dermatol. 2009;61:563–78.

Elder DE, Elenitsas R, Johnson BL, Murphy GF, Xu X. Lever's histopathology of the skin, edn 10. Philadelphia: Lippincott Williams and Wilkins; 2008.

Ferzli PG, Millett CR, Newman MD, Heymann WR. The dermatologist's guide to hereditary syndromes with renal tumors. Cutis. 2008;81:41–8.

Garg K, Tickoo SK, Soslow RA, Reuter VE. Morphologic features of uterine leiomyomas associated with hereditary leiomyomatosis and renal cell carcinoma syndrome: a case report. Am J Surg Pathol. 2011;35:1235–7.

Grimalt R, Ferrando J, Mascaro JM. Premature familial sebaceous hyperplasia: successful response to oral isotretinoin in three patients. J Am Acad Dermatol. 1997;37:996–8.

Handler MZ, Derrick KM, Lutz RE, et al. Prevalence of pilomatricoma in Turner syndrome: findings of a multicenter study. JAMA Dermatol. 2013;20:1–6.

Headington JT. Tumors of the hair follicle. A review. Am J Pathol. 1976;85:479–514.

Jackson EM, Cook J. Mohs micrographic surgery of a papillary eccrine adenoma. Dermatol Surg. 2002;28:1168–72.

James WD, Berger T, Elston D. Andrew's Diseases of the Skin: Clinical Dermatology, edn 11. China: Saunders Elsevier; 2011.

Kanitakis J. Adnexal tumours of the skin as markers of cancer-prone syndromes. J Eur Acad Dermatol Venereol. 2010;24:379–87.

Kazakov DV, Vanacek T, Zelger B, et al. Multiple (familial) trichoepitheliomas: a clinicopathological and molecular study including CYLD and PTCH gene analysis, of a series of 16 patients. Am J Dermatopathol. 2011;33:251–65.

Kazakov DV, Zelger B, Rütten A, et al. Morphologic diversity of malignant neoplasms arising in preexisting spiradenoma, cylindroma, and spiradenocylindroma based on the study of 24 cases, sporadic or occurring in the setting of Brooke-Spiegler syndrome. Am J Surg Pathol. 2009;33:705–19.

Laxmisha C, Thappa DM, Jayanthi S. Papillary eccrine adenoma. Indian J Dermatol Venereol Leprol. 2004;70:370–2.

Lee HJ, Chung KY. Erosive adenomatosis of the nipple: Conservation of nipple by Mohs micrographic surgery. J Am Acad Dermatol. 2002;47:578–80.

MacKie RM. Skin cancer: an illustrated guide to aetiology, clinical features, pathology and management of benign and malignant cutaneous tumors, edn 2. England: Martin Dunitz; 1996.

Martorell-Calatayud A, Sanz-Motilva V, Garcia-Sales MA, Calatayud-Blas A. Linear syringocystadenoma papilliferum: an uncommon event with a favorable prognosis. Dermatol Online J. 2011;17:5.

McDonald SK, Goh MS, Chong AH. Successful treatment of cyclosporine-induced sebaceous hyperplasia with oral isotretinoin in two renal transplant recipients. Australas J Dermatol. 2011;52:227–30.

Mentzel T, Kutzner H, Requena L, Hartmann A. Hauttumoren als Markerelaesionen hereditaerer Tumorsyndrome. Pathologie. 2010;31:489–96.

Michal M, Lamovec J, Mukensnabl P, Pizinger K. Spiradenocylindromas of the skin: tumors with morphological features of spiradenoma and cylindroma in the same lesion: report of 12 cases. Pathol Int. 1999;49:419–25.

Obaidat NA, Alsaad KO, Ghazarian D. Skin adnexal neoplasms - part 2: an approach to tumours of cutaneous sweat glands. J Cutan Pathol. 2007;60:145–59.

Obaidat NA, Awamleh AA, Ghazarian DM. Adenocarcinoma in situ arising in a tubulopapillary apocrine hidradenoma of the peri-anal region. Eur J Dermatol. 2006;16:576–8.

Pahwa P, Kaushal S, Gupta S, et al. Linear syringocystadenoma papilliferum: an unusual location. Pediatr Dermatol. 2011;28:61–2.

Patterson JW, Straka BF, Wick MR. Linear syringocystadenoma papilliferum of the thigh. J Am Acad Dermatol. 2001;45:139–41.

Petersson F, Mjörnberg PA, Kazakov DV, Bisceglia M. Eruptive syringoma of the penis. A report of two cases and review of the literature. Am J Dermatopathol. 2009;31:436–8.

Ponti G, Pellacani G, Seidenari S, et al. Cancer-associated genodermatoses: skin neoplasms as clues to hereditary tumor syndromes. Crit Rev Oncol Hematol. 2013;85:239–56.

Rajan N, Trainer AH, Burn J, Langtry JA. Familial cylindromatosis and Brooke-spiegler syndrome: a review of current therapeutic approaches and the surgical challenges posed by two affected families. Dermatol Surg. 2009;35:845–52.

Rütten A, Burgdorf W, Hügel H, et al. Cystic sebaceous tumors as marker lesions for the Muir-Torre syndrome: a histopathologic and molecular genetic study. Am J Dermatopathol. 1999;21:405–14.

Shalin SJ, Lyle S, Calonje E, Lazar AF. Sebaceous neoplasia and the Muir-Torre syndrome: important connections with clinical implications. Histopathology. 2010, 56:133–47.

Smith DR, Mathias CG, Mutasim DF. Multiple eccrine hidrocystoma treated with glycopyrrolate. J Am Acad Dermatol. 2008;59(5 Suppl):S122–3.

van Spaendonck-Zwarts KY, Badeloe S, Oosting SF, et al. Hereditary leiomyomatosis and renal cell cancer presenting as metastatic kidney cancer at 18 years of age: implications for surveillance. Fam Cancer. 2011;11:123–9.

Weedon D. Weedon's skin pathology, edn 3. China: Elsevier; 2010.

Weyers W, Nilles M, Eckert F, Schill WB. Spiradenomas in Brooke-Spiegler syndrome. Am J Dermatopathol. 1993;15:156–61.

Woolery-Lloyd H, Raipara V, Nijhavan RJ. Treatment of multiple periorbital eccrine hidrocystomas: botolinum toxin A. J Drugs Dermatol. 2009;8:71–3.

Yaghoobi R, Zadeh SH, Zadeh AH. Giant linear syringocystadenoma papilliferum on scalp. Indian J Dermatol Venereol Leprol. 2009;75:318–9.

Yazganoglu KD, Baykal C, Buyukbabani N. Spiradenocylindroma: rapid increase in size attributed to hemorrhage. J Dermatol. 2011;38:944–7.

Zhang XJ, Liang YH, He PP, et al. Identification of the cylindromatosis tumor-suppressor gene responsible for multiple familial trichoepithelioma. J Invest Dermatol. 2004;122:658–64.

Vascular Anomalies

Vascular anomalies comprise vascular tumors and vascular malformations. There are various classifications concerning these heterogeneous groups of diseases, and they are still changing. Vascular tumors, which are primarily the result of excess angiogenesis, can be benign or malignant. Benign vascular tumors are among the commonest benign cutaneous soft tissue neoplasms, but the malignant ones are rare. More than half of the benign vascular tumors are acquired and their association with congenital malformations is uncommon. Malignant vascular tumors will be discussed in a different chapter.

Vascular malformations are considered to occur as a result of a defect in vascular development and remodeling. Morphologic abnormalities in these malformations may involve one or more vessel types (e.g., capillaries, veins, arteries, and lymphatics). The great majority of vascular malformations are present at birth. They may show association with other congenital malformations and may appear in the setting of some syndromes. In some genodermatoses various types of vascular tumors and vascular malformations may occur concomitantly. Syndromes associated with vascular anomalies are mentioned in the related topics of the chapter. Lymphedema, which may be associated with lymphatic malformations, is also discussed in this chapter.

6.1 Benign Vascular Tumors

Benign vascular tumors constitute infantile hemangioma, congenital hemangioma, kaposiform hemangioendothelioma, tufted hemangioma, pyogenic granuloma, senile angioma, targetoid hemosiderotic hemangioma, glomeruloid hemangioma, angiolymphoid hyperplasia with eosinophilia, Kimura disease, intravascular papillary endothelial hyperplasia, and glomus tumor. The age of onset, evolution, clinical appearance, histopathologic features, complications, possibility of visceral involvement, associations and prognosis of these tumors vary widely. Therefore each should be considered separately. Glomus tumor and glomangioma (glomuvenous malformation) have been viewed as parts of the same spectrum in the past. However, they are considered separate tumors in the recent classifications of vascular anomalies. Glomus tumor and glomangioma are discussed together under the title of vascular malformations in this book.

6.1.1 Infantile Hemangioma (Capillary Hemangioma)

Infantile hemangioma is a vascular tumor of childhood, mostly benign in nature but at times associated with serious complications. In a great majority of cases it is localized to the skin, but it may rarely be associated with visceral involvement and structural anomalies. It may be present at birth or more commonly may arise in the first weeks of life; it grows rapidly in the early period followed by slow spontaneous involution. It is among the most common benign tumors of infancy and childhood and typically occurs sporadically. The prevalence of infantile hemangioma is estimated to be 3 to 10 percent of Caucasian infants. It is more common in girls than boys. Prematurity, placental anomalies, and low birth weight are the identified risk factors. Hypoxic stress during the intrauterine period is proposed to play a role in the pathogenesis, which is supported by the common occurrence of hemangiomas on pressure prone areas during gestation. However the exact etiopathogenesis is not known. Moreover, the role of genetic factors cannot be ruled out completely since, although rare, familial occurrence has been described.

Parents usually describe the typical evolution of the tumor. Infantile hemangioma is not fully developed at birth and can be noted as an ill-defined telangiectatic or bruise-like patch in the first several weeks of life (see Fig. 6.1). The lesion may be misdiagnosed as nevus flammeus in this period. It grows rapidly to a raised, protuberant, red nodule or mass (see Figs. 6.2 and 6.3) in 3 to 12 months (proliferative phase), follows a stable period during 12 to 36 months, and then shows a very slow regression (see Fig. 6.4a and b) over a period of 3 to 7 years (involutional phase). The fully developed tumor has a smooth or irregular surface. The color gets darker with time.

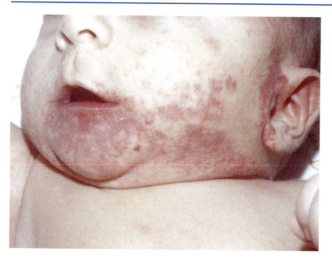

Fig. 6.1 Early lesion of infantile hemangioma presenting as a red telangiectatic patch in a newborn

The occurrence of grey streaks or white areas on the surface, flattening of the mass and lightening of the color are the early signs of the involutional phase (*see* Fig. 6.4b). At the end of the involutional phase, the skin may appear normal or redundant as a result of permanent atrophy and wrinkling (*see* Fig. 6.5). Telangiectases and dyspigmentation can also be observed. Fibro-fatty residual tissue occurring after the involution of deeply located hemangiomas appears as an elevated skin-colored mass (*see* Figs. 6.6 and 6.7). Sometimes regression may cause serious disfigurement.

Infantile hemangiomas may be classified into two variants, "superficial" and "deep," according to the depth of the vascular proliferation in the dermis. Superficial infantile hemangiomas, which are more common, involve the papillary dermis and deep hemangiomas involve the reticular dermis and subcutis. Superficial lesions are also called "strawberry" hemangiomas, and the deep ones are called "cavernous" hemangiomas. These forms have different clinical features and somewhat different prognoses. However, both components may appear concomitantly in one tumor.

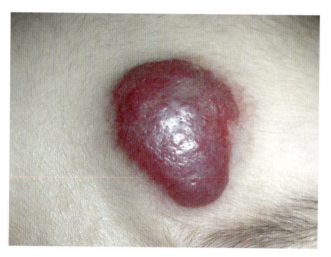

Fig. 6.2 Fully developed infantile hemangioma seen as a red raised nodule on the centrofacial area of a 2-year-old child. Involvement of the head is common

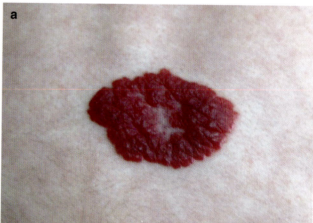

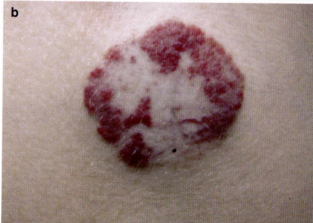

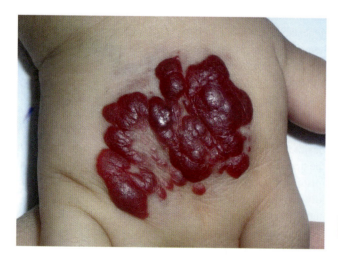

Fig. 6.3 Fully developed infantile hemangioma seen as a red-colored, lobulated, large tumor on the hand. These lesions are asymptomatic

Fig. 6.4 (**a**) Fully developed infantile hemangioma. (**b**) Involuting hemangioma. Note the flattening of the lesion and lightening of the color after two years

6.1 Benign Vascular Tumors

A superficial infantile hemangioma typically presents as a bright red, raised nodule or plaque with well-defined borders (*see* Figs. 6.2 and 6.8) and sometimes shows an irregular, lobulated surface (*see* Figs. 6.3 and 6.9). Some lesions have a patchy configuration (*see* Fig. 6.10). On the other hand, a deep infantile hemangioma presents as an ill-defined, skin-colored or bluish purple swelling, mostly with an intact skin surface. Dilated veins or telangiectases may be seen on the overlying skin (*see* Fig. 6.11). Infantile hemangiomas with both superficial and deep components have overlapping clinical features and are called combined hemangiomas (*see* Fig. 6.12).

Most patients have a solitary or a few tumors, but multiple lesions may also be observed. The head and neck are the most commonly involved sites (*see* Figs. 6.2, 6.8, and 6.10). However, any part of the body, including mucosal surfaces

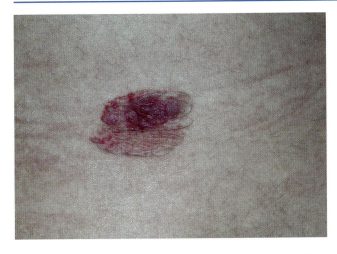

Fig. 6.5 Atrophy and wrinkling at the site of an infantile hemangioma at the end of the involutional phase

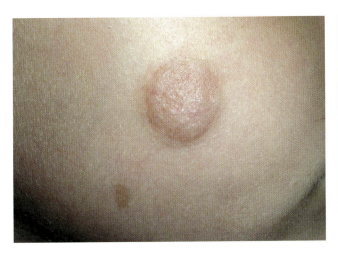

Fig. 6.6 Fibro-fatty residual tissue at the site of an infantile hemangioma after the involutional phase

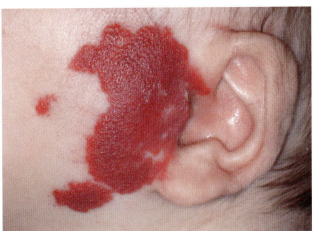

Fig. 6.8 A superficial infantile hemangioma on the preauricular area presenting as a bright red plaque with well-defined borders

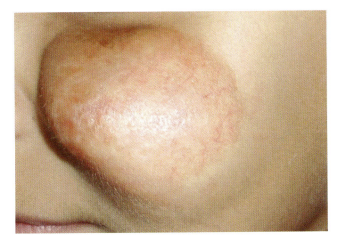

Fig. 6.7 Fibro-fatty residual tissue as a large elevated skin-colored mass at the site of a previous large infantile hemangioma

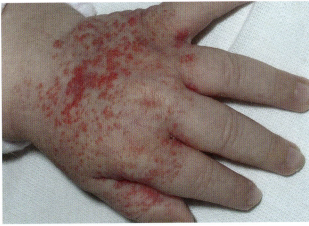

Fig. 6.9 An infantile hemangioma with a lobulated surface involving a broad anatomic area

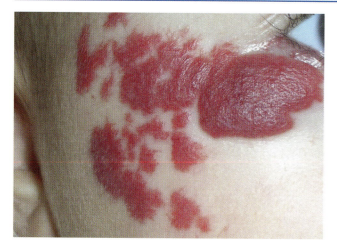

Fig. 6.10 Superficial infantile hemangioma with patchy configuration located on the face

(*see* Figs. 6.13 and 6.14), may be involved. The size of the tumor varies from a pinhead to a large mass (*see* Fig. 6.15). Infantile hemangioma is asymptomatic unless it is ulcerated.

Complications related to infantile hemangioma are closely associated with the size and location of the tumor. Location is also important in predicting the associations of the tumor, such as structural anomalies. Small lesions primarily localized on the centrofacial area (*see* Fig. 6.2) have no prognostic significance. Diffuse (plaque-like) lesions of the face with a segmental distribution (*see* Figs. 6.16 and 6.17) are prone to ulceration and can be part of PHACES syndrome. This acronym refers to posterior fossa brain abnormalities, hemangioma on a specific location, arterial abnormalities, coarctation of the aorta and other cardiac defects, eye anomalies, and sternal agenesia or supraumbilical raphae. Similar to cutaneous hemangiomas, the cerebral

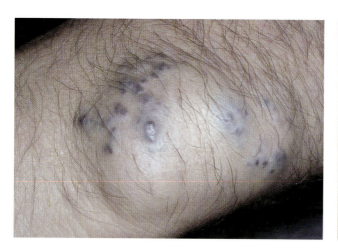

Fig. 6.11 Deep infantile hemangioma presenting as a skin-colored, elevated mass with overlying telangiectases

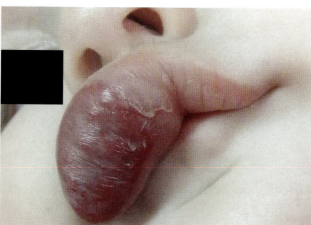

Fig. 6.13 Infantile hemangioma appearing as a raised red tumor on the upper lip. Involvement of the lips is not uncommon

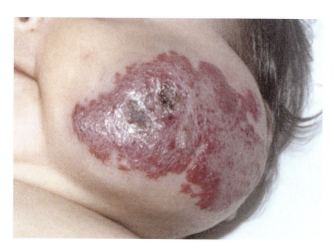

Fig. 6.12 Combined hemangioma showing clinical features of superficial and deep infantile hemangiomas concomitantly

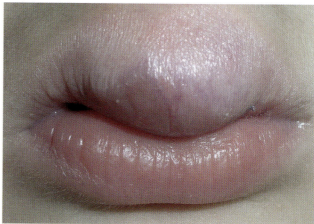

Fig. 6.14 Infantile hemangioma seen as a bluish deep nodule on the upper lip

6.1 Benign Vascular Tumors

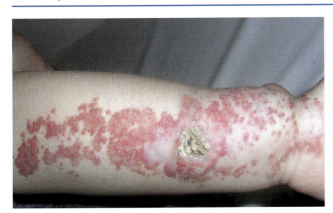

Fig. 6.15 Large infantile hemangioma with a linear shape located on the arm

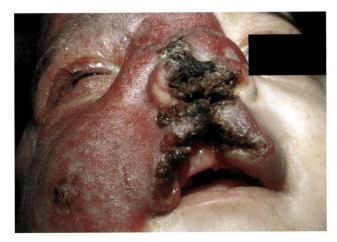

Fig. 6.16 Deeply ulcerated diffuse infantile hemangioma on the face with segmental distribution (With kind permission from Springer Science+Business Media: Baykal C, Yazganoğlu KD. Dermatological diseases of the nose and ears; 2010)

anomalies in these patients are also suggested to be related to hypoxia during the maternal period. Segmental hemangiomas are more common in females. The possibility of spontaneous regression is low with increased risk of residual disfigurement. In cases with large facial hemangiomas, imaging studies need to be performed in order to search for possible brain involvement. Hemangiomas of other organs may also accompany the cutaneous hemangiomas in this syndrome.

Deep infantile hemangiomas of the nasal tip may cause bulbous prominence of the nose that is called "Cyrano nose" (*see* Fig. 6.18). Hemangiomas on this location may invade the cartilage, leading to the development of fibrous tissue. Large hemangiomas of the nose may obstruct the nostrils and cause respiratory difficulties. Infantile hemangiomas on the beard area (preauricular area, chin, lower lip, and anterior neck) (*see* Fig. 6.19) may be associated with hemangiomas of the upper airways; this may cause obstruction resulting in life-threatening respiratory distress. Croup-like cough may be a sign of respiratory distress in such patients. Large hemangiomas on the external ear (*see* Fig. 6.17) can obstruct the external auditory canal and cause hearing loss. Preauricular infantile hemangiomas (*see* Fig. 6.8) may be associated with parotid involvement. Large hemangiomas on the eyelids (*see* Figs. 6.17 and 6.20) may occlude the visual axis and may compress the eyeball, resulting in strabismus, astigmatism, and permanent amblyopia. Moreover, a large infantile hemangioma around the mouth may interfere with feeding.

Large infantile hemangiomas covering almost the entire limb without a segmental distribution may also be found (*see* Fig. 6.21). Kaposiform hemangioendothelioma must be differentiated from these large lesions. However, lesions of kaposiform hemangioendothelioma are ill-defined,

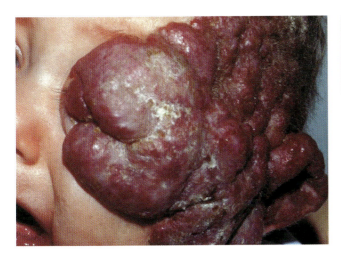

Fig. 6.17 Diffuse infantile hemangioma on the face with segmental distribution. This may be a marker of PHACES syndrome

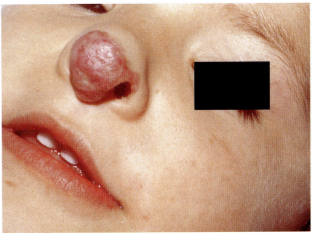

Fig. 6.18 Infantile hemangioma of the nasal tip causing a "Cyrano nose" appearance (With kind permission from Springer Science+Business Media: Baykal C, Yazganoğlu KD. Dermatological diseases of the nose and ears; 2010)

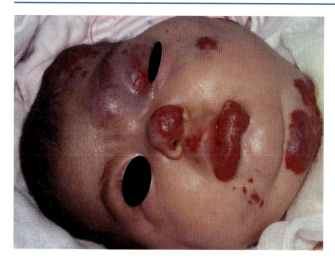

Fig. 6.19 Large infantile hemangioma on the face and neck. Deep lesions on the neck may cause obstruction of the upper airways

bruise-like patches or indurated plaques that may extend rapidly. Deep infantile hemangiomas of the breast may cause impairment of the development of mammary glands, causing breast asymmetry, mainly in females (*see* Fig. 6.22). Infantile hemangioma may also be located on the vulva (*see* Fig. 6.22) and penis. These lesions do not show different biological behavior. However, ulceration and bleeding may be a problem. Moreover, hemangiomas of the genitalia that do not regress may cause sexual dysfunction. Infantile hemangiomas on the perineal and lumbosacral regions (*see* Fig. 6.23) may be associated with spinal dysraphism, tethered cord syndrome, anogenital and cutaneous abnormalities, and renal and urologic anomalies. Neurologic symptoms may develop in later life. Central nerve system involvement or visceral hemangiomas leading to gastrointestinal bleeding may be life-threatening in some cases.

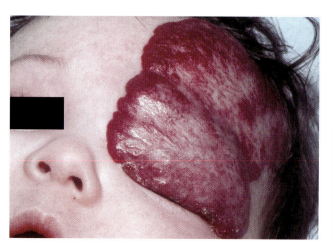

Fig. 6.20 Large infantile hemangioma around the eye, posing a high risk for ocular complications

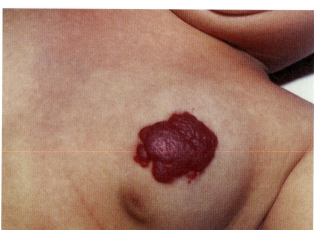

Fig. 6.22 Infantile hemangioma with superficial and deep components located on the breast

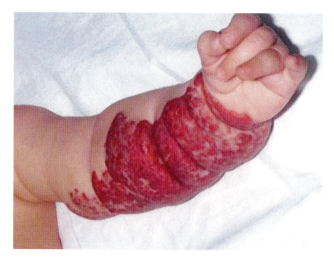

Fig. 6.21 Large infantile hemangioma covering the arm

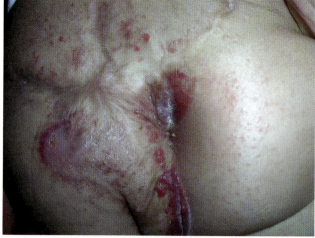

Fig. 6.23 Infantile hemangioma on the lumbosacral region. Note the scar of the operation for spinal dysraphism

Oral hemangiomas are mostly seen on the lips (see Figs. 6.13 and 6.14), tongue (see Figs. 6.24 and 6.25), palate, and buccal mucosa but may occur at any oropharyngeal location. They may be flat or slightly raised and are mostly ill-defined. The tumors are rubbery in texture. Reddish or slightly bluish lesions are asymptomatic. However, mucosal hemangiomas may ulcerate easily (see Fig. 6.16), and bleeding may be a problem. Some lesions extend into the underlying musculature. Rapidly progressing infantile hemangiomas on the oropharynx or lesions causing difficulties while feeding or airway obstruction need urgent intervention. Oral infantile hemangiomas may be confused with oral angiomatous lesions representing vascular malformations occurring sporadically or in the setting of syndromes such as Sturge-Weber (see Figs. 6.109 and 6.110), Klippel-Trenaunay, and Maffucci. Additionally, pyogenic granuloma (see Fig. 6.44) and lymphangioma circumscriptum (see Figs. 6.202 and 6.203) are differential diagnostic considerations in the oral mucosa.

Ulceration is a serious complication of infantile hemangioma (see Fig. 6.26), and it is more common on larger superficial lesions of the perineum and segmental facial lesions (see Fig. 6.16). It occurs mostly during the proliferative phase and may be very painful. Perineal ulcerated hemangiomas can cause painful defecation. Moreover, secondary bacterial infections may complicate the condition. Bleeding may occur and can cause anemia. Ulceration may result in regional permanent atrophy or scarring (see Fig. 6.27). Sensorial function may be impaired in these areas.

Infantile hemangiomas should primarily be differentiated from other benign vascular tumors and vascular malformations. The clinical features, age of onset, and typical history of the evolution of the tumor mostly allow an accurate

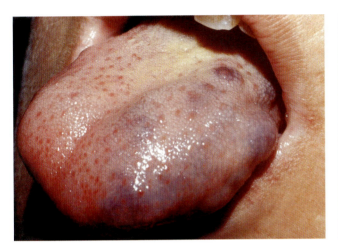

Fig. 6.24 Infantile hemangioma causing enlargement of the tongue

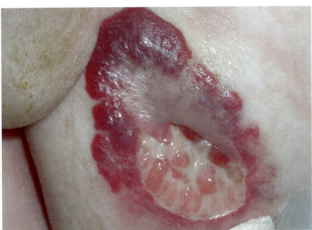

Fig. 6.26 Infantile hemangioma with a deep ulceration. These patients may suffer from recurrent bleeding

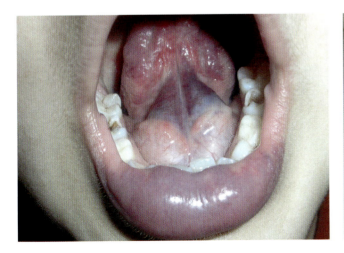

Fig. 6.25 Infantile hemangioma involving the lower lip and tongue concomitantly

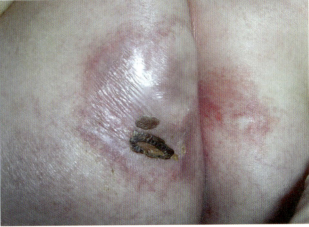

Fig. 6.27 Regional scarring at the site of an ulcerated infantile hemangioma after involution

diagnosis. A biopsy is rarely required. The main histopathologic features are vascular lumina lined by plump endothelial cells and a lobular architecture. The vascular channels are arranged in distinct lobules, separated by a delicate stroma. In involuted lesions the vascular lumina become more dilated, and the endothelial lining appears more flattened. Stromal fibrous tissue relatively increases, and microscopically this creates the impression that cellularity of the lesion has decreased. Glucose transporter-1 (GLUT 1), an erythrocyte-type glucose transporter protein, is expressed in endothelial cells in all phases of evolution and is a useful tool for distinguishing between infantile hemangioma and other vascular tumors such as kaposiform hemangioendothelioma, tufted angioma, congenital hemangioma, and vascular malformations.

Further examination is not routinely indicated in patients with infantile hemangiomas. Ultrasound may help to show the depth of deep tumors. However, especially patients with segmental facial and lumbosacral infantile hemangiomas should undergo additional investigation. Cranial magnetic resonance imaging (MRI), ophthalmologic examination, and echocardiography of the major cervical and thoracic vessels are indicated for facial segmental tumors, and medullar and pelvic MRI are indicated for lumbosacral hemangiomas. Furthermore, patients with multiple hemangiomas deserve special attention. Newborns with multiple infantile hemangiomas should be evaluated for diffuse neonatal hemangiomatosis, a distinct entity causing visceral involvement, with ultrasound or MRI of visceral organs.

Management. As most infantile hemangiomas show spontaneous involution with a satisfactory cosmetic result, therapeutic intervention is usually not necessary. Therefore, in solitary indolent lesions, the best approach is simple observation of spontaneous regression. Serial photography may be useful during this observation period. However, parents of the children are not always satisfied with the wait-and-see approach and may anticipate an immediate solution. It should be explained to the parents that aggressive therapy may cause morbidity, and surgical methods may result in scar formation. On the other hand, if permanent disfigurement is expected at the end of the involution period, such as in the presence of large lesions (*see* Fig. 6.28), then therapy can be applied. Furthermore, location, growth/involution rate, and ulceration of the tumor as well as hemorrhage and threatened interference with organ functions determine the therapeutic indications of infantile hemangiomas.

Different therapeutic alternatives are available for infantile hemangiomas, including a wide spectrum of medical therapies. Topical drugs (corticosteroids, beta-blockers, imiquimod), systemic drugs (corticosteroids, beta-blockers, interferon-alfa, vincristine), laser therapy, and radical surgery may be chosen in individual cases or a combination of different interventions may be required.

Although not routinely used, potent topical corticosteroids may be helpful in the therapy of small superficial infantile hemangiomas (*see* Fig. 6.29a and b). Cutaneous

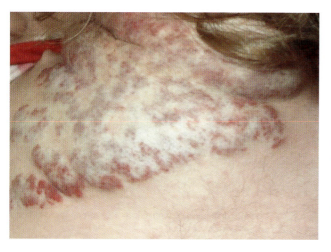

Fig. 6.28 Dyspigmentation and telangiectases after partial regression of large infantile hemangioma

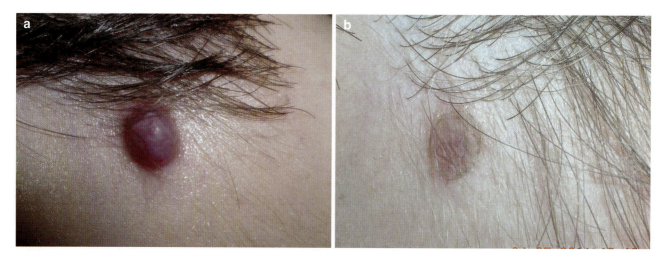

Fig. 6.29 (**a**) A small infantile hemangioma before treatment. (**b**) Regression after therapy with topical corticosteroid oinment

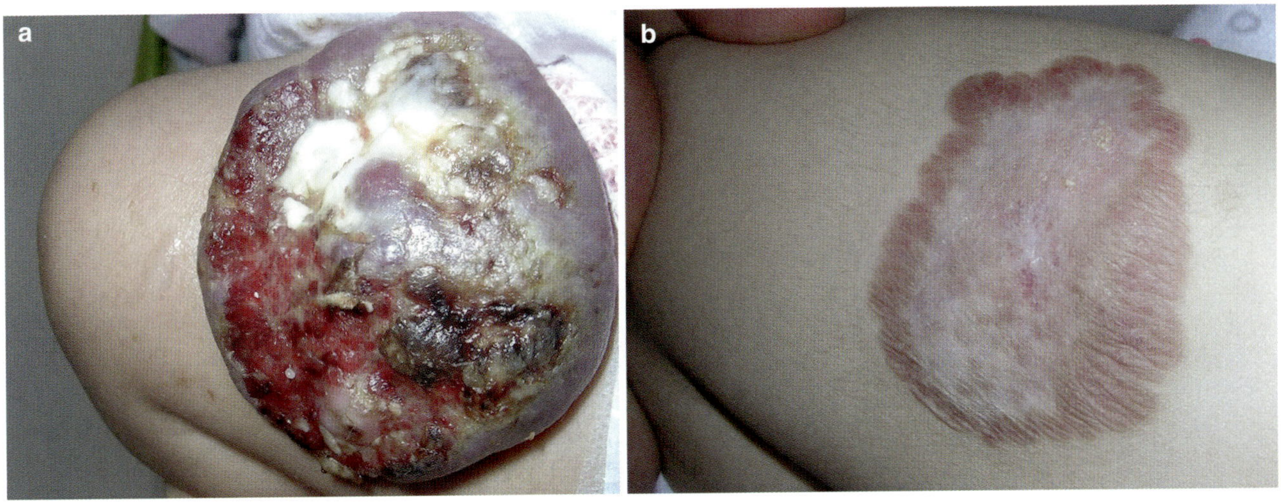

6.1 Benign Vascular Tumors

Fig. 6.30 (**a**) A large mass of ulcerated infantile hemangioma located on the leg. (**b**) Ulceration has healed and the lesion has flattened with central atrophy after six months of therapy with propranolol

atrophy and striae reflect adverse reactions to these drugs. Nonselective beta-blockers, such as propranolol and timolol, can be used topically for small nonulcerated infantile hemangiomas, especially those without a subcutaneous component. Topical administration of imiquimod can also be effective. Hemangiomas with small ulcers can initially be treated with wet compresses and topical antiseptics or antibiotics. But extensive and chronic ulcers, especially those associated with bleeding, should be managed with intralesional corticosteroids or flash lamp–pulsed dye laser. Intralesional injections (triamcinolone acetonide 10 to 20 mg/mL) are administered at several points of the tumor monthly for 2 to 3 months. This method is not preferred for periorbital hemangiomas because of the risk of serious ocular complications.

Systemic drugs should be used in segmental and multifocal infantile hemangiomas, lesions with high risk of permanent disfigurement, or hemangiomas at special locations that are prone to develop serious complications. Systemic corticosteroids were the mainstay of therapy for high-risk hemangiomas before the recently proved effectiveness of systemic beta-blockers. Propranolol also has a fast, dramatic initial effect in extensive infantile hemangiomas. Vasoconstriction of microvessels is the proposed mechanism of action. Ulcers heal initially. Regression in thickness and fading of color may be observed in months (*see* Fig. 6.30a and b). However, propranolol has side effects such as bronchospasm (wheezing), bradycardia, hypoglycemia, and insomnia; therefore patients should be followed carefully. Acebutolol and atenolol (hydrophilic beta-1 selective blocking agents) are other types of beta-blockers that can also be effective for these hemangiomas. After discontinuation of therapy, mild recoloration or relapse may occur. On the other hand, rare cases, especially deeper ones, show resistance to therapy with beta-blockers.

Systemic corticosteroids are employed at high initial doses (prednisolone 2 to 4 mg/kg/day) for 2 to 8 weeks during the proliferative period of infantile hemangiomas in selected cases. Then, the dose is tapered progressively, depending on the response. The mechanism of action of corticosteroids is poorly understood. Therapeutic effect appears within 2 to 3 weeks. Lesions may fade and become smaller (*see* Fig. 6.31a and b). Besides transient side effects, hypertension, hypertrophic cardiomyopathy, and adrenal insufficiency may occur during long-term therapy, limiting the use of systemic corticosteroids. On the other hand, the response rate is variable and recurrence is possible.

Interferon is a second-line therapeutic option used in severe complicated infantile hemangiomas. Both interferon alfa-2a and alfa-2b may be used because of their antiangiogenic effect. The drug is injected subcutaneously, and the duration of the therapy is usually long. There is a risk of neurotoxicity in childhood. Furthermore, the results are not always satisfactory. A chemotherapeutic agent, vincristine, is also a second-line choice in cases not responding to above-mentioned systemic drugs.

Some lasers (pulsed dye, Nd:YAG) based on the principle of selective photothermolysis, are especially effective in superficial variants of hemangiomas, but hemangiomas with a deep component are not usually responsive to these therapies. Therefore, the lasers are not routinely used for infantile hemangiomas. Early intervention does not always prevent the proliferation of hemangiomas and their invasion to deeper dermis or subcutis. On the other hand, telangiectasia and residual scarring that occur after the involution period may be treated with lasers.

Surgery may be used early in the proliferation phase and also for residual scarring. If medical therapy is contraindicated or not effective in complicated hemangiomas, excision can be

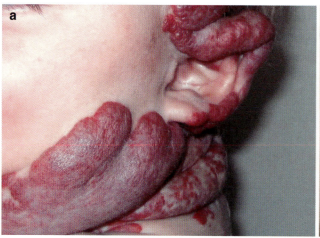
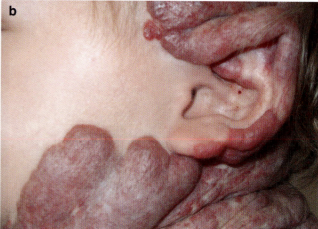

Fig. 6.31 (a) An extensive infantile hemangioma involving the scalp, auricle, and neck. (b) The lesion partially flattened and blanched after therapy with systemic corticosteroids

an alternative. When poor cosmetic results are expected, especially in cases with facial lesions, complete surgical removal can be planned after reducing the tumor size with beta-blocker or corticosteroid therapy. However, sometimes surgical scars may be worse than the postinvolutional results. Cosmetic surgery may be used for atrophic wrinkling and fibro fatty residual tissue that occur following natural involution of some hemangiomas in the late period (see Figs. 6.6 and 6.7).

6.1.1.1 Diffuse Neonatal Hemangiomatosis

Multiple infantile hemangiomas present at birth or appear in the first weeks of life have a special prognostic importance. In cases with only multiple cutaneous hemangiomas, the condition is called benign neonatal hemangiomatosis. However, if cutaneous hemangiomas are associated with visceral hemangiomas, the term diffuse neonatal hemangiomatosis is used. The skin lesions of both conditions are common. The number of hemangiomas is variable. Some patients have disseminated lesions (see Fig. 6.32). Any area of the body (see Figs. 6.33, 6.34 and 6.35), including mucosal surfaces (see Fig. 6.36a) may be involved. The lesions are typically infantile hemangiomas of the superficial type. Initial lesions may be 2 to 10 mm in diameter, clinically resembling senile angiomas. However these hemangiomas show a progressive course with rapid increase in the size of the lesions (see Figs. 6.36a and b, and 6.37a and b). The histopathology of these tumors is similar to that of classic infantile hemangiomas and the GLUT1 stain is also positive. Therefore, they are also called multifocal infantile hemangiomas.

All infants with multiple infantile hemangiomas should be screened for internal hemangiomas. The liver (most common), lungs, spleen, stomach, small intestine, large intestine and brain may be involved. Kidney and bone involvement are not expected. Radiologic examinations,

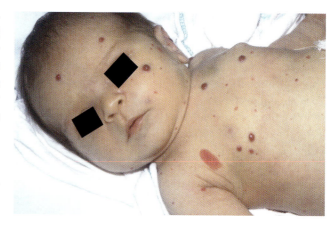

Fig. 6.32 Diffuse neonatal hemangiomatosis presenting as multiple lesions in a newborn. The patients should be evaluated about systemic involvement

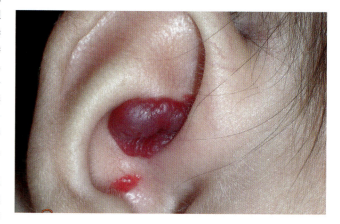

Fig. 6.33 Small hemangiomas on the ear of a patient with diffuse neonatal hemangiomatosis. Any body site may be involved

6.1 Benign Vascular Tumors

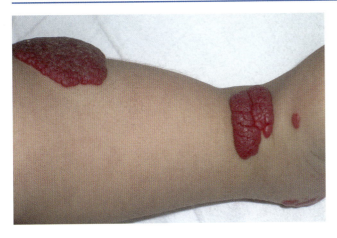

Fig. 6.34 Large hemangiomas on the leg of a patient with diffuse neonatal hemangiomatosis

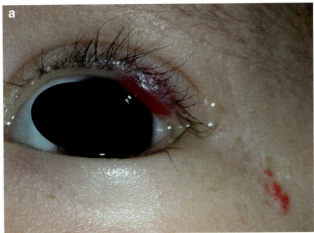

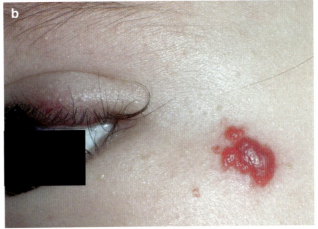

Fig. 6.36 (a) Hemangiomas on the periorbital skin and mucosa (conjunctiva) in an infant with diffuse neonatal hemangiomatosis. (b) Note the enlargement of the lesions in a few months

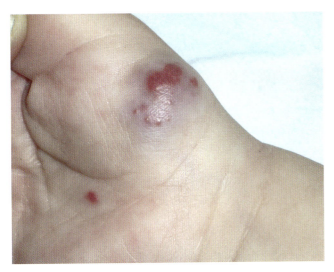

Fig. 6.35 Hemangiomas on palmoplantar area in a patient with diffuse neonatal hemangiomatosis

including ultrasonography and MRI, may be used for diagnosis and monitoring of internal hemangiomas. Hepatic hemangiomatosis has a high risk of cardiac failure. Gastrointestinal bleeding, visceral hemorrhage, and hydrocephaly are other complications of internal hemangiomas.

Management. Lesions of benign neonatal hemangiomatosis involute spontaneously in a few years (*see* Fig. 6.37a-c). The management of an individual lesion is similar to that of solitary infantile hemangioma. Large or ulcerated lesions are commonly treated (*see* Fig. 6.38a and b).

Diffuse neonatal hemangiomatosis may be a life-threatening disorder due to the severity of organ involvement that should be treated aggressively and monitored closely. High-dose systemic corticosteroids or propranolol may be used. Both cutaneous and internal hemangiomas usually respond well to these drugs but sometimes progression cannot be stopped. High-risk surgical interventions such as lobectomy, ligation, and arterial embolization may be required for hepatic hemangiomas.

6.1.2 Congenital Hemangioma

In contrast to infantile hemangiomas that proliferate after birth, congenital hemangiomas are fully formed at birth. They may be detected on prenatal ultrasound imaging. Congenital hemangiomas can be classified according to their biological behavior as rapidly involuting or noninvoluting congenital hemangiomas. Both types of tumor are sporadic.

Rapidly involuting congenital hemangioma is stable or shows little development in the postnatal period but spontaneously involutes within the 12 to 18 months of life. It is equally seen in girls and boys. It is predominantly located on the lower extremities and face as large violaceus superficial

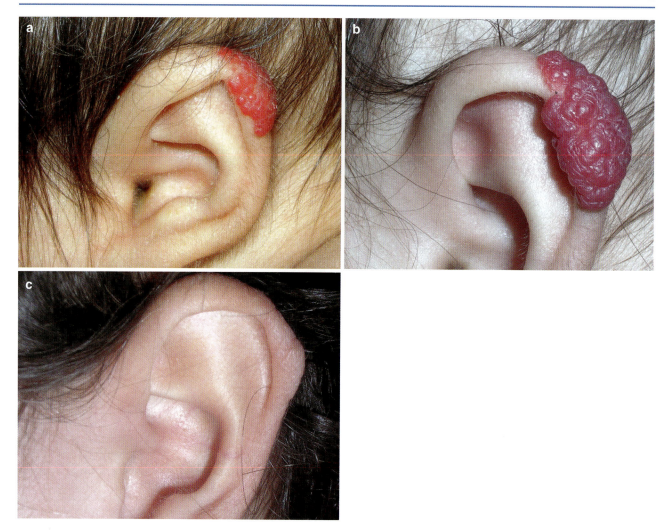

Fig. 6.37 (**a**) Hemangioma on the auricle in an infant with diffuse neonatal hemangiomatosis. This patient with multiple lesions did not have systemic involvement and has been considered as benign neonatal hemangiomatosis. (**b**) Enlargement of the lesion in a few months. (**c**) Spontaneous involution of the lesion after two years

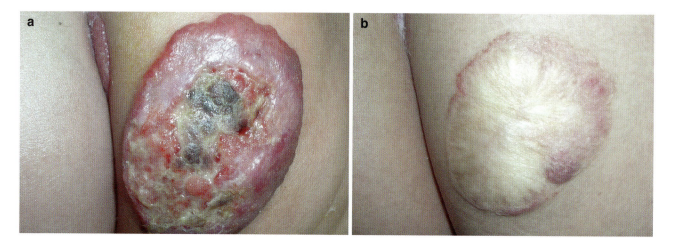

Fig. 6.38 (**a**) Large, ulcerated hemangioma on the gluteal region of a patient with benign neonatal hemangiomatosis. (**b**) The lesion was successfully treated with intralesional corticosteroid (triamcinolone acetonide) resulting with scarring as seen in the figure

tumors. Ulceration and necrosis may be observed. The tumor may regress, leaving loose skin or scarring (*see* Fig. 6.39).

The rare subtype of congenital hemangioma characterized by persistent lesions is called noninvoluting congenital hemangioma. It is present at birth and tends to grow in proportion to the child's growth. It is observed as a large pink to reddish purple tumor with overlying coarse telangiectases (*see* Fig. 6.40). It may be warm to the touch. Severe complications are not expected.

As opposed to the development of infantile hemangioma, a characteristic evolution period is absent in congenital hemangioma. Both tumors have similar histologic features. Infantile fibrosarcoma (*see* Fig. 13.66) may be another differential diagnostic challenge, but its histopathologic features are completely different.

Management. In congenital hemangiomas that spontaneously shrink, any unnecessary invasive diagnostic procedure and aggressive therapeutic intervention should be avoided. Close observation is essential. Medications are not very effective for noninvoluting congenital hemangioma, and excisional surgery and plastic reconstruction is the therapy of choice if necessary.

6.1.3 Kaposiform Hemangioendothelioma

Kaposiform hemangioendothelioma is an endothelial-derived spindle cell neoplasm of the skin, deep soft tissue, and bone. Spindle cells with slit-like vascular lumina forming this hemangioma are the reason for the term "kaposiform." It occurs nearly always in infants and young children, but is very rare in comparison with infantile hemangioma. The tumor has a predilection for the retroperitoneum and deep soft tissues of the extremities. But other body areas and the mediastinum may also be involved. The clinical features of cutaneous tumors are generally not distinctive. It has tendency to invade the neighboring tissue, causing ill-defined lesions. The clinical picture is also determined by the depth of the lesion. A variety of clinical presentations include purpuric, telangiectatic macules, ill-defined nodules, or infiltrated plaques that may be variable in color such as pink, purple, or red to brown. The diagnosis is based on histologic examination. The tumor is composed of nodules or sheets of bland spindle cells, lining slit-like or crescent-shaped narrow vascular channels. This tumor is negative for GLUT1 staining.

As opposed to infantile hemangioma and congenital hemangioma, kaposiform hemangioendothelioma is often associated with Kasabach-Merritt syndrome, which is a life-threatening complication causing consumption coagulopathy. Thrombocytes and clotting factors are consumed within the mass of this hemangioma. The coagulopathy mostly develops during the first year of life. When coagulopathy occurs, the tumor enlarges rapidly and becomes firm, tender, and hemorrhagic. Bleeding of the hemangioma or different sites including visceral organs should alert physicians to the possible development of Kasabach-Merritt syndrome. Thrombocytopenia, hemolytic anemia, and abnormalities of clotting markers are the hematologic findings of this reaction.

Lesions may show a stable course, and especially the small ones may regress in time. Larger lesions are more commonly associated with Kasabach-Merritt syndrome. Tumors may be very aggressive locally but have no metastatic potential. Kaposiform hemangioendothelioma may rarely be associated with lymphangiomatosis.

Management. Different therapeutic options mainly depending on the size and location of the hemangioma include interferon alfa, laser therapy (pulsed dye, argon),

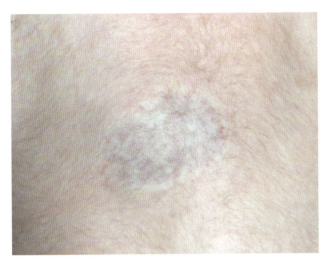

Fig. 6.39 Localized atrophy and telangiectases evident after regression of a rapidly involuting congenital hemangioma in an infant. The evolution of these lesions are different from infantile hemangiomas

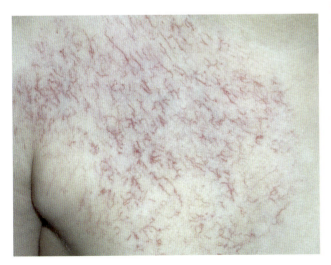

Fig. 6.40 Noninvoluting congenital hemangioma with overlying dense telangiectases in an adolescent

surgical excision, and arterial embolization. Sirolimus, a mTOR inhibitor drug, is a new therapeutic option.

The main consideration of aggressive treatment depends on the presence of Kasabach-Merritt syndrome. Vincristine, a vinca alkaloid, may be administered in patients with Kasabach-Merritt syndrome. Aspirin or other antiplatelet agents can be used to prevent coagulopathy.

6.1.4 Tufted Angioma

Tufted angioma is a rare type of benign vascular tumor localized to the skin and subcutaneous tissues. Most cases appear during the first 5 years of life, but it may also occur at birth or in adulthood. The tumor continues to enlarge slowly to a particular size in months to years and then remains stable. The upper trunk and neck are most commonly involved. It appears as a solitary, ill-defined, dull red or purple patch or infiltrated plaque and is clinically indistinguishable from kaposiform hemangioendothelioma. Some lesions may be tender. There may be superimposed angiomatous papules. Overlying hypertrichosis can be noted in some lesions. The size of the tumor varies from 2 to 5 cm. Histologic examination of the lesion reveals a cannonball pattern, which is described as distinct lobules of capillary vessels in the dermis and accompanying dilated small caliber vessels usually at their periphery. Tumoral cells are negative for GLUT1. Although not very often, Kasabach-Merritt syndrome may occur as a complication of this hemangioma.

Management. Spontaneous regression may occasionally be observed in tufted angioma. Clinical changes of the tumor and hematologic parameters for signs of Kasabach-Merritt syndrome should be closely monitored. Complete surgical excision, radiotherapy, and lasers have been tried for tufted angiomas with variable success.

6.1.5 Pyogenic Granuloma

Pyogenic granuloma is a common benign acquired capillary hemangioma occurring especially at sites of minor trauma. In contrast to its name, it is neither an infectious nor a granulomatous disease. It occurs more often in children and young adults as a solitary friable tumor. Its frequency is increased in pregnancy. However, pyogenic granuloma is not associated with any systemic disease. Lesions are more common on the hands (*see* Fig. 6.41) and head (*see* Fig. 6.42) but may occur anywhere on the skin and also on mucosal surfaces, especially the lips (*see* Fig. 6.43), gingivae, tongue (*see* Fig. 6.44), and nasal vestibule (*see* Fig. 6.45). Gingival lesions occurring during pregnancy are called granuloma gravidarum. The fingers are the most commonly involved sites (*see* Fig. 6.46). Patients typically describe the sudden onset and rapid growth

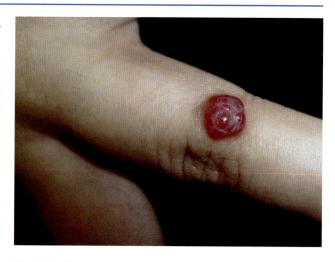

Fig. 6.41 Pyogenic granuloma on the hand manifesting as a solitary red dome-shaped nodule. Patients typically describe recent onset of these tumors

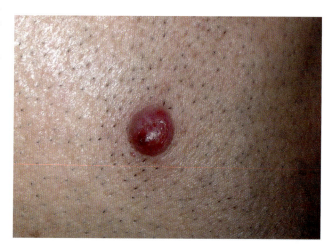

Fig. 6.42 Pyogenic granuloma on the face presenting as a small, sessile lesion

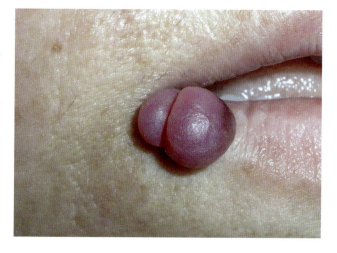

Fig. 6.43 A lobulated pyogenic granuloma on the lip. Besides skin, mucosae may also be involved

6.1 Benign Vascular Tumors

of the solitary exophytic tumor. Pyogenic granuloma expands rapidly in the first weeks and reaches a size of approximately 8 to 10 mm but then stabilizes. Multiple eruptive pyogenic granulomas distributed over the body (*see* Figs. 6.47 and 6.48) are extremely rare.

The typical lesion is a friable, red, sessile, dome-shaped nodule mostly with an eroded, moist surface (*see* Fig. 6.49). However, it may be stalky (*see* Figs. 6.50 and 6.51) or lobulated (*see* Figs. 6.52 and 6.53). The color of the tumor may sometimes be dirty yellow (*see* Fig. 6.49), and the surface may be intact (*see* Fig. 6.53) or crusted (*see* Figs. 6.54 and 6.55). A collarette of scale on the periphery of the tumor (*see* Fig. 6.56) is a diagnostic clue but is not always present. Oozing may be seen in eroded lesions. Tumors with an eroded surface tend to bleed easily at the slightest trauma, which may sometimes only be controlled with tampons.

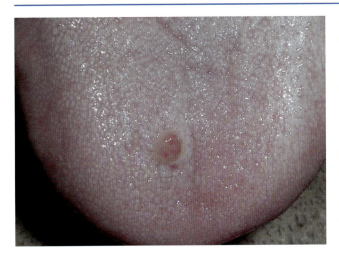

Fig. 6.44 Pyogenic granuloma on the tongue

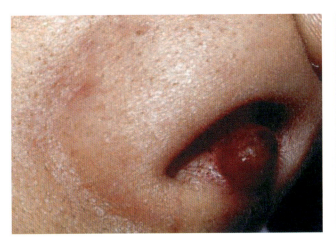

Fig. 6.45 Pyogenic granuloma on the nasal vestibule (With kind permission from Springer Science+Business Media: Baykal C, Yazganoğlu KD. Dermatological diseases of the nose and ears; 2010)

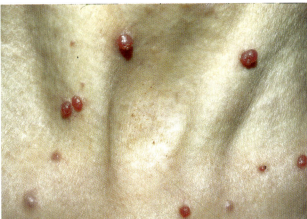

Fig. 6.47 Multiple eruptive pyogenic granulomas on the neck and upper trunk. This is an extremely rare presentation

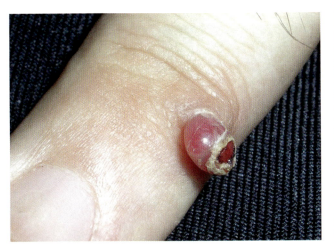

Fig. 6.46 Pyogenic granuloma on the finger presenting as a pedunculated nodule. Areas exposed to trauma are more commonly involved

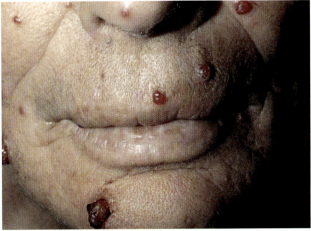

Fig. 6.48 Multiple eruptive pyogenic granulomas on the face appearing as numerous small angiomatous papules

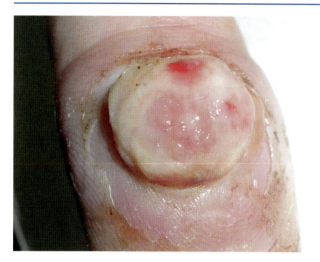

Fig. 6.49 Dome-shaped, glistening, dirty yellow-colored pyogenic granuloma with an eroded surface located on the finger

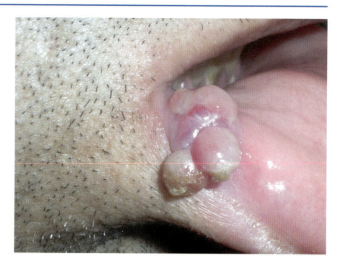

Fig. 6.52 Lobulated pyogenic granuloma with eroded surface located on the lip

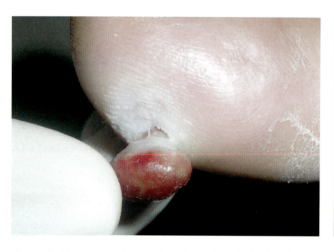

Fig. 6.50 Stalky pyogenic granuloma located on the heel. This morphology may be seen in some cases

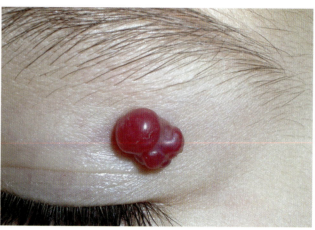

Fig. 6.53 Lobulated pyogenic granuloma with intact surface located on the eyelid

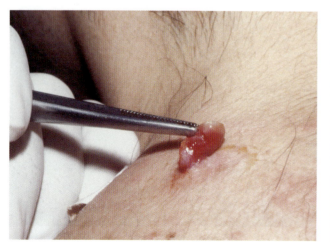

Fig. 6.51 Stalky pyogenic granuloma with eroded surface

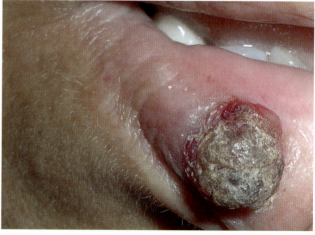

Fig. 6.54 Pyogenic granuloma on the lower lip with crusted surface

6.1 Benign Vascular Tumors

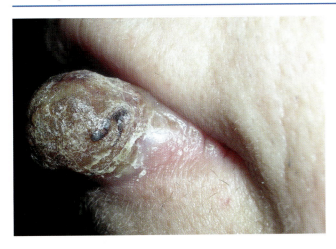

Fig. 6.55 Heavily crusted exophytic pyogenic granuloma on the lower lip. Bleeding is the main complaint related with this hemangioma

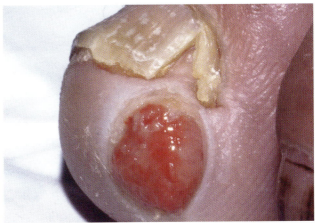

Fig. 6.57 Periungual pyogenic granuloma causing nail destruction

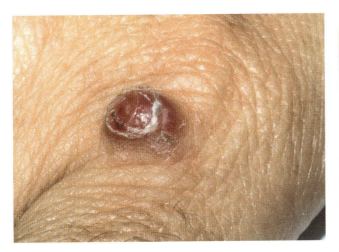

Fig. 6.56 Pyogenic granuloma with a collarette of scale at the periphery, a typical presentation

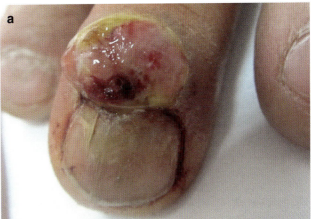

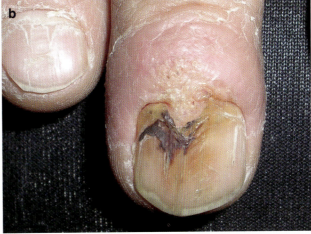

Fig. 6.58 (a) Pyogenic granuloma located on the proximal nailfold. (b) Nail destruction is remarkable after spontaneous healing of the lesion

Lesions located on periungual (*see* Fig. 6.57) and subungual areas may cause secondary nail destruction (*see* Fig. 6.58a and b) and onycholysis. Tumors may be asymptomatic or painful.

The rapid growth of the hemangioma may lead to concern about malignancy. Although it is a relatively slow-growing tumor, amelanotic melanoma (*see* Fig. 12.55) may be a diagnostic challenge and histopathologic confirmation is frequently necessary. Excess (hypertrophic) granulation tissue, which manifests as an exuberant irregular nodule with eroded surface, may also resemble pyogenic granuloma. Senile angioma with a relatively larger papule (*see* Figs. 6.67 and 6.69) may be similar to pyogenic granuloma, but its surface is typically intact. Palmoplantar lesions of pyogenic granuloma (*see* Fig. 6.59) may be similar to those of poroma (*see* Fig. 5.15) and Kaposi sarcoma (*see* Fig. 13.24). Bacillary angiomatosis, Bartonella infection motly seen in HIV-infected patients, is another differential diagnostic consideration. On histopathologic examination of pyogenic granuloma, an epidermal collarette encircles the lesion, composed of lobules

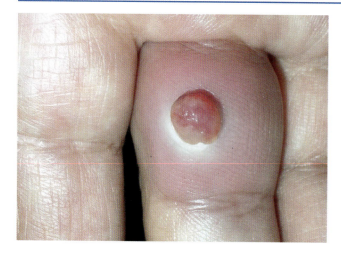

Fig. 6.59 Pyogenic granuloma on the volar aspect of the finger

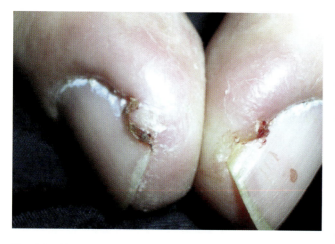

Fig. 6.60 Pyogenic granuloma-like lesions on the nailfolds that developed during therapy with an epidermal growth factor receptor inhibitor

A shaving biopsy may be preferred for confirmation of the diagnosis. Complete excision with primary closure, also providing a specimen for histopathological examination, can be performed in small lesions, especially on sites of low cosmetic importance such as the scalp. Surgery around the nail matrix may cause permanent nail dystrophy and is not recommended.

If there is no doubt about the diagnosis and lesions are located at sites where surgical procedures are difficult, treatment options other than excision may be preferred. These include topical application of silver nitrate (chemical cauterization), cryotherapy, lasers (pulsed dye, carbon dioxide), and imiquimod cream. Topical silver nitrate may be administered in several sessions with close follow-up (*see* Fig. 6.61a–c). Curettage combined with electrodesiccation may also be an option and cosmetic results are usually satisfactory. There is a risk of scar formation after destructive modalities.

Recurrence is possible after all methods but is low after surgical excision. Recurrence may be seen as regrowth of the primary lesion or of one or more satellite lesions around the site of the primary removed tumor. In recurrent primary tumors surgical excision is mostly required. Satellite lesions may occur in 1 to 4 months following surgery or destructive modalities (*see* Fig. 6.62). They are seen mostly on the trunk and scapula as small red papules or nodules. They are not associated with any complications and have a tendency toward spontaneous resolution. Further aggressive interventions are usually not necessary but persistent lesions are treated.

of capillary sized vessels. The stroma is usually edematous. A sparse inflammatory infiltrate is present in ulcerated cases. On the deep part of the lesion a feeding vessel of larger caliber is usually seen.

Some systemic drugs, including retinoids, capecitabine, or indinavir, may induce the formation of pyogenic granuloma-like lesions. Epidermal growth factor receptor inhibitors such as erlotinib and cetuximab may typically cause multiple periungual lesions (*see* Fig. 6.60).

Management. Pyogenic granuloma may heal spontaneously within 6 months (*see* Fig. 6.58a and b). Therefore, observation without any intervention may be preferred in some cases. However, most lesions are treated. Various treatment options exist. The possible occurrence of cosmetic sequelae should be taken into account when considering therapeutic modalities. The location and size of the tumor and the tendency to bleeding are also important factors in treatment decisions.

6.1.6 Senile Angioma (Cherry Angioma)

Senile angioma is one of the most common benign skin tumors. It is not a marker of senility, but it is mainly a tumor of adulthood. A great majority of adults have several senile angiomas. The cause of this hemangioma is unclear. Because of the bright red color of the tumor, it is also called cherry angioma. Lesions usually start to appear in the third decade. They present as multiple, petechiae-like macules or slightly elevated, firm papules less than 5 mm in diameter and are mostly seen on the trunk (*see* Fig. 6.63) and arms. Other parts of the limbs, face (*see* Fig. 6.64) and scalp may also be involved. Some lesions may be purplish in color (*see* Fig. 6.65). Sometimes relatively larger (*see* Fig. 6.66) or pedunculated (*see* Fig. 6.67) lesions that may be similar to pyogenic granuloma (*see* Fig. 6.42) are seen.

The number of the hemangiomas increases with age. Some elderly patients have numerous lesions (*see* Fig. 6.68). Sometimes innumerable senile angiomas may occur in an eruptive manner. The lesions are usually irregularly distributed but they may also appear in clusters (*see* Fig. 6.69). The surface of the tumor is intact and smooth, and it does not

6.1 Benign Vascular Tumors

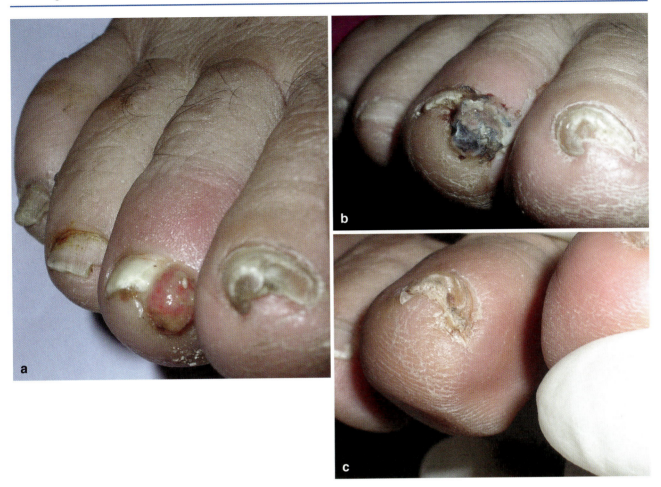

Fig. 6.61 (a) Pyogenic granuloma on the nail fold. (b) Crusted lesion after the first application of topical silver nitrate therapy. (c) Complete healing after the fourth application of silver nitrate

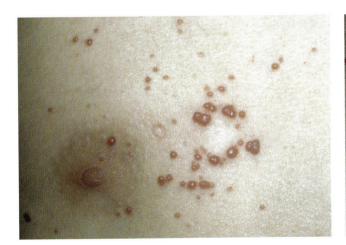

Fig. 6.62 Multiple small satellite pyogenic granulomas around the scar of a primary pyogenic granuloma treated with a destructive modality. They usually regress spontaneously

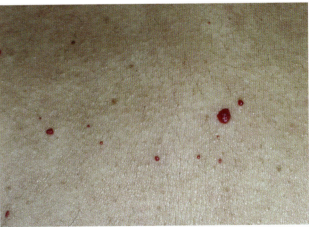

Fig. 6.63 Senile angioma presenting as multiple red papules on the trunk of an old patient. It is one of the most common benign tumors seen after middle age

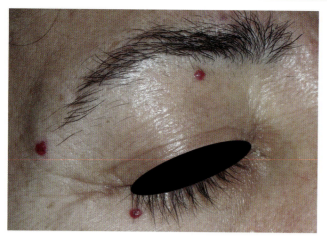

Fig. 6.64 Senile angioma on the face, an uncommon location

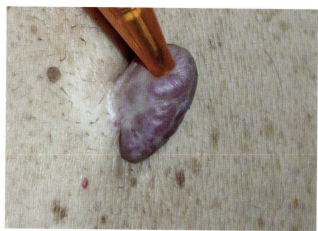

Fig. 6.67 Senile angioma seen as a pedunculated nodule and multiple small papules

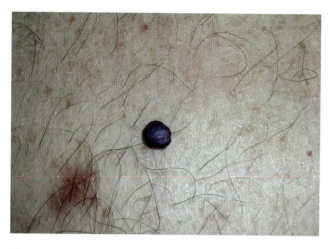

Fig. 6.65 Senile angioma presenting as a purplish round papule measuring 3–4 mm

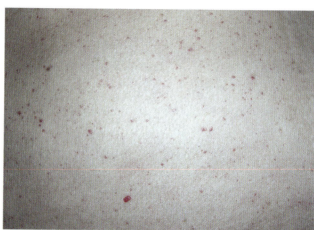

Fig. 6.68 Senile angioma presenting as scattered numerous tiny papules. They are asymptomatic

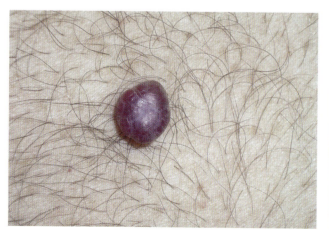

Fig. 6.66 A large (6–7 mm) papule of senile angioma is seen

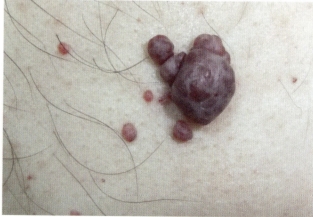

Fig. 6.69 Senile angioma presenting as grouped lesions in various sizes

6.1 Benign Vascular Tumors

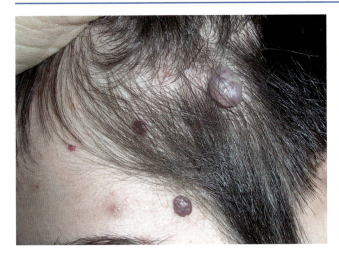

Fig. 6.70 Senile angiomas on the face and scalp of a young patient. Though rare, lesions may develop at early age

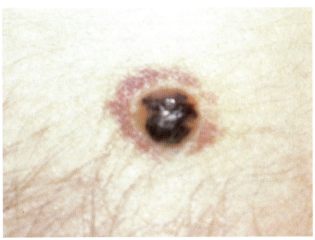

Fig. 6.71 Targetoid hemosiderotic hemangioma with target-like appearance

bleed easily. The diagnosis is nearly always based on clinical features. Histologically the lesion is composed of grouped and markedly dilated vascular channels in the dermis. Although uncommon, the tumor can be seen in young people (see Fig. 6.70); therefore the age of the patient is not sufficient to exclude a diagnosis of senile angioma. Multiple angiokeratomas seen in Fabry disease as small red papules (see Fig. 6.168) may be considered in the differential diagnosis, but they appear at a younger age and may also involve the genitalia, palms, and lips. Glomeruloid hemangioma (see Fig. 6.72) is another diagnostic consideration but is mostly associated with other manifestations of the POEMS syndrome. Cherry angiomas do not have any complications and do not show any association with systemic diseases.

Management. Reassurance of the patient about the benign nature of the tumor is the best approach for senile angiomas. Most patients do not request therapy for these asymptomatic small tumors. Treatment can rarely be administered for cosmetic reasons or for large tumors. Cryotherapy is not preferred for senile angioma. Laser ablation, shave excision, and light electrodesiccation can be performed, although there is a low risk of minor scarring.

6.1.7 Targetoid Hemosiderotic Hemangioma (Hobnail Hemangioma)

Targetoid hemosiderotic hemangioma is a rare benign vascular lesion with a distinct clinical appearance and pathognomonic histopathologic features. Trauma to a pre-existing hemangioma is suggested to play a role in the development of these lesions. However, there is strong evidence that these lesions originate from lymphatic vessels.

Targetoid hemosiderotic hemangioma is more frequent in young adults but can be seen in children and elderly patients as well. Lesions are usually located on the extremities and trunk. The size of a solitary lesion is generally about 1 cm in diameter. Larger lesions measuring up to 3 cm are also possible. There is a brown to pink, red or purple central papule that is surrounded by a peripheral ecchymotic ring forming a target-like appearance (see Fig. 6.71). Sometimes a thin, lighter area can be found between the papule and the ecchymotic ring. While the central papule is usually persistent, the ecchymotic ring may show a cyclic pattern, with alternating enlargement and resolution. The color of the ring may also show variations in time.

Targetoid hemosiderotic hemangioma can be clinically confused with a melanocytic nevus or an infantile hemangioma, especially in cases lacking the ecchymotic ring. On the other hand, thrombosed angiokeratoma (see Figs. 6.157 and 6.158a) may also show an ecchymotic halo, but its purpuric component resolves in a short time. Histopathologic examination of targetoid hemosiderotic hemangioma shows dermal ectatic vascular channels lined by protruding plump endothelial cells, named hobnail cells. These channels can exhibit a dissecting pattern in the deep dermis. Erythrocyte extravasation, stromal hemosiderin accumulation, and a mild inflammatory infiltrate are other findings. Kaposi sarcoma is the main histopathologic differential diagnosis.

Management. Targetoid hemosiderotic hemangioma does not show malignant transformation. The decision to remove the lesion depends on diagnostic purpose or cosmetic concern. Simple excision is usually curative. Recurrence after excision is not expected.

6.1.8 Glomeruloid Hemangioma

Glomeruloid hemangioma is a rare type of hemangioma with a distinct histopathology and is more commonly seen in patients with POEMS syndrome and sometimes with

Castleman disease. Very rarely, glomeruloid hemangioma is described in patients without any associated disease. The lesion is a pink to purple-red, dome-shaped papule or nodule with a smooth surface measuring less than 1 cm (*see* Figs. 6.72, 6.73 and 6.74) and clinically resembles a papular senile angioma (*see* Fig. 6.66). The term glomeruloid hemangioma is related to histologic features that consist of ectatic vascular spaces containing an aggregated proliferation of small capillaries, mimicking the appearance of a renal glomerulus.

Management. Therapy is not indicated for cutaneous lesions. Systemic examination for POEMS syndrome and Castleman disease is crucial.

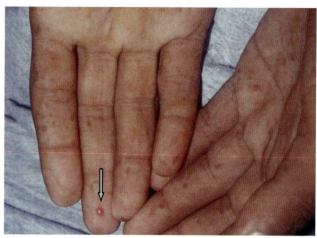

Fig. 6.74 Glomeruloid hemangioma on volar aspect of the finger (*arrow*) associated with palmar hyperpigmentation in a patient with POEMS syndrome

6.1.8.1 POEMS Syndrome (Crow-Fukase Syndrome)

POEMS syndrome is characterized by polyneuropathy, organomegaly (spleen, heart, kidneys), endocrinopathy, monoclonal plasma cell lymphoproliferative disorder, and skin changes. Glomeruloid hemangioma is seen approximately in one third of the patients in adulthood. They are usually multiple and mainly seen on the trunk and extremities. Hyperpigmentation covering large areas (*see* Figs. 6.73 and 6.74), hypertrichosis, increased sweating, sclerodermoid changes, nail clubbing, and leukonychia (*see* Fig. 6.73) are other skin findings of this rare syndrome. Severe sensorimotor polyneuropathy may be the predominant systemic finding. All patients should be screened for plasma cell disorders.

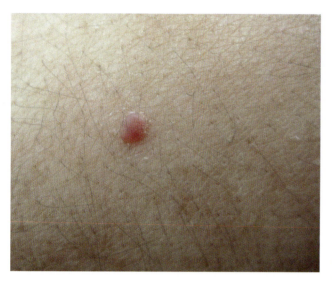

Fig. 6.72 Glomeruloid hemangioma seen as a reddish solitary papule on the trunk

6.1.9 Angiolymphoid Hyperplasia with Eosinophilia

Angiolymphoid hyperplasia with eosinophilia is a rare, benign, acquired inflammatory vascular proliferative disease of unknown origin presenting typically with a few papulonodular lesions. It most often occurs in young adults, predominantly in females. The pathogenesis of the disease is not clear. It may occur initially at pregnancy or be exacerbated during pregnancy.

Cutaneous lesions consist of 0.5 to 5 cm, tan, pink to dull red, brown or purple, dome-shaped papules or subcutaneous nodules mostly located on the head and neck region with a predilection for the ears, retroauricular area, and forehead (*see* Figs. 6.75, 6.76, 6.77 and 6.78). The predominantly involved site of the ear is the concha (*see* Fig. 6.79). Lesions may sometimes fill the auditory canal. Occasionally tumors

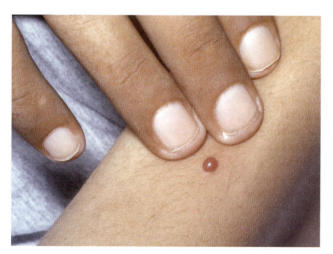

Fig. 6.73 Glomeruloid hemangioma associated with hyperpigmentation of the hand and leukonychia in a patient with POEMS syndrome

6.1 Benign Vascular Tumors

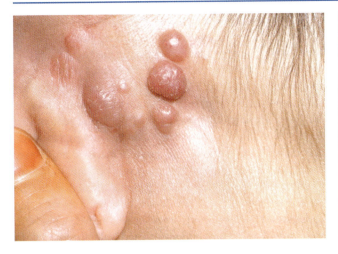

Fig. 6.75 Angiolymphoid hyperplasia with eosinophilia located on the retroauricular area, a typical localization

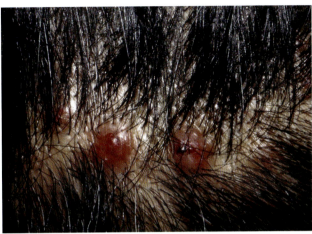

Fig. 6.78 Angiolymphoid hyperplasia with eosinophilia seen as red nodules on the scalp

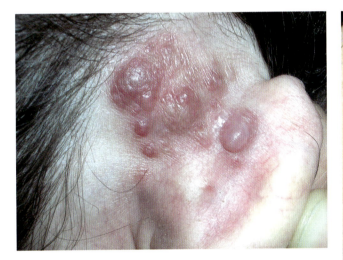

Fig. 6.76 Angiolymphoid hyperplasia with eosinophilia presenting as grouped, dome-shaped papules and nodules

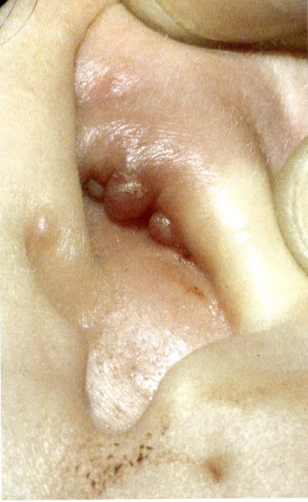

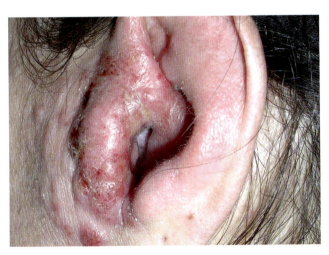

Fig. 6.77 Angiolymphoid hyperplasia with eosinophilia manifesting as an infiltrated plaque on the auricle. (With kind permission from Springer Science+Business Media: Baykal C, Yazganoğlu KD. Dermatological diseases of the nose and ears; 2010)

Fig. 6.79 Small papules of angiolymphoid hyperplasia with eosinophilia on the concha of the ear. (With kind permission from Springer Science+Business Media: Baykal C, Yazganoğlu KD. Dermatological diseases of the nose and ears; 2010)

may be seen on the trunk and distal extremities (*see* Figs. 6.80 and 6.81). There are usually few or multiple lesions. The surface of the tumors is usually smooth. However, erosion, ulceration, and bleeding may occasionally occur. They are mostly asymptomatic but pruritus, pain, and pulsatility may be found. Peripheral blood eosinophilia is reported in only approximately 20 percent of the patients. Differential diagnosis includes other tumors such as lymphocytoma cutis (*see* Fig. 14.193), Kaposi sarcoma (*see* Fig. 13.37), pyogenic granuloma (*see* Fig. 6.42), Kimura disease, and cutaneous metastasis (*see* Fig. 16.24). Histologic examination provides accurate diagnosis. There is a proliferation of thin- and thick-walled blood vessels lined by epithelioid, plump, and sometimes vacuolated endothelial cells. Perivascular lymphocytic and eosinophilic infiltration is also present. Lesions usually have a chronic course but do not show malignant degeneration.

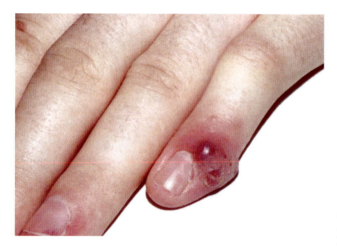

Fig. 6.80 Pregnancy-associated angiolymphoid hyperplasia with eosinophilia on the finger, an uncommon location

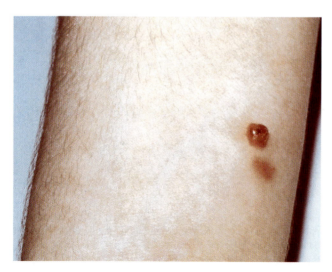

Fig. 6.81 Angiolymphoid hyperplasia with eosinophilia presenting as reddish papules on the arm

Management. Although the condition is benign and mostly persistent, spontaneous resolution has also rarely been noted. The appropriate therapeutic method depends on the location, number, and size of the lesions. Cryotherapy and lasers such as Nd:YAG, pulsed dye, and carbon dioxide can be used, but dyspigmentation and scarring may be seen after these procedures. In small localized tumors surgery is an effective choice (*see* Fig. 6.82a and b). However, it is difficult to determine the surgical margins and it may not be feasible on the ear. Recurrence is possible in incompletely excised tumors or in patients treated with the above-mentioned destructive modalities. Radiotherapy and intralesional corticosteroids are other alternative methods. In patients with refractory or disseminated lesions, medications such as corticosteroids (systemic, intralesional), interferon alfa, and vinblastine may be tried but the results are variable.

6.1.10 Kimura disease

Kimura disease is characterized by a deep hemangioma associated with systemic involvement. Angiolymphoid hyperplasia with eosinophilia and Kimura disease were formerly considered different stages of the same disease. However, currently they are classified as two distinct entities. Involvement of deeper tissue, intense peripheral blood eosinophilia, elevated serum IgE levels, lymphadenopathy, and involvement of internal organs are the key features of Kimura disease; these facilitate a distinction from angiolymphoid hyperplasia with eosinophilia. Moreover, Kimura disease occurs in average at a younger age than angiolymphoid hyperplasia with eosinophilia and is more common in men. Lesions are located predominantly in the head and neck region. The growth of the tumor is slowly progressive. Painless, soft, subcutaneous large nodules or masses are mainly seen on the preauricular area and commonly involve the salivary glands, especially the parotid gland. Lesions may be bilateral. Multiple regional lymph nodes especially the cervical and supraclavicular ones may be involved. Renal involvement may also rarely be present and resemble glomerulonephritis or nephrotic syndrome.

The diagnosis of Kimura disease is established with typical histopathologic features of subcutaneous tumor and lymph node in association with systemic involvement and laboratory findings. In contrast to angiolymphoid hyperplasia with eosinophilia, histologically newly formed vessels in Kimura disease do not have epithelioid endothelial cells, and there are much larger lymphoid follicles with germinal center formation. Dense eosinophilic infiltration with abscess formation is also seen. Radiologic examinations such as ultrasonography and MRI may be required to determine the limits of the tumor.

Management. A standard therapy has not yet been established. Surgical resection and radiotherapy are the main options. Systemic corticosteroids are effective in reducing

6.2 Vascular Malformations

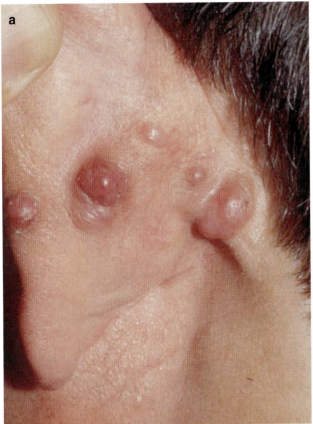

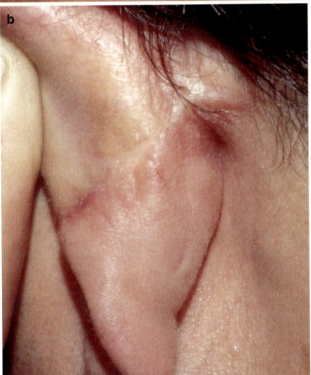

Fig. 6.82 (**a**) Angiolymphoid hyperplasia with eosinophilia restricted to a small area on the auricle. (With kind permission from Springer Science+Business Media: Baykal C, Yazganoğlu KD. Dermatological diseases of the nose and ears; 2010.) (**b**) Lesions cleared after excision

the size of the tumor, but recurrence occurs frequently after their cessation. Imatinib has also been used in some cases with success.

6.1.11 Intravascular Papillary Endothelial Hyperplasia (Masson Hemangioma)

Intravascular papillary endothelial hyperplasia is a rare type of acquired vascular tumor with unknown etiopathogenesis. It is suggested to be a reactive endothelial cell proliferation as a result of thrombosis followed by recanalization of a venule. It may be a primary lesion or may be associated with hemangiomas such as pyogenic granuloma. It is most commonly seen in adults. Clinical features are variable. The lesions are located predominantly on the skin but may also occur in visceral organs. The palmar surface of the fingers is the most commonly involved site, but the lesions may be seen anywhere on the skin. The solitary purplish nodule is variable in size (*see* Fig. 6.83) and may be painful. Because of the lack of specific clinical features, the tumor is usually diagnosed histopathologically. Microscopic examination generally shows an identifiable vascular wall, an organized thrombus or its remnants, and papillary projections lined by single-layered, protuberant endothelial cells. There is no multilayering, prominent atypia, or abnormal mitotic figures, which are important clues in the differential diagnosis of angiosarcoma.

Management. Complete excision is the therapy of choice.

6.2 Vascular Malformations

Vascular malformations are enlarged vessels without cellular proliferation related to the abnormalities in vascular formation during embryogenesis. Lesions that are usually present at birth typically expand proportionally with the child's growth. The tendency to spontaneous involution is low, and the enlarged vessels may progress later in life, causing serious complications. Malformations of the capillaries, veins, arteries, and lymphatics may be involved solely or in combination (e.g., capillaro-lymphaticovenous malformation). They are seen equally in females and males.

6.2.1 Capillary Malformations

Nevus flammeus and telangiectasia (including telangiectatic syndromes and angiokeratoma, which are completely different vascular lesions) will be discussed under the title of capillary malformations.

6.2.1.1 Nevus Flammeus

Nevus flammeus is a common type of capillary malformation characterized by congenital angiomatous patches or

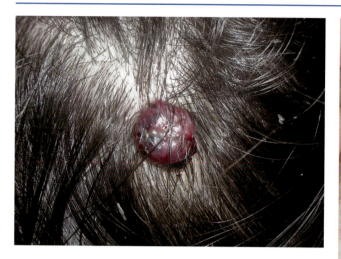

Fig. 6.83 Intravascular papillary endothelial hyperplasia presenting as a pyogenic granuloma-like nodule on the scalp

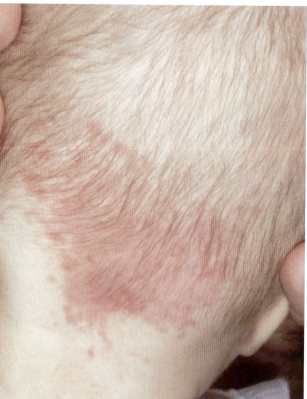

Fig. 6.85 Salmon patch on the nape of the neck of an infant. This common lesion heals usually spontaneously in early childhood

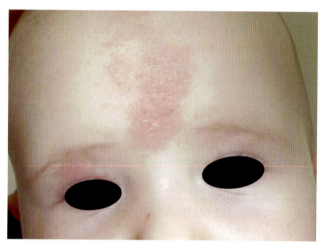

Fig. 6.84 Salmon patch presenting as a pink macule on the glabella and left upper eyelid in an infant. It is noticeable at birth

plaques on the skin and mucosal surfaces. The level of affected vessels in the dermis determines the subtypes of the lesion, which are salmon patch and port-wine stain.

Salmon Patch

Salmon patch is the superficial subtype of nevus flammeus. It is present in approximately half of the newborns. Dilated capillaries are restricted to the upper dermis in this malformation. The asymptomatic lesions are most commonly located on the face (forehead, glabella, upper eyelids, tip of the nose and philtrum) (see Fig. 6.84) and nape of the neck (see Fig. 6.85). In some patients more than one area is involved. Lesions on the nape of the neck, also called "stork bite", are typically located in the midline. Since this area is covered by hairs, it is not always noticed by parents. Typical lesions are irregular, pink or reddish macules with indistinct borders which are not usually large. They can easily be diagnosed clinically.

In contrast to the other types of vascular malformations, most of the lesions fade spontaneously within the first year of life. However, lesions on some areas, especially patches on the nape of the neck, may be persistent. Sometimes a persistent salmon patch of scalp is initially discovered when alopecia areata develops in adulthood (see Fig. 6.86). Salmon patch is a sporadic lesion and does not show any association with genodermatoses. There is no indication for therapy of salmon patch in infants. Parents should be counseled about the benign nature of the lesion.

Port-wine Stain

Port-wine stain is the deeper and permanent subtype of nevus flammeus and occurs in less than 1 percent of newborns. Unlike salmon patch, dilated capillaries are also seen in the reticular dermis in these lesions. Sometimes the terms nevus flammeus and port-wine stain are used synonymously. However, salmon patch, which is a transient superficial lesion, should be separated from port-wine stain. The initial lesions of the two conditions may look similar. In contrast to salmon patch, port-wine stain has a relatively deeper red or purple color when fully developed (see Figs. 6.87 and 6.88), and is always persistent. The number and size of the lesions are variable. Lesions that are not associated with a syndrome may be smaller. The involvement may be diffuse

6.2 Vascular Malformations

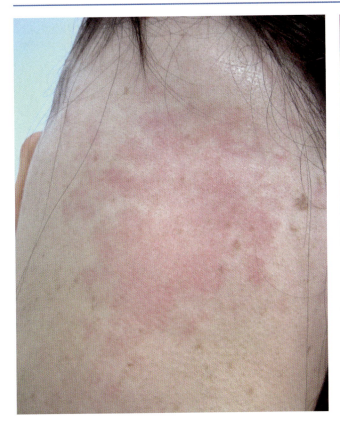

Fig. 6.86 Persistent salmon patch in an adult with alopecia areata. Lesion has been first noticed after the occurrence of alopecia areata

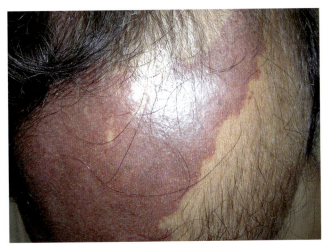

Fig. 6.87 Port-wine stain shown as a sharply demarcated, deep red macule on the scalp

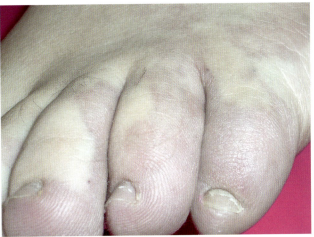

Fig. 6.88 Purplish port-wine stain located on the toes

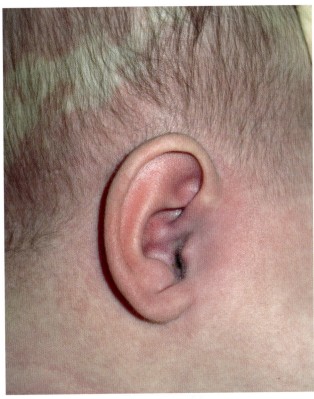

Fig. 6.89 Port-wine stain covering a large area of the face and scalp in a checkerboard pattern. Note the smooth surface of the lesion in a young patient

(see Fig. 6.87), but uninvolved areas on the patches or plaques (checkerboard pattern) may be observed (see Fig. 6.89). Some lesions have a reticulated appearance (see Fig. 6.90).

The congenital well-demarcated smooth macules expand proportionally with the child's growth. At an older age, the color of the lesion may become darker (see Fig. 6.91). Additionally, the lesion may become elevated and infiltrated, and papulonodular (pyogenic granuloma-like) lesions may occur on the surface owing to the involvement of the deeper reticular dermis (see Fig. 6.92). Sometimes the surface of elder lesions may be warty. Furthermore, large nodules may develop on the surface of some port-wine stains, especially those located on the face and scalp (see Fig. 6.93). Underlying structures like muscles are not involved in this capillary vascular malformation.

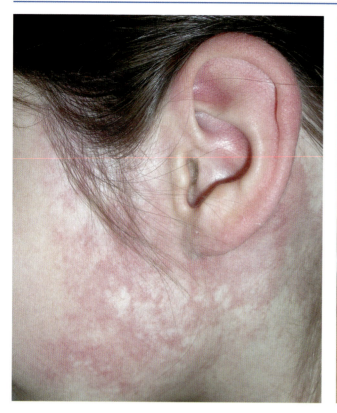

Fig. 6.90 Port-wine stain on the face demonstrating a reticulated pattern

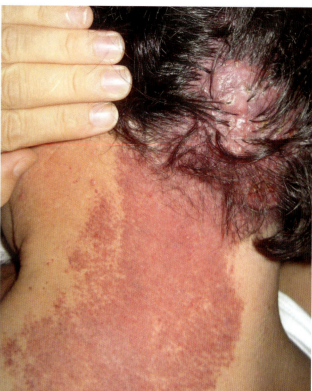

Fig. 6.92 Port-wine stain extending from the nape of the neck to the scalp in an adult patient; note the papulonodular component on the scalp

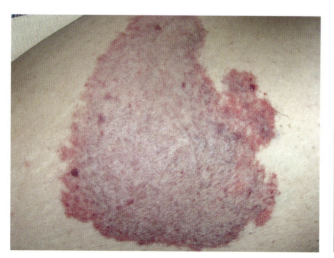

Fig. 6.91 Port-wine stain on the trunk of an otherwise healthy adult. This lesion was slightly raised

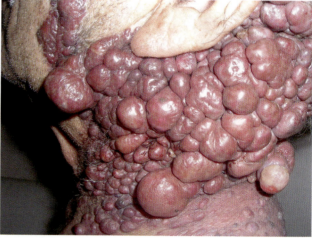

Fig. 6.93 Port-wine stain on the head covered with multiple large nodules. Surface of the lesions may become irregular with advancing age as seen in the elderly patient

Port-wine stain is most common on the face but may be seen elsewhere on the skin (*see* Fig. 6.94) and on mucosal surfaces (*see* Fig. 6.95). Large macules may show a segmental distribution (*see* Figs. 6.96 and 6.97) but do not follow the lines of Blaschko. Some large lesions involve both sides of the body (*see* Fig. 6.98). Segmental lesions on the face are mostly unilateral and appear in three types according to the area supplied by the divisions of the branches of the

6.2 Vascular Malformations

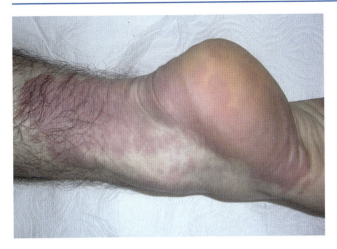

Fig. 6.94 Port-wine stain located on the foot and lower leg

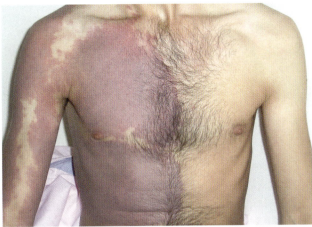

Fig. 6.97 Unilateral large port-wine stain on the trunk of an adult. Note that the lesion does not exceed the midline

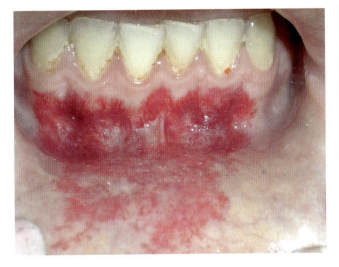

Fig. 6.95 Port-wine stain located on the lower lip and gum in an adult

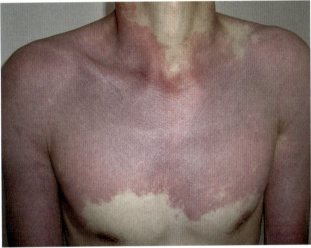

Fig. 6.98 Large port-wine stain involving the chest and arms bilaterally

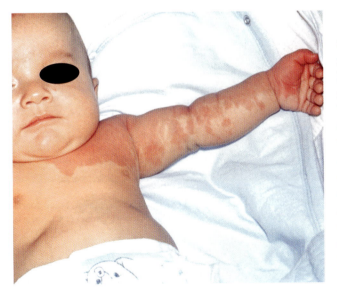

Fig. 6.96 Large port-wine stain on one side of the trunk and ipsilateral arm in an infant

trigeminal (fifth) cranial nerve. Cranial nerve V1 (ophthalmic branch) innervates the forehead and upper eyelids (*see* Fig. 6.99), cranial nerve V2 (maxillary) innervates the maxillary region (*see* Figs. 6.100 and 6.101) and cranial nerve V3 (mandibular) innervates the mandibular region (*see* Figs. 6.102 and 6.103). Sometimes more than one neighboring region is involved by port-wine stain (*see* Figs. 6.99 and 6.104). Dilated conjunctival vessels on the ipsilateral eye may accompany the eyelid lesions. Port-wine stain on the extremities may be large (*see* Fig. 6.96) and may sometimes involve nearly the whole extremity (*see* Fig. 6.105). Overlying papulonodular lesions commonly develop on the facial lesions of port-wine stain (*see* Figs. 6.106 and 6.107) but rarely on the trunk and limb lesions.

Port-wine stain may be an isolated condition or it may be associated with a variety of syndromes (genodermatoses). The location of the capillary malformation may be

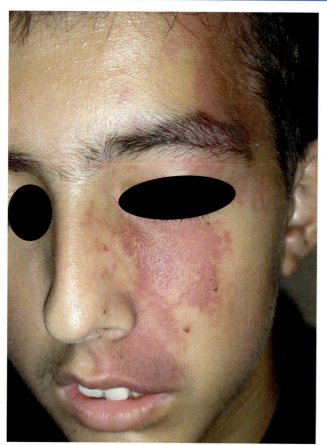

Fig. 6.99 Unilateral facial port-wine stain localized on the area innervated by V1 (ophthalmic) and V2 (maxillary) branches of the trigeminal cranial nerve. There is a high risk of association with Sturge-Weber syndrome in this location

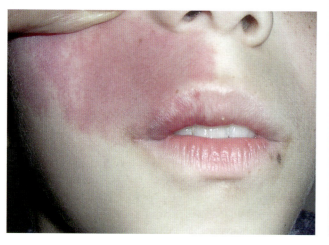

Fig. 6.100 Unilateral port-wine stain located on the region of the face innervated by the V2 (maxillary) branch of the trigeminal cranial nerve

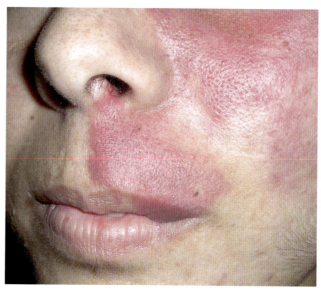

Fig. 6.101 Port-wine stain on the upper lip and cheek innervated by the V2 (maxillary) branch of the trigeminal cranial nerve. Note the midline demarcation and the lip involvement

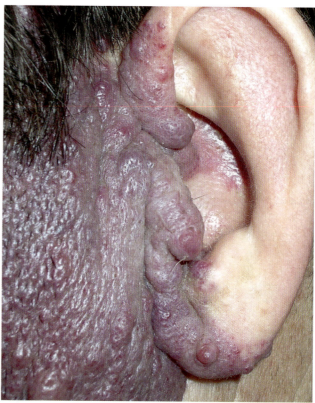

Fig. 6.102 Port-wine stain on the preauricular area and chin innervated by the V3 (mandibulary) branch of the trigeminal cranial nerve, including also the ears

6.2 Vascular Malformations

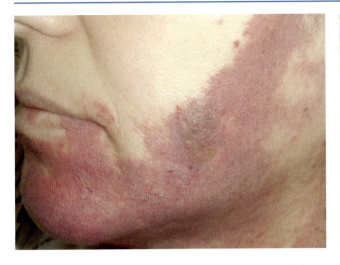

Fig. 6.103 Port-wine stain restricted to the lower lip and chin innervated by the V3 (mandibulary) branch of the trigeminal cranial nerve. Association with Sturge-Weber syndrome is not expected in this location

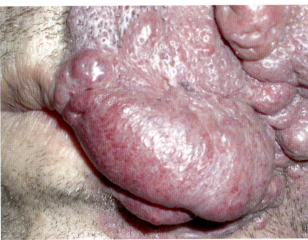

Fig. 6.106 Port-wine stain on the area innervated by the V2 (maxillary) branch of the trigeminal cranial nerve. Note the papulonodular lesions causing enlargement of the lower lip in the adult patient

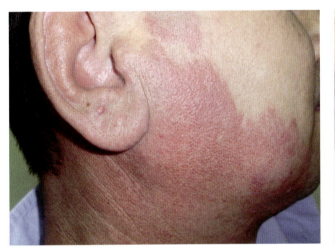

Fig. 6.104 Port-wine stain on the chin innervated by the V3 (mandibulary) branch of trigeminal cranial nerve together with involvement of the neck is shown

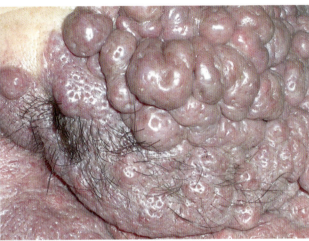

Fig. 6.107 An adult patient with Sturge-Weber syndrome. Note the nodular component of port-wine stain on the area innervated by the V1 (ophthalmic) branch of the trigeminal cranial nerve

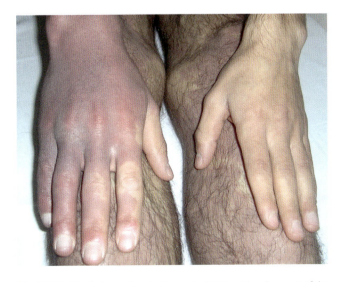

Fig 6.105 Flat lesions of port-wine stain. Bilateral involvement of the hands and legs are noticeable

an indicator for the related disorder. Sturge-Weber syndrome, Klippel-Trenaunay syndrome, Cobb syndrome, Proteus syndrome, and phakomatosis pigmentovascularis are among the various syndromes associated with nevus flammeus. Moreover, when nevus flammeus is located on the midline of the back, it may be associated with spinal dysraphism.

Sturge-Weber Syndrome (Encephalotrigeminal Angiomatosis)

Sturge-Weber syndrome is mostly sporadic, but familial cases have been reported. The main defect of this syndrome is the persistence of primitive vascular plexus around the cephalic neural tube beneath the part of the ectoderm destined to be the facial skin. In Sturge-Weber syndrome

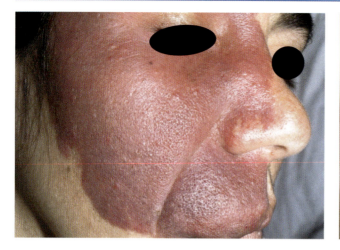

Fig. 6.108 Port-wine stain involving the regions innervated by the V1 (ophthalmic) and V2 (maxillary) branches of the trigeminal cranial nerve in a patient with Sturge-Weber syndrome

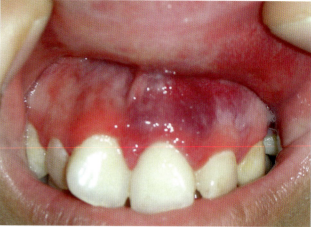

Fig. 6.110 Port-wine stain on the lip and gingivae in a patient with Sturge-Weber syndrome

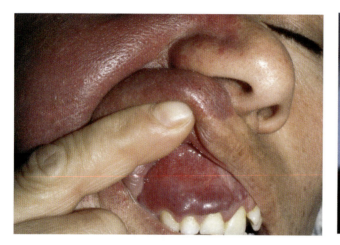

Fig. 6.109 Port-wine stain involving the regions innervated by the V1 (ophthalmic) and V2 (maxillary) branches of the trigeminal cranial nerve in a patient with Sturge-Weber syndrome. Note the involvement of the gingivae

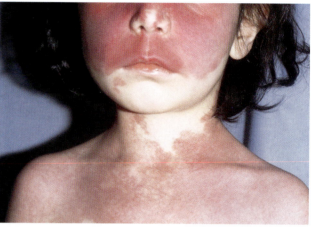

Fig. 6.111 Bilateral port-wine stain involving the regions innervated by the V1 (ophthalmic) and V2 (maxillary) branch of the trigeminal cranial nerve together with extensive involvement of the upper trunk in a patient with Sturge-Weber syndrome

port-wine stain is typically located unilaterally on the face with respect to cranial nerve V1 region (see Figs. 6.107 and 6.108). But not all nevi flammeus showing this typical distribution are associated with Sturge-Weber syndrome. Port-wine stain may extend into the regions of V2 and V3 branches. When only the latter two regions are involved, there is no increased risk for Sturge-Weber syndrome. Involvement of the oral mucosa, especially lesions on the lips (see Figs. 6.106 and 6.108), gingivae (see Figs. 6.109 and 6.110), and tongue with ipsilateral distribution may be seen in some cases. Although rare, port-wine stains located on the trunk, extremities, and bilaterally on the face may also be encountered in Sturge-Weber syndrome (see Fig. 6.111). Hypertrophy of underlying soft tissue and bone may occur. Facial asymmetry may appear due to the growth of the maxilla and jaw. Vascular malformation of the leptomeninges and brain ipsilateral to the port-wine stain is present in some patients. Convoluted calcification occurs in cortical areas, mostly in the temporal and occipital lobes. Thus, epilepsy, hemiplegia, hemisensory defects, and homonymous hemianopsia may appear. Most patients are mentally normal; however, mental retardation develops in patients with uncontrolled epilepsy. Vascular malformations on conjunctiva, iris, choroid, and retina typically ipsilateral to the port-wine stain may have complications, including congenital glaucoma (buphthalmos), retinal abnormalities and even blindness.

Klippel-Trenaunay syndrome

In Klippel-Trenaunay syndrome, nevus flammeus is mostly located on the lower limbs extensively (see Figs. 6.112 and 6.113). Upper extremity and other areas including the genitalia

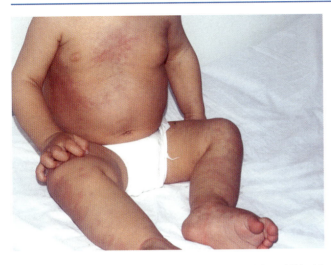

Fig. 6.112 Port-wine stain on the extremities and trunk in a child with Klippel-Trenaunay syndrome

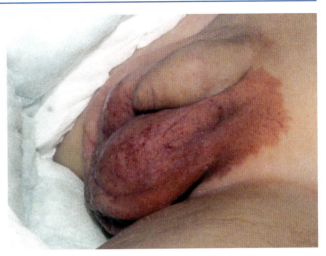

Fig. 6.114 Port-wine stain located on the genitalia in a patient with Klippel-Trenaunay syndrome

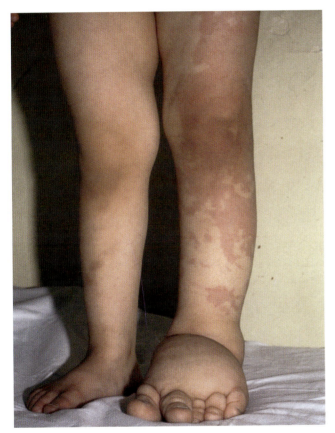

Fig. 6.113 Unilateral port-wine stain associated with pronounced ipsilateral hypertrophy of the soft tissue and bones on the affected limb (hemihypertrophy) in a child with Klippel-Trenaunay syndrome

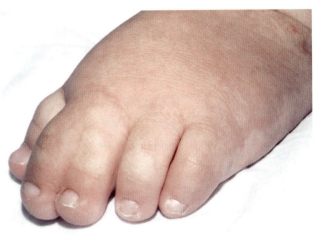

Fig. 6.115 Port-wine stain associated with underlying soft tissue hypertrophy and syndactyly in a patient with Klippel-Trenaunay syndrome. Various anomalies of digits may be seen in this syndrome

(*see* Fig. 6.114) may also be involved. Most patients have unilateral port-wine stain (*see* Fig. 6.113), but bilateral involvement is also possible. Lesions are well-demarcated and are dark in color. Underlying soft tissue, muscle, and bone may be slightly hypertrophic at birth but this overgrowth become more apparent as the child grows (*see* Fig. 6.113). Asymmetric length and/or girth of the affected limbs are typical, which may lead to functional problems in time. Pathologic fractures are also possible. Anomalies such as syndactyly (*see* Fig. 6.115) and polydactyly (*see* Fig. 6.116) may be present in some patients. Other vascular lesions such as angiokeratomas (*see* Figs. 6.117 and 6.118), hemangiomas, superficial venous varicosities (*see* Figs. 6.118 and 6.119), deep venous malformations, lymphangiomas, and lymphatic anomalies leading to lymphedema (*see* Fig. 6.120) may be seen in this syndrome. It is also known as capillaro-lymphaticovenous malformation. Recurrent cellulitis, phlebitis, deep venous thrombosis, and chronic ulcers accompanying lymphedema may be observed in some patients. The severity of the disease is variable. Symptoms may worsen with age. Klippel-Trenaunay syndrome and Parkes-Weber syndrome have common clinical features, but arteriovenous malformations are present in

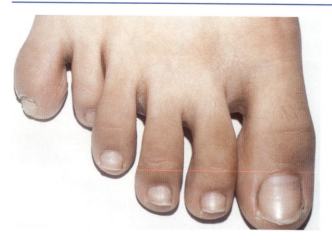

Fig. 6.116 Polydactyly in a patient with Klippel-Trenaunay syndrome

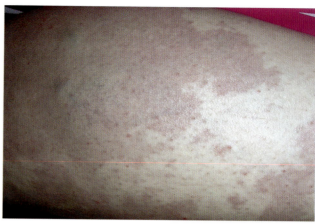

Fig. 6.119 Port-wine stain and superficial venous varicosities on the lower leg of a patient with Klippel-Trenaunay syndrome

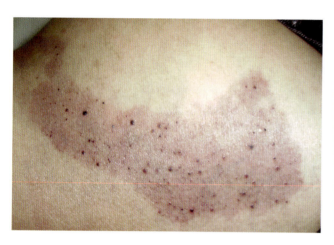

Fig. 6.117 Port-wine stain on the trunk of a patient with Klippel-Trenaunay syndrome. Note the overlying angiokeratomas presenting as small violaceous papules

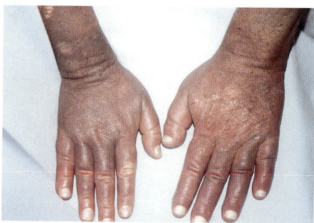

Fig. 6.120 Bilateral port-wine stain associated with lymphedema of the hands and arms in an adult patient with Klippel-Trenaunay syndrome

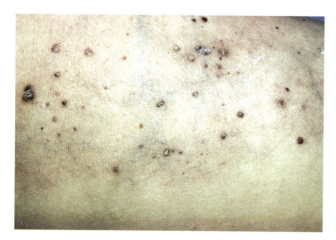

Fig. 6.118 Port-wine stain, angiokeratomas, and superficial venous varicosities are shown in a patient with Klippel-Trenaunay syndrome

the latter one. Moreover, nevus flammeus is not observed in all patients, and serious complications may arise such as the development of high-output heart failure or auto-amputations caused by persistent skin ulcers.

Cobb Syndrome (Cutaneous Meningospinal Angiomatosis)

Cobb syndrome is characterized by port-wine stain located in a dermatomal distribution associated with underlying spinal septal malformations and meningeal angiomatosis. Angiokeratomas and lymphangioma circumscriptum may be rarely seen. Paralysis, hemiplegia, and other neurologic symptoms may develop as a result of spinal defects. If any doubt about Cobb syndrome emerges, imaging studies and neurologic consultation are mandatory.

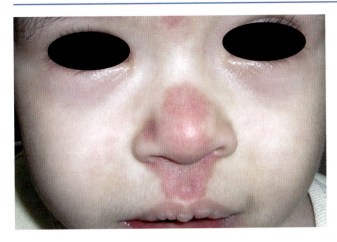

Fig. 6.121 Port-wine stain on the midface in a patient with Proteus syndrome

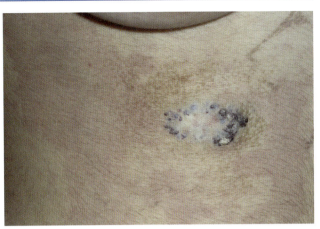

Fig. 6.123 Port-wine stain associated with a venous malformation (bluish red papules) and epidermal nevus (hyperkeratotic brownish papules) in a patient with Proteus syndrome

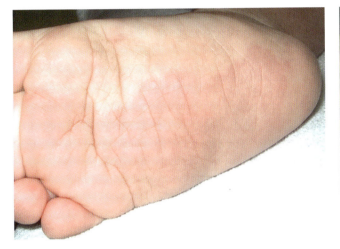

Fig. 6.122 Port-wine stain associated with a plantar cerebriform collagen nevus in a child with Proteus syndrome

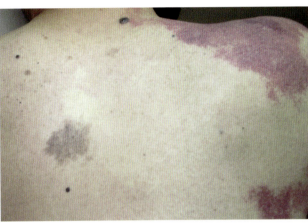

Fig. 6.124 Port-wine stain (reddish patches) associated with multiple blue nevi (dark papules) and other dermal melanocytic tumors (dark patches) representing the main manifestations of phakomatosis pigmentovascularis

Proteus Syndrome

Port-wine stain may also be seen in Proteus syndrome but as a minor sign. The red vascular patches are in varying sizes and distributed at random sites of the body (*see* Figs. 6.121 and 6.122). The main clinical features of this rare syndrome which are not present at birth are asymmetric overgrowth of extremities, macrodactyly, macrocephaly, cranial hemihypertrophy, scoliosis, soft subcutaneous masses, cerebriform connective tissue nevus on the palmoplantar area (plantar hyperplasia) (*see* Figs. 6.122 and 8.92), and epidermal nevus (*see* Fig. 1.89). Lipomas, hyperpigmented macules, patchy dermal hypoplasia, venous malformations (*see* Fig. 6.123), lymphatic malformations and bullous lung alterations may also be seen. The disease has a slowly progressive course, and the extremities of some patients may become gigantic in time. CLOVES syndrome may be considered in the differential diagnosis. It is characterized by congenital lipomatous overgrowth, epidermal nevi, vascular malformations and skeletal abnormalities.

Phakomatosis Pigmentovascularis

Phakomatosis pigmentovascularis is characterized by concomitant occurrence of various benign skin tumors or hamartomas. These include port-wine stain, cutis marmorata telangiectatica, nevus spilus, nevus anemicus (*see* Fig. 3.225), and dermal melanocytic tumors. Different types of phakomatosis pigmentovascularis have been proposed according to the combination of these lesions. Port-wine stain is usually extensive and asymmetrically distributed. Nevus spilus and dermal melanocytic tumors may also be multiple and extensive (*see* Figs. 3.44, 6.124 and 6.125).

Spinal Dysraphism

Nevus flammeus localized on the midline of the back (*see* Fig. 6.126), especially in combination with other paraspinal lesions such as lipomas, tail-like hairy patches (*see* Fig. 6.127), and dimples, may be associated with underlying

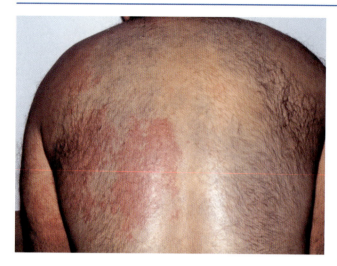

Fig. 6.125 A patient with phakomatosis pigmentovascularis. A large port-wine stain and diffuse macular dermal melanocytic tumor are seen concomitantly on the trunk

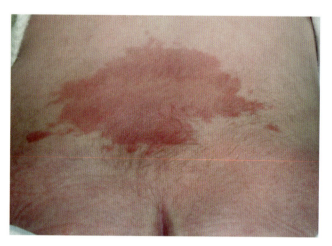

Fig. 6.126 Port-wine stain localized on the midline of the back. This location may indicate an association with spinal dysraphism

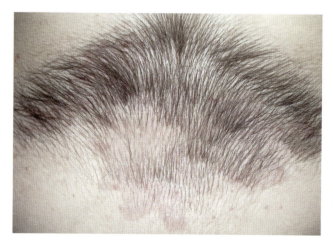

Fig. 6.127 Port-wine stain associated with tail-like hypertrichosis limited to the midline of the back in a patient with spinal dysraphism

spinal dysraphism. Neurologic findings and urinary incontinence may be present in these patients. MRI must be performed to detect underlying abnormalities.

Management. The first step of the approach to nevus flammeus is to differentiate between salmon patch and port-wine stain. Routine systemic investigations and therapy are not indicated for salmon patch. However, children with large port-wine stains, especially in specific locations, should be further evaluated. A complete dermatologic examination can reveal other cutaneous manifestations of the above-mentioned syndromes. Ocular examination, imaging studies such as computed tomography, MRI, or positron emission tomography (PET) of the brain are indicated to diagnose Sturge-Weber syndrome. Color Doppler ultrasonography (ultrasound) and MRI are useful to show vascular anomalies and involvement of soft tissue and bones in Klippel-Trenaunay syndrome.

Port-wine stains or persistent salmon patches may be treated, especially in patients with cosmetic concerns. Lesions on the face may be the source of social problems and depression. While cosmetic camouflage is helpful in some locations, patients may also request therapy. Moreover, some untreated port-wine stains may gradually raise up, and nodules occurring on the surface worsen the cosmetic appearance. Accordingly, early treatment of all port-wine stain lesions can be considered. The flash lamp–pulsed dye laser is commonly used for this capillary malformation. It is mostly effective in small flat lesions, leading to good cosmetic appearance. The lesions may fade but may not always disappear, especially the large ones. The risk of atrophic or hypertrophic scars and dyspigmentation is not high with this method. Medical therapies including beta-blockers are not effective in nevus flammeus.

6.2.1.2 Telangiectasia

Telangiectases are permanent dilatations of superficial vessels of the dermis and are not related to vascular proliferation. Most patients have multiple, nonpulsatile, dull red, usually nonpalpable, and sometimes slightly raised short lines that are approximately 0.5 to 1 mm wide. Lesions blanch on slight compression, e.g., with diascopy examination. Telangiectases may occur anywhere on skin and mucosal surfaces, but the face, especially the nose (*see* Fig. 6.128) and the cheeks (*see* Fig. 6.129) are more commonly involved; the lips are the typical location of mucosal telangiectases (*see* Figs. 6.130 and 6.131). Most lesions are acquired and can be seen at any age. In some patients no triggering factor can be detected. Many adults have idiopathic fine telangiectases on alae nasi (*see* Fig. 6.128).

Telangiectasia may be an isolated finding on normal skin or may overly other cutaneous lesions. Poikiloderma, which may be seen in mycosis fungoides, dermatomyositis, or in various genodermatoses appears as a combination

6.2 Vascular Malformations

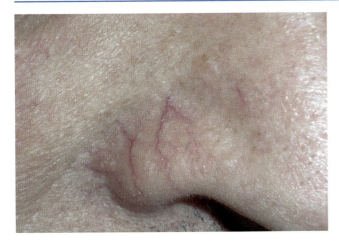

Fig. 6.128 Idiopathic telangiectasia on ala nasi. It is very common in adults

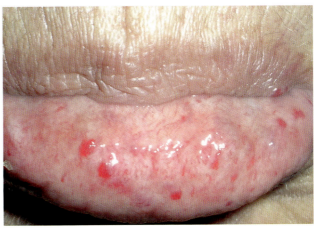

Fig. 6.131 Telangiectases on the lower lip shown as red tiny papules

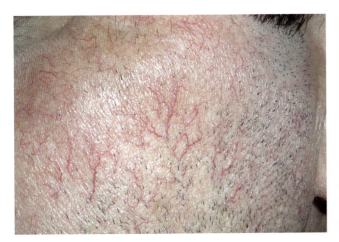

Fig. 6.129 Telangiectases on the cheek presenting as short red lines

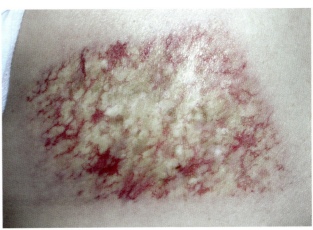

Fig. 6.132 Telangiectases overlying a hypopigmented and sclerotic area representing typical features of chronic radiodermatitis

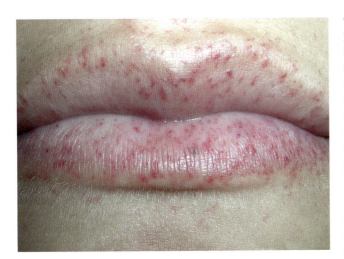

Fig. 6.130 Telangiectases on the lips. Mucosal telangiectases may be associated with syndromes but this patient was otherwise healthy

of telangiectases, atrophy, and dyspigmentation. Rosacea patients usually have facial erythema accompanied by a varying amount of telangiectases. Long-term use of topical corticosteroids may also lead to telangiectasia associated with erythema, especially on the face. Telangiectases may be observed on the surface of some inflammatory cutaneous disorders or tumors such as necrobiosis lipoidica diabeticorum, chronic radiodermatitis (see Fig. 6.132), keloid (see Fig. 8.98), epidermoid cyst (see Fig. 4.17), congenital hemangioma (see Fig. 6.40), and basal cell carcinoma (see Fig. 11.28).

Telangiectases may arise secondarily as complication of some treatment modalities such as cryotherapy, laser, or radiotherapy. Chronic sun damage and heat or cold exposure are common causes of facial telangiectasia. Hyperestrogenemia, cirrhosis of the liver (see Fig. 6.133), carcinoid syndrome, and connective tissue disorders such as systemic lupus erythematosus, dermatomyositis,

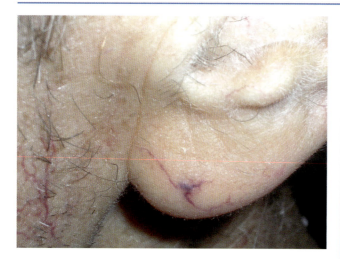

Fig. 6.133 Telangiectases on the face and ears in a patient with cirrhosis of the liver

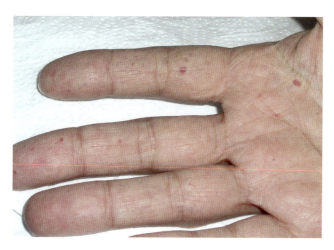

Fig. 6.134 Mat-like telangiectases on the palmar area. This location is typical for CREST syndrome

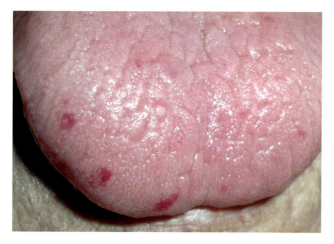

Fig. 6.135 Telangiectases on the tongue in a patient with CREST syndrome

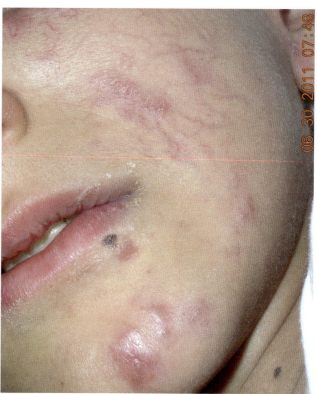

Fig. 6.136 Telangiectasia on the face in a patient with ataxia telangiectasia. These lesions typically appear in childhood

scleroderma, and CREST syndrome are among the systemic diseases associated with telangiectases. Periungual telangiectasia is a common finding of connective tissue disorders. Mat-like telangiectasia on palms may be observed in CREST syndrome (see Fig. 6.134). Telangiectases may also be seen on the tongue in this disease (see Fig. 6.135). HIV infection, mastocytosis (telangiectasia macularis eruptiva perstans), and pregnancy are among other factors in the development of telangiectases. Intravascular lymphoma may present with diffuse telangiectases, which may be relatively wide, long, and slightly raised (see Fig. 14.181). Involuting infantile hemangioma may end up with telangiectases (see Fig. 6.39).

Some genetic diseases such as ataxia telangiectasia (Louis-Bar syndrome), hereditary hemorrhagic telangiectasia (Osler-Weber-Rendu syndrome), and Bloom syndrome may also manifest with telangiectases as the major finding.

Ataxia Telangiectasia

Thin and relatively long telangiectases may show a butterfly pattern on the face in ataxia telangiectasia (see Fig. 6.136), and they are also observed on the ears and eyes (bulbar conjunctiva) (see Fig. 6.137). The neck, upper chest, and flexor sites of the forearms may also be involved. Progeric facies, granulomatous skin lesions, and premature canities are other

6.2 Vascular Malformations

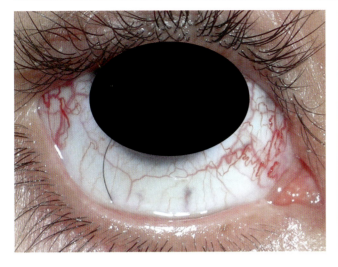

Fig. 6.137 Prominent telangiectasia on the eye of a patient with ataxia telangiectasia

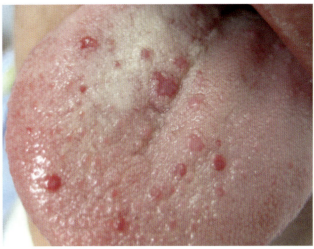

Fig. 6.139 Multiple papular telangiectases on the tongue in a patient with Osler-Weber-Rendu syndrome

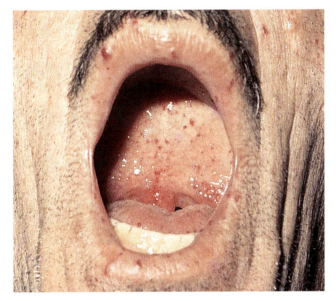

Fig. 6.138 Papular telangiectases on the lips and tongue seen in a patient with Osler-Weber-Rendu syndrome

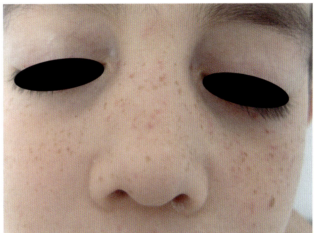

Fig. 6.140 Mat-like telangiectases on the face in a patient with Osler-Weber-Rendu syndrome

dermatologic findings. The syndrome leads to increased mortality and morbidity resulting from neurologic manifestations such as cerebellar ataxia and associated systemic lymphomas.

Osler-Weber-Rendu Syndrome (Hereditary Hemorrhagic Telangiectasia)

Diffuse telangiectases especially localized on the lips (see Fig. 6.138), tongue (see Fig. 6.139), conjunctivae, face (see Fig. 6.140), ears (see Fig. 6.141), and fingertips may suggest Osler-Weber-Rendu syndrome. These telangiectases are relatively papular (see Figs. 6.138 and 6.141) and mat-like. Recurrent epistaxis due to nasal telangiectases is usually the initial manifestation seen in childhood. Intermittent gastrointestinal and sometimes genitourinary bleeding, secondary iron deficiency anemia, hepatic arteriovenous malformations, and pulmonary arteriovenous fistulas are among other manifestations of this syndrome that occur later in life.

Management. Telangiectasia is only a cosmetic problem. Bleeding is very rare, and there are no serious complications. However, it may be a sign of the underlying disorder, especially in patients with extensive telangiectases. A thorough medical or sometimes laboratory evaluation is necessary in these patients. Telangiectases are nearly always diagnosed clinically. In intravascular lymphoma, biopsy of the telangiectasia will

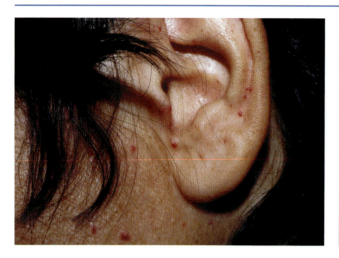

Fig. 6.141 Slightly raised (papular) telangiectases on the ears in a patient with Osler-Weber-Rendu syndrome. (With kind permission from Springer Science+Business Media: Baykal C, Yazganoğlu KD. Dermatological diseases of the nose and ears; 2010)

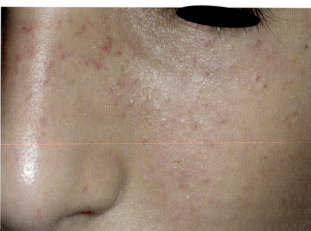

Fig. 6.142 Unilateral nevoid telangiectasia presenting as fine facial telangiectases located on the area innervated by the trigeminal cranial nerve

usually reveal neoplastic lymphoid cells confined to the vascular lumen.

Telangiectasia is mostly not treated other than cosmesis. Electrocautery or laser therapy (pulsed dye laser, argon laser, Nd:YAG laser, KTP laser) may be applied and have good cosmetic outcome.

Unilateral Nevoid Telangiectasia

Unilateral nevoid telangiectasia is a rare disorder characterized by unilateral fine telangiectases in a dermatomal distribution. Trigeminal (*see* Fig. 6.142), cervical, and upper thoracic dermatomes are the most commonly involved sites. The disorder may be congenital or acquired. Hyperestrogenism and increased sensitivity of target tissues toward hormones are suggested as etiologic factors. Pregnancy, puberty, chronic hepatic diseases, and hormonal contraceptive therapy are among the associated conditions in the acquired cases. Neurologic disorders may accompany unilateral nevoid telangiectasia in some patients. Lesions are usually permanent. Unilateral localization may be similar to that of angioma serpiginosum (*see* Fig. 6.144), but the latter disease manifests with punctate vascular papules without a segmental distribution.

Generalized Essential Telangiectasia

Widespread telangiectases without an underlying cause is called generalized essential telangiectasia. It is more common in women and may sometimes be familial. Telangiectases begin mostly in adult life and show a progressive course starting mostly in the extremities, later spreading to the trunk and sometimes to the face; they may involve large areas (*see* Fig. 6.143). The patients are otherwise healthy. Telangiectases on the skin do not show a tendency to bleeding. Lesions are permanent and constitute only a cosmetic problem. These

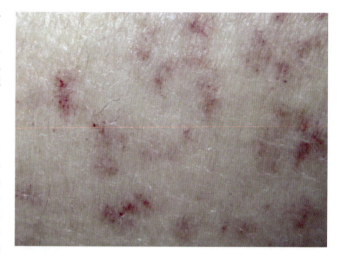

Fig. 6.143 Numerous lesions of generalized essential telangiectasia on the trunk. Generalized lesions occur typically in adulthood

patients should be investigated to exclude diseases such as collagen vascular disorders, which can also induce telangiectases on different areas of the body.

Angioma Serpiginosum

Angioma serpiginosum is a rare idiopathic disorder characterized by numerous, persistent minute vascular lesions arising as a result of dilation of capillaries. It occurs mostly sporadically in the first decades of life and is predominant in females. Lesions are most commonly located unilaterally on the extremities, sparing the palmoplantar area. Bilateral and extensive lesions are uncommon. Grouped, nonpalpable, deep red punctate lesions (*see* Figs. 6.144 and 6.145) show a slow progressive course. A serpiginous or annular pattern is

6.2 Vascular Malformations

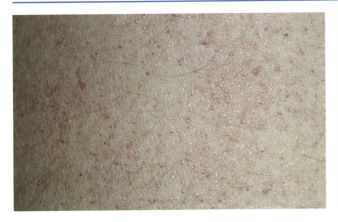

Fig. 6.144 Angioma serpiginosum presenting as multiple pinpoint vascular papules on the arm

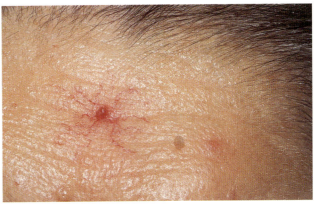

Fig. 6.146 Spider angioma formed by a central tiny red papule surrounded by radiating thin tortuous telangiectases

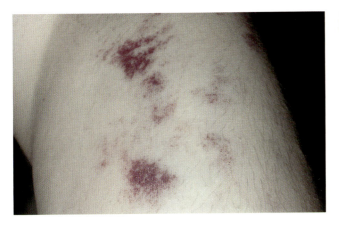

Fig. 6.145 Angioma serpiginosum manifesting as tiny vascular papules located on the upper arm unilaterally

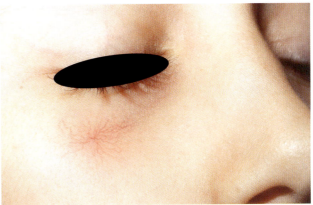

Fig. 6.147 Idiopathic solitary spider angioma on the cheek of a child. If there is a solitary lesion there is no need for any detailed examinations to search for a systemic disease

usually remarkable, attributable to the occurrence of new lesions at the periphery, while the central lesions may slightly fade. Slight erythema may be seen in the background. Lesions of angioma serpiginosum do not fade upon compression. Mucosal surfaces are not involved, and there is no well-described systemic association. Unlike unilateral nevoid telangiectasia (see Fig. 6.142), a segmental pattern is not present. The diagnosis is usually established clinically. Histopathologic examination reveals single or grouped ectatic, congested capillaries in the papillary dermis.

Management. Angioma serpiginosum may sometimes be cosmetically disfiguring. Vascular laser therapy such as pulsed dye laser is a therapeutic option for these cases.

Spider Angioma (Nevus Araneus)

Spider angioma is formed by an arteriole ending with radiating branches of capillaries in the papillary dermis. It occurs as a single lesion (see Figs. 6.146 and 6.147) or as a few small lesions in 10 to 15 percent of people who are otherwise normal. However, multiple and relatively larger lesions may be observed during pregnancy or in patients with chronic liver failure or who are using oral contraceptives. Increased estrogen concentration is considered to trigger these vascular lesions. They are seen more commonly in young children and adults. The face, especially the nose and cheeks, neck, upper trunk, and arms are more commonly involved. In children, hands and finger lesions are also not rare.

Centrally, a slightly elevated reddish papule of several millimeters in diameter represents the dilated superficial arteriole (see Fig. 6.146). Thin tortuous telangiectases radiating outward from the central papule represent dilated capillaries. This appearance looks like the body and legs of a spider. In rare cases the central papule measures up to 8 to 10 mm (see Fig. 6.148). Lesions may be pulsatile at the center. Bleeding is rare. The diagnosis is nearly always established clinically. If the central papule is compressed, the radiating telangiectases bleach temporarily as a result of emptying of capillaries but refill in a short time beginning at the center.

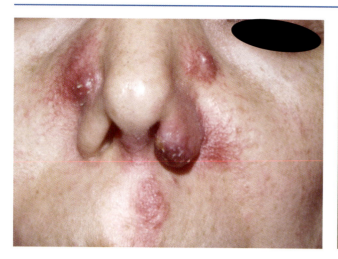

Fig. 6.148 Multiple spider angiomas in a pregnant woman. Note the unusual presence of large red nodules. They resolved spontaneously in a few months after delivery in this case. (With kind permission from Springer Science+Business Media: Baykal C, Yazganoğlu KD. Dermatological diseases of the nose and ears; 2010)

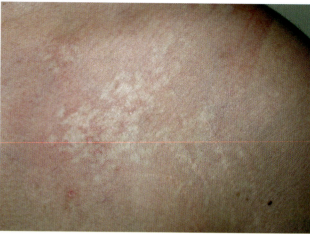

Fig. 6.149 Nevus anemicus presenting as a solitary white patch with irregular margins on the upper trunk

Management. There is no indication to search for systemic diseases in patients with solitary lesions. However, patients with multiple lesions should be evaluated for underlying causes. As the lesions may be permanent, treatment can be applied for cosmetic purposes. Gentle cautery in the central arteriole and pulsed dye laser are mostly effective. There is a low risk of small pit-like scars after therapy. Recurrence rarely occurs. Pregnancy-associated lesions may resolve spontaneously in a few months after delivery.

Nevus Anemicus

Nevus anemicus is a sporadic, congenital, persistent, pale patch developing secondary to vasoconstriction. Permanent vasoconstriction is caused by local blood vessel hypersensitivity to endogenous catecholamines. Therefore, the lesion is also called pharmacologic nevus. The trunk is the major site, followed by the limbs. An asymptomatic, white, well-defined, 5 to 10 cm macule with an irregular border and surrounding smaller white macules is the typical clinical appearance (*see* Fig. 6.149). There are no accompanying epidermal changes such as scaling.

Nevus depigmentosus, vitiligo, ash-leaf of tuberous sclerosis, and hypopigmented mycosis fungoides (*see* Fig. 14.66) may be considered in the differential diagnosis. Some of these may be differentiated by clinical examination. In contrast to vitiligo, nevus anemicus does not become evident on Wood light examination. Diascopy examination reveals normal skin color quite indistinguishable from the surrounding skin. Friction or hot or cold application on the lesion cannot induce reflex erythema but borders become hyperemic. Histopathologic examination is usually not necessary and if performed is normal. However, it may sometimes be helpful to exclude other diseases.

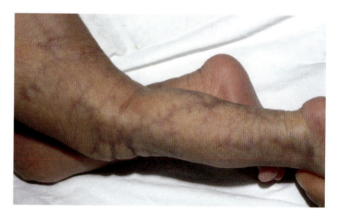

Fig. 6.150 Cutis marmorata telangiectatica congenita causing reticulated erythema on the legs

Management. Nevus anemicus is mostly an isolated disorder but may sometimes be associated with port-wine stain type of nevus flammeus or develop as a component of phacomatosis pigmentovascularis (*see* Fig. 3.225). Systemic examination is not necessary in patients with nevus anemicus. There is no effective treatment. Cosmetic camouflage can be helpful.

Cutis Marmorata Telangiectatica Congenita

Cutis marmorata telangiectatica congenita is a rare vascular disorder with congenital reticulated erythema (cutis marmorata) associated with extracutaneous findings. It is usually sporadic, but rare familial occurrence has also been described. It may be a component of phacomatosis pigmentovascularis.

Cutaneous findings are mostly present at birth and include reticulated erythematous (*see* Fig. 6.150), sometimes atrophic (*see* Fig. 6.151) skin patches that may be localized, segmental, or generalized. The persistent patches have a

6.2 Vascular Malformations

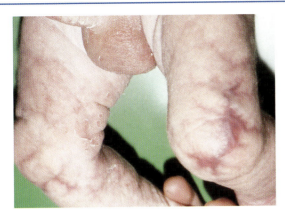

Fig. 6.151 Cutis marmorata telangiectatica congenita manifesting as reticulated erythema and cutaneous atrophy

reddish-blue hue. Ulceration and localized necrosis may rarely be observed overlying the cutaneous lesions. The most common affected sites are the extremities, especially the legs. Involvement may be more prominent on one side. The trunk and face may also be involved. The surface of the lesions may be hyperkeratotic and crusted. Telangiectases may also be seen in some cases. Other vascular malformations may be associated. Differential diagnoses include physiologic cutis marmorata, aplasia cutis congenita, neonatal lupus erythematosus, and Rothmund-Thomson syndrome. In contrast to physiologic cutis marmorata, reticulated erythematous patches are persistent, become prominent in the cold, and do not respond to local heat.

In approximately half of the cases, there are accompanying extracutaneous findings. Ipsilateral hemiatrophy or hemihypertrophy of the affected site leading to body asymmetry and discrepancy of limb length or circumference can be seen. Other possible associated findings include glaucoma, macrocephaly, mental retardation, hypospadias, and cardiovascular problems. Glaucoma is especially detected in cases with periocular skin involvement. In some cases, other vascular malformations such as port-wine stain and superficial varicose veins may be found. These findings may be located within the same area of cutis marmorata telangiectatica congenita or may be at other areas.

The diagnosis of the disorder is clinical and a biopsy is rarely performed. Histologic findings are not specific. Dilated capillaries and veins are seen in the dermis.

Management. There is no effective treatment of cutaneous manifestations, but one must search for the associated findings after arriving at the diagnosis of cutis marmorata telangiectatica congenita. Ulcerated lesions may be treated symptomatically. Regular measurement of limb length or circumference is advised. Cutaneous findings, especially erythema, usually improve with age, particularly within the first few years. Secondary postinflammatory hypo- and hyperpigmentation may develop. The discrepancy of limb length or circumference may also improve over time. In cases with prominent atrophy, cosmetic concern is high. Associated systemic anomalies may require therapy.

6.2.1.3 Angiokeratoma

Angiokeratoma is a benign vascular lesion characterized by prominent, cavernous ectasia of capillaries in the papillary dermis associated with mild hyperkeratosis and irregular acanthosis of the overlying epidermis, generally forming a collarette embracing the tumor. Several types of angiokeratomas are described in varying sizes, with different predilection areas, and in association with systemic disease. Different types are not expected to appear concomitantly in the same patient.

Solitary Angiokeratoma

Typically this idiopathic variant of angiokeratoma is a solitary, dark blue, bluish-red or bluish-purple papule or nodule on the limbs of young adults (*see* Figs. 6.152, 6.153 and 6.154). However, lesions may be located anywhere (*see* Fig. 6.155), and sometimes there may be more than one lesion. It more commonly occurs in childhood and adolescence. The lesion may resemble a pyogenic granuloma (*see* Fig. 6.46) because of its tendency to bleeding. Necrotic crusts may overlie lesions (*see* Fig. 6.153). The dark color of angiokeratoma and the occurrence of a sudden enlargement may raise a suspicion for malignant melanoma. Dermoscopy may be useful in the differentiation of these cases without performing a biopsy. Some lesions have a warty surface (*see* Fig. 6.156) resembling verruca vulgaris or a papillomatous melanocytic nevus (*see* Fig. 3.127). A purpuric halo around solitary angiokeratomas may be observed as a result of thrombosis, probably induced by a recent exogenous trauma. This target-like appearance of traumatic angiokeratoma (*see* Figs. 6.157 and 6.158a) may clinically be confused with targetoid hemosiderotic hemangioma (*see* Fig. 6.71). Thrombosis resolves spontaneously without any therapeutic intervention and the purpuric halo bleaches (*see* Fig. 6.158a and b).

Angiokeratoma of Fordyce

Angiokeratoma of Fordyce is a relatively common variant. The distinctive features of this type are the typical locations and the presence of multiple lesions. The scrotum (*see* Fig. 6.159) is the most commonly involved site in the male, but the penis (*see* Fig. 6.160) and the labium majus in females may also be involved. Scattered red to dark blue papules that are 2 to 5 mm in size are observed on the genital area of middle-aged or elderly adults. Multiple lesions may form a diffuse reddish appearance on the scrotum (*see* Fig. 6.161). Hyperkeratosis is not prominent in this type of angiokeratoma. Although usually asymptomatic, lesions may occasionally be itchy. Bleeding may rarely occur due to

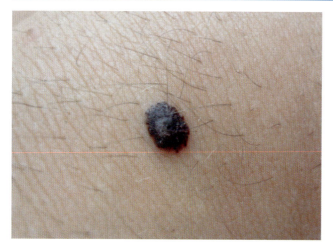

Fig. 6.152 Solitary angiokeratoma presenting as a bluish-red nodule

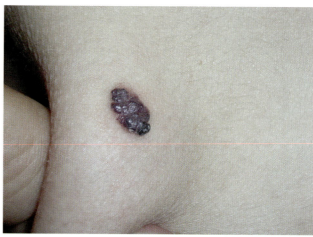

Fig. 6.155 Solitary angiokeratoma presenting as a lobulated nodule on the ear

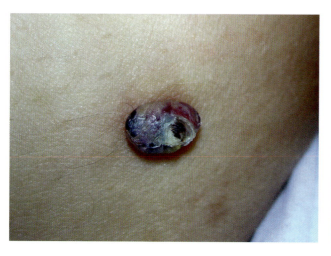

Fig. 6.153 Solitary angiokeratoma with a crusted surface on the leg

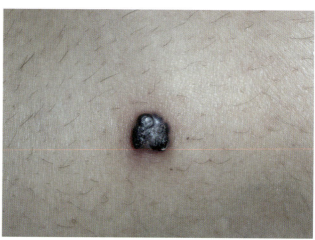

Fig. 6.156 Solitary angiokeratoma with hyperkeratotic surface

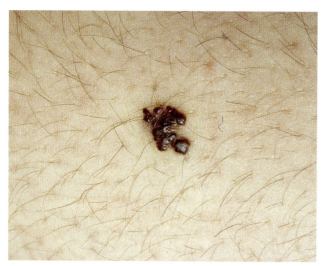

Fig. 6.154 Solitary angiokeratoma with a lobulated appearance

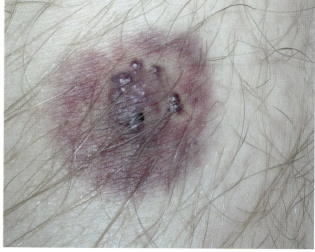

Fig. 6.157 Traumatic angiokeratoma on the leg. Note the purpuric halo around the central papule

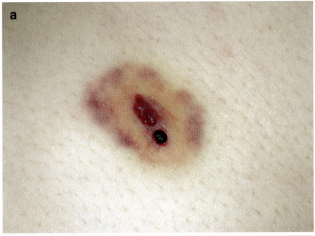

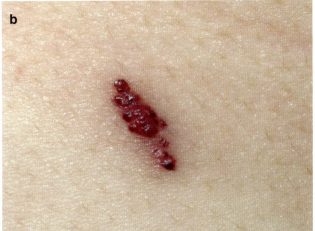

Fig. 6.158 (a) Traumatic angiokeratoma with a target-like appearance. (b) Purplish halo around the papular lesion has resolved spontaneously in fifteen days

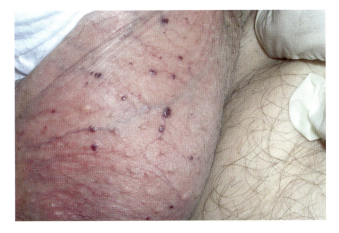

Fig. 6.159 Angiokeratoma of Fordyce presenting as multiple papules located on the scrotum, a characteristic site

trauma. Angiokeratomas of Fabry disease may also involve the genital area, but these patients also have diffuse lesions on the trunk and extremities.

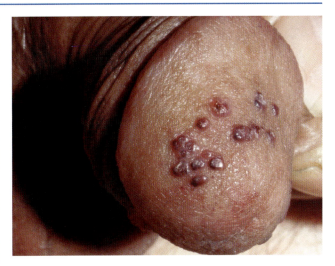

Fig. 6.160 Reddish penile papules representing angiokeratoma of Fordyce

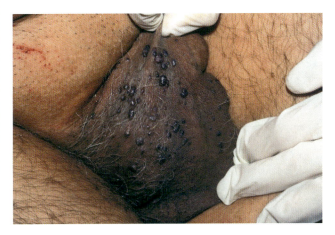

Fig. 6.161 Numerous lesions of angiokeratoma of Fordyce causing diffuse redness on the scrotum

Angiokeratoma of Mibelli

This is a rare type of angiokeratoma presenting with 1 to 5 mm, dark red or dark blue papules predominantly located on the dorsum of the fingers and toes. Hands, feet, elbows, and knees (*see* Fig. 6.162) may also be affected. The surface of the lesions may show verrucous changes. Affected individuals are mainly adolescent girls. An autosomal dominant inheritance may be present. Cold intolerance is a typical feature and may cause acrocyanosis and chilblains. A tendency to spontaneous healing is not expected. On the contrary, lesions may show gradual progression.

Angiokeratoma Circumscriptum

This is one of the rarest types of angiokeratomas, appearing with unilaterally distributed plaques most commonly on the lower leg (*see* Figs. 6.163 and 6.164) and sometimes on other parts of the limbs, buttock or trunk. Small hyperkeratotic papules may be present at birth or appear in childhood. These papules have a tendency to coalesce into a solitary large verrucous plaque. Congenital appearance is a distinguishing feature from other types of angiokeratomas. Patients are otherwise healthy. It probably represents the same entity described as verrucous hemangioma. Bleeding easily occurs with trauma.

Fabry Disease

Multiple angiokeratomas on different sites of the body may be a part of Fabry disease as well as some other rare storage disorders like fucosidosis and sialidosis. Angiokeratomas may accompany coarse facies, growth and mental retardation, dysostosis multiplex, and neurologic deterioration in fucosidosis. On the other hand, in some patients with multiple angiokeratomas of variable size and location, no associated systemic manifestations may be detected (*see* Figs. 6.165, 6.166 and 6.167).

Fabry disease is a lysosomal storage disorder caused by the deficiency of α-galactosidase A (GLA) and resulting

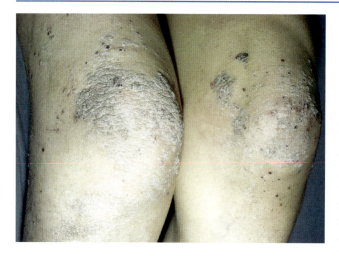

Fig. 6.162 Angiokeratoma of Mibelli presenting as multiple hyperkeratotic lesions on the knees

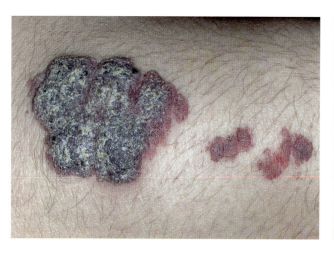

Fig. 6.163 Angiokeratoma circumscriptum presenting with a large reddish verrucous plaque together with smaller lesions on the leg

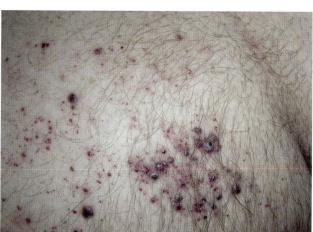

Fig. 6.165 Multiple angiokeratomas on the buttocks in an otherwise healthy patient

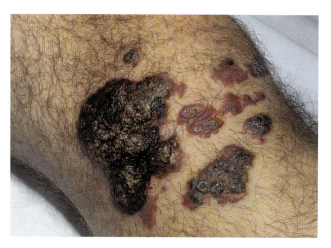

Fig. 6.164 Angiokeratoma circumscriptum formed by multiple reddish verrucous plaques on a localized area on the leg

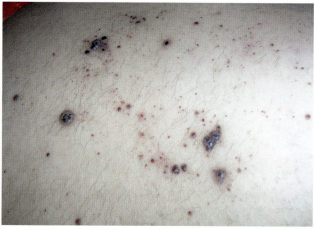

Fig. 6.166 Angiokeratomas presenting as tiny reddish papules widely distributed on the trunk in an otherwise healthy patient

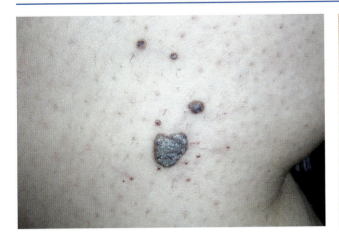

Fig. 6.167 Multiple angiokeratomas of variable size in an otherwise healthy patient

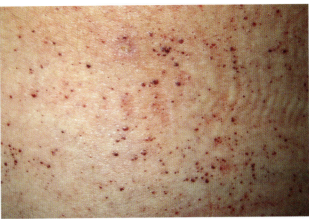

Fig. 6.168 Numerous angiokeratomas on the abdomen typical of Fabry disease. This multysystem disease was first diagnosed with cutaneous findings in depicted case

in an accumulation of globotriaosylceramide in the vascular endothelium of various tissues affecting multiple organ systems. It has a progressive course, leading to organ failure and premature death. The X-linked recessive disease is caused by mutation of *GLA* gene. Clinical features are most commonly prominent in males but females can also be affected. The onset of symptoms of classic Fabry disease is usually in childhood. Neurologic and gastrointestinal symptoms usually appear early in childhood and adolescence. Episodic acral paresthesia, acral/abdominal pain, heat intolerance, headache, and hearing impairment are main systemic symptoms. Ocular abnormalities may also be detected in childhood. Corneal opacities (cornea verticillata) are the diagnostic finding of ocular involvement. Retinal vessel tortuosity and cataract are other ophthalmologic features. Renal, cerebrovascular, and cardiovascular involvements usually start later in life and worsen gradually. Mild proteinuria may be the first sign of renal involvement and can also be detected in some of the children with Fabry disease. Renal failure, cardiomyopathy, ischemic attacks, and stroke are the late manifestations of the disease. Osteopenia and osteoporosis also occur in adulthood. Untreated male patients typically die between the ages of 40 to 50.

The main cutaneous manifestation of Fabry disease is diffuse angiokeratomas measuring 1 to 2 mm that are usually located on the lower trunk (*see* Fig. 6.168). The genital area (*see* Fig. 6.169), femoral area, umbilicus, and buttocks are typically involved. The palms, perioral area, and lips (*see* Fig. 6.170) are other frequently affected sites. Lesions mainly appear in the first 5 to 10 years of life and increase in number over the years. In an adult patient there may be hundreds of angiokeratomas. Hypohidrosis or anhidrosis, telangiectasia, hypotrichosis, and lymphedema are other cutaneous findings of this disorder. Coarse facial features may be detected in some cases.

Management. The size and type of the angiokeratoma mainly designate the choice of therapy. Special management

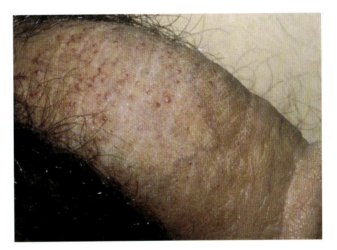

Fig. 6.169 Minute angiokeratomas on the penis in a patient with Fabry disease

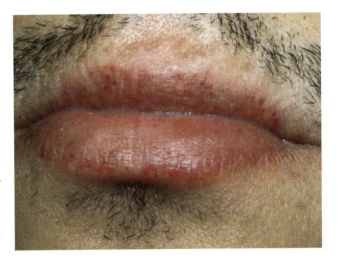

Fig. 6.170 Multiple tiny angiokeratomas on the lips of a patient with Fabry disease

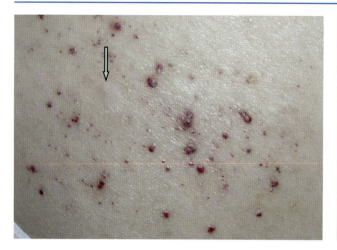

Fig. 6.171 Multiple angiokeratomas are shown. Scar formation may be observed after treatment with destructive modalities; in this case scars (*arrow*) were caused by cryotherapy

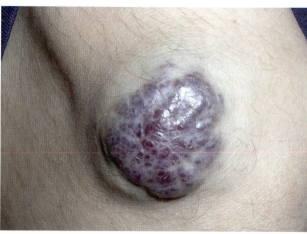

Fig. 6.172 Large bluish persistent nodule representing a vascular malformation typical for blue rubber bleb nevus syndrome

is required for syndromes associated with angiokeratomas. Surgical excision or laser can be applied for solitary angiokeratomas. Recurrence is not expected after surgery. Ablative laser methods (e.g., carbon dioxide, Er:YAG), in combination with vascular types of lasers, may be helpful in hyperkeratotic lesions. However, results are not always satisfactory. In the presence of multiple Fordyce angiokeratomas surgery is not feasible, and cauterization may lead to bleeding and scar formation. Laser therapy (argon) may be helpful in these cases. However, therapy is not obligatory. Cauterization, cryotherapy, laser, or surgery may be effective in angiokeratoma of Mibelli. Neither of these therapies prevents the occurrence of new lesions, particularly in patients with multiple angiokeratomas such as those with Fabry disease (*see* Fig. 6.171).

A multidisciplinary approach is necessary in the management of Fabry disease. The progression of the disorder can be reduced or stabilized by enzyme replacement therapy, namely, agalsidase alfa and beta. Initiation of enzyme replacement therapy must be considered in young patients before the development of any significant organ damage. Moreover, in patients with established organ damage, concomitant treatments are indicated. Management of angiokeratomas of Fabry disease is not different from that of other types of angiokeratomas.

6.2.2 Venous Malformations

Venous malformations are deep-seated vascular malformations causing blue or bluish-purple soft nodules or masses. They occur sporadically or are inherited. They may be an isolated finding or part of a syndrome. Syndromic lesions are typically multifocal. Lesions may appear at birth or early in childhood and usually have a progressive course. In contrast to capillary malformations, deeper structures such as subcutaneous tissue, muscles, joints, and bones may be involved. Histologically, widely dilated vein-like structures extending from the dermis to the subcutis may be observed. These vascular structures have thin, hyalinized walls and are lined by flat endothelium. Venous malformations may cause serious complications related to the locations. Lesions on the extremities may cause muscle weakness. Large lesions on the face can lead to serious cosmetic concerns and functional impairment. Sleep apnea syndrome may develop as a result of pharyngeal and laryngeal venous malformations. Involvement of muscles and joints can cause pain. Gastrointestinal venous malformations with recurrent bleeding may result with anemia.

Multiple lesions of venous malformations can be associated with rare syndromes such as blue rubber bleb nevus syndrome and Maffucci syndrome.

6.2.2.1 Blue Rubber Bleb Nevus Syndrome

Venous malformations are major findings of blue rubber bleb nevus syndrome and are observed as multiple, asymmetrically distributed, angiomatous papules and nodules of varying sizes (*see* Figs. 6.172 and 6.173). They may appear at birth or in childhood. They are commonly located on the extremities (*see* Figs. 6.173 and 6.174), especially on the palms and soles and the trunk but may be observed anywhere on the body, including the oral mucosa. Lesions may be painful. The size and number of vascular lesions increase with age. Large lesions measuring 3 to 5 cm can be observed. There is no increase in skin temperature and thrill is absent. In contrast to the red and relatively harder papulonodular lesions of

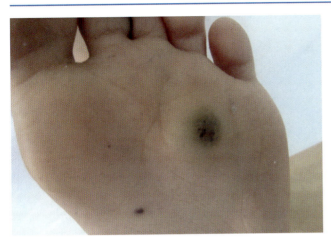

Fig. 6.173 Multiple bluish nodules on the sole of a patient with blue rubber bleb nevus syndrome. These vascular malformations are typically soft on palpation

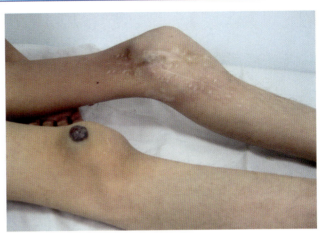

Fig. 6.175 Bluish vascular nodule in a patient with blue rubber bleb nevus syndrome. This patient was operated on for vascular malformation involving bones

6.2.2.2 Maffucci Syndrome

Venous malformations on multiple sites are associated with enchondromatosis in this rare syndrome. Recently, mutations on the gene encoding *IOH1* and *IOH2* have been detected in these patients. Some lesions may be congenital, but they usually appear in early childhood and have a progressive course until the third decade. Enchondromas are benign cartilaginous tumors that usually occur on the extremities. Swelling of the fingers and dorsum of the hands and feet is usually the first sign of this syndrome (*see* Fig. 6.176a). However, enchondromas can be present anywhere on the body. Both enchondromas and vascular lesions are distributed asymmetrically and enlarge gradually (*see* Fig. 6.176b). Vascular malformations may be superficial or deep. They may occur as bluish soft subcutaneous nodules on any part of the body with a predilection for the extremities (*see* Figs. 6.176a and b, and 6.177). Histologically some lesions are spindle cell hemangiomas. Cutaneous lesions resemble those of blue rubber bleb nevus syndrome (*see* Fig. 6.172), but the presence of enchondromas confirms the diagnosis of Maffucci syndrome. The face (*see* Fig. 6.178) and trunk are other common locations of vascular lesions. Visceral and central nervous system involvement caused by vascular malformations may also be seen in some patients.

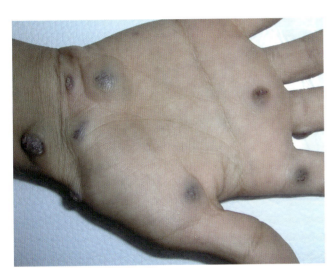

Fig. 6.174 Blue rubber bleb nevus syndrome presenting as multiple bluish vascular nodules on the palm, a characteristic site

diffuse neonatal angiomatosis (*see* Fig. 6.32), these tumors are blue (*see* Fig. 6.172), soft, and compressible. Deep infantile hemangiomas that may also be blue in color, glomuvenous malformation (*see* Fig. 6.193), and venous lake (*see* Fig. 6.186) are other differential diagnostic considerations.

Involvement of the gastrointestinal tract may cause chronic bleeding leading to iron-deficiency anemia. Initial diagnosis of this rare syndrome can be made during investigations for anemia. Venous malformations of other visceral organs such as the brain, lungs, bones (*see* Fig. 6.175), heart, and liver may be also encountered. Neurologic deficits are possible. Patients usually experience a normal life span.

Different complications of bone and vascular lesions may occur in the course of Maffucci syndrome. Thrombosis, phleboliths, and calcifications may develop within vascular malformations. In rare instances, aneurysms of major vessels may be detected. While extremity enchondromas may lead to fractures and deformities, cranial and vertebral enchondromas may lead to neurologic sequelae. Malignant transformation of enchondromas, namely chondrosarcomas, occur in about one fifth of the patients. Rare associated malignancies include angiosarcoma, fibrosarcoma, osteosarcoma, lymphangiosarcoma, and adenocarcinoma. Patients usually have a normal life span if no malignancy develops.

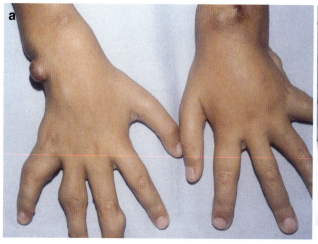
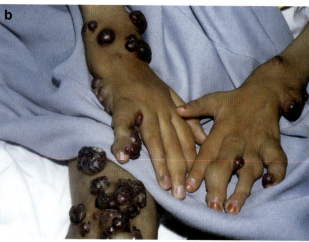

Fig. 6.176 (a) A child with Maffucci syndrome. Fusiform swellings on the fingers representing enchondromas and bluish nodules representing venous malformations are seen concomitantly. (b) Note the increase in the number and size of the vascular nodules on the hands in 4 years' time. Additionally, multiple large venous malformations are also seen on the legs

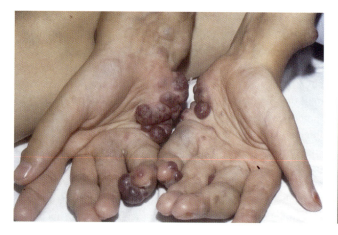

Fig. 6.177 Venous malformation on the palms associated with enchondromas of the fingers in a patient with Maffucci syndrome

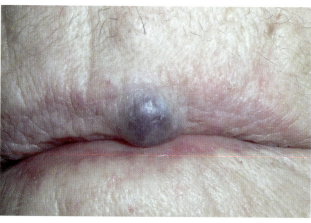

Fig. 6.179 Venous lake presenting as a solitary violaceous nodule on the midline of the upper lip in an adult

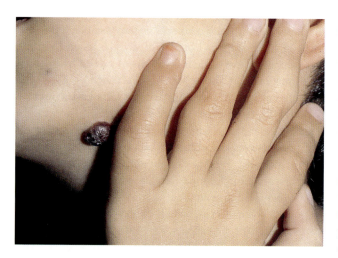

Fig. 6.178 Venous malformation on the chin and enchondromas on the fingers are shown in a patient with Maffucci syndrome

Management. Patients with venous malformations should be examined for systemic findings of possible associated syndromes. Therapy of venous malformation is difficult. Satisfactory cosmetic and functional results may be obtained with sclerotherapy combined with surgery. Aggressive surgical intervention including amputation may be mandatory in Maffucci syndrome. Patients should be followed for the risk of malignant transformation. Treatment of anemia is necessary in blue rubber bleb nevus syndrome.

6.2.2.3 Venous Lake (Phlebectasia)

Venous lake is an idiopathic acquired superficial varix that leads to violaceous (*see* Fig. 6.179) or dark blue (*see* Fig. 6.180) papules or nodules on skin and mucosae. It occurs mostly in elderly patients and is more common in men. The vermilion border of the lips is the most typical location (*see* Fig. 6.181). Face, ears (*see* Fig. 6.182), and neck (*see* Fig. 6.183) are

6.2 Vascular Malformations

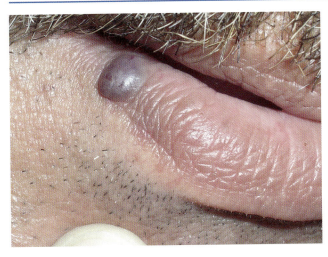

Fig. 6.180 Venous lake seen as a solitary blue nodule on the vermilion border of the lower lip. Softness of the lesion is a helpful diagnostic clue

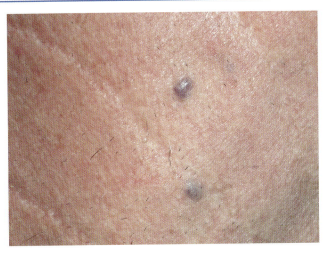

Fig. 6.183 Bluish papules on the neck representing venous lake

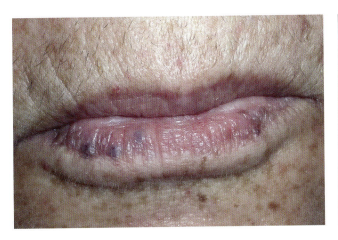

Fig. 6.181 A few small violaceous papules on the vermilion border of the lower lip representing venous lake

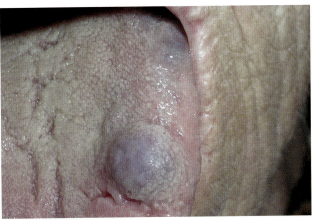

Fig. 6.184 Venous lakes located on the lateral side of the tongue; a small one on the upper part of the figure and a large one on the bottom are seen

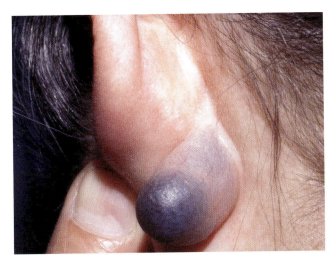

Fig. 6.182 Venous lake presenting as a large dark blue nodule on the ear, a characteristic site. (With kind permission from Springer Science+Business Media: Baykal C, Yazganoğlu KD. Dermatological diseases of the nose and ears; 2010)

other commonly affected sites. The tongue may also be involved (see Fig. 6.184). Most patients have solitary (see Figs. 6.179 and 6.180) or a few (see Figs. 6.181, 6.185, and 6.186) lesions. Blue nevus (see Fig. 3.71), nodular melanoma (see Fig. 12.42), pigmented basal cell carcinoma (see Fig. 11.72), venous malformations (see Fig. 6.172), and glomuvenous malformation are the main clinical diagnostic challenges. Venous lake on the lips and tongue may be confused with Kaposi sarcoma. Soft, easily compressible, slightly elevated, smooth-surfaced swellings less than 1 cm point to venous lake. Moreover, the lesion fades on pressure from glass (diascopy) owing to the dispersion of the blood content (see Fig. 6.187a and b). Dermoscopy is useful in differentiating venous lake from melanocytic tumors. A biopsy is rarely performed. A large dilated vein in the papillary dermis, filled with erythrocytes and sometimes containing a thrombus, is the main histopathologic feature.

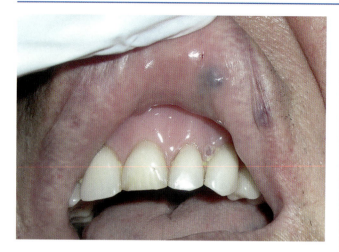

Fig. 6.185 Venous lake located on the mucosa of the upper lip as a few compressible lesions

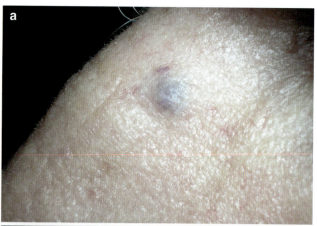

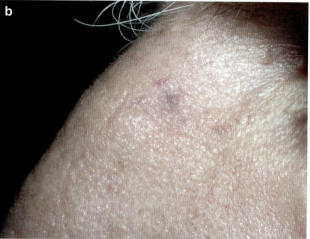

Fig. 6.187 (a) Slightly raised lesion of venous lake. (b) Visible flatting and blanching of the lesion after diascopy

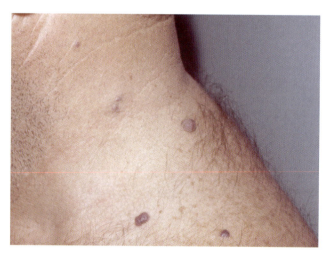

Fig. 6.186 Multiple lesions of venous lake located on the nape and upper back

Management. Even though the lesions are persistent, they are asymptomatic and do not lead to any serious complication. Bleeding by trauma is rare. Cosmetic concern and recurrent bleeding may underlie treatment decisions. Electrodesiccation, various types of laser therapy, and surgical excision can be performed.

6.2.3 Glomus Tumor and Glomuvenous Malformation (Glomangioma)

Glomus tumor and glomuvenous (glomulovenous) malformation have some common histopathologic features, but recently they are considered separate entities. The former is regarded as a benign tumor and the latter as a special type of malformation.

Glomus tumor is a painful hamartomatous tumor that arises from the modified vascular smooth muscle cells found in specialized arteriovenous shunts called Sucquet-Hoyer canals. These shunts play a role in temperature regulation and are mostly present in acral sites. Therefore, the characteristic location of glomus tumor is the fingertips, primarily the subungual part. It should be considered within the painful tumors of nail unit. But a glomus tumor may also occur on the hands, forearms, knee, and elsewhere. It usually arises in adulthood. The tumor nearly always appears as a solitary, skin-colored, purple or deep blue papule or nodule less than 1 cm in diameter (*see* Fig. 6.188). Larger tumors are rarely seen. The typical presentation includes bluish or reddish spots of the nail bed (*see* Fig. 6.189), nail dystrophy including distal notching (*see* Figs. 6.190 and 6.191), and in some cases, pain and tenderness upon tactile stimulation. Pain irradiating proximally may be precipitated by pressure and cold. The tumor usually has an intact surface, but subungual tumors may sometimes cause ulceration. Glomangiomyoma is a rare clinicopathologic variant of glomus tumor (*see* Fig. 6.192). Ultrasonography and high-resolution MRI may

6.2 Vascular Malformations

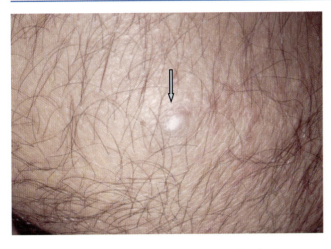

Fig. 6.188 Glomus tumor presenting as a skin-colored subcutaneous nodule on the leg

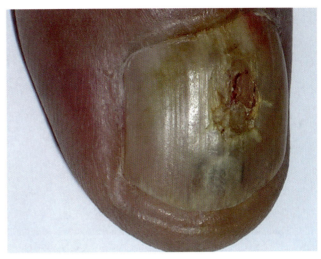

Fig. 6.191 Glomus tumor associated with nail dystrophy

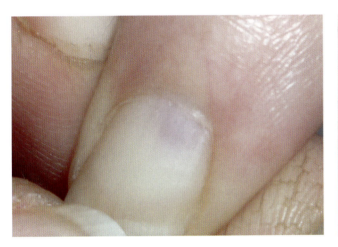

Fig. 6.189 Glomus tumor causing a bluish discoloration on the nailbed. The patients typically complain of pain

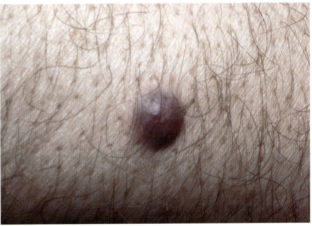

Fig. 6.192 Glomus tumor presenting as a solitary reddish elevated nodule. This patient was histopathologically diagnosed as having glomangiomyoma

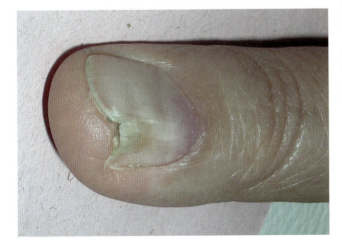

Fig. 6.190 Glomus tumor on the nailbed as purplish color change associated with localized nail dystrophy and distal notching

be helpful to support the clinical diagnosis and define the limits of the subungual tumor before surgery is performed.

Glomuvenous malformation (glomangioma) is rare and may be sporadic or inherited in an autosomal dominant pattern caused by loss of function mutations in *glomulin*. The lesions more commonly appear in infants and children. In contrast to the solitary and painful lesions of glomus tumor, glomangioma is usually painless, and typically multiple lesions are seen. The upper extremities are frequently involved (*see* Fig. 6.193), but lesions may occur elsewhere on the skin (*see* Fig. 6.194) and rarely on mucosal surfaces. They may sometimes be grouped in one area and occasionally show segmental distribution. Disseminated lesions may also occur. Reddish-blue or violaceous macules, nodules, or plaques may be seen. Different from venous lake (*see* Fig. 6.186), they are not compressible. Syndromes causing venous malformations such as blue rubber bleb nevus syndrome (*see* Fig. 6.172) could be considered

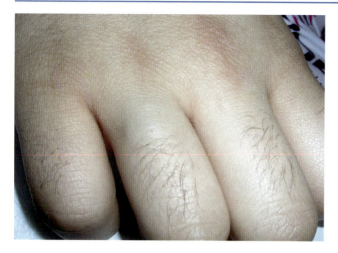

Fig. 6.193 Glomuvenous malformation presenting as multiple bluish papules on the dorsum of the hand

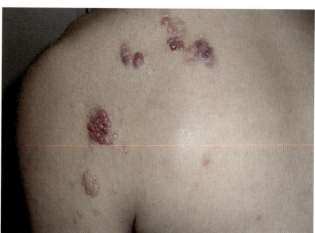

Fig. 6.195 Typical appearance of lymphangioma circumscriptum, including the clustered vesicle-like lesions in a herpetiform pattern. Location on the trunk is common

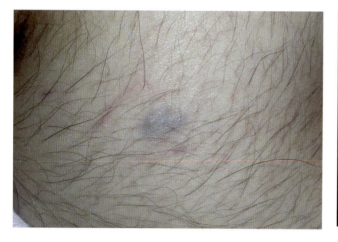

Fig. 6.194 Glomuvenous malformation presenting as violaceous flat lesions on the buttock

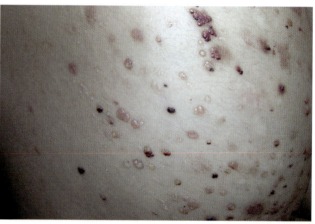

Fig. 6.196 Scattered vesicle-like lesions of lymphangioma circumscriptum on the buttocks. Clear and hemorrhagic lesions are seen

in the clinical differential diagnosis but histopathology distinguishes the two conditions. Moreover, visceral involvement is not seen in patients with glomangioma.

Cutaneous lesions of glomus tumor and glomuvenous malformation are diagnosed by biopsy. Glomus tumor is composed of glomus cell aggregates surrounding small vessels. Glomus cells are uniform, rounded with centrally located dark stained nuclei. The tumor is well circumscribed. Glomuvenous malformations are composed of dilated vascular channels surrounded by a single row or a few layers of glomus cells. The large thin-walled vascular spaces, the relatively scarce glomus cell content, and the poor circumscription are the main differences from glomus tumor.

Management. A therapeutic intervention is usually required for glomus tumor because of pain. Surgical removal is preferred for a solitary lesion. In incompletely excised tumors, recurrence with typical symptoms is not rare. Multiple lesions of glomuvenous malformation are not easy to remove surgically. Sclerotherapy may be a choice in the therapy of these lesions.

6.2.4 Lymphatic Malformation

Lymphatic malformations are developmental abnormalities of the lymphatic system. They can be classified as microcystic lymphatic malformations (lymphangioma circumscriptum), macrocystic lymphatic malformations (cystic hygroma, cavernous lymphangioma), and a combined form.

6.2.4.1 Lymphangioma Circumscriptum

Lymphangioma circumscriptum is the most common type of lymphatic malformation. It is usually present at birth but sometimes occurs later in life. The trunk (see Fig. 6.195), buttocks (see Figs. 6.196 and 6.197), genital area, limbs, and oral mucosa are the most commonly involved areas. However, it can occur anywhere, including the acral sites of the digits (see Fig. 6.198). The typical appearance is tiny, clear (see Fig. 6.195), and/or hemorrhagic vesicle-like lesions (see Figs. 6.196 and 6.197) clustered in a herpetiform pattern (see Fig. 6.195) or scattered in one region (see Fig. 6.196). Unlike classic vesicles, these lesions that

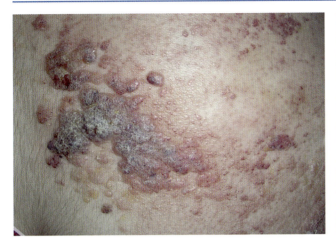

Fig. 6.197 Grouped and confluent lesions of lymphangioma circumscriptum on the buttocks. Note most of them are hemorrhagic

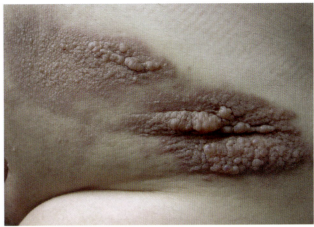

Fig. 6.199 Lymphangioma circumscriptum forming a large plaque with a verrucous surface

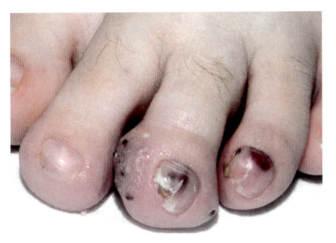

Fig. 6.198 Lymphangioma circumscriptum located on the toe, an unusual location

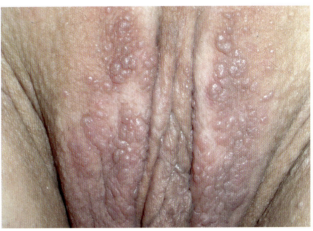

Fig. 6.200 Lymphangioma circumscriptum presenting as multiple papules on the vulva

represent dilated lymphatic channels are hard on palpation and do not easily rupture.

The invasion of the lesion is variable; it may involve deeper layers. Sometimes the surface of the lesions may be verrucous (see Fig. 6.199). The affected area may be swollen or enlarged in some patients suggesting a deeper involvement. MRI can be used to detect the extent of the involvement.

Lymphangioma circumscriptum sometimes occurs on the vulva and penis, causing typical papules (see Fig. 6.200) or indurated plaques and regional swelling (see Fig. 6.201). One of the most common locations of lymphangioma is the oral mucosa. The tongue, buccal mucosa, and floor of the mouth may be affected. Grouped vesicle-like lesions with serous or hemorrhagic content (see Fig. 6.202) or exophytic masses (see Fig. 6.203) localized on the dorsum of the tongue are typical. Lymphangioma circumscriptum is an important cause of macroglossia, especially in children. Mucosal lesions may infiltrate deep tissues such as the parotid gland and the muscles of the tongue. Intermittent leakage of the clear lymphatic fluid is another feature.

The lesions may sometimes expand or contract in response to the flow of lymphatic fluid. Inflammation or intralesional bleeding may also contribute to the size of the lesions. Most lesions are asymptomatic, but inflammation may occur in the event of secondary infections. Recurrent bacterial infections such as cellulitis may be seen in patients with widespread lesions (see Fig. 6.204a and b). Secondarily infected mouth lesions may be malodorous. Secondary ulcerations are rarely encountered (see Fig. 6.205).

The differential diagnosis mainly includes secondary lymphangiectases, which may be misnamed "acquired lymphangiomas." Secondary lymphangiectases (see Fig. 6.222) may arise as a result of lymphatic damage caused by radiation therapy, surgery, or chronic inflammation. Sometimes they may be associated with persistent lymphedema. Histologically lymphangioma circumscriptum is composed of dilated lymphatic spaces generally situated at superficial

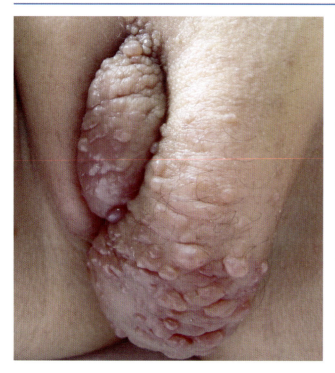

Fig. 6.201 Lymphangioma circumscriptum causing asymmetric enlargement with overlying vesicle-like lesions on the vulva

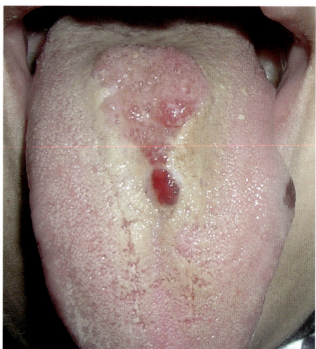

Fig. 6.203 Lymphangioma circumscriptum presenting as a raised mass on the tongue

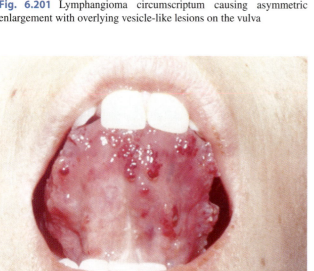

Fig. 6.202 Lymphangioma circumscriptum presenting as multiple vesicle-like lesions on the tongue. Note that some have hemorrhagic content

and deep dermis. The lumina contain eosinophilic lymph and sometimes erythrocytes. Vessels in deep tissue may contain muscular tissue in their walls.

6.2.4.2 Cystic Higroma

Cystic higroma (macrocystic lymphatic malformation) is distinct variant of lymphangioma which may be observed on various locations, most commonly the neck and axilla. Symptoms of the tumor is related with its location. It is typically a painless, soft, large, diffuse swelling that transilluminates (*see* Fig. 6.206). It is not warm and no thrill is present. Cystic higroma shows large dilated cavernous lymphatic channels filled with eosinophilic fluid and sometimes erythrocytes. Accompanying lymphoid aggregates may be seen.

Management. Involution is not expected in lymphatic malformations. Most patients are observed without any intervention because of the lack of an effective therapeutic modality. Treatment decisions are usually made according to the size, location, and symptoms of the lymphatic malformations. The main causes of treatment include recurrence of secondary infections, persistent oozing, and painful or ulcerated lesions. Cosmetic concern or functional disabilities are other important indications for therapy. Surgical removal and/or sclerotherapy are the main treatment modalities of lymphatic malformations. However, extensive lesions and lesions localized near vital structures are difficult to treat with surgery. Recurrences are common, especially if the deep component cannot be removed by surgery (*see* Fig. 6.207). In cases with relapsing cellulitis prophylactic use of penisilin may be necessary.

6.2.4.3 Lymphedema

Lymphedema is a localized persistent swelling of soft tissue caused by lymph fluid retention in turn resulting from failure of lymphatic drainage. Capillary filtration is unaffected. The legs are most commonly involved, but the arms, head, neck, and genitalia can also be affected.

Lymphedema may occur primarily, as an isolated condition due to the developmental anomaly of lymphatic vessels

6.2 Vascular Malformations

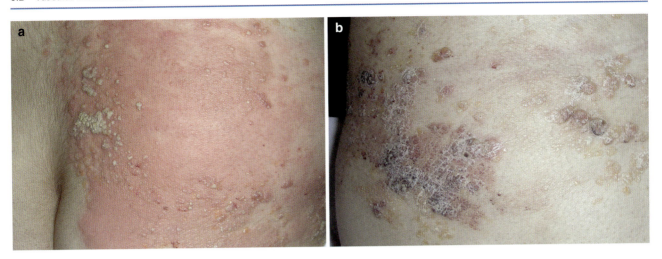

Fig. 6.204 (a) Lymphangioma circumscriptum infected secondarily (cellulitis). (b) The same lesion after treatment of secondary bacterial infection with systemic antibiotics

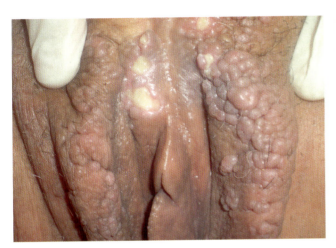

Fig. 6.205 Lymphangioma circumscriptum on the vulva associated with secondary ulcerations

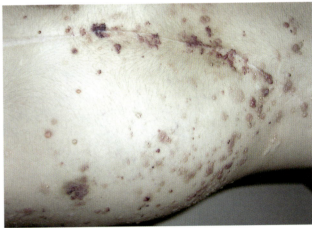

Fig. 6.207 Relapse of lymphangioma circumscriptum on the operation site. Relapse is not rare unless a radical surgery has been performed

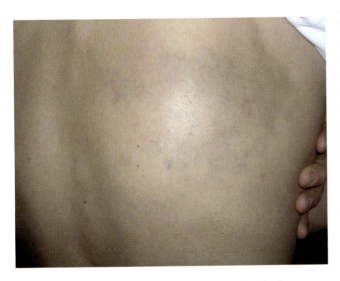

Fig. 6.206 Cystic higroma presenting as an ill-defined subcutaneous mass on the back (*upper right*). The diagnosis was established with imaging studies in this case

or in the setting of some syndromes, or secondarily, caused by injury of the lymphatic vessels. Primary lymphedema may be present at birth (Milroy disease) (*see* Fig. 6.208), develop at puberty (lymphedema praecox, Meige disease) (*see* Fig. 6.209), or in adulthood (lymphedema tarda) (*see* Fig. 6.210). There may be a history of lymphedema in other family members. Primary lymphedema may also be seen in the setting of other syndromes such as yellow-nail syndrome (*see* Fig. 6.211), Turner syndrome, Noonan syndrome, lymphedema-distichiasis syndrome, and Klippel-Trenaunay syndrome (*see* Fig. 6.120).

Secondary lymphedema may be associated with various diseases causing damage to the lymphatics. It may occur at any age. Lymphedema develops frequently in patients with breast cancer after mastectomy and axillary lymph node dissection or radiotherapy, and it is usually seen on the arm of the affected side (*see* Fig. 6.212). Postsurgical lymphedema may also be seen in the setting of some other malignancies at the sites of surgery. External compression of lymphatics by tumors is also

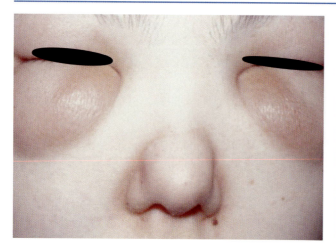

Fig. 6.208 Milroy disease causing lymphedema of the eyelids in a child

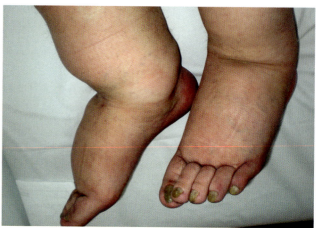

Fig. 6.211 Lymphedema involving both lower extremities in a patient with yellow-nail syndrome. Note the typical nail changes

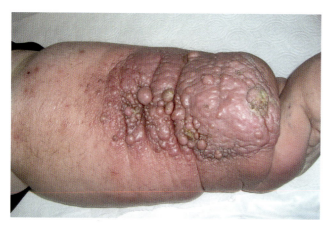

Fig. 6.209 Lymphedema precox causing lymphedema on the foot and leg in a middle-aged adult. In this case lymphedema has started in the second decade

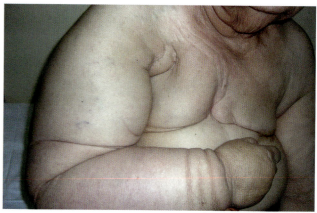

Fig. 6.212 Lymphedema involving one arm and hand in a patient who has been treated for cancer of the ipsilateral breast with mastectomy, radiotherapy, and chemotherapy

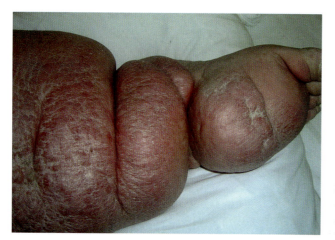

Fig. 6.210 Lymphedema tarda in an adult patient. In this case lymphedema has started in the fourth decade and has shown a rapidly progressive course. The overlying erythema is related with secondary infection

possible. Some malignancies, especially Kaposi sarcoma, may cause lymphedema of the limbs by neoplastic infiltration leading to obstruction of the lymphatic vessels (see Fig. 13.15). Filariasis is an infectious disease causing lymphedema. Another presentation of secondary lymphedema is the postinflammatory type that develops after recurrent attacks of cellulitis. Rosacea may also cause lymphedema of the face.

Lymphedema presents with nonpitting edema, especially on the dorsum of the feet, lower legs, dorsum of the hands, and forearms. The circumference of the affected limb is widened to a varying extent. The swollen region may be discolored, and skin creases are pronounced. Progressive fibrosis results in localized hardening of the tissues and skin. In contrast to primary lymphedema, secondary lymphedema of the extremities is usually unilateral (see Fig. 6.213). Primary lymphedema mostly begins on one extremity but in the course of the disease both extremities may be involved (see Fig. 6.214). Primary lymphedema may also occur on the face, especially on periorbital regions (see Fig. 6.208). The affected sites vary according to the underlying cause in secondary lymphedema. Lymphedema on the genitalia may cause enlargement of these organs (see Figs. 6.215 and 6.216). The diagnosis of lymphedema is usually clinical.

6.2 Vascular Malformations

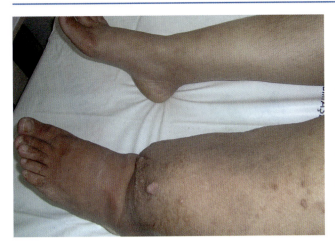

Fig. 6.213 Unilateral lymphedema causing pronounced discrepancy of the size of the lower legs

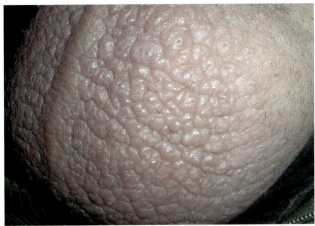

Fig. 6.215 Scrotal lymphedema associated with secondary surface changes

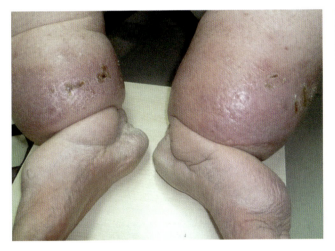

Fig 6.214 Primary lymphedema involving both legs symmetrically in an elder patient. Severe lymphedema may restrict the movements

Lymphangiography or lymphoscintigraphy may be helpful in demonstrating the underlying malformation.

Severe hyperkeratosis and a verrucous appearance may develop on the surface of the long-standing lesions and is called elephantiasis nostras verrucosa (see Fig. 6.217). Xanthomatous deposits as yellow nodules may rarely appear in patients with hereditary lymphedema (xanthomatosis and chylous lymphedema) (see Fig. 6.218). In these cases, chylous discharge may be associated. Lymphedema on the feet may cause secondary nail dystrophy (see Fig. 6.219). Recurrent cellulitis is a common complication of lymphedema (see Figs. 6.210, 6.220, and 6.221) and may cause painful and malodorous lesions. Chronic ulcers may also occur in the setting of lymphedema. Lymphangiosarcoma (Stewart-Treves syndrome) is a rare malignancy developing in chronic lymphedema, particularly after mastectomy. Purplish-red papules or nodules may be the initial clinical sign of this sarcoma (see Fig. 13.55).

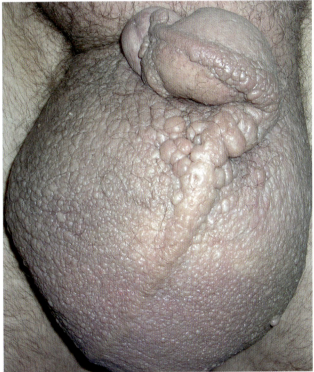

Fig. 6.216 Genital lymphedema causing enlargement of male genitalia

Management. Lymphedema is a chronic problem necessitating a multidisciplinary approach. Underlying causes need to be identified and treated. In patients with lymphedema developing as a result of recurrent secondary bacterial infections, prophylactic treatment with antibiotics may be beneficial. The severity of edema and the degree of fibrosis are important decisions in choosing the appropriate therapy. Compression therapies such as bandaging, manual compression, lymphatic massage, or pneumatic pumps are mostly used but are not very effective in cases with pronounced fibrosis. Various surgical

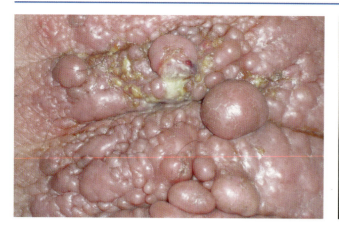

Fig. 6.217 Severe hyperkeratosis and a verrucous appearance (elephantiasis nostras verrucosa) developing on the surface of the long-standing lymphedema

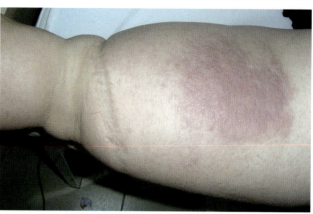

Fig. 6.220 Cellulitis on chronic lymphedema presenting as a flat reddish patch that was tender to the touch

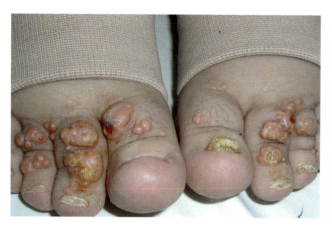

Fig. 6.218 Xanthomas on the dorsum of toes in a child with hereditary lymphedema (xanthomatous and chylous lymphedema)

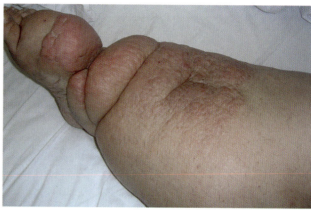

Fig. 6.221 Cellulitis covering a large area in a patient with primary lymphedema. Recurrence of streptococcal infections on the affected area is one of the major complaints of the patients

6.2.4.4 Lymphangiectasia

Lymphangiectasia usually presents with acquired grouped papular lesions caused by dilated cutaneous lymph vessels. Clinical and histopathologic features are similar to those of lymphangioma circumscriptum, but lymphangiectasia usually occurs in the setting of underlying lymphedema. The major pathogenic factor is disruption of the normal structure of lymphatic channels leading to dilatation. "Acquired lymphangioma" is a misnomer, as these are not real neoplasms.

Typical lesions are translucent or flesh-colored, dome-shaped, firm papules measuring 2 to 5 mm (*see* Fig. 6.222). Initial lesions are commonly misdiagnosed as viral warts. Some translucent papules may look like vesicles mimicking herpes zoster. Drainage of lymph fluid or chyle may be observed spontaneously or upon trauma. Lesions may be complicated by recurrent secondary infections such as cellulitis.

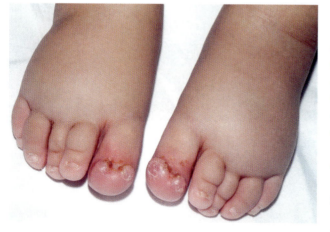

Fig. 6.219 Secondary nail dystrophy on both big toes due to primary lymphedema (Milroy disease)

techniques could be used in severe cases for the lymphatic malformation, but these have a transient effect without inducing a cure. Low-level laser therapy is also an alternative.

6.2 Vascular Malformations

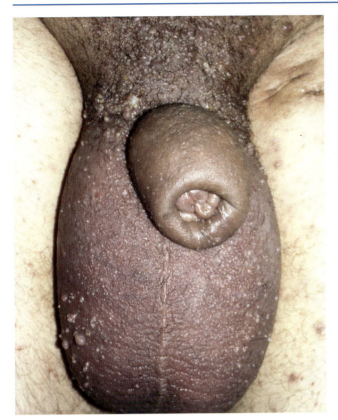

Fig. 6.222 Lymphangiectasia presenting as translucent, flesh-colored, dome-shaped, small papules. This condition has developed on long-standing scrotal and penile lymphedema

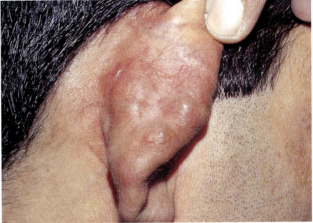

Fig. 6.223 A red patch and papules on the ear representing early stage of arteriovenous malformation (With kind permission from Springer Science+Business Media: Baykal C, Yazganoğlu KD. Dermatological diseases of the nose and ears; 2010)

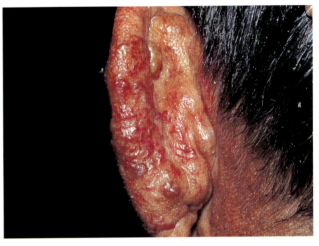

Fig. 6.224 Arteriovenous malformation forming a plaque with overlying telangiectases on the ear (With kind permission from Springer Science+Business Media: Baykal C, Yazganoğlu KD. Dermatological diseases of the nose and ears; 2010)

Management. Since lymphangiectases are caused by certain factors that lead to lymphedema, the underlying factors must be treated first. In the presence of extensive involvement, excision of the lesions is an alternative option. Sclerotherapy, cryotherapy, and carbon dioxide laser may be applied with varying success, but recurrence is common.

6.2.5 Arteriovenous Malformation

Arteriovenous malformation is a rare type of vascular malformation with a progressive course and serious complications. Direct communication among arteries and veins forming a nidus is the underlying mechanism of an arteriovenous malformation. It may present at birth or appear later. The most common location of arteriovenous malformations is the head. Arteriovenous malformations on the ears are mostly unilateral. Along with the pinnae, lateral aspects of the scalp and neck may also be involved. Initial lesions are small, red, asymptomatic macules or flat plaques. At this stage the lesions may be misdiagnosed as port-wine stain or infantile hemangioma. Consequently, they may be mistreated unsuccessfully. Lesions may be stable in childhood but proliferate and enlarge in advancing years, forming reddish raised masses (*see* Figs. 6.223, 6.224 and 6.225). The lesions are not compressible but warm and pulsatile. Dilated vessels may be seen on the surface. A thrill-like sound, which can be heard at auscultation, is helpful for diagnosis. Induration and necrosis of the underlying structures and persistent ulcers occur later. Hemorrhage and secondary infections may be life-threatening. Cardiac decompensation is a late complication of arteriovenous malformation.

Several syndromes have been described that are mostly related to the location of arteriovenous malformations. Bonnet-Dechaume-Blanc syndrome (congenital retinocephalic vascular malformation) consists of arteriovenous mal-

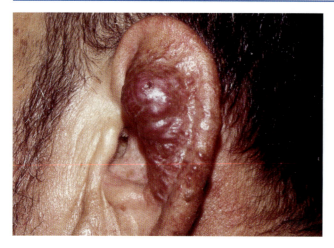

Fig. 6.225 Reddish pulsatile mass on the ear due to arteriovenous malformation. (With kind permission from Springer Science+Business Media: Baykal C, Yazganoğlu KD. Dermatological diseases of the nose and ears; 2010)

formations mainly located in the midface (maxillofacial and mandibular). In the late stages of this syndrome, epistaxis, nasal congestion and symptoms owing to ocular (retinal) and brain involvement, can occur.

When clinical features are not sufficient for the diagnosis of an arteriovenous malformation, imaging studies such as Doppler ultrasound, MRI, angiography or percutaneous venogram may be helpful.

Management. Although they progress slowly, arteriovenous malformations may be life-threatening. Therefore, therapy is indicated before any serious complications occur. Radical surgery is the optimal treatment. Embolization followed by surgical removal is usually preferred. In the advanced stages, amputation may sometimes be indicated for lesions of the extremities.

Suggested Reading

Akcay A, Karakas Z, Saribeyoglu ET, et al. Infantile hemangiomas, complications and follow-up. Indian Pediatr. 2012;49:805–9.

Akman-Karakaş A, Kandemir H, Senol U, et al. Unilateral nevoid telangiectasia accompanied by neurological disorders. J Eur Acad Dermatol Venereol. 2011;25:1356–9.

Batta K, Goodyear H M, Moss C, et al. Randomised controlled study of early pulsed dye laser treatment of uncomplicated childhood hemangiomas: results of a 1-year analysis. Lancet. 2002; 360:521–7.

Bolognia JL, Jorizzo JL, Schaffer JV. Dermatology, edn 3. London: Mosby; 2012.

Bond J, Basheer MH, Gordon D. Lymphangioma circumscriptum: pitfalls and problems in definitive management. Dermatol Surg. 2008;34:271–5.

Burgdorf WHC, Plewig G, Wolff HH, Landthaler M. Braun-Falco's Dermatology, edn 3. Italy: Springer-Verlag; 2009.

Caputo R, Tadini G. Atlas of genodermatoses. Spain: Taylor and Francis; 2006.

Dispenzieri A. POEMS syndrome: update on diagnosis, risk-stratification and management. Am J Hematol. 2012;87:804–14.

Drolet BA, Frommelt PC, Chamlin SL, et al. Initiation and use of propranolol for infantile hemangioma: report of a consensus conference. Pediatrics. 2013;13:128–40.

Fernández Y, Bernabeu-Wittel M, García-Morillo JS. Kaposiform hemangioendothelioma. Eur J Intern Med. 2009;20:106–13.

Fernández-Guarino M, Boixeda P, de Las Heras E, et al. Phakomatosis pigmentovascularis: clinical findings in 15 patients and review of the literature. J Am Acad Dermatol. 2008;58:88–93.

Glick ZR, Frieden IJ, Garzon MC, et al. Diffuse neonatal hemangiomatosis: an evidence-based review of case reports in the literature. J Am Acad Dermatol. 2012;67:898–903.

González-Guerra E, Haro MR, Fariña MC, et al. Glomeruloid haemangioma is not always associated with POEMS syndrome. Clin Exp Dermatol. 2009;34:800–3.

Khunger N. Lymphatic malformations: current status. J Cutan Aesthet Surg. 2010;3:137–8.

Krol A, MacArthur CJ. Congenital hemangiomas: rapidly involuting and noninvoluting congenital hemangiomas. Arch Facial Plast Surg. 2005;7:307–11.

Léauté-Labrèze C, Prey S, Ezzedine K. Infantile haemangioma: part I. Pathophysiology, epidemiology, clinical features, life cycle and associated structural abnormalities. J Eur Acad Dermatol Venereol. 2011;25:1245–53.

Léauté-Labrèze C, Prey S, Ezzedine K. Infantile haemangioma: part II. Risks, complications and treatment. J Eur Acad Dermatol Venereol. 2011;25:1254–60.

Lee BB, Lardeo J, Neville R. Arterio-venous malformation: how much do we know? Phlebology. 2009;24:193–200.

Lee J, Sinno H, Tahiri Y, Gilardino MS. Treatment options for cutaneous pyogenic granulomas: a review. J Plast Reconstr Aesthet Surg. 2011;64:1216–20.

Marcum CB, Zager JS, Bélongie IP, et al. Profound proliferating angiolymphoid hyperplasia with eosinophilia of pregnancy mimicking angiosarcoma. Cutis. 2011;88:122–8.

Mehta A, Beck M, Eyskens F, et al. Fabry disease: a review of current management strategies. QJM. 2010;103:641–59.

Metry D, Heyer G, Hess C, et al. Consensus statement on diagnostic criteria for PHACE syndrome. Pediatrics. 2009;124:1447–56.

Miest RY, Comfere NI, Dispenzieri A, et al. Cutaneous manifestations in patients with POEMS syndrome. Int J Dermatol. 2013;52:1349–56.

Mittal R, Aggarwal A, Srivastava G. Angiokeratoma circumscriptum: a case report and review of the literature. Int J Dermatol. 2005;44:1031–4.

North PE, Waner M, Mizeracki A, Mihm MC Jr. GLUT1: a newly discovered immunohistochemical marker for juvenile hemangiomas. Hum Pathol. 2000;31:11–22.

Redondo P, Aguado L, Martínez-Cuesta A. Diagnosis and management of extensive vascular malformations of the lower limb: part I. Clinical diagnosis. J Am Acad Dermatol. 2011;65:893–906.

Requena L, Sangueza OP. Cutaneous vascular proliferation. Part II. Hyperplasias and benign neoplasms. J Am Acad Dermatol. 1997;37:887–919.

Schopp JG, Sra KK, Wilkerson MG. Glomangioma: a case report and review of the literature. Cutis. 2009;83:24–7.

Schumacher WE, Drolet BA, Maheshwari M, et al. Spinal dysraphism associated with the cutaneous lumbosacral infantile hemangioma: a neuroradiological review. Pediatr Radiol. 2012; 42:315–20.

Schwartz RA, Sidor MI, Musumeci ML, Lin RL, Micali G. Infantile haemangiomas: a challenge in paediatric dermatology. J Eur Acad Dermatol Venereol. 2010;24:631–8.

Verma SB. Lymphangiectasias of the skin: victims of confusing nomenclature. Clin Exp Dermatol. 2009;34:566–9.

Weedon D. Weedon's Skin Pathology, edn 3. China: Elsevier; 2010.

Wong SN, Tay YK. Tufted angioma: a report of five cases. Pediatr Dermatol. 2002,19:388–93.

Zaraa I, Mlika M, Chouk S, et al. Angiolymphoid hyperplasia with eosinophilia: a study of 7 cases. Dermatol Online J. 2011;17:1.

Neural Skin Tumors

Neural skin tumors constitute only a small part of benign cutaneous soft tissue neoplasms. The skin has a rich supply of sensory nerves of the peripheral nervous system that are located in the dermis. Benign tumors of the nerve sheath, which is composed of Schwann cells and endoneural and perineural fibroblasts are the main topic of this chapter. Axonal hyperplasia-related lesions are also discussed. Malignant peripheral nerve sheath tumor, which is closely related to benign neural neoplasms, is discussed in the section of cutaneous sarcomas.

7.1 Neurofibroma

Neurofibroma is the most common neural skin tumor. It is a benign neoplasm of the nerve sheath presenting typically as nodules of variable size. This tumor is composed of proliferation of all elements of the nerve sheath. Two major subtypes of the tumor are defined according to their depth of involvement: dermal neurofibroma and plexiform neurofibroma.

7.1.1 Dermal Neurofibroma

Dermal neurofibroma is the classic subtype of the tumor and constitutes the predominant part in clinical practice. It may occur as a solitary lesion or as multiple lesions. While solitary tumors are mostly sporadic, multiple lesions are mainly part of neurofibromatosis, a relatively common genodermatosis transmitted as an autosomal dominant trait. Sporadic lesions may initially appear in early adulthood. However, in neurofibromatosis type 1 (NF-1; von Recklinghausen disease), dermal neurofibromas usually arise in the second decade. Many patients have a history of another neurofibromatosis patient in the family. In patients with neurofibromatosis, café-au-lait macules are generally the initial cutaneous finding. However, neurofibromas increase slowly in number and size, and in adulthood they are the predominant type of the skin lesions (see Fig. 7.1). Neurofibromas may occur anywhere on the body in varying numbers (see Figs. 7.2, 7.3 and 7.4). Some adult patients have hundreds of neurofibromas extending over the trunk, extremities, or face (see Fig. 7.5). The size of the tumors ranges from a few millimeters to several centimeters (see Figs. 7.6, 7.7, 7.8 and 7.9). Sessile (see Fig. 7.7) or pedunculated (see Figs. 7.8 and 7.10) lesions are randomly distributed. Most lesions are flesh-colored (see Figs. 7.11 and 7.12) but sometimes a violaceous hue or slight brownish pigmentation occurs (see Fig. 7.6). The surface of the neural tumor is smooth and may sometimes be flaccid or slightly folded (see Fig. 7.13). Tumors are soft or rubbery on palpation.

Lesions located on the scalp may be alopecic (see Fig. 7.14). The areola of the breast is also a typical involvement site of neurofibromas in neurofibromatosis patients (see Figs. 7.15 and 7.16). Neurofibromas may sometimes appear as flat or slightly atrophic, light brownish or hypopigmented patches (see Figs. 7.17 and 7.18). Dermal neurofibromas are usually asymptomatic, but a mild pruritus may be present in patients with numerous lesions.

Neurofibromas may also arise on oral mucosa as submucosal soft papules or nodules with a smooth surface (see Figs. 7.19 and 7.20). The tongue and buccal mucosa are predominantly involved, but lesions may appear anywhere on the mouth. Since mucosal neurofibromas are usually asymptomatic, most lesions are initially noticed during physical examination. Rarely, pain and parasthesia may occur as a result of compression of large tumors on cranial nerves.

Schwannoma (see Fig. 7.35), intradermal nevus (see Fig. 3.109), lipoma (see Fig. 10.3) and acrochordon (see Fig. 8.74) are the possible differential diagnostic challenges of neurofibromas on the skin. The clinical diagnosis is relatively easier in patients with multiple lesions

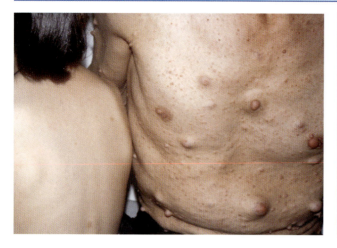

Fig. 7.1 Café-au-lait macules on the back of a boy and multiple neurofibromas on the abdomen of his father; familial occurrence of neurofibromatosis. The number of neurofibromas gradually increase throughout life

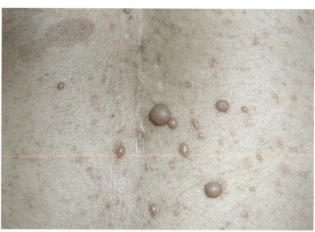

Fig. 7.3 Multiple small neurofibromas on the back. The size of the tumors may be variable

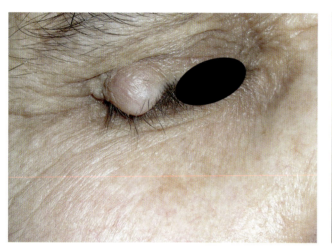

Fig. 7.2 Neurofibroma on the upper eyelid. This neural tumor may occur anywhere on the skin

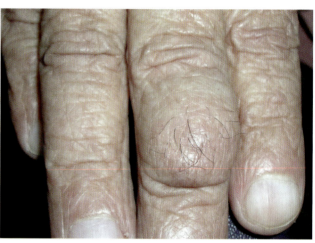

Fig. 7.4 A flesh nodule of neurofibroma on the dorsum of the finger

(*see* Fig. 7.21) and in those whose lesions are associated with café-au-lait macules (*see* Figs. 7.22 and 7.23), axillary freckling (*see* Figs. 3.38 and 7.11), or extracutaneous findings such as skeletal (*see* Fig. 7.24) and endocrine manifestations including hirsutism (*see* Fig. 7.25) suggestive of neurofibromatosis. Invagination of the elevated lesion of neurofibroma by the pressure of the fingertip is called the buttonhole sign. This is related to the underlying dermal defect of the tumor. Buttonhole sign is usually a helpful clinical clue in diagnosis, although a biopsy is performed in most patients with solitary lesions. The histology of a dermal neurofibroma reveals a circumscribed but not encapsulated spindle cell proliferation among thin collagen fibers. Components of the peripheral nerve (axons) are present. The cells have wavy nuclei. The stroma may be fibrotic, vascular, or myxoid and usually contains mast cells.

7.1.2 Plexiform Neurofibroma

Plexiform neurofibroma is the rare subtype of neurofibroma presenting as larger, deeper, and disfiguring masses located anywhere on the skin (*see* Figs. 7.26 and 7.27). It commonly involves subcutaneous and deeper tissues, and occurs along the course of peripheral nerves, which are transformed into thickened, tortuous nerves forming large masses. Plexiform neurofibroma is always a marker of neurofibromatosis type 1. It may be congenital or may appear at an early period of life and grow progressively in childhood but then mostly remain unchanged. Lesions may cause asymmetric overgrowth of the extremities (*see* Figs. 7.28, 7.29 and 7.30), ears, or other parts of the body. The tumor may sometimes reach huge dimensions, may be pendulous, and may have a surface that is excessively folded (*see* Fig. 7.30), similar to that of cutis laxa. Even large masses of neurofibroma are

7.1 Neurofibroma

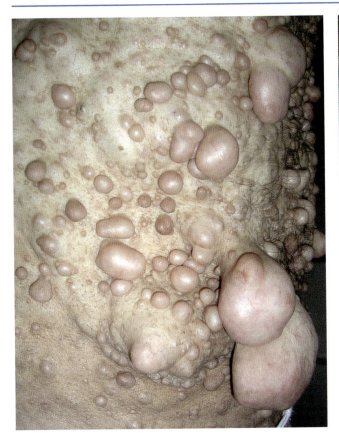

Fig. 7.5 Innumerable neurofibromas on the trunk of an adult with neurofibromatosis. Cosmesis is the main concern in this case

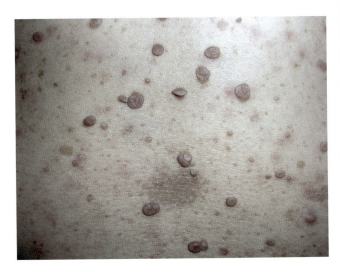

Fig. 7.6 Multiple small brownish neurofibromas. Some lesions are similar to acrochordons in this case

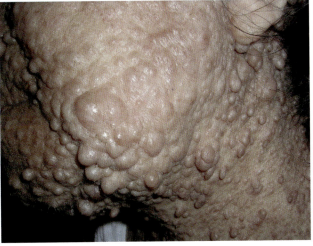

Fig. 7.7 Numerous neurofibromas in different sizes on the face and neck in a patient with neurofibromatosis. Most of the lesions are sessile in this case

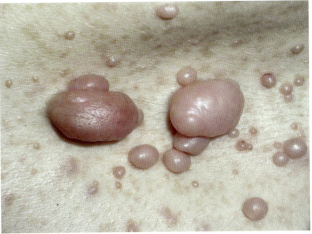

Fig. 7.8 Sessile and pedunculated neurofibromas of variable size are seen concomitantly. They are typically soft on palpation

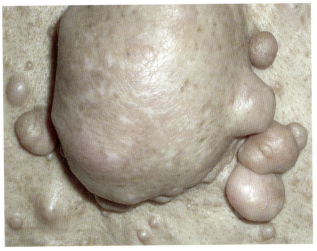

Fig. 7.9 A large tumor of neurofibroma surrounded by smaller lesions

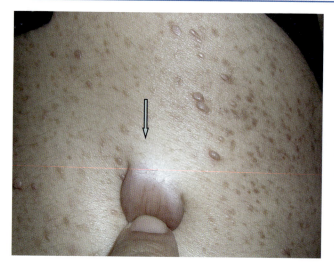

Fig. 7.10 Pedunculated neurofibroma on the back

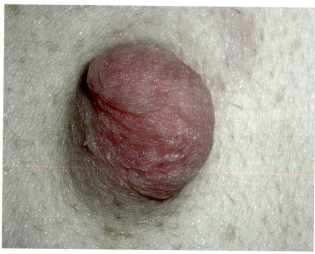

Fig. 7.13 Pinkish brown neurofibroma with folded surface

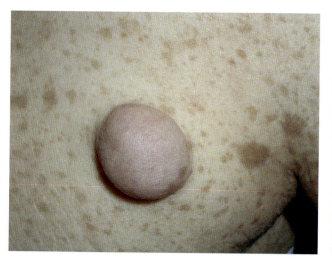

Fig. 7.11 A flesh-colored neurofibroma. Note also the numerous café-au-lait macules and axillary freckling in a patient with neurofibromatosis type 1

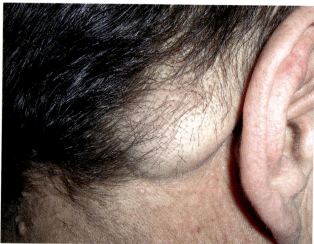

Fig. 7.14 Neurofibroma on the scalp. Note the mild alopecia on the surface of the tumor

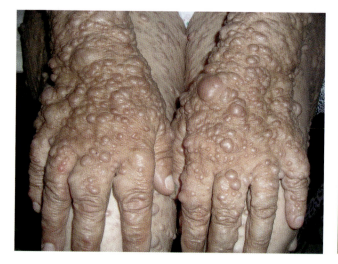

Fig. 7.12 Multiple skin-colored neurofibromas on both hands

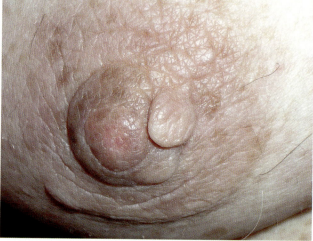

Fig. 7.15 Pedunculated neurofibroma on the areola of the breast, a typical location

7.1 Neurofibroma

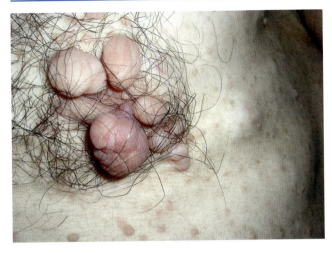

Fig. 7.16 Multiple neurofibromas on the nipple and areola of the breast in a male patient with neurofibromatosis

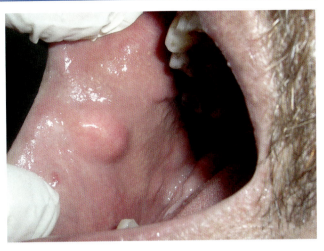

Fig. 7.19 Neurofibroma on the buccal mucosa. Note the flesh-colored nodule

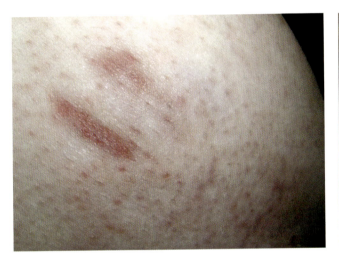

Fig. 7.17 Brownish-colored flat neurofibromas

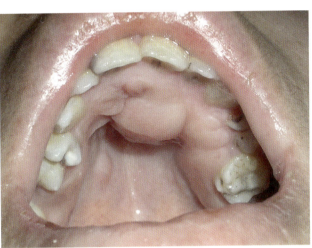

Fig. 7.20 Neurofibroma on the hard palate presenting as submucosal nodules with smooth surface

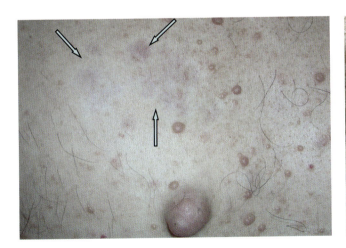

Fig. 7.18 Multiple atrophic neurofibromas with a pale hue are shown (*arrows*). The patient also has typical sessile neurofibromas

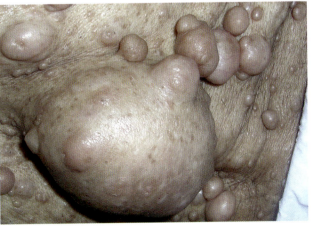

Fig. 7.21 Multiple neurofibromas of varying sizes in a patient with neurofibromatosis type 1

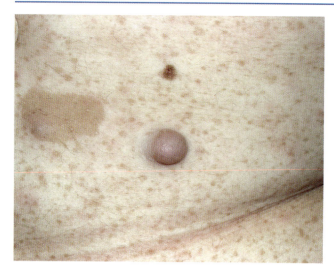

Fig. 7.22 Neurofibroma associated with multiple café-au-lait macules in a patient with neurofibromatosis type 1

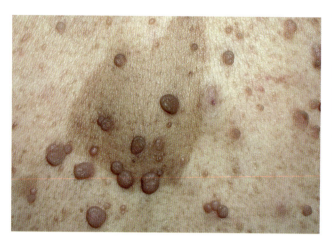

Fig. 7.23 Multiple neurofibromas associated with café-au-lait macules. Both types of lesions may overlap, as seen in the figure

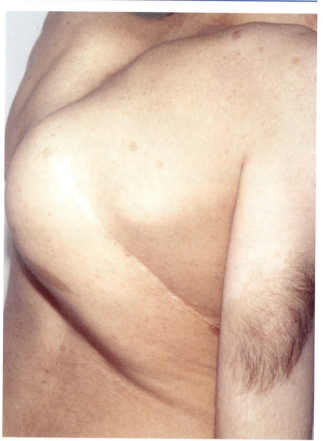

Fig. 7.24 Skeletal deformity in a patient with neurofibromatosis. A plexiform neurofibroma is also seen on the upper arm

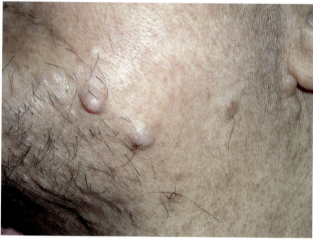

Fig. 7.25 A female with hirsutism related to endocrinological abnormalities of neurofibromatosis. Neurofibromas are also noticeable

soft. Overlying hyperpigmentation and localized hypertrichosis are additional features of some tumors (*see* Fig. 7.31). Thus plexiform neurofibroma may be considered in the differential diagnosis of large congenital melanocytic nevi (*see* Fig. 3.175). The oral mucosa is a rare location of plexiform neurofibroma (*see* Fig. 7.32). Histologically plexiform neurofibromas are characterized by their tortous plexiform architecture reminiscent of a tortous nerve. Cellular content is the same as in diffuse neurofibromas.

Morbidity of plexiform neurofibroma is high when compared with that of dermal neurofibromas. In addition to severe cosmetic disturbance, muscle weakness, skeletal deformities, and visceral problems may occur in relation to the location of plexiform type lesions.

In contrast to the dermal type, a small percentage of plexiform neurofibromas may show malignant degeneration to malignant peripheral nerve sheath tumors. Sudden growth of the mass and development of nodularity, pain, and neurologic symptoms may be indicators of malignancy.

Nodular plexiform neurofibroma is a rare variant of plexiform neurofibroma and is mostly diagnosed after childhood. It is more deeply located and does not cause superficial skin changes. Multiple lesions may be restricted to one area. The subcutaneous nodules may be tender or painful and are typically arranged along a nerve plexus (*see* Fig. 7.33).

7.2 Schwannoma (Neurilemmoma)

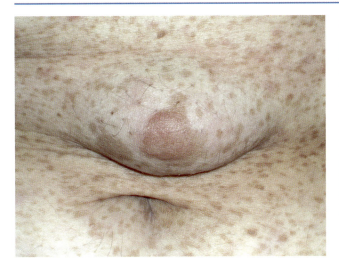

Fig. 7.26 Plexiform neurofibroma presenting as a subcutaneous mass on the trunk. This subtype of neurofibroma may become rather large and disfiguring

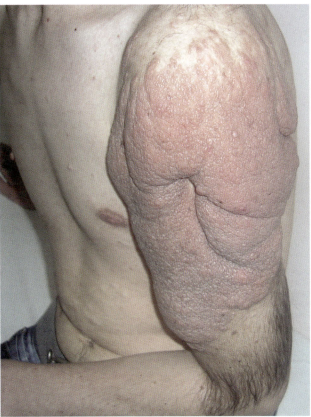

Fig. 7.28 Plexiform neurofibroma involving a broad anatomic area on the upper arm. Note the hypertrichosis around the elbow

examination) and neurologic and endocrinologic consultations can be performed. The prognosis of neurofibromatosis is not associated with dermal neurofibromas as there is no risk of malignant degeneration. However, they may be a serious cosmetic problem. Solitary lesions may be excised, but in patients with multiple lesions, surgical intervention is not feasible. Antihistaminic drugs may be used for the relief of pruritus.

Because plexiform neurofibromas are usually large and show deep invasion, they are more difficult to treat surgically and unsightly scars may occur (*see* Fig. 7.34). Due to the risk of malignant transformation patients should be followed closely.

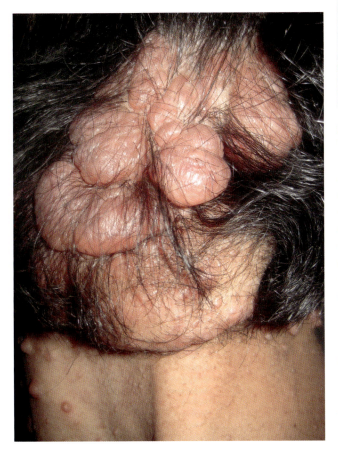

Fig. 7.27 Plexiform neurofibroma on the scalp. Note the lobulated pattern of the large mass

Management. Patients with one plexiform or more than one dermal neurofibroma should be evaluated for other manifestations of neurofibromatosis. In addition to dermatologic examination directed to other skin findings of the syndrome, ophthalmologic examination for Lisch nodules (slit-lamp

7.2 Schwannoma (Neurilemmoma)

Schwannoma is a nerve sheath tumor occurring as a result of proliferation of periaxonal or endoneural Schwann cells. It is less common than neurofibroma. Cutaneous schwannomas are predominantly seen in adults but may occur at any age. Women are more commonly affected than men. Most lesions are solitary but multiple lesions may occur infrequently, and they may be associated with neurofibromatosis, especially neurofibromatosis type 2 (NF-2). Café-au-lait macules are

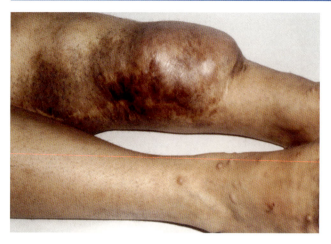

Fig. 7.29 Plexiform neurofibroma on the leg causing overgrowth of the extremity. A discrepancy in size of extremities is remarkable

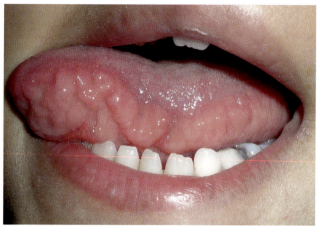

Fig. 7.32 Plexiform neurofibroma on one side of the tongue

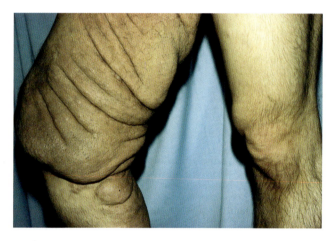

Fig. 7.30 Plexiform neurofibroma seen as a pendulous, folded large mass on the leg

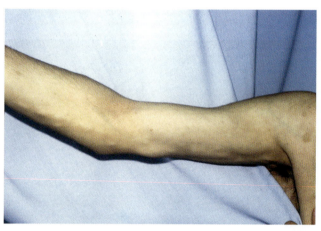

Fig. 7.33 Nodular plexiform neurofibroma with linearly arranged subcutaneous nodules on the arm

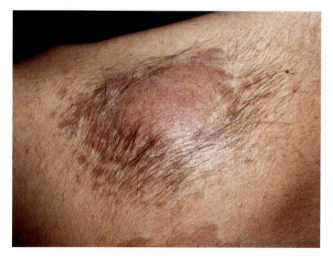

Fig. 7.31 Plexiform neurofibroma with localized hypertrichosis and hyperpigmentation on the periphery

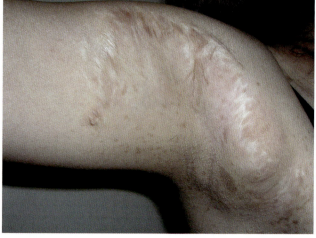

Fig. 7.34 A large scar on the excision site of a plexiform neurofibroma

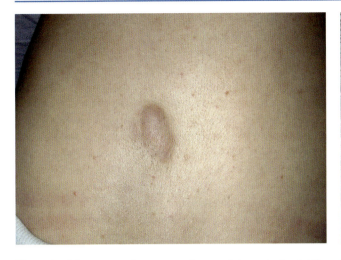

Fig. 7.35 Schwannoma shown as a solitary nodule on the trunk. The patient was otherwise healthy

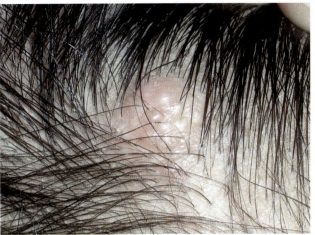

Fig. 7.37 Schwannoma located on the head, a typical area

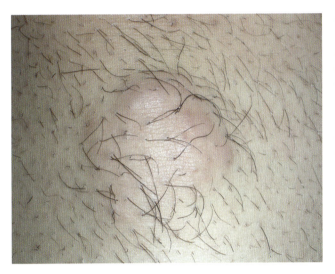

Fig. 7.36 Schwannoma seen as a solitary nodule with a smooth surface

not expected to occur in this type of neurofibromatosis. However, acoustic neuromas which are schwannomas of the vestibular division of the cranial nerve are indicators of NF-2. There are also patients with multiple cutaneous schwannomas but who lack acoustic neuromas. The term schwannomatosis is used for these cases.

Schwannoma mostly appears as a yellowish- or pinkish-colored, 0.5 to 3 cm soft dermal or subcutaneous papule or nodule with a smooth surface (*see* Figs. 7.35 and 7.36). The main location of the tumor is the flexural surfaces of the extremities followed by the head and neck (*see* Fig. 7.37). Although they are usually asymptomatic, tumors may sometimes be painful and tender as a result of pressure on the nerve. Motor dysfunction and paresthesias are rare complications of cutaneous schwannomas.

A schwannoma can often be clinically confused with a dermal neurofibroma (*see* Fig. 7.12) but also with a lipoma (*see* Fig. 10.3), angiolipoma, spiradenoma (*see* Fig. 5.25), epidermoid cyst (*see* Fig. 4.1), leiomyoma (*see* Fig. 5.73), and ganglion cyst (*see* Fig. 4.58). Histopathologic examination is required to confirm the diagnosis. It reveals an encapsulated deep dermal or subcutaneous tumor consisting of spindle cell proliferation. Tumor usually does not contain axons. Two different types of tissue are present: Antoni A and B. Antoni A type tissue is hypercellular and consists of cells with palisading nuclei and characteristic Verocay bodies. Antoni B type tissue is hypocellular and shows degenerative changes. There are different histopathologic variants such as cellular, ancient, epithelioid, myxoid, plexiform, and psammomatous melanotic schwannoma. The presence of psammomatous melanotic subtype may be an indicator for the Carney complex.

Most schwannomas are benign. However, on rare occasions they may show malignant degenerative change resulting in malignant schwannoma (malignant peripheral nerve sheath tumor).

Management. Excision of the tumor is usually preferred because schwannomas may be associated with pain or rare complications including malignant degeneration. Simple excision of the tumor without sacrificing the associated nerve is effective. Enucleation can also be performed. The tendency to recurrence is relatively higher in plexiform schwannomas.

7.3 Neuromas

Neuromas are nerve sheath tumors composed of Schwann cells and many axons. Multiple mucosal neuromas, cutaneous neuroma, palisaded encapsulated neuroma, and traumatic neuroma are well-known variants of this neural tumor.

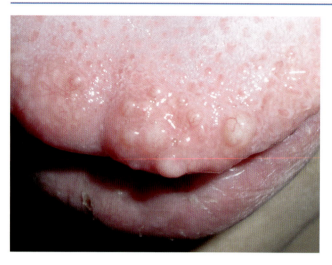

Fig. 7.38 Multiple mucosal neuromas in a patient with MEN-2B syndrome. Note the flesh-colored smooth small papules on the tip of the tongue

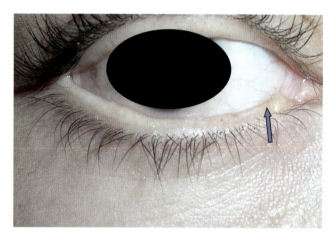

Fig. 7.39 Mucosal neuroma on the eyelid seen as a small papule in a patient with MEN-2B syndrome

7.3.1 Multiple Mucosal Neuromas

Mucosal neuroma presenting as multiple lesions of the mouth and eye is a manifestation of multiple endocrine neoplasia type 2B (MEN-2B), an autosomal dominantly inherited syndrome that is associated with tumors of the endocrine glands such as the adrenal and the thyroid glands. Marfanoid habitus and intestinal ganglioneuromatosis are other manifestations of this syndrome. Mutation of the *RET proto-oncogene* is identified in this rare disease. Mucosal neuromas are seen in all the patients and usually occur in the first decade as an early sign of the syndrome. Multiple yellowish white- or skin-colored, dome-shaped, or pedunculated asymptomatic papules that are 2 to 4 mm in size are typically located on the tongue (*see* Fig. 7.38) and lips. Neuromas may also be seen on other surfaces of the oral mucosa, on the eyelids (*see* Fig. 7.39), sclera, and rarely around the nose. Eyelid tumors may cause eversion of the eyelids while neuromas on the lip may cause thickened, enlarged lips and asymmetric appearance. Oral fibroma (*see* Fig. 8.46) may be considered in the differential diagnosis, but it presents mostly as a solitary lesion. Biopsy may sometimes be required, especially in patients without any known endocrinologic manifestations. Mucosal neuromas are partially encapsulated tumors composed of either Schwann cell fascicles resembling palisaded encapsulated neuromas or a more prominent axonal component. There are also tortuous hyperplastic nerve bundles surrounded by a thickened perineurium.

Mucosal neuromas are benign and do not have a risk of malignant degeneration. However, when the diagnosis of mucosal neuroma is confirmed by histology, patients should be screened for MEN-2B syndrome and accompanying endocrine gland tumors. Identifying the presence of *RET proto-oncogene* is also helpful for the diagnosis.

Medullary thyroid carcinoma and pheochromocytoma usually occur after puberty. Medullary thyroid carcinoma has a highly aggressive course and the potential for metastasis. Therefore, early diagnosis of the syndrome is crucial. Increased serum and urine levels of calcitonin confirm the diagnosis of medullary thyroid carcinoma. Patients with pheochromocytoma commonly have hypertension and increased levels of serum catecholamines as well as urinary vanillylmandelic acid and an altered epinephrine/norepinephrine ratio.

Management. Family members of patients should also be screened for MEN-2B syndrome. Mucosal neuromas do not require therapy but may be excised for aesthetic purposes if surgery is feasible. The main challenge after diagnosis of this syndrome is the decision regarding prophylactic thyroidectomy, as almost all patients develop medullary thyroid carcinoma. Patients need to be followed for life for the associated endocrine problems.

7.3.2 Cutaneous Neuroma

Cutaneous neuroma is a rare benign neural tumor that can be observed in MEN-2B syndrome in the perinasal area, pinnae, face, and less often the trunk. We have followed a patient with multiple skin-colored, smooth-surfaced, linear papules of cutaneous neuromas on the trunk and extremities (see Fig. 7.40). The lesions persisted during a follow-up period of 15 years. The patient also had medullary thyroid carcinoma. The diagnosis of cutaneous neuroma is usually confirmed with biopsy. In the overmentioned case, histopathologic study showed tortuous hyperplastic nerve bundles surrounded by a thickened perineurium.

Management. Therapy is not necessary for the asymptomatic lesion.

7.3 Neuromas

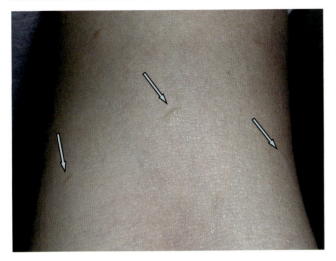

Fig. 7.40 Multiple cutaneous neuromas shown as linear small, skin-colored papules. This exceptional case was associated with medullary thyroid carcinoma

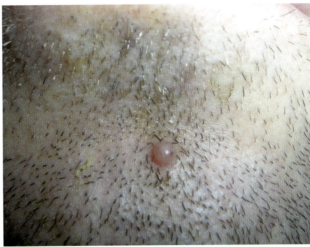

Fig. 7.41 Palisaded encapsulated neuroma shown as a skin-colored solitary papule on the face, a typical location

7.3.3 Palisaded Encapsulated Neuroma

Palisaded encapsulated (solitary circumscribed) neuroma is a rare benign neural neoplasm mostly seen as a solitary facial papule. It usually occurs in middle-aged individuals. The favored sites of the tumor are mid-face (see Fig. 7.41), especially the nose and nasolabial folds, followed by the cheek and chin. The trunk (see Fig. 7.42), extremities, genitalia, and oral mucosa, especially the hard palate, are rarely affected. The typical lesion is an asymptomatic, slow-growing, flesh- or pinkish-colored, dome-shaped, rubbery, pearly papule with a smooth surface measuring 2 to 6 mm.

Clinical differentiation of palisaded encapsulated neuroma from fibrous papule of the nose (see Fig. 8.16), intradermal melanocytic nevus (see Fig. 3.114), neurofibroma (see Fig. 7.2), trichoepithelioma (see Fig. 5.38), and early nonulcerated lesions of basal cell carcinoma (see Fig. 11.23) may sometimes be difficult. Surface alterations such as telangiectasia, increased hairs, and ulceration are absent or minimal on palisaded encapsulated neuroma. Most lesions are diagnosed by histopathologic examination. Histologic findings include a well-circumscribed, round to oval, partially encapsulated dermal nodule composed of Schwann cell fascicles usually containing axons. The thin capsule composed of perineurial cells surrounds the deep dermal border of the nodule. There is no well-known association with systemic diseases. Therefore, further examination is not necessary.

Management. There is no risk of malignant degeneration, and therefore no therapeutic intervention is needed. Excision may be performed for cosmetic concerns or for confirmation of the diagnosis by means of histopathologic examination. Recurrence is not expected.

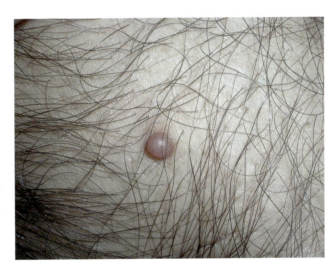

Fig. 7.42 Palisaded encapsulated neuroma seen as a dome-shaped solitary papule on the leg. This rare neural tumor is mostly misinterpreted as intradermal nevus from clinical point of view

7.3.4 Traumatic Neuroma

Traumatic neuroma is a reactive lesion occurring at sites of amputation or injury and is caused by hyperproliferation of the nerve fibers at the injured sites of a nerve. The ones occurring as a result of amputation are more commonly seen on the extremities. This type of neuroma is a solitary, skin-colored, firm, tender or painful papule or nodule with a broad base occurring typically at the sites of previous trauma and surgical interventions. Histology reveals

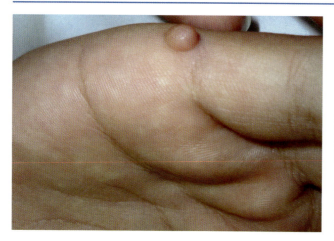

Fig. 7.43 Rudimentary digit at the base of the lateral side of the fifth finger, the most typical location

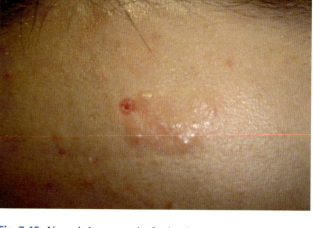

Fig. 7.45 Neurothekeoma on the forehead

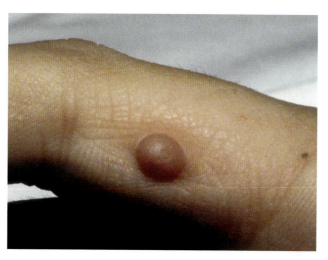

Fig. 7.44 Rudimentary digit shown as a congenital skin-colored papule with a smooth surface

proliferation of nerve fascicles in a fibrous or fibromyxoid stroma. The proliferated nerve fascicles are in varying sizes and shapes and are irregularly arranged.

The rudimentary digit represents a variant of amputation neuroma resulting from intrauterine autoamputation of intact supernumerary digits. The sequela of the congenital anomaly is typically observed at the base of the lateral side of the fifth digit of newborns (see Fig. 7.43). It may be bilateral. There may be one lesion on each hand or foot. Rarely, it can be observed on the radial side of the thumb. Smooth-surfaced, skin-colored, usually asymptomatic papules or nodules of the rudimentary digit (see Fig. 7.44) may be confused with acquired digital fibrokeratoma (see Fig. 8.56), but this latter condition is not present at birth. Histology of the rudimentary digit shows features similar to those of traumatic neuromas of other causes.

Management. Traumatic neuroma is a benign but persistent lesion. Simple excision is curative and mostly performed in patients with symptomatic lesions. Rudimentary digits causing a cosmetic problem may also be removed.

7.4 Neurothekeoma

Neurothekeoma has been a controversial entity. In the past, nerve sheath myxoma and neurothekeoma (cellular neurothekeoma) were considered tumors of neural origin. The contemporary point of view considers only nerve sheath myxoma as a tumor of neural origin, whereas neurothekeoma is regarded as a tumor unrelated to the former and of disputed cellular origin.

Nerve sheath myxoma is more common in middle-aged adults. Head, neck, and extremities, especially the hands and pretibial areas, are the usual involved sites. A solitary, slow-growing, pink or flesh-colored, dome-shaped asymptomatic papule or nodule measuring 0.5 to 2.5 cm is seen. The tumor may be multinodular. Histopathologic examination shows a multilobulated, nonencapsulated tumor, composed of a myxoid stroma and spindle-shaped, stellate, or epithelioid cells, which express S100 protein. The cells are arranged in a concentric or lamellar pattern.

Cellular neurothekeoma is more commonly found in females, typically on the head and neck region. Children and young adults are more commonly involved. The lesion is usually solitary; on rare occasions multiple lesions may be observed. A dome-shaped papule or nodule varying in size between 0.5 and 2 cm can be observed (see Fig. 7.45). The lesion may be firm. The color can be red-brown, resembling a dermatofibroma. Neurothekeoma may also be confused with intradermal melanocytic nevus (see Fig. 3.115) and other dermal tumors. Histopathologically cellular neurothekeoma has a multilobular appearance. Whorling or concentric spindle cells form nests. Tumoral cells have a sometimes striking epithelioid morphology;

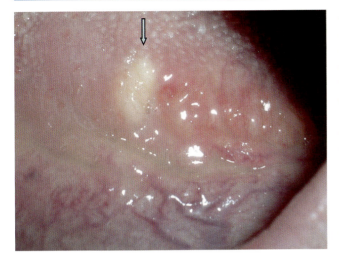

Fig. 7.46 Granular cell tumor on the tongue, a typical location

hence the name of the entity is "cellular." They do not express S100 as occurs in nerve sheath myxoma but are positive for NKI/C3, which is frequently positive in histiocytic tumors.

Management. Malignant degeneration is not reported. Complete excision is curative, but recurrence may be seen after incomplete excision.

7.5 Granular Cell Tumor (Granular Nerve Sheath Tumor)

Granular cell tumor is a rare neoplasm of adults that is considered to be of Schwann cell origin. Women and the black population are more commonly affected. Although the tumor is usually solitary, multiple lesions may also be seen, predominantly in black people. Any site can be involved, including mucosal surfaces and internal organs. The tongue is among the most common sites (*see* Fig. 7.46). Skin lesions appear most often on the head and neck region.

Granular cell tumor is a slow-growing, skin-colored or brownish red, 0.5 to 3 cm firm papule or nodule with smooth, rough, verrucous, or rarely ulcerated surface. While most tumors are asymptomatic, patients may sometimes complain about pruritus or tenderness. Because of variety of clinical features, the diagnosis is mostly established by biopsy. Histologic examination of the lesion reveals a poorly defined tumor with pale, large, polygonal cells and eosinophilic granular cytoplasm. Pseudoepitheliomatous hyperplasia is a common accompanying feature if the tumor is located close to the epidermis or to mucosal surfaces. Owing to epidermal hyperplasia, superficial biopsy of the lesion may lead to confusion with squamous cell carcinoma. The tumor must also be differentiated from a variety of tumors showing granular cell change.

Most granular cell tumors remain benign. On very rare occasions, the deep-seated tumors may show malignant transformation. Malignant granular cell tumors are mostly larger than the benign ones. Cytologic atypia, mitoses, necrosis, spindling of the cells, and infiltrative growth are histopathologic markers of malignant tumors.

Management. Total excision with tumor-free margins is curative and helpful in preventing the recurrence of a granular cell tumor. However, local recurrence may be a marker of malignant degeneration.

Suggested Reading

Baykal C, Buyukbabani N, Boztepe H, et al. Multiple cutaneous neuromas and macular amyloidosis associated with medullary thyroid carcinoma. J Am Acad Dermatol. 2007;56 (2 Suppl):S33–7.

Benbenisty KM, Andea A, Metcalf J, Cook J. Atypical cellular neurothekeoma treated with Mohs micrographic surgery. Derm Surg. 2006;32:582–7.

Boyd KP, Korf BR, Theos A. Neurofibromatosis type 1. J Am Acad Dermatol. 2009;61:1–14.

Burgdorf WHC, Plewig G, Wolff HH, Landthaler M. Braun-Falco's dermatology, edn 3. Italy: Springer-Verlag; 2009.

Caputo R, Tadini G. Atlas of genodermatoses. Spain: Taylor and Francis; 2006.

Elder DE, Elenitsas R, Johnson BL, Murphy GF, Xu X. Lever's histopathology of the skin, edn 10. Philadelphia: Lippincott Williams and Wilkins; 2008.

James WD, Berger T, Elston D. Andrew's diseases of the skin: clinical dermatology, edn 11. China: Saunders Elsevier; 2011.

Jung Lee M, Hun Chung K, Soo Park J, et al. Multiple endocrine neoplasia type 2B: early diagnosis by multiple mucosal neuroma and its DNA analysis. Ann Dermatol. 2010;22:452–5.

LeBoit PE, Burg G, Weedon D, Sarasin A. Pathology and genetics of skin tumours. World Health Organization classification of tumours. France: IARC Press; 2006.

Nascimento AF, Fletcher CD. The controversial nosology of benign nerve sheath tumors: neurofilament protein staining demonstrates intratumoral axons in many sporadic schwannomas. Am J Surg Pathol. 2007;31:1363–70.

Russo L, Falaschini S, Cincione R, et al. Granular cell tumour of the tongue in a 14-year-old boy: case report. The Open Otorhinolaryngology Journal. 2001;5:15–7.

Weedon D. Weedon's skin pathology, edn 3. China: Elsevier; 2010.

Benign Fibrohistiocytic Tumors and Proliferations

8

Fibroblasts are the main cell type of dermal connective tissue in addition to scarce histiocytes and mast cells. The major function of fibroblasts is collagen synthesis. A subset of benign tumors and reactive processes show an increase of fibroblasts and histiocytes in addition to collagen and elastic fibers. A great number of benign tumors and proliferations of fibrous tissue of skin and tendons will be discussed in this chapter. Some of them, such as acrochordon and keloid, are very common. Most show benign biological behavior without malignant transformation, but some tumors may be locally invasive. Perfollicular fibroma, which may also be evaluated as an adnexal (hair follicle) tumor due to its origin, is included in this chapter. Juvenile hyaline fibromatosis, which clinically presents as tumoral lesions, is in fact not a neoplasm but related to the deposition of an extracellular matrix substance. It is also mentioned in this chapter. Diseases characterized by mast cell proliferation will be discussed in another chapter.

8.1 Dermatofibroma (Histiocytoma)

Dermatofibroma is a common type of fibrohistiocytic tumor causing acquired papulonodular lesions. The etiopathogenesis is not known. It has been suggested that it may be a reactive process to triggering factors such as insect bite. Although it is named also histiocytoma, it is not a type of histiocytoses. This benign tumor has a slight female predominance and is seen mostly in young adults. It occurs sporadically as a solitary lesion (*see* Fig. 8.1) or as a few but less than five lesions (*see* Fig. 8.2). Rarely, patients with human immunodeficiency virus (HIV) infection, systemic lupus erythematosus, and those undergoing immunosuppressive therapy may have more than 15 dermatofibromas.

The most common location of dermatofibroma is the limbs, particularly the anterior surface of the legs (*see* Fig. 8.2). The shoulders and buttocks are other commonly involved sites. However, it can occur anywhere on the skin, including the digits (*see* Fig. 8.3) and the palmoplantar area. Typical lesions are round or ovoid, firm, slowly growing pap-

ules or nodules, 5 to 10 mm in diameter (*see* Figs. 8.4, 8.5 and 8.6). Whereas some lesions are flat and on the skin level (*see* Fig. 8.7), some are slightly raised above the skin surface, and some appear as markedly elevated dome-shaped

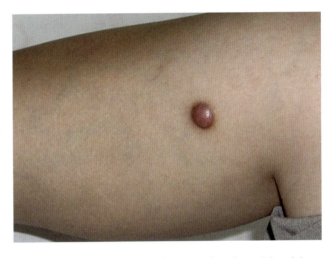

Fig. 8.1 Dermatofibroma presenting as a solitary brownish nodule on the lower leg. Most patients have solitary or a few lesions

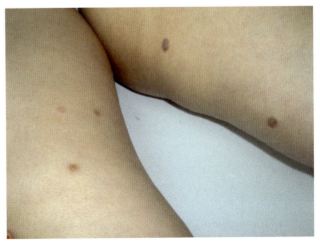

Fig. 8.2 Several lesions of dermatofibroma located on both legs

C. Baykal, K.D. Yazganoğlu, *Clinical Atlas of Skin Tumors*,
DOI 10.1007/978-3-642-40938-7_8, © Springer-Verlag Berlin Heidelberg 2014

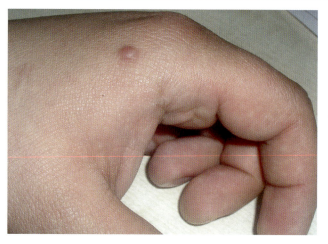

Fig. 8.3 Dermatofibroma on the finger, a rare location

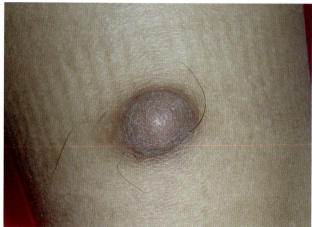

Fig. 8.6 Dermatofibroma presenting as a round, elevated nodule with smooth surface

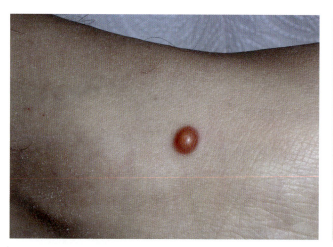

Fig. 8.4 Dermatofibroma presenting as a small, round, well-defined papule

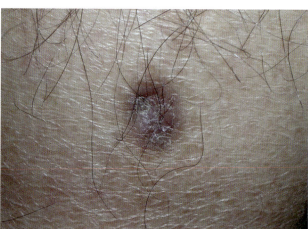

Fig. 8.7 Dermatofibroma manifesting as a flat nodule. Lesion is firm on palpation

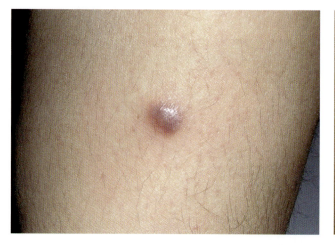

Fig. 8.5 Dermatofibroma seen as an ovoid pink-brown nodule. Asymptomatic lesions may be initially detected by dermatologic examination

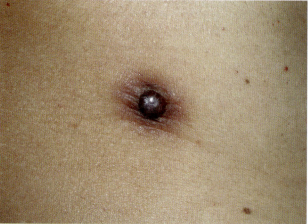

Fig. 8.8 Dermatofibroma presenting as a dome-shaped indurated nodule

8.1 Dermatofibroma (Histiocytoma)

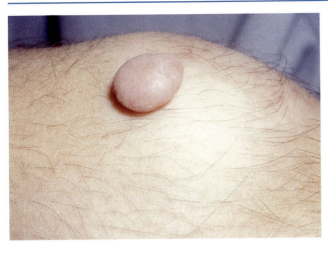

Fig. 8.9 Dermatofibroma shown as a protuberant, skin-colored nodule. This is not a common presentation

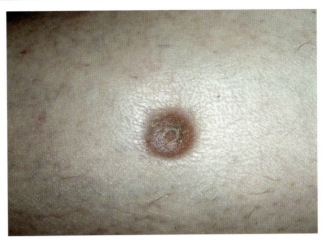

Fig. 8.11 Dermatofibroma with a mild scaly surface

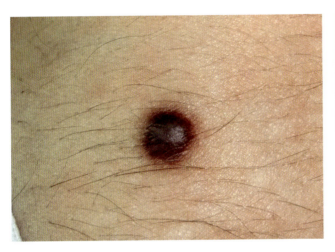

Fig. 8.10 Hyperpigmented dermatofibroma. Nodular melanoma may be considered in the differential diagnosis of darkly pigmented lesions

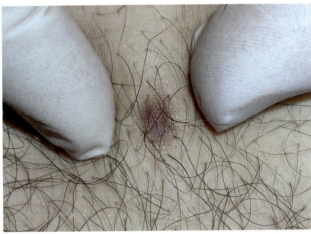

Fig. 8.12 Dimple sign in dermatofibroma on lateral pressure of the fingers

nodules (*see* Fig. 8.8). Protuberant (*see* Fig. 8.9) or plaque-like lesions may also be observed. Occasionally, large lesions up to 3 cm are seen. The color of the tumors is variable. In light-skinned individuals slight yellow, pink-brown (*see* Fig. 8.5) or skin-colored (*see* Fig. 8.9) lesions are more common, whereas in patients with relatively darker skin, deeply pigmented lesions (*see* Fig. 8.10) are typical. In addition to classic lesions with uniform color, some tumors have a pale center and peripheral hyperpigmentation mimicking a compound melanocytic nevus of cocarde pattern (*see* Fig. 3.100). The surface of dermatofibroma is mostly smooth but occasionally rough or mildly scaly (*see* Fig. 8.11). Most lesions are asymptomatic but some patients experience slight pruritus.

Dermatofibroma is usually diagnosed clinically. The dimple sign is helpful for diagnosis. This sign is characterized by tumor retraction (dimpling) beneath the skin on lateral pressure of the fingers (*see* Fig. 8.12). Dermatofibroma can easily be misdiagnosed for an intradermal melanocytic nevus. The presence of hairs is in favor of melanocytic nevus, but nevi may also be hairless. Nevi are typically softer than dermatofibromas. Furthermore it may be difficult to differentiate dermatofibromas from nodular malignant melanoma (*see* Fig. 12.43) and dermatofibrosarcoma protuberans (*see* Fig. 13.59). Dermatofibrosarcoma has usually a more irregular appearance. Dermoscopy may be helpful in differentiating dermatofibroma from melanocytic nevi and melanoma. Histopathologic examination may be required to confirm the diagnosis of some lesions. Histopathologic patterns may differ among various subtypes. Typically, epidermal hyperplasia and hyperpigmentation of the basal layer are accompanied by poorly circumscribed tumor tissue in the reticular dermis composed of a variable mixture of spindle cells, histiocytes, and blood vessels.

Some clinical subtypes of dermatofibroma have been described. Angiomatous and atrophic dermatofibromas are among these rare variants. Angiomatous dermatofibroma has

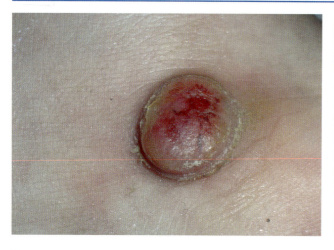

Fig. 8.13 Dome-shaped nodule with reddish areas located on the foot; it was histologically diagnosed as angiomatous dermatofibroma

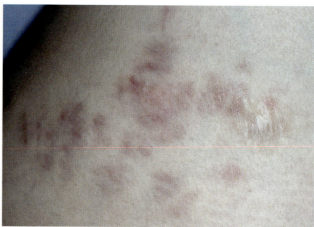

Fig. 8.15 Dermatofibroma presenting as a large atrophic plaque. Though clinical features are not typical, histopathologic examination confirmed the diagnosis in this case

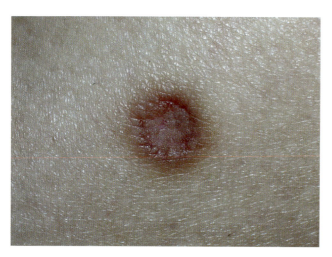

Fig. 8.14 Atrophic dermatofibroma seen as a small depressed area

a prominent vascular component and abundant hemosiderin pigment in the dermis. Therefore, this type of tumor has a dull red color (see Fig. 8.13). Atrophic dermatofibroma may present as an anetodermic or depressed but infiltrated plaque (see Fig. 8.14) on the upper trunk, usually on the shoulder girdle, resembling non-neoplastic dermatoses like anetoderma, atrophoderma, or atrophic scars. Atrophic plaques may occasionally be large (see Fig. 8.15), resembling atrophic dermatofibrosarcoma protuberans.

Management. Dermatofibroma is in general a persistent tumor without malignant potential. It may infrequently regress spontaneously. Hence, therapeutic intervention is not necessary in many cases. Destructive modalities, including cryotherapy and lasers, are usually not effective. Excision can be preferred for cosmetic reasons or can be performed for histopathologic examination to exclude malignant tumors. Although excision with narrow margins is sufficient, deep location of the tumor requires excision of superficial subcutaneous tissue. Therefore the resultant scars may be worse than the initial appearance of the tumor. Patients should be informed before surgery about the risk of unsightly scar formation.

8.2 Fibrous Papule of the Nose

Fibrous papule of the nose is an idiopathic benign papular lesion, most commonly located on the nose. The pathogenesis is not known. It is more commonly observed in middle-aged people. Most patients do not consult physicians about this asymptomatic small lesion, but it can be detected during dermatologic examination. The lesion is mostly located on the tip of the nose or on the alae (see Fig. 8.16) and is a skin-colored, 2 to 6 mm, dome-shaped papule, usually with a smooth surface (see Fig. 8.17). While most are solitary (see Figs. 8.16 and 8.17), there may sometimes be more than one lesion (see Figs. 8.18 and 8.19). Rarely, it can be observed on other parts of the face such as the cheeks and chin (see Fig. 8.20) or on the neck. Therefore it has also been named fibrous papule of the face. The papules may sometimes be pedunculated.

The differential diagnosis includes mainly perifollicular fibroma (see Fig. 8.39), palisaded encapsulated neuroma (see Fig. 7.41), angiofibroma (see Fig. 8.24), and intradermal nevus (see Fig. 3.114), which may also appear as skin-colored papules on the face. Early lesions of basal cell carcinoma (see Fig. 11.24) may be misdiagnosed as fibrous papules of the nose, but the lesions of basal cell carcinoma have a slightly translucent appearance. Histopathologic examination of the fibrous papule shows a sclerotic or hyalinized stroma, ectatic small-caliber vessels, and dendritic/stellate or sometimes multinuclear fibroblasts. Differentiation

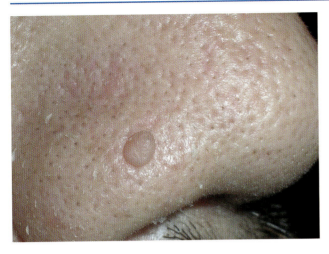

Fig. 8.16 Solitary fibrous papule of the nose located on ala nasi. The asymptomatic lesion may be initially detected during physical examination

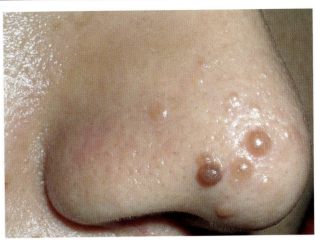

Fig. 8.19 Multiple fibrous papules of the nose located on the tip of the nose

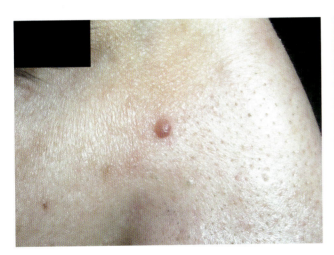

Fig. 8.17 Solitary fibrous papule of the nose presenting as a skin-colored, dome-shaped papule

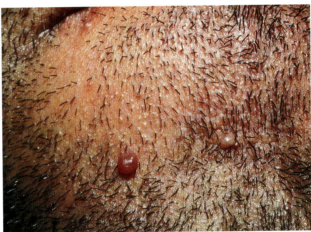

Fig. 8.20 Fibrous papule of the nose involving a different area (fibrous papule of the face). Two lesions located on the chin are shown

from facial angiofibromas encountered in tuberous sclerosis can sometimes be difficult.

Management. There is no risk of malignant transformation and overgrowth of lesions; therefore therapy is not necessary. However, patients may request therapy for cosmetic reasons. Surgical excision is curative.

8.3 Angiofibroma

Angiofibroma is a benign fibrohistiocytic tumor that may be associated with a few syndromes. Multiple angiofibromas of the face are usually a part of tuberous sclerosis. Rarely, tumors with the histopathologic appearance of angiofibroma may also be seen in multiple endocrine neoplasia type 1 (MEN 1).

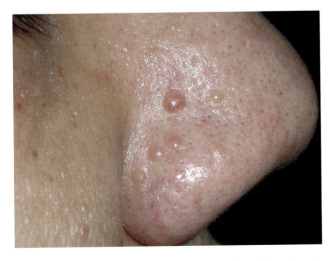

Fig. 8.18 Multiple fibrous papules of the nose located on ala nasi. Some patients have more than one lesion

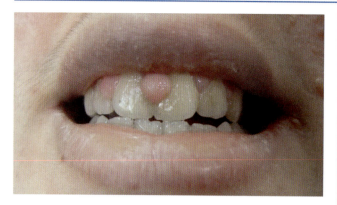

Fig. 8.21 Gingival fibromatosis in a patient with tuberous sclerosis. It occurs typically in childhood

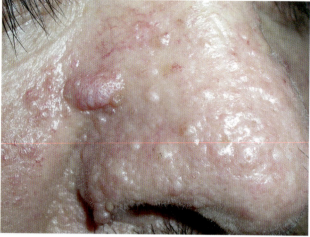

Fig. 8.22 Small skin-colored papules of angiofibromas typically located on the nose and nasolabial fold in tuberous sclerosis

8.3.1 Tuberous sclerosis

Tuberous sclerosis is a relatively common genodermatosis presenting with multiple types of benign fibrohistiocytic tumors and proliferations, including angiofibroma, connective tissue nevus (shagreen patch or forehead plaque) (*see* Figs. 8.85 and 8.89), acrochordon (*see* Fig. 8.68), periungual fibroma (Koenen tumor) (*see* Fig. 8.33), and gingival fibromatosis (*see* Fig. 8.21) accompanied by hypopigmented macules (ash leaf patch), and systemic involvement of various organs. One of the most frequent manifestations of tuberous sclerosis is angiofibromas. They are not present at birth and occur between the ages of 2 and 6 years. Angiofibromas increase in number during childhood. The typical presentation is numerous, smooth-surfaced, dome-shaped, 1 to 3 mm symmetrically distributed, firm papules on the face, especially on the nose, nasolabial folds (*see* Fig. 8.22), and cheeks (*see* Fig. 8.23). Some lesions may be larger (*see* Fig. 8.24). The tumor may be skin-colored (*see* Fig. 8.21), pink, reddish-brown, or rarely red (*see* Fig. 8.25). Papules may be grouped, especially in the nasolabial folds and alae nasi, and may become confluent evolving into elevated nodules (*see* Fig. 8.26). The eyelids (*see* Fig. 8.27), forehead, chin (*see* Fig. 8.28), and sometimes the external ear (*see* Figs. 8.29 and 8.30) may also be involved. Angiofibromas are asymptomatic but may be disfiguring, especially when they increase in size and number. Sometimes, hundreds of lesions may be seen in tuberous sclerosis patients.

Although the clinical features of a solitary angiofibroma are not specific, typical location and symmetric distribution of multiple lesions on the face are usually helpful for the diagnosis. "Adenoma sebaceum symmetricum" is an old term for angiofibroma that is not widely used today because of the lack of any change in the sebaceous glands. Fibrous

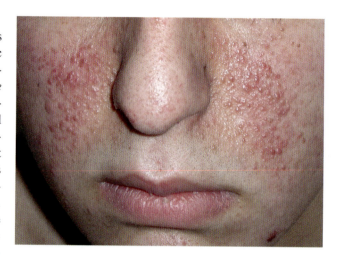

Fig. 8.23 Angiofibromas symmetrically located on the cheeks in tuberous sclerosis; a characteristic appearance

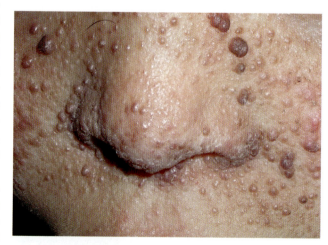

Fig. 8.24 Small and relatively large papules of facial angiofibroma in tuberous sclerosis

8.3 Angiofibroma

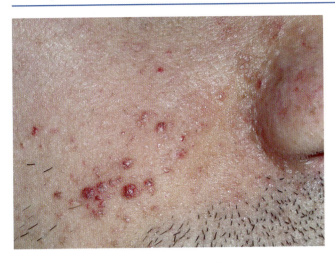

Fig. 8.25 Red angiofibromas in a tuberous sclerosis patient

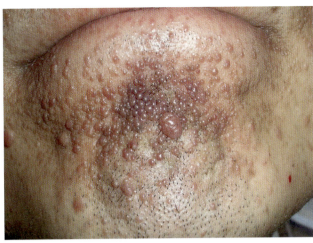

Fig. 8.28 Confluent angiofibromas in a tuberous sclerosis patient on the chin, a common location

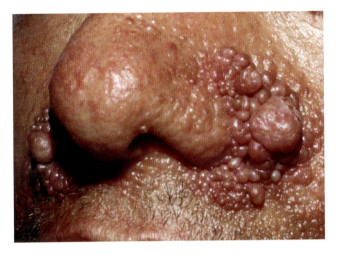

Fig. 8.26 Confluent angiofibromas forming an elevated nodule in a tuberous sclerosis patient

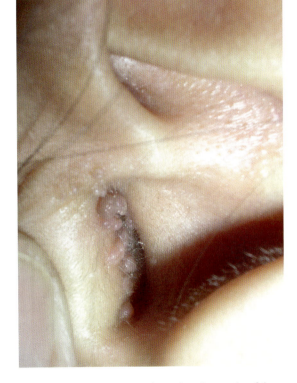

Fig. 8.29 Multiple angiofibromas located on the concha of the ear

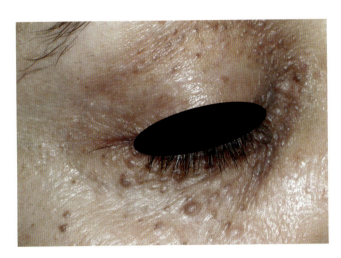

Fig. 8.27 Multiple angiofibromas on the eyelid in a tuberous sclerosis patient

tissue proliferation around numerous small vessels in the papillary dermis is the typical histopathologic appearance of this lesion. Some of these vessels are dilated and have an irregular outline.

When patients have one of the cutaneous findings of tuberous sclerosis, a detailed dermatologic examination should be performed to look for other accompanying features. None of the skin tumors have a prognostic significance, but they allow the diagnosis of this multisystem

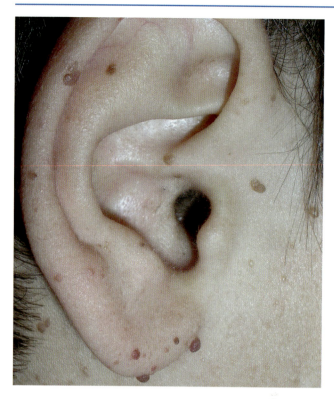

Fig. 8.30 Multiple angiofibromas on the auricle of a tuberous sclerosis patient. (With kind permission from Springer Science+Business Media: Baykal C, Yazganoğlu KD. Dermatological diseases of the nose and ears; 2010)

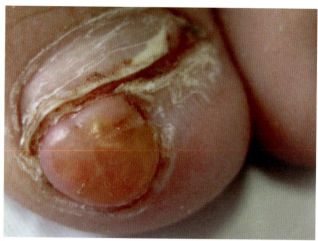

Fig. 8.31 Solitary periungual fibroma in an otherwise healthy individual

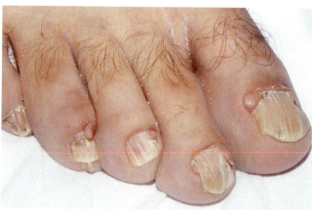

Fig. 8.32 Multiple periungual fibromas around the toenails in tuberous sclerosis (Koenen tumor)

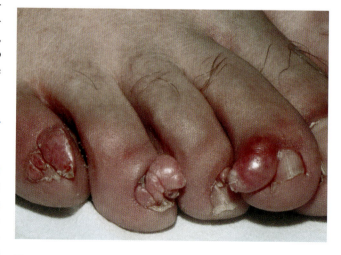

Fig. 8.33 Periungual fibromas presenting as pink projectile papules arising from proximal nailfolds and extending over the nails in tuberous sclerosis

disorder. Systemic manifestations include central nervous system involvement (e.g., infantile spasms, mental retardation, and subependymal nodules) as well as retinal hamartomas, renal angiomyolipomas, cardiac rhabdomyomas, and lymphangiomyomatosis of the lung.

Management. Angiofibromas are not associated with any complications. But multiple persistent facial lesions may be a serious cosmetic problem. Destructive therapeutic modalities, including dermabrasion, shave excision, and a combination of carbon dioxide laser and dye laser, can be helpful, but the relapse rate is high. Rapamycin (sirolimus) may also be effective when used topically in the treatment of mutiple angiofibromas seen in tuberous sclerosis.

8.4 Periungual Fibroma (Koenen Tumor)

Peri- or subungual fibromas are acquired benign nailfold tumors. They are among the distinctive features of tuberous sclerosis. Rarely, they may occur sporadically (*see* Fig. 8.31) without any association with this genodermatosis. They usually arise after puberty. In tuberous sclerosis, multiple toenails or fingernails may be involved bilaterally, and there may be multiple tumors on one nail (*see* Figs. 8.32 and 8.33). The clinical appearance of the tumor may be subtle in some

8.4 Periungual Fibroma (Koenen Tumor)

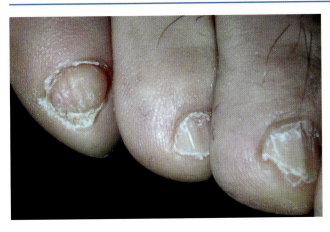

Fig. 8.34 A skin-colored, round papule with a smooth surface on the little toenail representing periungual fibroma in a tuberous sclerosis patient

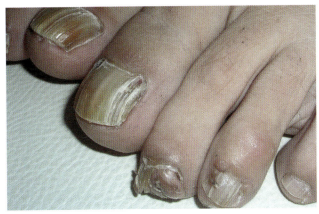

Fig. 8.36 Multiple periungual fibromas and secondary nail changes such as longitudinal grooves typical of tuberous sclerosis

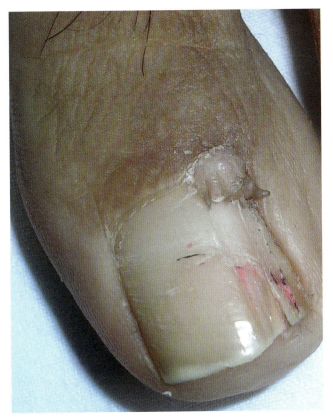

Fig. 8.35 A longitudinal groove of the nail is aligned with a periungual fibroma on the nailfold in a tuberous sclerosis patient

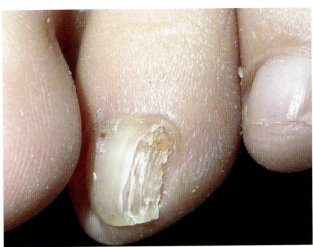

Fig. 8.37 Severe nail destruction associated with periungual fibroma in a patient with tuberous sclerosis

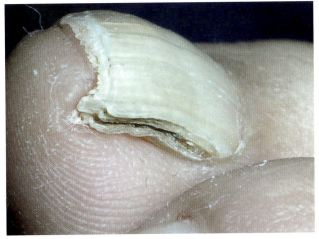

Fig. 8.38 Linear nail plate destruction on the big toe without associated visible periungual fibroma in a patient with tuberous sclerosis

cases. Firm, skin- or pink-colored, smooth papules or finger-like projections usually arising from the distal part of the nailbed or from the skin of the nailfold are typical (see Figs. 8.33, 8.34, 8.35 and 8.36). Tumors associated with tuberous sclerosis are more common on the toenails. Although these fibromas are generally thin and long, thicker tumors may also be observed. Nail destruction may sometimes be a prominent feature (see Fig. 8.37). Rarely, subungual tumors may present solely with destruction of the nail plate (*see* Fig. 8.38). Alterations of the nail plate, such as longitudinal depressions or grooves due to the compression of the tumor on the nail matrix, may be observed (*see* Figs. 8.35 and 8.36). Tumors are usually painless, but destruction of the periungual tissue may be disturbing.

Periungual fibromas may be misdiagnosed as viral warts, but smooth surface and associated nail findings are diagnostic findings. In patients with tuberous sclerosis, association with other dermatologic manifestations of this syndrome facilitates the diagnosis. Biopsy is rarely used for the diagnosis of these tumors. Histologically, the periungual fibromas show fibrosis and sometimes capillary dilatation like angiofibromas.

Management. As most lesions are asymptomatic and there is no risk of malignant transformation, therapy is not necessary. On the other hand, surgical excision can be helpful in relieving the symptoms of large destructive tumors. But recurrence is possible. Electrodesiccation and carbon dioxide laser have also been used in the treatment. However, complications of these procedures, such as destruction of the nailfold and nail plate, are possible. Shaving followed by matrix phenolization is an alternative treatment modality.

8.5 Perifollicular Fibroma

Perifollicular fibroma, fibrofolliculoma, and trichodiscomas are acquired benign tumors of the fibrous root sheath of the hair follicle. They typically manifest as asymptomatic, skin- or grey- to yellow-colored, 2 to 3 mm, dome-shaped, smooth, firm papules (*see* Figs. 8.39 and 8.40). The lesion may be solitary or can appear as many scattered papules on the face (*see* Fig. 8.39), scalp, neck, or upper trunk. Perifollicular fibroma, fibrofolliculoma, and trichodiscoma are thought to originate from the mantle of the hair follicle and considered to be part of the same clinicopathologic spectrum representing the same entity in different periods of development. Thus, clinical distinction between these tumors is usually impossible. Multiple trichilemmomas seen in Cowden syndrome (*see* Fig. 5.46) and angiofibromas seen in tuberous sclerosis (*see* Fig. 8.25) are the main differential diagnostic challenges. Histologically, perifollicular fibroma or fibrofolliculoma is associated with a central follicular structure, peripherally radiating epithelial chords and loose connective tissue in adjacent dermis. Trichodiscoma is slightly different histologically. It is a fibrovascular tumor of the superficial dermis, with mucinous ground substance, which is usually associated with a hair follicle at the periphery of the lesion.

8.5.1 Birt-Hogg-Dubé Syndrome

The presence of multiple perifollicular fibromas, fibrofolliculomas, or trichodiscomas, together with a family history, should arouse a suspicion of Birt-Hogg-Dubé

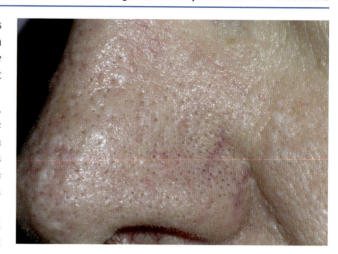

Fig. 8.39 Perifollicular fibroma presenting as multiple tiny papules on the face

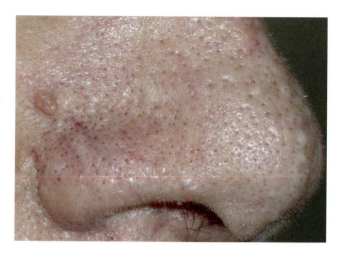

Fig. 8.40 Perifollicular fibroma seen as multiple dome-shaped papules. A pendulous lesion and smaller whitish lesions are seen concomitantly

syndrome. It is inherited in an autosomal dominant trait and mutations in the *folliculin* (*FLCN*) gene play a role in pathogenesis. The number of skin tumors may increase with age, and some adults may have hundreds of fibrofolliculomas or trichodiscomas, especially on the scalp, face (*see* Figs. 8.41 and 8.42), neck, and upper trunk (*see* Fig. 8.43). Acrochordon is another benign tumor seen in this syndrome. Small acrochordons may be seen on the neck (*see* Fig. 8.44), axillae, face, and upper trunk. In addition to cutaneous manifestations, visceral involvement and high risk of internal malignancies increase the importance of this syndrome. Benign and malignant tumors of the kidney and thyroid, parathyroid, and parotid glands can be seen. Renal cell carcinoma occurs at a young age and may be bilateral. Bilateral lung cysts are common and they may remain asymptomatic for a long time. Recurrent spontaneous pneumothorax, bronchiectasis, emphysema, and chorioretinopathy are other systemic manifestations.

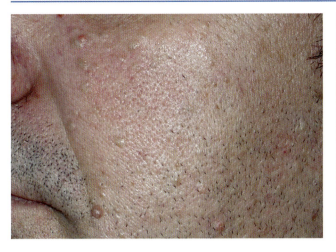

Fig. 8.41 Perifollicular fibroma appearing as dome-shaped, scattered facial papules in a patient with Birt-Hogg-Dubé syndrome

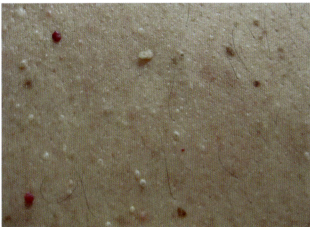

Fig. 8.43 Numerous perifollicular fibromas scattered on the trunk in a patient with Birt-Hogg-Dubé syndrome

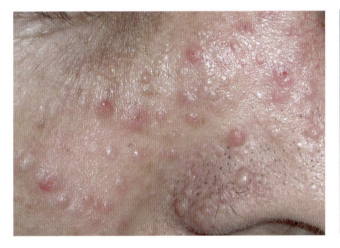

Fig. 8.42 Multiple perifollicular fibromas in a patient with Birt-Hogg-Dubé syndrome. The lesions are asymptomatic

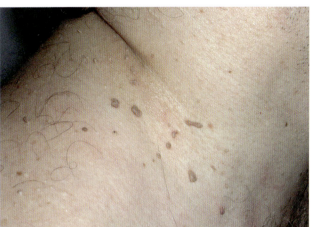

Fig. 8.44 Perifollicular fibromas and acrochordons are seen concomitantly on the neck of a patient with Birt-Hogg-Dubé syndrome

Rarely, the disease manifests only with visceral findings without associated skin tumors.

Management. Perifollicular fibroma may be cosmetically disturbing and therefore surgical excision can be performed for solitary lesion. Laser ablation and dermabrasion are feasible therapeutic options for multiple lesions. However, recurrence may be a problem. The diagnosis of Birt-Hogg-Dubé syndrome is important in order to allow early detection of internal malignancies. A careful lifelong follow-up for the development of accompanying malignancies is recommended for these patients. Other risk factors for pneumothorax such as smoking should be avoided. Dermatologic and oncologic screenings of family members are also indicated.

8.6 Oral Fibroma

Oral fibroma is one of the most common benign tumoral lesions of the oral cavity, presenting as a solitary papule or nodule. It has been accepted as a reactive scar-like condition caused by chronic local irritation or repeated trauma in the oral cavity. Therefore, it is also called irritation fibroma. Most of the patients are adults. As cheek or lip biting are possible etiologic factors, the lesion is commonly located on the buccal mucosa, especially along the closure line where maxillary and mandibular teeth meet (*see* Fig. 8.45). The sides (see Fig. 8.46) and dorsum of the tongue (*see* Fig. 8.47) gingivae, and mucosal side of the lower lip are other predilection sites. The typical lesion

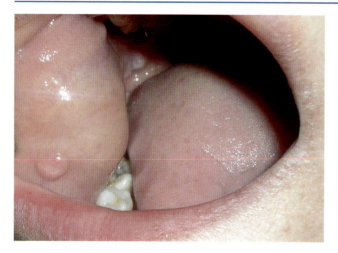

Fig. 8.45 Oral fibroma located at the closure line on the buccal mucosa

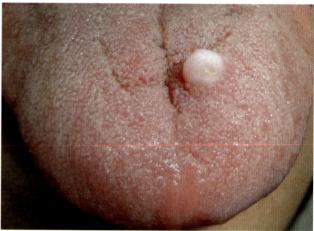

Fig. 8.47 Oral fibroma seen as a white, dome-shaped, solitary nodule on the dorsum of the tongue

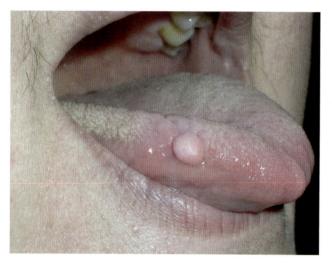

Fig. 8.46 Oral fibroma presenting as a pinkish solitary nodule on the side of the tongue

is a dome-shaped or pedunculated, pinkish or white, firm, noninflammatory papule or nodule smaller than 1 cm (see Figs. 8.46 and 8.47). It has usually a smooth surface but may also be hyperkeratotic and may rarely ulcerate secondarily. The painless lesion grows to reach a certain size and then remains unchanged.

Oral verrucae, mucocele, neurofibroma (see Fig. 7.19), and many other oral tumors may be clinically considered in the differential diagnosis of oral fibroma. Biopsy may be performed to exclude these conditions. Histologically a nodule composed of hyalinized collagen bundles with relatively few cells is typical. The overlying mucosa can show hyperkeratosis.

Management. Oral fibroma is a persistent lesion but does not show malignant degeneration. Therefore, therapeutic intervention is not obligatory. Surgical removal with narrow clear margins is the single treatment option in lesions causing discomfort, and this also allows histopathologic examination. On the other hand, recurrence may be seen if underlying etiologic factors cannot be eliminated.

8.7 Acquired Digital Fibrokeratoma

Acquired digital fibrokeratoma is an uncommon benign tumor of fibrous tissue appearing mostly as a solitary, skin-colored papule on the hands and feet of adults. It is more often seen in men. Although the tumors may typically be located on fingers (see Fig. 8.48) or toes (see Fig. 8.49) (as the name "digital" implies), they may also be seen on other sites of the body, such as the palm, dorsum of the hand, elbow (see Figs. 8.50 and 8.51), wrist, ankle, calf, sole, or prepatellar area. The etiology is unknown. Trauma has been suggested as a triggering factor, but a history of trauma is absent in most cases.

The typical presentation is a solitary, dome-shaped (see Figs. 8.52 and 8.53), or finger-like (see Fig. 8.54), smooth-surfaced, skin-colored, firm papule or nodule. Most of the lesions are smaller than 1 cm. Lesions may be sessile (see Fig. 8.51) or pedunculated (see Fig. 8.55). A hyperkeratotic (see Fig. 8.53) or verruciform surface can be noticed in some lesions. One of the most important differentiating features of acquired digital fibrokeratoma can be noticed at the base of the lesion in the form of slightly elevated skin causing a collarette (see Figs. 8.53 and 8.56). Periungual fibrokeratoma may cause secondary nail changes (see Fig. 8.57).

Acquired digital fibrokeratoma can easily be misdiagnosed for other common benign lesions such as verruca vulgaris or filiform verrucae, which usually are not subject to routine histopathologic examination. Rudimentary digit (see Fig. 7.44), periungual fibroma (see Fig. 8.31), pyogenic granuloma (see Fig. 6.46), poroma (see Fig. 5.17), cutaneous horn (see

8.7 Acquired Digital Fibrokeratoma

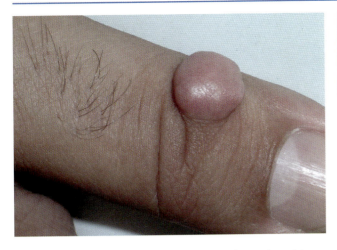

Fig. 8.48 Acquired digital fibrokeratoma on the finger of an adult

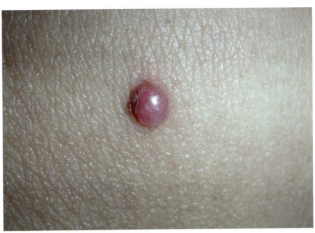

Fig. 8.51 Acquired digital fibrokeratoma manifesting as a sessile nodule on the elbow

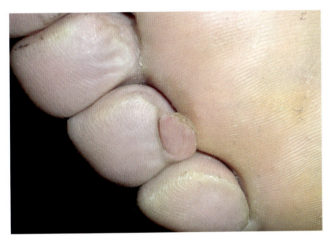

Fig. 8.49 Acquired digital fibrokeratoma seen as a solitary lesion on the volar surface of the toe

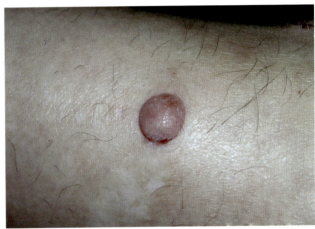

Fig. 8.52 Acquired digital fibrokeratoma presenting as a solitary dome-shaped nodule

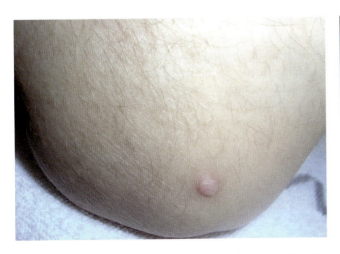

Fig. 8.50 Acquired digital fibrokeratoma on the elbow, a rare location

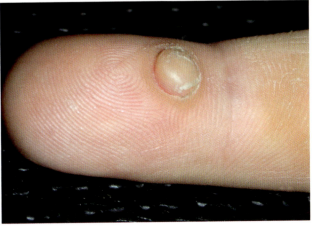

Fig. 8.53 Acquired digital fibrokeratoma shown as a skin-colored, dome-shaped nodule with a perilesional collarette and hyperkeratotic surface

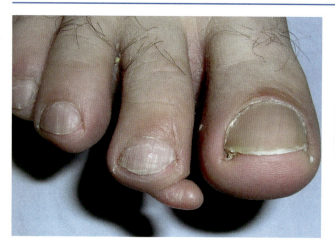

Fig. 8.54 Acquired digital fibrokeratoma manifesting as a finger-like projectile nodule

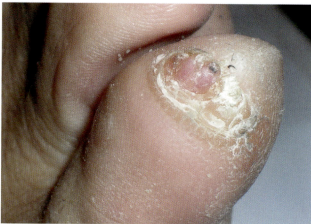

Fig. 8.57 Periungual acquired digital fibrokeratoma causing secondary nail destruction

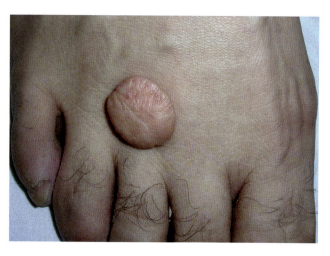

Fig. 8.55 Acquired digital fibrokeratoma presenting as a pedunculated nodule

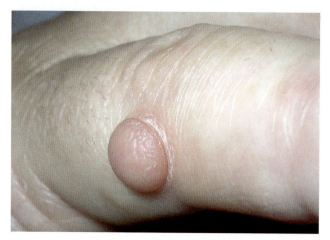

Fig. 8.56 Dome-shaped acquired digital fibrokeratoma with perilesional collarette

Fig. 2.57), acrochordon (*see* Fig. 8.80), and neurofibroma (*see* Fig. 7.4) are among the other lesions included in the differential diagnosis. A mamillated surface can frequently be noticed on verruca vulgaris. The rudimentary digit is a type of amputation neuroma that is usually congenital and located at the base of the fifth finger, and an epidermal collarette is absent. On the other hand, an epidermal collarette may be present in pyogenic granuloma, but this reddish vascular tumor has a sudden onset and often an eroded surface. Periungual fibromas (Koenen tumors) are usually located on the fingernails or toenails and are usually multiple in contrast to the solitary lesion of acquired digital fibrokeratoma. They are mostly a part of tuberous sclerosis. Acrochordons are softer and more common on intertriginous sites and the trunk.

If there is any doubt about the diagnosis, a biopsy can be performed. Although there are some subtle histologic differences concerning the clinical shapes of the tumors, hyperkeratosis and acanthotic epidermis with an underlying connective tissue proliferation are common features of all lesions. Collagen bundles are thick, closely packed, and oriented along the vertical axis of the lesion.

Management. Acquired digital fibrokeratoma is an asymptomatic tumor with no potential for malignant transformation. However, lesions are persistent and spontaneous regression is not expected. Surgical excision can be performed for cosmetic reasons or to enable histopathologic examination, and recurrence is rare.

8.8 Epithelioid Cell Histiocytoma

Epithelioid cell histiocytoma is a rare benign fibrous tissue tumor considered to be a variant of dermatofibroma. It is more common in adults. The trunk and limbs are the favored locations. It typically presents as a solitary, reddish, firm, sessile

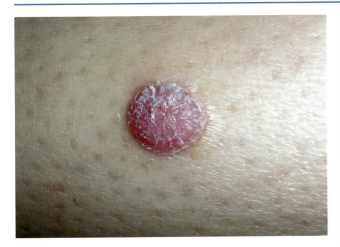

Fig. 8.58 Epithelioid cell histiocytoma presenting as a sessile reddish nodule

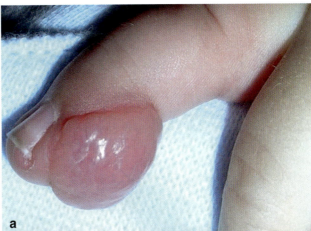

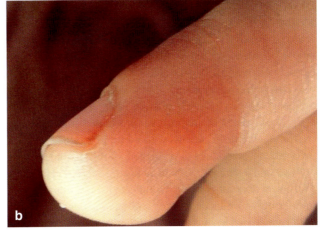

Fig. 8.59 (**a**) Infantile digital fibromatosis presenting as a large solitary nodule on the finger of an infant. (**b**) Spontaneous healing of the lesion in two years

or polypoid nodule smaller than 2 cm (*see* Fig. 8.58). It may be confused clinically with angiomatous dermatofibroma (*see* Fig. 8.13), desmoplastic Spitz nevus (*see* Fig. 3.218), and pyogenic granuloma (*see* Fig. 6.46). Histopathologic examination shows angulated epithelioid cells with abundant eosinophilic cytoplasm that bear a close resemblance to Spitz nevus. However, these cells are negative for S100 and positive for factor XIIIa, a marker considered to point to dermal dendrocytic origin.

Management. Lesions are usually asymptomatic and therapy is not obligatory. Recurrence is rare after surgical removal.

8.9 Infantile Digital Fibromatosis

Infantile digital fibromatosis is a benign, idiopathic fibro/myofibroblastic proliferation that occurs primarily on acral regions. It involves the fingers or toes and has a predilection for the third, fourth, and fifth digits. The thumb and big toe are almost always spared. The tumor usually occurs in the first year of life but may also be present at birth. Less commonly, it may occur later in childhood. There is often a solitary lesion, but sometimes two tumors may be seen. An individual lesion is approximately 1 to 2 cm, firm, slightly erythematous, pinkish or skin-colored tumor with a smooth surface, and generally is located on the lateral or dorsal site of the distal phalanges (*see* Fig. 8.59a). Especially large tumors may cause pain, interfere with the function of the digit, and cause deformities of adjacent joints. Tumors may also lead to secondary nail dystrophy.

The differential diagnosis includes various benign tumors such as acquired digital fibrokeratoma (*see* Fig. 8.48), dermatofibroma (*see* Fig. 8.3), giant cell tumor of the tendon sheath (*see* Fig. 8.110), keloid and multicentric reticulohistiocytosis, which are mostly seen later in life. A tumor in a typical location with history of early-onset is usually suggestive of infantile digital fibromatosis. However, a biopsy is usually indicated for confirmation of the diagnosis. Irregularly arranged and interlacing spindle-shaped myofibroblasts and collagen bundles in the dermis and subcutis, and the presence of eosinophilic cytoplasmic inclusion bodies are the main histopathologic features. Ultrasonography and magnetic resonance imaging studies are used to determine the limits of the tumor, especially its depth.

Management. The tumor's growth stabilizes in a short time, and the lesion shows a tendency to spontaneous healing during early childhood (*see* Fig. 8.59a and b). However, tumors causing functional problems or growing aggressively may be excised. On the other hand, large tumors may not be technically easy to remove because of their location. Undesirable scars after excision are possible, and the relapse rate is high. Intralesional corticosteroids (triamcinolone acetonide) and 5-flourouracil have been used with variable results. If there is no diagnostic suspicion and the function of the digit is not affected, the best approach appears to be observation without intervention.

8.10 Infantile Myofibromatosis

Infantile myofibromatosis is a tumor of infants and early childhood occurring as a result of proliferation of fibroblasts and myofibroblasts. The tumor appears as solitary or multiple, well-defined, firm dermal nodules or masses that also involve subcutaneous tissue and are usually located on the head and neck areas. The size of the lesions is variable. In cases with disseminated skin lesions, tumors also may involve visceral organs and bone, and may be life-threatening. Infantile fibrosarcoma and desmoid tumor may be considered in the differential diagnosis. The diagnosis can be established with a biopsy of cutaneous tumors. Histologically there is usually a dermal nodule formed by fascicles of somewhat plump spindle cells with features of myofibroblasts. Small vessels with a hemangiopericytoma-like pattern is another typical finding. The spindle cells are positive for smooth muscle actin.

Management. In patients with multiple lesions, systemic involvement should be investigated. Solitary tumors may regress spontaneously without requiring therapy. However, excision with wide margins is indicated for solitary lesions interfering with function or for multiple lesions. In patients with generalized lesions and visceral involvement, radiotherapy and chemotherapy are indicated. Recurrence may occur.

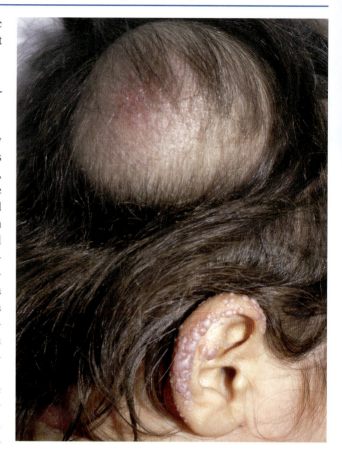

Fig. 8.60 Confluent papules on the pinna and a large mass on the scalp in juvenile hyaline fibromatosis

8.11 Juvenile Hyaline Fibromatosis

Juvenile hyaline fibromatosis is a rare autosomal recessive genodermatosis characterized by progressive papulonodular lesions and joint and bone involvement. A defect on *capillary morphogenesis gene-2* (*CMG2*) also known as *ANTXR2* gene is found. Skin lesions appear in the first years of life. Skin-colored or translucent papules or nodules that show a tendency to confluence may be seen on the hands and face, especially on the nose and ears (*see* Fig. 8.60). However other regions like perianal area may also be involved. Large subcutaneous nodules or masses may be seen on the scalp (*see* Fig. 8.60), trunk, and extremities. The number of lesions increases in time and may interfere with joint function. Progressive joint contracture is a common complication of the disease (*see* Fig. 8.61). Myopathy, osteolytic lesions, and gingival hypertrophy (see Fig. 8.62), the last of which may result in misaligned teeth and caries, are other findings of the disease. Infantile systemic hyalinosis is another genetic disease with similar cutaneous findings but with severe visceral involvement and a poor prognosis.

Tuberous sclerosis and infantile myofibromatosis are challenging differential diagnoses. The typical histologic appearance of juvenile hyaline fibromatosis is dermal

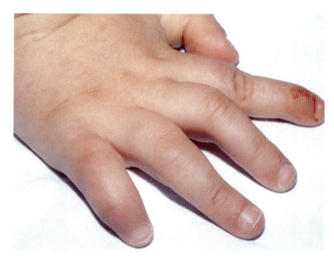

Fig. 8.61 Contracture of the finger joints in juvenile hyaline fibromatosis

deposition of amorphous, hyaline substance with a few embedded fibroblastic cells.

Management. There is no effective treatment for juvenile hyaline fibromatosis. Because lesions are multiple, surgical excision is mostly not feasible. Furthermore, recurrence after surgery is common. Systemic corticosteroids and orthopedic interventions may be required for joint contractures.

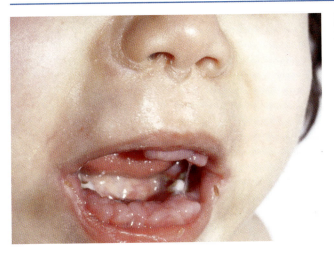

Fig. 8.62 Small papules around the nose and gingival hypertrophy in a patient with juvenile hyaline fibromatosis

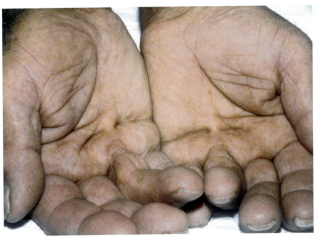

Fig. 8.64 Bilateral Dupuytren contracture causing dimpling and finger deformity

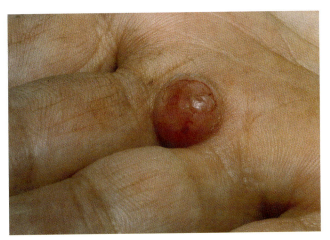

Fig. 8.63 Calcifying aponeurotic fibroma shown as a large nodule on the palm

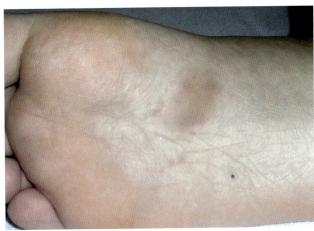

Fig. 8.65 Superficial plantar fibromatosis presenting as a solitary subcutaneous nodule on the sole of the foot of a child

8.12 Calcifying Aponeurotic Fibroma

Calcifying aponeurotic fibroma (juvenile aponeurotic fibroma) is a rare, soft tissue tumor manifesting as a solitary, slow-growing subcutaneous nodule on the hands or feet. It is seen in children and adolescents. Involvement of the palms is typical (*see* Fig. 8.63), but it may also occur on the soles or fingers. Involvement of other parts of the body is unusual. The deeply located, infiltrating, hard mass may be adherent to the underlying tendon, fasciae, or rarely bone. However, it does not metastasize. It should be differentiated from palmar and plantar fibromatoses (*see* Figs. 8.64 and 8.65), which may also occur at the same locations, but these tumors lack a myofibroblastic component. Plantar collagenoma (*see* Fig. 8.93), nodular fasciitis, fibrosarcoma (*see* Fig. 13.67), and giant cell tumor of the tendon sheath (*see* Fig. 8.109) are other differential diagnostic challenges. Histologically, myofibroblastic cells form a poorly circumscribed cellular mass invading subcutaneous tissue and muscle accompanied by calcifications. The calcification may also be seen radiologically. Tumors may be persistent or regress spontaneously.

Management. Surgery with wide margins is the therapy of choice in persistent lesions but recurrence commonly occurs.

8.13 Fibromatoses

Fibromatoses are a group of benign tumors or proliferations of connective tissue with unknown etiology that may be locally aggressive but do not metastasize. They may be localized superficially (fasciae) or involve deeper soft tissues, including muscles. Various types of these tumor groups have been described according to their specific location. They grow slowly but may be progressive, causing functional impairment or discomfort.

8.13.1 Palmar Fibromatosis

Palmar fibromatosis (Dupuytren contracture) is a type of fibromatosis of the palmar fasciae seen unilaterally or bilaterally on the palms of adults. It is the most common type of superficial fibromatoses. It may appear as a dimple or lump on the palmar area, and local skin blanching can be noticed upon extension of the fingers (see Fig. 8.64). A firm, fixed subcutaneous nodularity or fibrous band can be palpated. It has a slow progressive course, causing flexion contractures of the fourth and fifth fingers in severe cases.

8.13.2 Plantar Fibromatosis

Plantar fibromatosis is composed of different entities. Ledderhose disease is the plantar counterpart of palmar fibromatosis seen in adults. Both diseases may be seen in the same patient. Involvement is mostly bilateral. One or more subcutaneous nodules or masses are mostly located on the medial aspect of the sole. As opposed to palmar fibromatosis, contraction deformities of the feet are unusual. Most lesions are asymptomatic, but enlarged tumors may cause pain in walking and tumors involving neurovascular bundles and tendons may also be painful. Superficial plantar fibromatosis is an uncommon subtype of plantar fibromatosis mostly encountered in childhood. One or a few subcutaneous nodules in varying sizes may be seen (see Fig. 8.65). The lesions are mostly asymptomatic. They may be persistent after reaching a certain size or may involute spontaneously.

Calcifying aponeurotic fibroma (see Fig. 8.63), plantar collagenoma (see Fig. 8.93), lipoma, keloid (see Fig. 8.101), epidermoid cyst (see Fig. 4.5), and ganglion cyst may be considered in the differential diagnosis of palmar and plantar fibromatoses. The histopathology of palmar and plantar fibromatoses is similar. In the early stages cellular nodules of myofibroblastic cells are seen. Especially in palmar fibromatosis, these tend to transform into poorly cellular, hyalinized collagenous nodules and bundles as the lesion gets older.

8.13.3 Knuckle Pads

Knuckle pads are localized fibromatous lesions presenting as firm, flat plaques overlying the interphalangeal and metacarpophalangeal joints (see Fig. 8.66). Trauma has been suggested as a possible etiologic factor. They may be associated with other fibromatoses and some genodermatoses (epidermolytic palmoplantar keratoderma, Bart-Pumphrey syndrome).

8.13.4 Penile Fibromatosis (Peyronie Disease)

Penile fibromatosis is a rare acquired condition affecting the fibrous septae between the corpus spongiosum and the

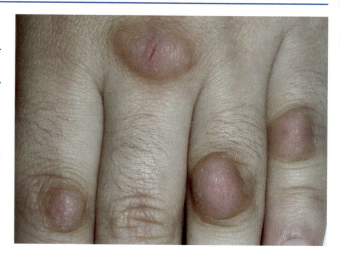

Fig. 8.66 Knuckle pads seen as well-circumscribed flat plaques on the dorsum of finger joints. They are asymptomatic

corpus cavernosum on the dorsal aspect of the penis that causes localized hardening. It may be painful. Urination is not affected, but erectile dysfunction may occur.

Management. Observation may be the preferred method in Dupuytren contracture and Ledderhose disease, as some lesions may heal spontaneously. Intralesional corticosteroids can be injected into the fibromatous nodules, but this creates a risk of atrophy. Radiotherapy can be applied in the early stages of these diseases. In patients with severe painful lesions, significant disability, or serious contractures, surgical excision is the therapy of choice. Fasciotomy or fasciectomy can be performed. However, recurrence is possible after surgery. A conservative approach should be chosen for superficial plantar fibromatosis because of the possibility of spontaneous regression. Similarly, penile fibromatosis may be observed for a period with only symptomatic measures for pain, since spontaneous resolution is possible. Corporal plication is a surgical technique used in persistent cases of Peyronie disease.

8.14 Acrochordon (Skin Tag)

Acrochordon is the most common benign fibrohistiocytic tumor of the skin. Approximately 50 percent of humans have one or more acrochordons in their lifetimes. Although it was formerly suggested, an association of these skin tumors with gastrointestinal polyps could not be shown. The high frequency of the tumor is an additional clue that it could not be a distinct marker of any systemic disease. However, it should be noted that it is more commonly observed in obese individuals. Furthermore, acrochordons may be seen in some diseases such as tuberous sclerosis (see Figs. 8.67 and 8.68), Birt-Hogg-Dubé syndrome (see Fig. 8.44), and acanthosis nigricans (see Fig. 8.69). Acrochordons in tuberous sclerosis are associated with other fibrohistiocytic tumors and may appear at a younger age. Acrochordons in Birt-Hogg-Dubé syndrome are associated with skin appendage tumors like

8.14 Acrochordon (Skin Tag)

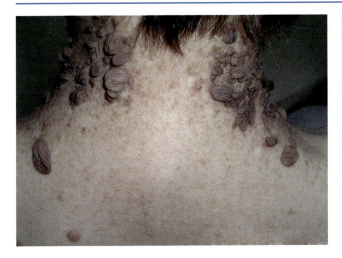

Fig. 8.67 Multiple acrochordons on the nape of the neck seen in a child with tuberous sclerosis

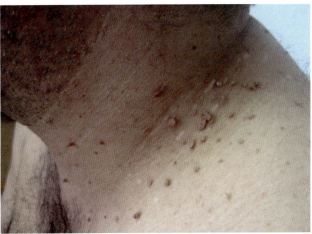

Fig. 8.69 Acanthosis nigricans associated with multiple acrochordons

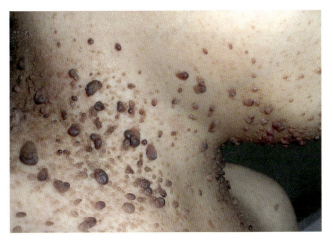

Fig. 8.68 Profuse acrochordons on the neck and upper chest in a child with tuberous sclerosis

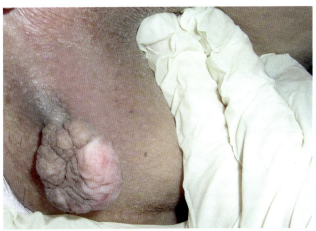

Fig. 8.70 A large solitary acrochordon located on the groin

perifollicular fibroma presenting as papular lesions. Multiple acrochordons located on the flexures may overlap with acanthosis nigricans on the same site.

Acrochordons do not show gender preponderance. The lesions begin mostly in the second or third decade and increase gradually in number. They are most commonly seen in the axillae and neck (*see* Fig. 8.67), followed by other major flexural areas such as the groin (*see* Fig. 8.70). The eyelids and trunk may also be involved. Typical pedunculated lesions are skin-colored (*see* Figs. 8.71 and 8.72) or slightly hyperpigmented. They are soft on palpation and may have a folded surface (*see* Fig. 8.72). The stalk is usually narrow (*see* Figs. 8.73 and 8.74). The size of the lesions is variable. Although lesions on the eyelids are tiny (1 to 2 mm) (*see* Fig. 8.75), classic lesions on the flexures range from 3 to 10 mm and truncal lesions may be larger (*see* Fig. 8.76). Some tumors may be lobulated (*see* Fig. 8.77). The number of lesions also varies in individuals. While some individuals have solitary or a few lesions, some have profuse lesions. Truncal lesions are mostly solitary and have a bag-like appearance (*see* Fig. 8.76). Multiple lesions on more than one site may also be observed. The nipple is an unusual location of the acrochordon (*see* Figs. 8.78 and 8.79).

The acrochordon is an asymptomatic lesion without any malignant potential. Therefore it is just a cosmetic problem. However, occasionally trauma may induce torsion of the stalk, which enhances the blood supply of the tumor and results in slight or severe inflammation (*see* Fig. 8.80), hemorrhage (*see* Fig. 8.81), and sometimes partial or complete necrosis (*see* Fig. 8.82). These lesions may be transiently painful.

The differential diagnosis usually constitutes skin-colored, pedunculated intradermal nevi (*see* Fig. 3.129) and pedunculated neurofibromas (*see* Fig. 7.15). Acrochordon-like multiple basal cell carcinomas may be observed in Gorlin syndrome (*see* Figs. 11.82 and 11.86). Some seborrheic keratoses with stalks (*see* Fig. 1.31) may also be confused with acrochordons. The papillomatous surface with embedded tiny cysts and a relatively darker color of seborrheic

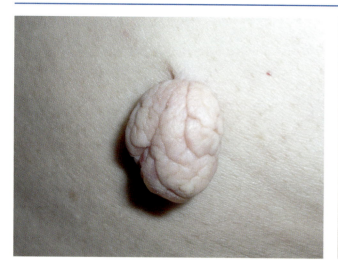

Fig. 8.71 An acrochordon presenting as a skin-colored pedunculated nodule with a narrow stalk

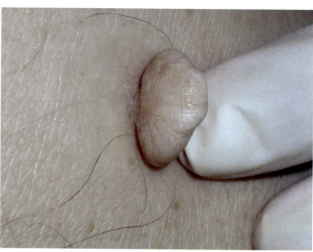

Fig. 8.74 Acrochordon with a narrow stalk that is mobile on palpation

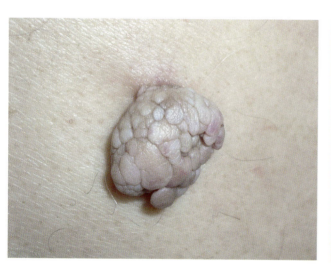

Fig. 8.72 Acrochordon with a folded surface

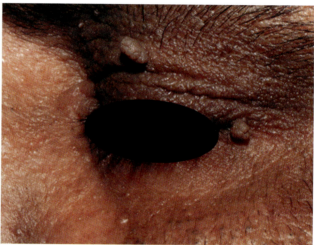

Fig. 8.75 Tiny acrochordons on the eyelids. Some patients have multiple lesions

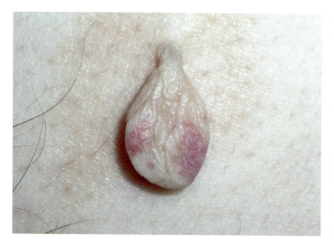

Fig. 8.73 Acrochordon with a narrow stalk. This lesion was soft

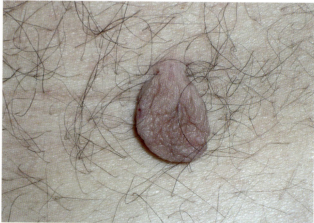

Fig. 8.76 Large skin-colored acrochordon on the trunk

8.14 Acrochordon (Skin Tag)

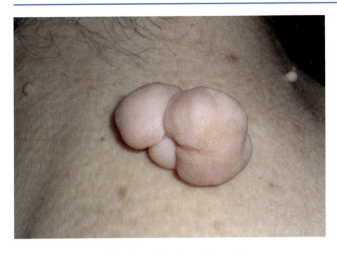

Fig. 8.77 Large lobulated acrochordon on the neck

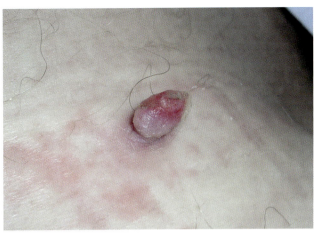

Fig. 8.80 Inflamed acrochordon; note the reddish color

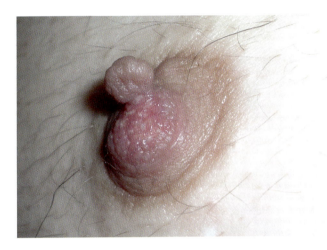

Fig. 8.78 Acrochordon on the nipple, an unusual localization

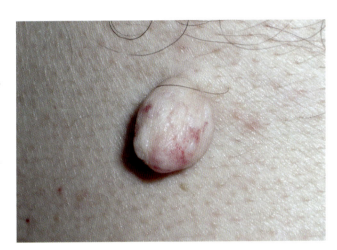

Fig. 8.81 Acrochordon showing slight hemorrhage

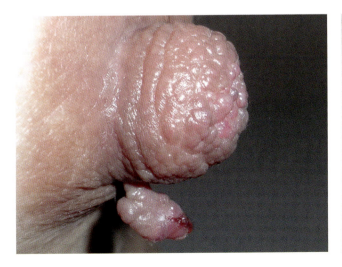

Fig. 8.79 Acrochordon with a narrow stalk located on the nipple

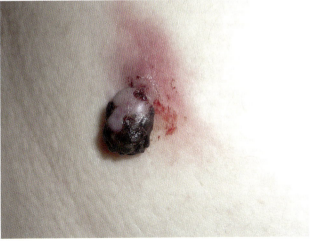

Fig. 8.82 Acrochordon showing complete necrosis

keratosis, and the presence of the button-hole sign in neurofibroma are clinical distinguishing features. The histopathology of an acrochordon reveals a fibroadipous central core, rich in small caliber vessels, covered with an epidermis that is sometimes papillomatous.

Management. Therapy is not obligatory. On the other hand, frequently traumatized lesions and the ones causing cosmetic disturbance may all be treated. Small tumors can be cauterized easily. Larger lesions may be removed with scissors or tangential excision. The risk of scar formation on the excision site is minimal.

8.15 Connective Tissue Nevus (Collagenoma)

Connective tissue nevus is a rare hamartoma of dermal connective tissue components. It may be an isolated tumor or may be associated with a systemic disease or a genodermatosis. The number of lesions and clinical presentations vary primarily according to the clinical type and associated condition. In some cases connective tissue nevus may be observed as small papules, while in others as large plaques. Familial cutaneous collagenoma and connective tissue nevi seen in tuberous sclerosis, Buschke-Ollendorff syndrome, and Proteus syndrome are the hereditary types of connective tissue nevus. Sporadic types include isolated collagenoma and eruptive collagenoma.

8.15.1 Tuberous Sclerosis

Connective tissue nevus is most commonly associated with tuberous sclerosis. It can be seen in this genodermatosis in two distinctive presentations: shagreen patch and forehead plaque. Shagreen patch occurs nearly in half of the tuberous sclerosis patients. It may be present at birth, but more commonly appears around the age of 2. It is often localized on the lower back, typically on one side of the lumbosacral area (*see* Figs. 8.83, 8.84 and 8.85). However, upper back (*see* Fig. 8.86), flanks (*see* Fig. 8.87), and thighs may also be involved. We observed a connective tissue nevus of fingers in a patient with tuberous sclerosis (*see* Fig. 8.88). Multiple skin-colored or yellowish, firm, irregularly distributed papules, nodules, or plaques may occur. Some papules may coalesce to form plaques (*see* Fig. 8.84). The size of the plaques may reach up to 10 to 15 cm (*see* Figs. 8.85, 8.86 and 8.87). The uneven cobblestoned surface (*see* Fig. 8.85) resembling shagreen leather and prominent follicular openings are further clues in the clinical diagnosis. The asymptomatic subtle lesions may initially be noticed during routine dermatologic examination. Isolated papular

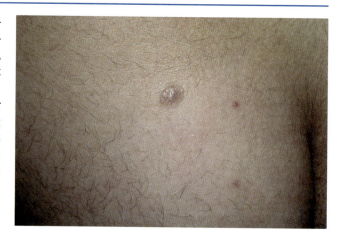

Fig. 8.83 Connective tissue nevus presenting as an isolated nodule located on the lumbosacral area of a patient with tuberous sclerosis

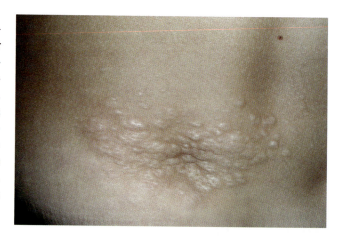

Fig. 8.84 Connective tissue nevus seen as a large plaque on the lumbosacral area of a patient with tuberous sclerosis

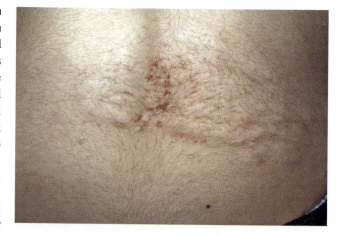

Fig. 8.85 Connective tissue nevus in a patient with tuberous sclerosis. Note the typical cobblestone surface of the skin-colored large plaque

lesions (*see* Fig. 8.83) may easily be misdiagnosed as intradermal melanocytic nevi (*see* Fig. 3.108). Nevus lipomatosus superficialis (*see* Fig. 10.9) is another differential

8.15 Connective Tissue Nevus (Collagenoma)

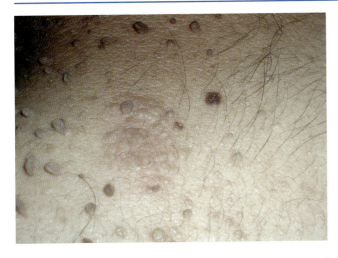

Fig. 8.86 Connective tissue nevus and multiple acrochordons located on the upper back of a patient with tuberous sclerosis

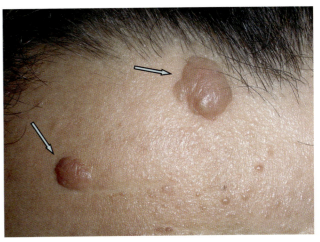

Fig. 8.89 Two skin-colored nodules on the face representing forehead plaques in a patient with tuberous sclerosis

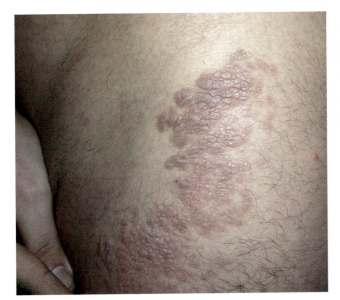

Fig. 8.87 Connective tissue nevus presenting as a large plaque on the flank in a patient with tuberous sclerosis. Even large lesions are asymptomatic

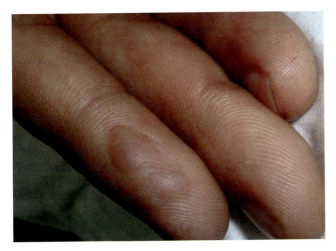

Fig. 8.88 Connective tissue nevus in tuberous sclerosis located on the fingers, an unusual site

diagnostic consideration, especially in cases with large plaques. All patients with connective tissue nevus should be examined for other cutaneous and systemic manifestations of tuberous sclerosis.

Forehead plaque typically seen in tuberous sclerosis (*see* Fig. 8.89) as a skin-colored nodule or flat plaque on the forehead is also a clinical subtype of connective tissue nevus. It may also be located on other regions of the face and rarely on the scalp (*see* Fig. 8.90). It is usually seen together with facial angiofibromas.

8.15.2 Buschke-Ollendorff syndrome

Buschke-Ollendorff syndrome is an autosomal dominantly inherited rare disorder characterized mainly by connective tissue nevus (dermatofibrosis lenticularis disseminata) associated with bone findings (osteopoikilosis). The connective tissue nevi, which are usually multiple, appear in early life as asymmetric, yellow, or skin-colored papules or plaques on the trunk (*see* Fig. 8.91) and limbs. Skeletal manifestations of the syndrome such as increased bone density as circumscribed sclerotic areas in the long and flat bones are clinically asymptomatic but may be diagnosed radiologically.

8.15.3 Proteus syndrome

Connective tissue nevus, epidermal nevus (*see* Fig. 1.89), and vascular malformations (*see* Fig. 6.123) are the main dermatologic manifestations seen in Proteus syndrome. Connective tissue nevus is typically located on the plantar area, and is called plantar collagenoma (cerebriform connective tissue nevus). It is less commonly seen on the pal-

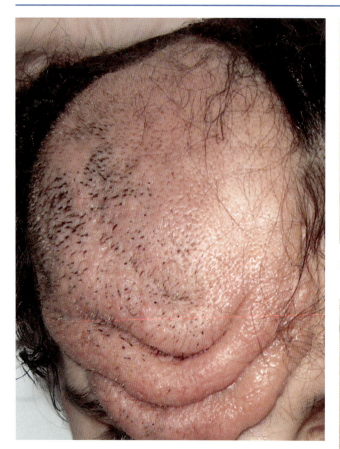

Fig. 8.90 A giant connective tissue nevus on the scalp of a patient with tuberous sclerosis. The large mass shown here is an extreme presentation

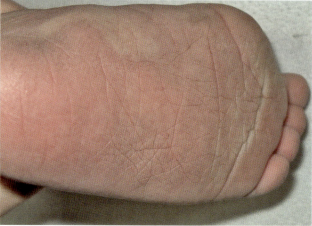

Fig. 8.92 Plantar collagenoma in a child with Proteus syndrome

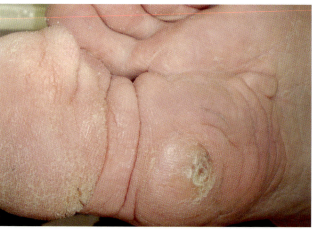

Fig. 8.93 Plantar collagenoma in an adult patient with Proteus syndrome. Note the cerebriform surface

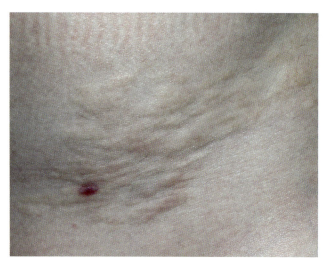

Fig. 8.91 Connective tissue nevus presenting as a large plaque on the trunk in a child with Buschke-Ollendorff syndrome (dermatofibrosis lenticularis disseminata)

mar area. It appears as a skin-colored, sharply demarcated, firm, rugose, cerebriform plaque of variable sizes (*see* Figs. 8.92 and 8.93). The lesion grows throughout childhood but thereafter remains stable. Lesions on the sole are prone to secondary hyperkeratosis, ulceration, and crusting. Palmoplantar localization is unusual for other types of connective tissue nevus. Cerebriform lesions may be rarely seen on the trunk.

8.15.4 Familial Cutaneous Collagenoma

Familial cutaneous collagenoma is characterized by numerous symmetrically distributed papulonodular connective tissue nevi on the upper trunk. Lesions usually appear in adolescence. Some cases have associated cardiologic problems.

8.15.5 Eruptive Collagenoma and Isolated Collagenoma

Eruptive collagenoma is described as generalized multiple 2 to 5 mm papular lesions (*see* Fig. 8.94) without any association or familial occurrence, whereas isolated collagenoma is a localized lesion in otherwise healthy patients (*see* Fig. 8.95).

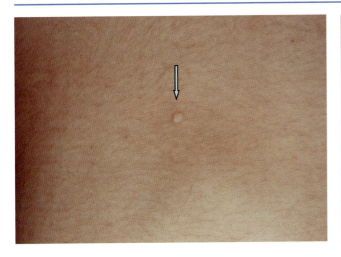

Fig. 8.94 Eruptive collagenoma shown as a small papule on the trunk (*arrow*) in an otherwise healthy adult

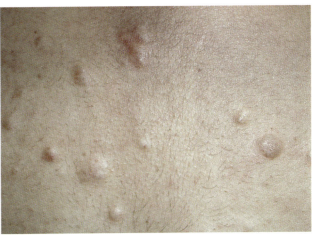

Fig. 8.96 Papular elastorrhexis seen as multiple whitish papules on the trunk

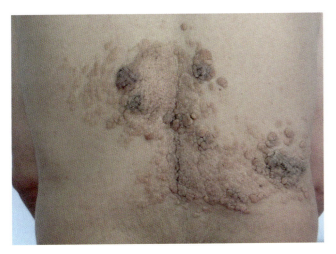

Fig. 8.95 Isolated collagenoma presenting as a giant lesion on the trunk. The patient was otherwise healthy

Most connective tissue nevi are diagnosed clinically, but clinical types cannot always be differentiated from each other. Epidermal nevus (*see* Fig. 1.70), nevus lipomatosus superficialis (*see* Fig. 10.9), and cutaneous leiomyoma are considered among the differential diagnosis of large lesions. Histologic features may slightly differ according to the clinical type. Dermal changes such as altered amounts of collagen and elastic tissue without the proliferation of fibroblasts characterize this lesion.

8.15.6 Papular Elastorrhexis

Papular elastorrhexis is a malformation of connective tissue seen as multiple white papules on the trunk and shoulders (*see* Fig. 8.96). The condition clinically resembles connective tissue nevus but has different histopathologic features. Most patients are women. Sporadic occurrence is more commonly observed, but there are also familial cases. Elastic fibers are decreased and fragmented in histopathologic examination.

Management. Patients diagnosed with collagenomas should be examined for the possible associated syndromes. All types of connective tissue nevi are persistent but do not show malignant transformation. Trunk lesions are usually considered cosmetically unimportant, so treatment is not necessary. Destructive methods are ineffective. Undesirable scars may occur after excision of large lesions. While lesions on the sole of the foot may interfere with walking, excision of palmoplantar lesions may lead to functional problems.

8.16 Keloid and Hypertrophic Scar

Keloid is a hyperproliferative response of connective tissue to dermal injury occurring especially in predisposed individuals. It is more common among dark-skinned people. Pathogenesis is not fully understood. An exaggerated repair process of the injury develops, resulting in the formation of large collagen bundles that replace the normal tissue of the dermis. The process may begin in the early period of injury but may also occur later. It usually arises in the second and third decades. Some keloids occur spontaneously (*see* Fig. 8.97).

Keloids present as raised, firm, irregularly shaped, pink, reddish-brown, skin-colored or white nodules or plaques with smooth and shiny surfaces (*see* Fig. 8.98). The size of the lesions is variable and mostly related to the underlying injury. Symptoms such as itching, tenderness, or pain may be present in some instances. Enlarging beyond the injury site (*see* Fig. 8.99) and irregular extensions on the border of the plaque (*see* Fig. 8.99) are typical for a keloid. The epidermis on the surface is thin. Telangiectasia may be prominent, and ulceration may develop easily. Keloids occurring in childhood,

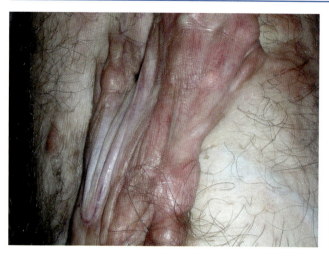

Fig. 8.97 Large keloids with a history of spontaneous occurrence

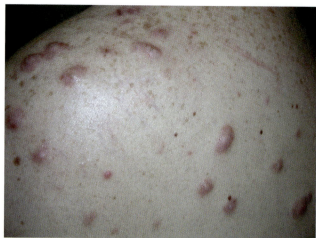

Fig. 8.100 Multiple keloids on the shoulder and upper back occurring after severe acne vulgaris

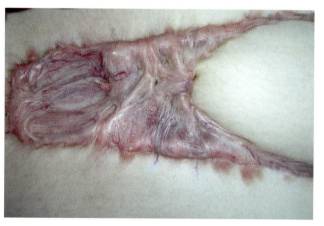

Fig. 8.98 Keloid presenting as an irregular plaque with telangiectases on the surface

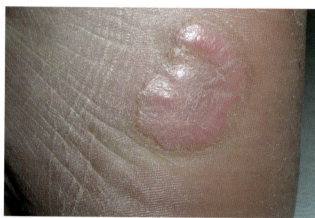

Fig. 8.101 Keloid on the sole of the foot. Lesions on this location may be a management problem

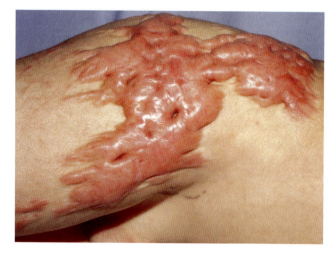

Fig. 8.99 Keloid caused by second-degree burn. Note extensions beyond the injury site

especially around the joints, may result in contractures and restrict the motion of that site.

Risk factors associated with the formation of keloid include anatomic site, skin tension, the type of scar, and the presence of secondary bacterial infections. It may occur anywhere on the body, but the shoulders, chest, and ears are more commonly involved. The sternum and ankle are common sites where skin tension is higher. In patients with severe acne vulgaris, multiple scattered keloids may develop on the upper trunk (*see* Fig. 8.100). Extensive keloids forming elevated irregular masses may be seen after second degree burns (*see* Fig. 8.99). Sometimes local infections may also be causative factors. Keloid may rarely occur on the sole of the foot (see Fig. 8.101) and may be painful.

The earlobe is one of the most common locations of keloid. Ear piercing is a major cause of earlobe keloids. Most

8.16 Keloid and Hypertrophic Scar

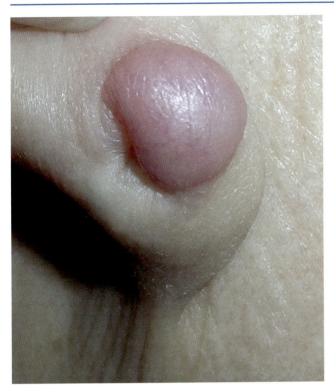

Fig. 8.102 Earlobe keloid presenting as an elevated solitary nodule with a smooth surface. The earlobe is one of the most frequent locations of this reactive process

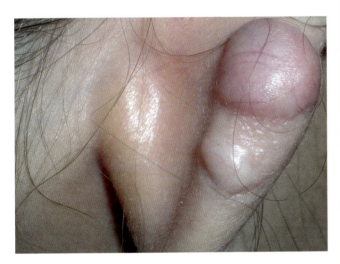

Fig. 8.103 Two nodules of keloid on unusual ear piercing sites. Telangiectases seen on the surface are common features

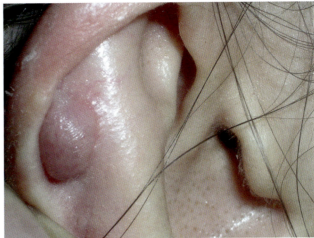

Fig. 8.104 Keloid after piercing on the antihelix, an unusual site

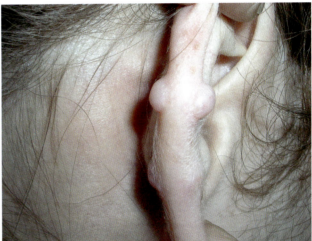

Fig 8.105 Multiple papulonodular lesions of keloid on the ear piercing sites

are located on the back side of the earlobes and appear as elevated smooth-surfaced nodules (*see* Fig. 8.102) and may sometimes be bilateral. They may be seen on other areas of the ears, developing secondary to piercing in atypical locations (*see* Figs. 8.103 and 8.104) and may be multiple (*see* Fig. 8.105).

Hypertrophic scars are differentiated from keloids by being confined to the original injury site. Various surgical procedures may cause hypertrophic scars. Linear configuration of the lesion is typical (*see* Fig. 8.106). Unlike keloids, hypertrophic scars improve spontaneously in about one year. Clinical features and a history of previous injury are mostly diagnostic for hypertrophic scar. Dermatofibroma (*see* Fig. 8.9), dermatofibrosarcoma protuberans (*see* Fig. 13.59), fibromatoses, and scar sarcoidosis should be considered in the differential diagnosis of keloid and hypertrophic scar. Biopsy may result in further keloid formation. Therefore it should not be performed if the clinical diagnosis is obvious. The histopathologic appearance of keloid typically shows hyalinized collagen bundles arranged in large

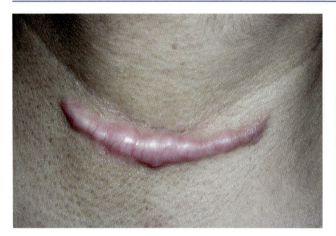

Fig. 8.106 Hypertrophic scar with linear configuration on the operation site

acellular nodules. Hypertrophic scar is very similar, although collagen bundles and nodules are slightly more cellular.

Management. Lesions of keloid are persistent, and their management is often challenging, including both preventing the occurrence of new lesions and therapy. People with a tendency to develop keloid should be warned against the higher risk after tissue traumas such as ear piercing and cosmetic interventions (such as removal of nevi or other nonessential surgical procedures). Acne vulgaris should be treated aggressively in these patients. Continuous pressure may be applied for months to years with pressure bandages following burns and operations in those who are prone to develop aggressive keloids.

Topical corticosteroids, intralesional corticosteroids (triamcinolone acetonide), topical silicone gel or silicone gel sheeting, topical onion extract, pressure dressings, and intralesional cryotherapy are the main alternative methods in the therapy. High potency topical corticosteroids, especially those used under occlusion, may be effective (*see* Fig. 8.107a and b). Flattening and softening of the lesion may be observed after several injections of intralesional corticosteroids. However there is a risk of telangiectasia and regional atrophy if they are used inadequately (*see* Fig. 8.108).

Intralesional treatment with 5-flourouracil, bleomycin, interferon, and verapamil (a calcium channel blocker) are other alternative methods in the treatment of keloids. Various combination options such as intralesional corticosteroids plus pulsed dye laser, cryotherapy, silicone gel or pressure dressings can also be used.

Simple excision of keloidal tissue is not recommended because it may result in larger scar formation. Excision can be combined with periodical intralesional corticosteroid administration into the wound edges, radiotherapy, or imiquimod cream following surgery. Recurrence may be seen following any of the above-mentioned therapies.

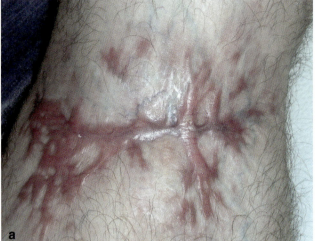
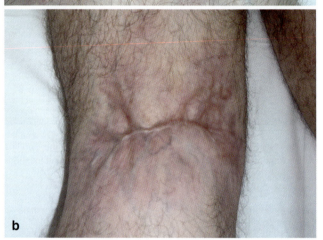

Fig. 8.107 (a) Keloid on the site of pyoderma gangrenosum. (b) Healing of the lesion after therapy with highly potent topical corticosteroids

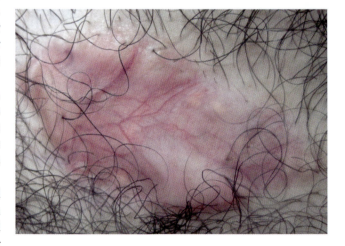

Fig. 8.108 Atrophy and telangiectasia on the site of a keloid after inadequate treatment with intralesional corticosteroids

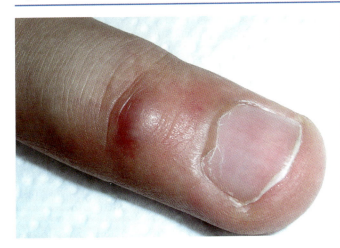

Fig. 8.109 Giant cell tumor of the tendon sheath on the finger

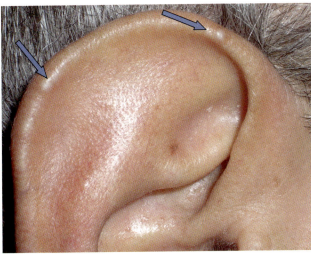

Fig. 8.111 Weathering nodules of the ear shown as multiple tiny papules on the helix

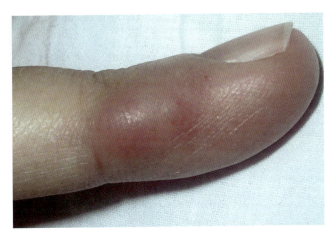

Fig. 8.110 Giant cell tumor of the tendon sheath presenting as an ill-defined, skin-colored nodule on the lateral side of the finger

8.17 Giant Cell Tumor of The Tendon Sheath

Giant cell tumor of the tendon sheath is a benign soft tissue tumor of the hands mostly seen on the volar aspect of the fingers. Lesions may also occur on the dorsal aspect of the fingers (see Fig. 8.109), wrists, and rarely on the toes or knees. Most of the patients are middle aged. Solitary or a few lesions may be seen. Firm, painless, ill-defined, skin-colored subcutaneous nodules grow slowly and are 1 to 3 cm at diagnosis (see Figs. 8.109 and 8.110). Calcifying aponeurotic fibroma (see Fig. 8.63) and infantile digital fibromatosis (see Fig. 8.59a) are the main differential diagnoses. Histopathologic appearance shows a collagenous, hyalinized stroma and more or less cellular areas composed of spindle-shaped and polygonal cells, respectively. The hallmarks of the tumor are lipidized histiocytes, multinuclear giant cells, and hemosiderin deposition. Giant cells can sometimes be numerous.

Management. Surgery can be performed in disturbing cases but the rate of local recurrence is high.

8.18 Weathering Nodules of the Ear

Weathering nodules of the ear are 2 to 3 mm, white- or skin-colored, slightly elevated firm papules covered with intact skin, which are mostly observed on the free edge of the helix (see Fig. 8.111). They are more common in elder Caucasian males who have had dense solar damage. The patients have solitary or a few lesions. Bilateral involvement may also be seen. The papules are generally small in contrast to the term "nodule" in the title. Different from chondrodermatitis nodularis helicis, inflammation is not observed during the course of the disease, and it is asymptomatic. It is usually diagnosed clinically. Histologically, an extension of fibrous tissue containing a focus of cartilage is seen.

Management. In patients with multiple lesions, weathering nodules of the ear may be regarded as a cosmetic problem. However, therapy is not necessary.

Suggested Reading

Akpinar F, Dervis E. Association between acrochordons and the components of metabolic syndrome. Eur J Dermatol. 2012;22:106–10.

Baykal C, Buyukbabani N, Yazganoglu KD, Saglik E. Acquired digital fibrokeratoma. Cutis. 2007;79:129–32.

Bolognia JL, Jorizzo JL, Schaffer JV. Dermatology, edn 3. London: Mosby; 2012.

Boza JC, Trindade EN, Peruzzo J, et al. Skin manifestations of obesity: a comperative study. Eur J Dermatol. 2012;26:1220–3.

Burgdorf WHC, Plewig G, Wolff HH, Landthaler M. Braun-Falco's dermatology, edn 3. Italy: Springer-Verlag; 2009.

Calonje JE, Brenn T, Lazar AJ, McKee PH. McKee's pathology of the skin, edn 4. China: Elsevier; 2012.

Caputo R, Tadini G. Atlas of genodermatoses. Spain: Taylor and Francis; 2006.

Chang SE, Choi JH, Sung KJ, et al. Subcutaneous dermatofibroma showing a depressed surface. Int J Dermatol. 2001;40:77–8.

Collins GL, Somach S, Morgan MB. Histomorphologic and immunophenotypic analysis of fibrofolliculomas and trichodiscomas in Birt-Hogg-Dube syndrome and sporadic disease. J Cutan Pathol. 2002;29:529–33.

Elder DE, Elenitsas R, Johnson BL, Murphy GF, Xu X. Lever's histopathology of the skin, edn 10. Philadelphia: Lippincott Williams and Wilkins; 2008.

Finch J, Berke A, McCusker M, Chang MW. Congenital multiple clustered dermatofibroma in a 12-year-old girl. Pediatr Dermatol. 2014;31:105–6.

Gauglitz GG, Korting HC, Pavicic T, et al. Hypertrophic scarring and keloids: pathomechanisms and current and emerging treatment strategies. Mol Med. 2011;17:113–25.

Gauglitz GG. Management of keloids and hypertrophic scars: current and emerging options. Clin Cosmet Investig Dermatol. 2013;6:103–14.

Goldsmith LA, Katz SI, Gilchrest BA, Paller AS, Leffell J, Wolff K. Fitzpatrick's dermatology in general medicine, edn 8. New York: McGraw-Hill Publishing; 2007.

James WD, Berger T, Elston D. Andrew's diseases of the skin: Clinical Dermatology, edn 11. China: Saunders Elsevier; 2011.

Kawaguchi M, Mitsuhashi Y, Hozumi Y, Kondo S. A case of infantile digital fibromatosis with spontaneous regression. J Dermatol. 1998;25:523–6.

Kluger N, Giraud S, Coupier I, et al. Birt-Hogg-Dubé syndrome: clinical and genetic studies of 10 French families. Br J Dermatol 2010;162:527–37.

Koenig MK, Hebert AA, Roberson J, et al. Topical rapamycin therapy to alleviate the cutaneous manifestations of tuberous sclerosis complex: a double-blind, randomized, controlled trial to evaluate the safety and efficacy of topically applied rapamycin. Drugs R D. 2012;12:121–6.

López V, Jordá E, Monteagudo C. Birt-Hogg-Dubé syndrome: an update. Actas Dermosifiliogr. 2012;103:198–206.

Mazaira M, del Pozo Losada J, Fernández-Jorge B, et al. Shave and phenolization of periungual fibromas, Koenen's tumors, in a patient with tuberous sclerosis. Dermatol Surg. 2008;34:111–3.

Menko FH, van Steensel MA, Giraud S, et al. Birt-Hogg-Dubé syndrome: diagnosis and management. Lancet Oncol. 2009;10:1199–206.

Niiyama S, Katsuoka K, Happle R, Hoffmann R. Multiple eruptive dermatofibromas: a review of the literature. Acta Derm Venereol (Stockh) 2002;82:241–4.

Rosser T, Panigrahy A, McClintock W. The diverse clinical manifestations of tuberous sclerosis complex: a review. Semin Pediatr Neurol. 2006;13:27–36.

Sears JK, Stone MS, Argenyi Z. Papular elastorrhexis: a variant of connective tissue nevus. Case reports and review of the literature. J Am Acad Dermatol. 1988;19(2 Pt 2):409–14.

Vincent A, Farley M, Chan E, James WD. Birt-Hogg-Dubé syndrome: a review of the literature and the differential diagnosis of firm facial papules. J Am Acad Dermatol. 2003;49:698–705.

Weedon D. Weedon's skin pathology, edn 3. China: Elsevier; 2010.

Mastocytosis

Mastocytosis is characterized by the increase and accumulation of mast cells in the skin and visceral organs. The etiopathogenesis of the proliferation of mast cells is not known, but it has been suggested that mastocytosis is a clonal disease. Mast cells are among the cells of the dermis, but they may also be seen in different organs. They play an important role in type 1 hypersensitivity reactions owing to their rich supply of different intracytoplasmic mediators, especially histamine. The disease can be classified as cutaneous and systemic mastocytosis, according to the locations of the proliferated cells. Cutaneous mastocytosis is more common. In general, the skin is the most commonly involved site in mastocytosis, and most patients are diagnosed at dermatology clinics. Bone marrow, bones, the gastrointestinal system, liver, spleen, lymph nodes, and any site other than the central nerve system can be involved. Occurrence of mastocytosis is mostly sporadic and rarely familial.

9.1 Cutaneous Mastocytosis

Cutaneous mastocytosis is characterized by skin lesions that may be associated with systemic symptoms. Urticaria pigmentosa, diffuse cutaneous mastocytosis, and isolated mastocytoma are the clinical types of cutaneous mastocytosis with childhood onset. The skin findings show differences according to the clinical type. Telangiectasia macularis eruptive perstans is also a variant of cutaneous mastocytosis, but it is mostly seen in adults. Cutaneous involvement may also be present in systemic mastocytosis, but in these cases the onset of skin lesions usually occurs in adults (adult systemic mastocytosis). Like systemic mastocytosis, various types of cutaneous mastocytosis may also be associated with a rich spectrum of systemic symptoms as a result of the release of several mediators (e.g., histamine, prostaglandin D2, tryptase, kinase, TNF-alpha, and heparin) from granules of skin mast cells. The severity of these symptoms is variable and can even be life-threatening. Flushing and pruritus are common. Other symptoms such as urticaria; headache; fatigue; respiratory symptoms; cardiovascular symptoms such as tachycardia, hypotension, and syncope; and gastrointestinal symptoms such as nausea, vomiting, and diarrhea may also be seen. Liver fibrosis, bone pain, and osteopenia or osteoporosis may also develop in patients with mastocytosis due to the effects of different mediators.

9.1.1 Urticaria Pigmentosa

Urticaria pigmentosa, also called maculopapular cutaneous mastocytosis, is the most common type of mastocytosis in childhood. It is usually limited to the skin but can be associated with systemic symptoms, although visceral involvement is usually not present. The onset is usually during the first 6 months of life, but in some cases this period may extend into adulthood. The upper trunk, neck, and extremities are the most commonly involved cutaneous sites (see Fig. 9.1). The scalp may also be affected (see Fig. 9.2). Facial (see Fig. 9.3) and palmoplantar involvement are

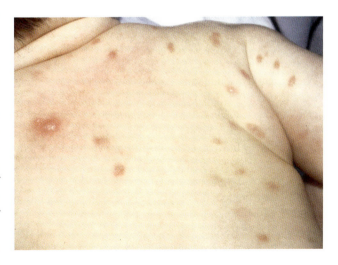

Fig. 9.1 Multiple maculopapular lesions of urticaria pigmentosa on upper trunk of an infant. These lesions are persistent in the early years of life

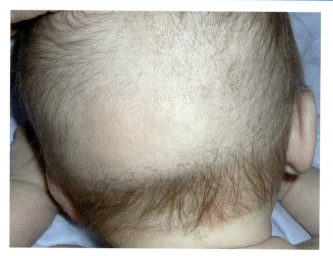

Fig. 9.2 Urticaria pigmentosa presenting as a large yellowish plaque on the scalp

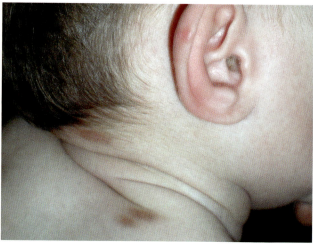

Fig. 9.4 Patients with a few scattered lesions of urticaria pigmentosa, a not uncommon occurrence

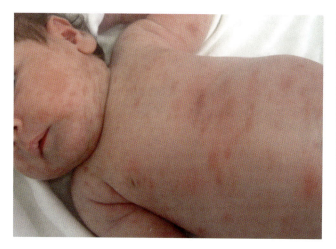

Fig. 9.3 Urticaria pigmentosa with facial and truncal involvement

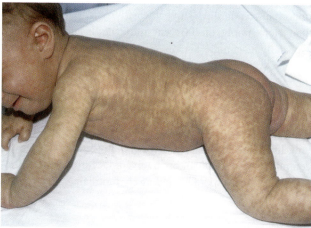

Fig. 9.5 A child with profuse papulonodular and plaque lesions of urticaria pigmentosa

mainly seen in cases with disseminated lesions. Mucosal involvement is very rare. The amount of skin lesions shows great variability. While some patients have only a few lesions (*see* Fig. 9.4), others may have several to hundreds of scattered lesions (*see* Fig. 9.5). The number of lesions may increase in the early period of the disease but then remains stable. Pink, yellowish, or reddish to brown macules, papules, or more rarely nodules measuring 0.5 to 1 cm (*see* Fig. 9.6) are asymmetrically distributed. Whereas some patients have predominantly plaque type lesions since onset, in other cases papules may be grouped, forming a plaque (*see* Fig. 9.2). Petechiae and telangiectasia are very rare features of the disease. Although different clinical presentations are possible, most patients have a monomorphic eruption. Because of secondary melanocyte hyperplasia, lesions may become hyperpigmented in time (*see* Fig. 9.7). Mild to severe pruritus accompanies most of the cases.

A helpful finding in the clinical diagnosis is the Darier sign, which can be observed in different types of cutaneous mastocytosis and can be looked for in suspected cases during dermatologic examination. It is an acute response to slight trauma such as rubbing or scratching the lesion sites. Trauma causes degranulation of mast cells of the skin and release of histamine, which initially leads to pruritus followed by transient reddening and urticarial swelling that can even exceed the lesion site (*see* Fig. 9.8). Lesions may also spontaneously show this changes without any manipulation. Vesicles or bullae may be seen overlying the maculopapular lesions, especially in children under the age of three. Dermatographism, a type of physical urticaria, can be induced on normal skin

9.1 Cutaneous Mastocytosis

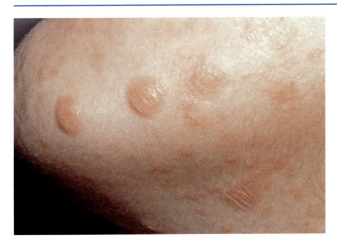

Fig. 9.6 Papulonodular lesions of urticaria pigmentosa on the face of an adolescent

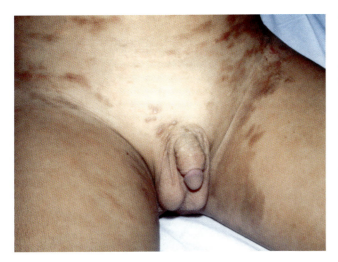

Fig. 9.7 Lesions of urticaria pigmentosa with prominent hyperpigmentation

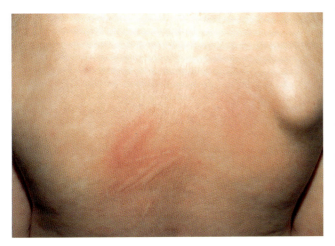

Fig. 9.8 Darier sign (transient urticarial swelling) around the lesion site, a characteristic finding in urticaria pigmentosa

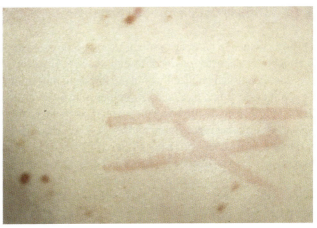

Fig. 9.9 Dermatographism induced on normal skin in a patient with urticaria pigmentosa. It is more common than the normal population

in nearly half of the patients with urticaria pigmentosa (*see* Fig. 9.9).

Systemic symptoms may occur in the course of urticaria pigmentosa as a result of activated skin mast cell degranulation and subsequent release of mediators. In the presence of associated systemic symptoms such as flushing, dyspnea, diarrhea, and syncope, mastocytosis can be misdiagnosed as carcinoid syndrome.

Other differential diagnoses of urticaria pigmentosa include non-Langerhans cell histiocytoses such as benign cephalic histiocytosis (*see* Fig. 15.36), generalized eruptive histiocytosis (*see* Fig. 15.38) and xanthoma disseminatum (*see* Fig. 15.42), neoplastic infiltrations of skin such as cutaneous leukemia (*see* Fig. 14.213), and benign skin tumors like leiomyoma (*see* Fig. 5.69). The clinical diagnosis of mastocytosis can be confirmed with biopsy. Perivascular mast cell infiltration and an increase in melanin in the epidermis are the main histopathologic findings of cutaneous mastocytosis. The degree and severity of mast cell infiltration are variable in different clinical types of the disease and are not markers of systemic involvement. Mast cell infiltration in urticaria pigmentosa is moderate and limited to the perivascular area of small vessels in the papillary dermis. Scattered eosinophils are usually present. Tryptase is a protein on the secretory granules of mast cells and is considered to show the burden of mast cells. The serum tryptase level may be elevated in some types of mastocytosis but is usually found to be normal in urticaria pigmentosa.

The prognosis of urticaria pigmentosa in childhood is good. Systemic involvement is not usual at this age. Therefore, there is generally no need for routine bone marrow biopsy in children with urticaria pigmentosa. Spontaneous regression is seen in most around puberty. Rare cases have persistent lesions that continue in adulthood.

9.1.2 Diffuse Cutaneous Mastocytosis

Diffuse cutaneous mastocytosis is a rare type of cutaneous mastocytosis characterized by diffuse mast cell infiltration of the skin. It is usually noticed within the first 6 months of life or at birth. The trunk, face, and extremities may be involved. The typical well-defined maculopapular or plaque type lesions of urticaria pigmentosa are absent. The skin may be infiltrated extensively with a dough-like consistency leading to a thickened and edematous appearance that may be flesh- or yellowish to orange-colored (*see* Figs. 9.10 and 9.11). Widespread vesiculobullous lesions and erosions overlying infiltrated areas may appear spontaneously from time to time (*see* Figs. 9.12, 9.13 and 9.14). Manipulation of the skin may also trigger the development of bullous lesions and cause systemic symptoms. In infants with diffuse blistering, the condition is also called bullous mastocytosis. This condition, which manifests with large and sometimes hemorrhagic

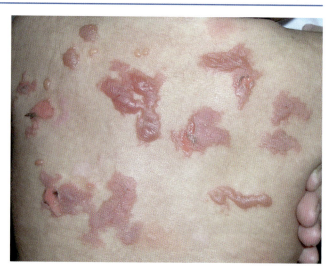

Fig. 9.12 Vesiculobullous lesions in a patient with diffuse cutaneous mastocytosis. They do not have any prognostic significance and heal without scarring

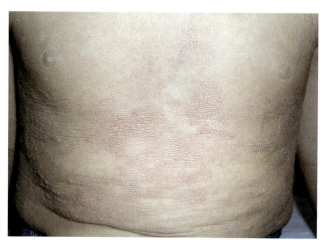

Fig. 9.10 Diffuse cutaneous mastocytosis. Note diffuse flesh-colored involvement of the trunk of a child

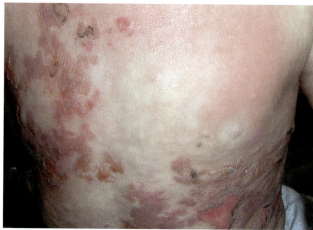

Fig. 9.13 Widespread vesiculobullous lesions and erosions overlying other lesions of diffuse cutaneous mastocytosis

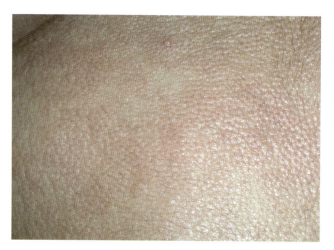

Fig. 9.11 Diffuse cutaneous mastocytosis leading to thickened and edematous appearance of the skin. Discrete papules and nodules cannot be seen in this type of cutaneous mastocytosis

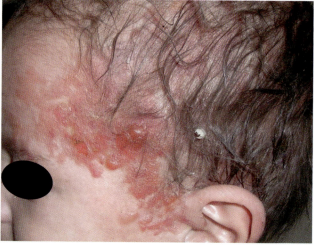

Fig. 9.14 Vesiculobullous lesions on the scalp of a child with diffuse cutaneous mastocytosis. Note that some of them are hemorrhagic

bullae (*see* Fig. 9.14), may be clinically misdiagnosed as autoimmune bullous disorders of infancy or erythema multiforme. The bullae heal without scarring.

As a result of the diffuse involvement of skin with mast cells, systemic symptoms such as flushing, diarrhea, and abdominal hypotension are more frequently seen and may be more severe than in other types of cutaneous mastocytosis of childhood. The main histopathologic features of diffuse cutaneous mastocytosis are similar to those of urticaria pigmentosa. The blisters form subepidermally. The serum tryptase level is usually high.

Disease activity, including the development of bullous lesions, decreases in time but a leather-like diffuse infiltration and slight hyperpigmentation persist in childhood. The prognosis of diffuse cutaneous mastocytosis is favorable, and progression to systemic mastocytosis is not usual. However, the risk of anaphylaxis is high, which increases the morbidity of this type of mastocytosis.

Pseudoxanthomatous mastocytosis is a rare subtype of cutaneous mastocytosis that is suggested to be a variant of diffuse cutaneous mastocytosis. Yellow-colored papules and nodules that are a few millimeters in size may clinically resemble xanthomas. This subtype of mastocytosis does not have a special prognostic significance but is a challenging diagnosis from a clinical point of view.

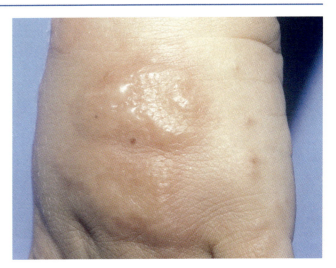

Fig. 9.15 Isolated mastocytoma on the dorsum of the hand. Most patients have a solitary lesion or a few

9.1.3 Isolated (Solitary) Mastocytoma

The second most common type of cutaneous mastocytosis is isolated mastocytoma, which generally presents as a solitary lesion usually larger than the ones observed in urticaria pigmentosa. Most lesions of so-called "isolated type of mastocytosis" are congenital or appear in the first few months of life, but childhood- or adult-onset may be seen occasionally. Any skin site can be involved, but the trunk, extremities (especially the dorsum of the hands) (*see* Fig. 9.15), and the neck are most commonly involved. The palms and soles are spared. A typical lesion is a sharply defined, dirty yellow, orange, red, or brown nodule or infiltrated plaque that is generally smaller than 1 cm but can reach 5 cm (*see* Figs. 9.16 and 9.17). Sometimes a few lesions can be found. Some plaques may be annular or linear in configuration (*see* Fig. 9.18). They have a rubbery consistency. The surface may be smooth (*see* Fig. 9.19) or rough, revealing the appearance of peau d'orange (*see* Fig. 9.20). Lesions usually urticate upon manipulation, showing a positive Darier sign. Pruritus and even systemic symptoms related to mast cell degranulation may be seen in some cases. However, these symptoms are usually less severe than those observed in urticaria pigmentosa because of less mediator release. As an exception, in some patients generalized flushing may occur. Vesicles or blisters may develop on the lesion (*see* Fig. 9.21),

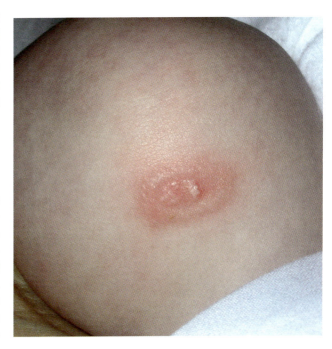

Fig. 9.16 Isolated mastocytoma presenting as a solitary yellowish-red infiltrated plaque on the trunk

either spontaneously or by manipulation. Eroded areas may be observed on the surface of the nodules. Patients rarely have multiple lesions, namely, disseminated mastocytoma, those are clinically the same as solitary mastocytoma (*see* Fig. 9.22). Differential diagnosis with urticaria pigmentosa (*see* Fig. 9.3) may be difficult in these cases.

While a solitary lesion of yellowish or reddish color in a child may be confused with juvenile xanthogranuloma (*see* Fig. 15.20) or Spitz nevus (*see* Fig. 3.219), darker lesions may be mistaken for congenital melanocytic nevi (*see* Fig. 3.142). The positive Darier sign or a history of generalized

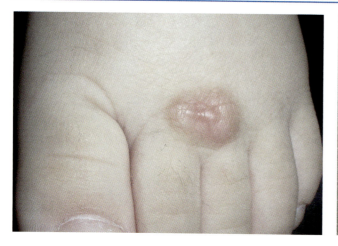

Fig. 9.17 Isolated mastocytoma manifesting as a yellowish-brown nodule on the dorsum of the foot

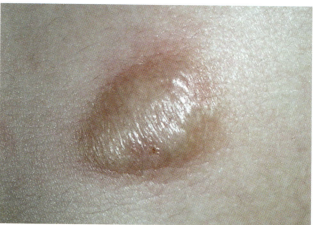

Fig. 9.19 Isolated mastocytoma presenting as an elevated round plaque, with smooth surface. These lesions are firm on palpation

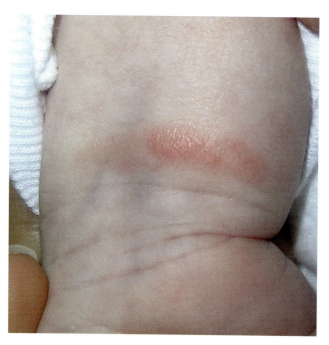

Fig. 9.18 Isolated mastocytoma seen as a linear plaque

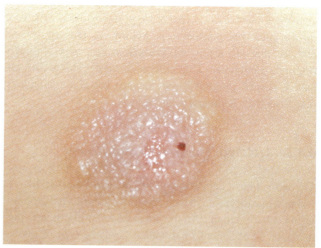

Fig. 9.20 Isolated mastocytoma on the trunk. Note the typical peau d'orange appearance

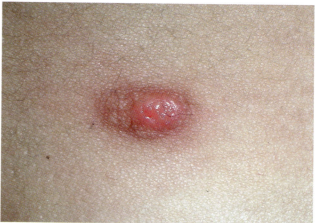

Fig. 9.21 Blistering on isolated mastocytoma. They mostly change to erosions in a short time

flushing attacks is usually supportive of the diagnosis of isolated mastocytoma. Melanocytic tumors may be excluded with the use of dermoscopy. A histopathologic examination will confirm the diagnosis, revealing dense mast cell infiltration of the dermis. In isolated mastocytoma, cellular infiltration is dense compared to that of urticaria pigmentosa, and it involves the reticular dermis. The serum tryptase level is almost always within normal range.

The prognosis of this type of cutaneous mastocytosis is very good. Visceral involvement is not expected. Lesions usually regress spontaneously in years, mostly in childhood before the age of 10.

9.2 Adult Systemic Mastocytosis

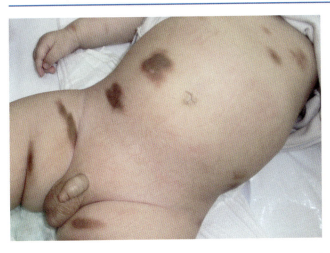

Fig. 9.22 Multiple lesions of isolated mastocytoma: this rare clinical presentation is called disseminated mastocytoma

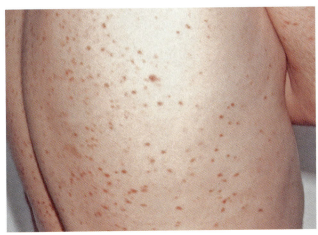

Fig. 9.23 Numerous small erythematous papular lesions on the trunk of a young adult patient. This is not an uncommon presentation of mastocytosis in adulthood and most patients have systemic involvement

9.1.4 Telangiectasia Macularis Eruptiva Perstans

Telangiectasia macularis eruptiva perstans is an uncommon subtype of cutaneous mastocytosis clinically resembling urticaria pigmentosa, but it is mainly seen in adulthood. Persistent, multiple, brown-to-red small macules and a few telangiectases, mostly located on the trunk, are observed. Bullae are not expected. Darier sign cannot usually be elicited. It may be confused with secondary syphilis or diseases presenting with diffuse telangiectases. The prognosis of this type of mastocytosis is good, with relatively rare systemic involvement. The serum tryptase level is usually found to be normal. Mast cell infiltration and dilated capillaries in the dermis, and epidermal pigmentation are observed histopathologically.

9.2 Adult Systemic Mastocytosis

Systemic mastocytosis is mainly characterized by mast cell infiltration of bone marrow and/or other extracutaneous sites. In general it is typically seen in adulthood. Therefore it is also called adult systemic mastocytosis. In addition to visceral organs, it may involve the skin. On the other hand, urticaria pigmentosa beginning in childhood may rarely progress into adulthood.

Systemic mastocytosis has been classified into four variants: indolent systemic mastocytosis, systemic mastocytosis with an associated clonal hematologic non–mast cell lineage disorder, aggressive systemic mastocytosis, and mast cell leukemia.

Skin lesions are seen especially in indolent mastocytosis, which is the most common form and has a relatively better

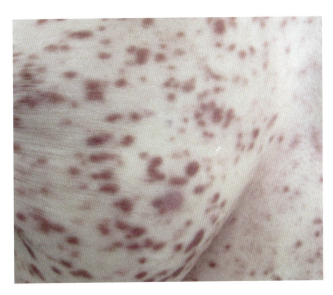

Fig. 9.24 Mastocytosis presenting as multiple discrete papules in an adult patient

prognosis than the other three. Typically, multiple brown-colored, slightly elevated, small papules are scattered throughout the trunk and extremities of the patients (see Figs. 9.23, 9.24 and 9.25). On the other hand, large plaques (see Figs. 9.26, 9.27 and 9.28) may also be encountered. Skin lesions do not have a tendency toward spontaneous resolution. Therefore it must be considered as an entirely separate entity from urticaria pigmentosa.

Multiple organs may be involved. Lymphadenopathy, hepatosplenomegaly, weight loss, and ascites in the abdomen are among the systemic manifestations. Gastrointestinal involvement may be noticed, with diarrhea and abdominal pain. Bone involvement may cause bone pain. Systemic involvement must be looked for in all patients with adult-onset cutaneous mastocytosis. A complete blood count must

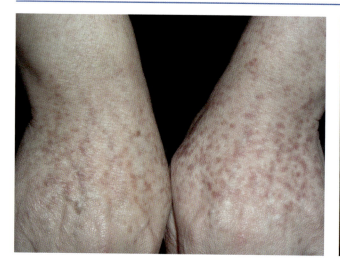

Fig. 9.25 Multiple brownish-colored papules on the dorsum of the hands in an adult patient with mastocytosis

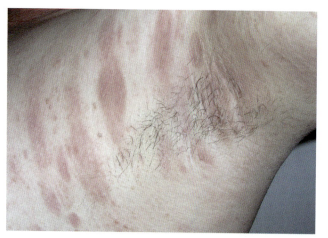

Fig. 9.26 Mastocytosis manifesting as linear red plaques in an adult patient with systemic involvement

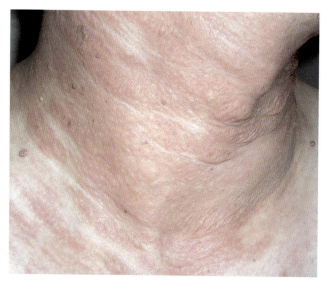

Fig. 9.27 An adult mastocytosis patient presenting with large erythematous plaques on the upper trunk and neck

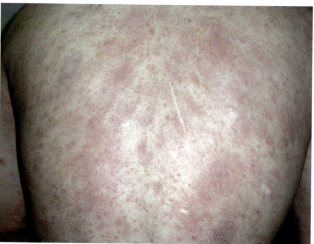

Fig. 9.28 Disseminated plaques on the trunk in an adult patient with mastocytosis. Different from childhood mastocytosis, investigations regarding systemic involvement should be performed in adulthood

be obtained and examined in all patients. A peripheral blood smear and bone marrow examination are usually required. Plain bone x-ray, scintigraphy, endoscopic examination, abdominal ultrasonography, and intestinal biopsy may be required in searching for internal involvement according to the presence of systemic symptoms. The persistently increased level of serum tryptase is a typical laboratory finding of systemic mastocytosis. Adult patients with cutaneous mastocytosis must be followed up by both dermatologists and hematologists.

Management. Management of mastocytosis depends on the clinical type, severity of systemic symptoms, and the presence of systemic involvement. A specific therapy leading to permanent cure does not exist, but many childhood-onset types of cutaneous mastocytosis have a tendency to spontaneous healing. On the other hand, release of mediators may sometimes cause life-threatening systemic problems in children. Therefore all patients with cutaneous mastocytosis and their parents must be warned about the triggering factors that can cause mediator release and subsequent severe systemic symptoms such as hypotension and anaphylaxis. Arthropod bite, extreme cold and heat, alcohol consumption, physical exercise, and manipulations such as friction or massage are among risk factors that can trigger systemic symptoms via mediator release. Some drugs like aspirin, opiates, reserpine, morphine, and polymyxin B may also cause mast cell degranulation. These drugs must be avoided until remission occurs. Patients should also inform their surgeons or anesthesiologists about their disease. An emergency set that includes injectable epinephrine should be carried in daily life, especially by patients with frequent and severe symptoms.

Treatment is utilized mainly in symptomatic patients with cutaneous mastocytosis. Long-term administration of systemic antihistamines, mainly H1 blockers, may be helpful for alleviating flushing attacks and pruritus. However, severe pruritus may sometimes be difficult to treat. Topical corticosteroids may be helpful in localized lesions of urticaria pigmentosa. PUVA or UVA1 therapy may produce temporary relief in generalized cutaneous lesions and systemic symptoms but is mainly preferred in adult patients. Extensive blistering in diffuse cutaneous mastocytosis may be treated with systemic corticosteroids for a short period.

Follow-up without therapy and waiting for spontaneous resolution is mostly preferred for isolated mastocytoma. Potent topical corticosteroids can be administered in pruritic cases but they carry a risk of atrophy. Solitary lesions that cause severe systemic symptoms may be excised if it is technically feasible.

In patients with frequent or severe systemic symptoms, long-term use of mast cell stabilizers like sodium cromoglycate and ketotifen, calcium-channel blockers such as nifedipine, or leukotriene antagonists like montelukast may also be indicated. Gastrointestinal symptoms may be controlled with H1 and H2 blockers or proton pump inhibitors. In the case of anaphylactic shock systemic corticosteroids and epinephrine are the main options.

The approach to adult patients with systemic mastocytosis is quite different. Interferon-alpha with or without systemic corticosteroids, imatinib, or cladribine (2-chlorodeoxyadenosine) may be used for systemic involvement. Splenectomy or even bone marrow transplantation may be required in some cases.

Suggested Reading

Akoglu G, Erkin G, Cakir B, et al. Cutaneous mastocytosis: demographic aspects and clinical features of 55 patients. J Eur Acad Dermatol Venereol. 2006;20:969–73.

Burgdorf WHC, Plewig G, Wolff HH, Landthaler M. Braun-Falco's dermatology, edn 3. Italy: Springer-Verlag; 2009.

Elder DE, Elenitsas R, Johnson BL, Murphy GF, Xu X. Lever's histopathology of the skin, edn 10. Philadelphia: Lippincott Williams and Wilkins; 2008.

Heide R, Beishuzen A, De Groot H, et al. Dutch National Mastocytosis Work Group. Mastocytosis in children: a protocol for management. Pediatr Dermatol. 2008;25:493–500.

Lange M, Niedoszytko M, Nedoszytko B, et al. Diffuse cutaneous mastocytosis: analysis of 10 cases and a brief review of the literature. J Eur Acad Dermatol Venereol. 2012;26:1565–71.

Lange M, Niedoszytko M, Renke J, et al. Clinical aspects of paediatric mastocytosis: a review of 101 cases. J Eur Acad Dermatol Venereol. 2013;27:97–102.

Pardanani A. Systemic mastocytosis in adults: 2012 Update on diagnosis, risk stratification, and management. Am J Hematol. 2012;87: 401–11.

Valent P, Horny HP, Escribano L, et al. Diagnostic criteria and classification of mastocytosis: a consensus proposal. Leuk Res. 2001;25: 603–25.

Neoplasms of Subcutaneous Fat

Adipocytic tumors have a wide spectrum from benign to aggressive sarcomas. A very common benign tumor of adipose tissue—namely lipoma—and its subtypes will be discussed in this chapter. Nevus lipomatosus superficialis, which is characterized by adipose tissue in the dermis, is also included. Sarcomas originating from fat tissue are discussed in the chapter on cutaneous sarcomas.

10.1 Lipoma

Lipoma is a common benign soft tissue tumor containing adipose tissue and developing on skin and visceral organs. Cutaneous lipoma is usually seen incidentally in otherwise healthy individuals but may sometimes be associated with a syndrome. It commonly arises in adults between ages 40 and 60. Arms (*see* Fig. 10.1), shoulders, nape of the neck, trunk, proximal parts of the lower extremities and buttocks are most commonly affected. The face (*see* Fig. 10.2) and scalp may also be involved, as may any other skin site. Many patients have a solitary tumor, but multiple lesions (*see* Fig. 10.1) are not uncommon. Typical lesions are round to oval, soft subcutaneous swellings without any surface change (*see* Figs. 10.3 and 10.4). Most lipomas are 1 to 2 cm, but sometimes through gradual growth they may reach a size of 8 to 10 cm (*see* Fig. 10.5). In rare instances, they may be larger. Some lesions are multilobular. They are slightly movable on palpation (*see* Fig. 10.6). Small lipomas are usually asymptomatic, but large lesions may induce regional pain as a result of nerve compression.

Most lipomas are diagnosed clinically. Differential diagnosis includes mainly benign cutaneous tumors or cysts. Lipoma can be confused with epidermoid cyst (*see* Fig. 4.3), which is also among other common causes of round masses located elsewhere. However, epidermoid cysts are harder, more elevated and commonly show surface changes such as a central pore or telangiectasia. Trichilemmal cysts on the scalp may be considered another differential diagnostic challenge, but these cysts are usually mildly alopecic (*see* Fig. 4.43) and firm. A neurofibroma (*see* Fig. 7.11) can be differentiated from a lipoma, with its typical button-hole sign detected on palpation. A pilomatricoma is also distinct because of its hard consistency and various colors (*see* Fig. 5.53). Eccrine spiradenoma (*see*

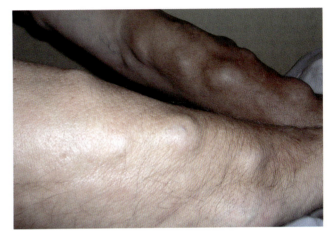

Fig. 10.1 Multiple lipomas on the arms of an adult patient

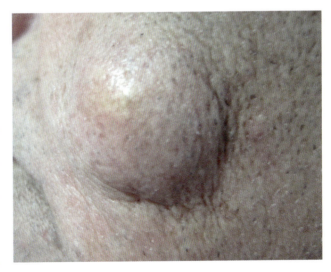

Fig. 10.2 Solitary lipoma on the face, not a common location

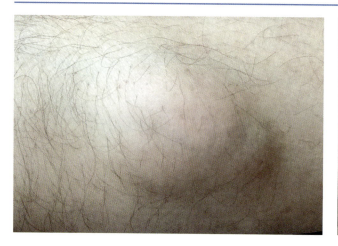

Fig. 10.3 Solitary lipoma presenting as a subcutaneous swelling without any surface change. This tumor is not very hard on palpation

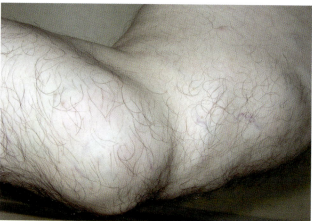

Fig. 10.5 A large lipoma on the arm

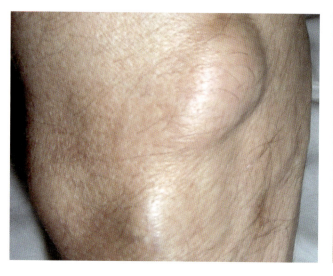

Fig. 10.4 Multiple lipomas manifesting as subcutaneous swellings without any surface change

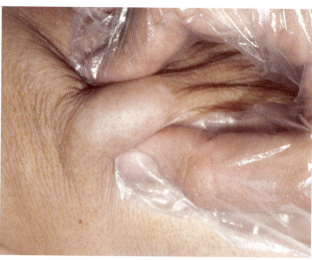

Fig. 10.6 Lipomas are slightly movable tumors on palpation

Fig. 5.25) is typically painful. It is also important that some malignant tumors should be considered in the differential diagnosis of lipoma. Initial lesions of soft tissue sarcomas, including liposarcoma, may be misdiagnosed as lipoma. However, sarcomas may grow rapidly. Eruptive occurrence of multiple hard subcutaneous lesions is typical for cutaneous metastasis. Ultrasonographic examination may be used to support the clinical diagnosis or to detect the depth of the lipoma. When any doubt of a malignancy exists, a biopsy should be performed. Histologically, a lipoma is an encapsulated lesion composed of mature fat cells usually situated in the subcutaneous tissue.

In some patients with multiple lipomas, a family history may be present (familial multiple lipomatosis). This rare disease has an autosomal dominant inheritance. There may be hundreds of lipomas, usually found on the forearms and thighs. They usually develop in the third decade of life without any other associated finding. Adiposis dolorosa (Dercum disease) and benign symmetric lipomatosis (Madelung disease) are rare syndromes defined with multiple lipomas and other associated manifestations. Adiposis dolorosa is mostly seen in obese adult women. Symmetrically distributed lipomas are mostly encountered on the lower trunk, lower extremities, and periarticular areas (see Fig. 10.7). They may be painful. Fatigue and psychiatric symptoms may also be associated.

Benign symmetric lipomatosis is seen in adult males and is mostly associated with alcoholism. Symmetric large swellings owing to fat deposition are seen on the neck, abdomen, and shoulder girdle. Diffuse lipomatosis is another disease manifesting with lipomas, but there is diffuse infiltration of mature adipose tissue involving a large part of the trunk or an extremity. The lesions are mostly found in children under 2 years of age.

10.2 Nevus Lipomatosus Superficialis

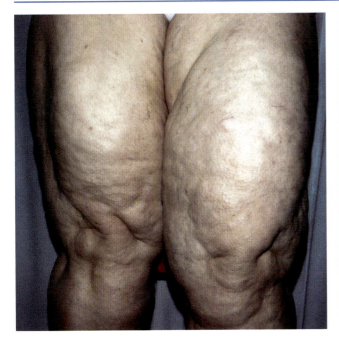

Fig. 10.7 Lipomas appearing as bilateral large masses on the legs in a patient with adiposis dolorosa

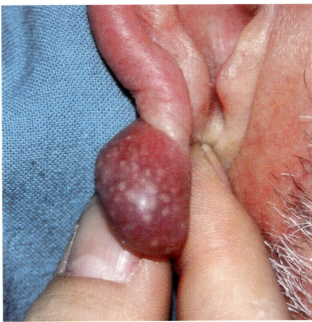

Fig. 10.8 Angiolipoleiomyoma (angiomyolipoma) on the earlobe. Note the reddish nodule

A lipoma on the lumbosacral area over the spinal column may be the sign of spinal dysraphism. It may also be associated with other regional cutaneous manifestations, such as nevus flammeus and infantile hemangioma. Lipomas may also be a minor sign of some syndromes such as Gardner syndrome, Proteus syndrome, Cowden syndrome, and Bannayan-Zonana syndrome. Epidermoid cysts, desmoid tumors and osteomas are manifestations of Gardner syndrome, which is characterized by colonic polyposis. Bannayan-Zonana syndrome, caused by mutations in the *PTEN* gene, is associated with multiple lipomas, hemangiomas, lymphangiomas, and macrocephaly. Some drugs such as protease inhibitors that are used in the treatment of HIV infection have been suggested to induce the development of lipomas.

Several clinicopathologic variants of lipoma have been described, such as angiolipoma, angiolipoleiomyoma, pleomorphic lipoma, spindle cell lipoma, and intramuscular lipoma. Angiolipoma has an excessive vascular component in addition to increased fatty tissue; thus its color is reddish or bluish, simulating hemangiomas. It is more common in young adults, and the forearm is the typical location. It may appear as multiple small nodules. This subtype of lipoma is usually painful. Angiolipoleiomyoma (angiomyolipoma) is a rare type of lipoma that may be seen in the kidney and also on the skin, especially on acral regions, including the nose and ears (*see* Fig. 10.8). They are slow growing, painless, firm nodules. Spindle cell lipoma is usually a solitary, painless nodule measuring 3 to 5 cm and is mostly located on the nape of the neck and upper back, seen most often in the older population. It is composed of spindle-shaped mature fat cells. Intramuscular lipoma is a deep-seated tumor with frequent recurrence, and complete excision may be difficult.

Lipomas may also be located in visceral organs such as the lung, gastrointestinal tract, and genitourinary tract. Large internal lipomas may be associated with serious complications. Gastrointestinal tract lesions may cause obstruction and bleeding.

Management. Most cutaneous lipomas do not require any therapy. Because they are skin-colored, their cosmetic importance is negligible. After reaching a certain size, lipomas do not change. Moreover, lipomas are not expected to show malignant degeneration; therefore prophylactic excision is not indicated. However, lesions with a history of rapid growth can be removed for histopathologic examination to rule out liposarcoma. If treatment is desired, surgical excision is preferred for small lesions. The recurrence rate is usually low, but unsightly scars may occur. Larger lipomas or benign symmetric lipomatosis may be treated with liposuction, which causes less scarring. Multiple painful angiolipomas may also be a therapeutic challenge.

10.2 Nevus Lipomatosus Superficialis

Nevus lipomatosus superficialis is a rare developmental disorder of fat causing localized papulonodular lesions. Ectopic adipose tissue composed of mature adipocyte aggregates are found in the dermis. It is usually present at birth or appears during childhood. The lower back, especially the pelvic girdle (*see* Fig. 10.9), is the preferred site of this hamartomatous lesion.

The upper thighs, abdomen, chest, and face (*see* Fig. 10.10) are rarely involved. The hamartoma is classified into two types, presenting as either multiple or solitary lesions. The classic form (Hoffman-Zurhalle) with multiple lesions is usually restricted to one area. Flesh-colored or yellowish, soft papules and nodules mostly coalesce to form plaques in a linear shape. The surface may be wrinkled or cerebriform (*see* Fig. 10.9). The other form of nevus lipomatosus superficialis is defined as a solitary papule (*see* Fig. 10.11) or nodule (*see* Fig. 10.12). These asymptomatic lesions are persistent but cause only cosmetic concern.

The initial clinical appearance of the classic form may resemble connective tissue nevi, such as shagreen patch (*see* Fig. 8.85), but plaques of nevus lipomatosus superficialis are more elevated and partially pedunculated. It may also be confused with focal dermal hyoplasia (Goltz syndrome) or plexiform neurofibroma. Solitary papules or nodules may be misdiagnosed as dermal neurofibroma. Cases with multiple lesions occurring in typical locations are usually clinically diagnosed. Biopsy may be required to confirm the diagnosis in some cases. In solitary lesions, the diagnosis is nearly always established after biopsy. Histopathologic examination reveals large masses of mature adipocytes in the dermis. Differentiation from acrochordon or old melanocytic nevi that may also contain adipocytes can sometimes be difficult.

Management. As the lesion shows no malignant degeneration, therapy is not necessary. If technically possible and better cosmetic result is anticipated, surgical excision is the single alternative. Recurrence is rare.

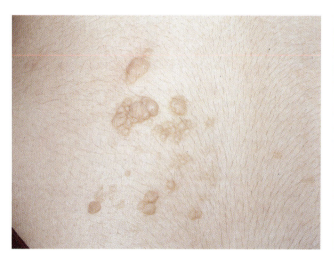

Fig. 10.9 Nevus lipomatosus superficialis with multiple lesions on the lower back. Note the typical cerebriform surface

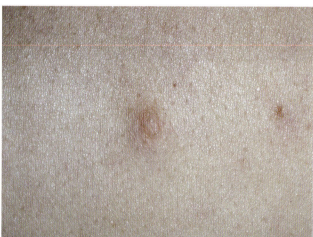

Fig. 10.11 Nevus lipomatosus superficialis evident as a solitary papule. The diagnosis is mostly established with biopsy in such lesions

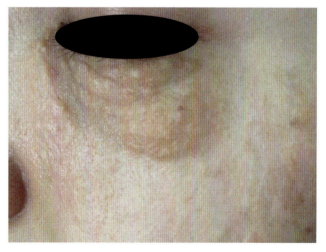

Fig. 10.10 Nevus lipomatosus superficialis on the face, a rare location

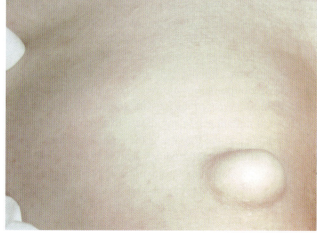

Fig. 10.12 Nevus lipomatosus superficialis shown as a solitary nodule on the gluteal region

Suggested Reading

Balestreire E, Haught JM, English JC 3rd. Multiple subcutaneous lipomas induced by HAART in the absence of protease inhibitors. Arch Dermatol. 2007;43:1596–7.

Bolognia JL, Jorizzo JL, Schaffer JV. Dermatology, edn 3. London: Mosby; 2012.

Burgdorf WHC, Plewig G, Wolff HH, Landthaler M. Braun-Falco's dermatology, edn 3. Italy: Springer-Verlag; 2009.

Caputo R, Tadini G. Atlas of genodermatoses. Spain: Taylor and Francis; 2006.

Elder DE, Elenitsas R, Johnson BL, Murphy GF, Xu X. Lever's histopathology of the skin, edn 10. Philadelphia: Lippincott Williams and Wilkins; 2008.

Enzi G. Multiple symmetric lipomatosis: an updated clinical report. Medicine (Baltimore). 1984;63:56–64.

James WD, Berger T, Elston D. Andrew's diseases of the skin: clinical dermatology, edn 11. China: Saunders Elsevier; 2011.

Jones EW, Marks R, Pongsehirun D. Naevus superficialis lipomatosus. A clinicopathological report of twenty cases. Br J Dermatol. 1975;93:121–33.

Reece PH, Wyatt M, O'Flynn P. Dercum's disease (adiposis dolorosa). J Laryngol Otol. 1999;113:174–6.

Shinde GB, Viswanath V, Torsekar RG. Multiple yellowish plaques in cerebriform pattern on the right elbow. Nevus lipomatosus cutaneous superficialis (NLCS)—classical type of Hoffmann and Zurhalle. Int J Dermatol. 2012;51:662–4.

Part II
Malignant Tumors

Malignant Epithelial Tumors

11

Malignant cutaneous tumors arising from epithelial cells, including malignant adnexal neoplasia are the topics of this chapter. Malignant melanoma that derives from epidermal melanocytes is the subject of another chapter. Basal cell carcinoma and squamous cell carcinoma are referred to as non–melanoma skin cancers. Both tumors compose the great majority of skin cancers and cause significant health concerns. They have typical features that will be discussed broadly. Their morbidity can be significantly reduced with early diagnosis. In addition, there are many types of malignant adnexal skin tumors including the ones with high metastatic potential. But all of them are rare. Most malignant adnexal tumors present as nonspecific bizarre nodules, plaques, or ulcerations and are usually difficult to diagnose clinically. While some of these tumors (syringocystadenocarcinoma papilliferum, spiradenocarcinoma, malignant cylindroma, pilomatrix carcinoma) are only mentioned in the chapter regarding their benign counterparts, most are discussed here. Additionally, Merkel cell carcinoma is also included in this chapter.

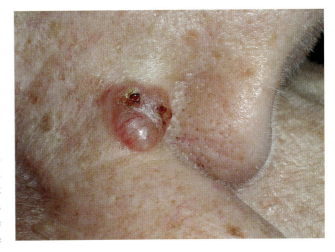

Fig. 11.1 Noduloulcerative basal cell carcinoma on the nasolabial fold

11.1 Basal Cell Carcinoma

Basal cell carcinoma has been thought to develop from the basal cells in the epidermis. However, this concept is subject to debate, since according to some authors, the tumor originates from the hair follicle epithelium. It is a slow-growing skin cancer with an extremely low metastatic potential. It is the most common malignancy in humans. Therefore it is among the most important health problems. Ultraviolet radiation is the predominant but not the single etiologic factor. The tumor is more common in fair-skinned individuals with blond or red hair who are unable to tan. It is rare in the black population. Basal cell carcinoma arises mostly in older individuals, probably as a result of cumulative sun damage. However, it may also be seen in younger patients, especially in the setting of some genodermatoses.

The face, the most commonly sun-exposed area, is the major location of basal cell carcinoma (see Figs. 11.1 and 11.2).

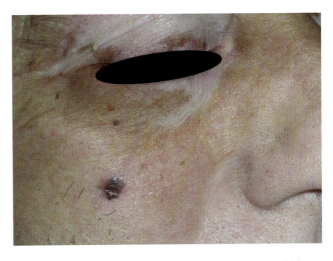

Fig. 11.2 Basal cell carcinoma on the face of a patient with vitiligo

The lesions have a predilection for sun-damaged skin. The scalp may be frequently affected in bald men (see Fig. 11.3). On the other hand, this cancer is not common on the dorsum of the hands (see Fig. 11.4) and forearms, other areas with dense sun exposure, but may frequently be located on minimally sun-exposed or non–sun-exposed areas such as

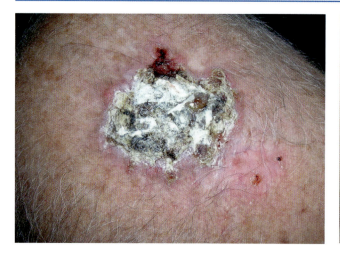

Fig. 11.3 Basal cell carcinoma on the scalp of a bald male, in a densely sun-exposed area. Other features of sun damage are also noticable

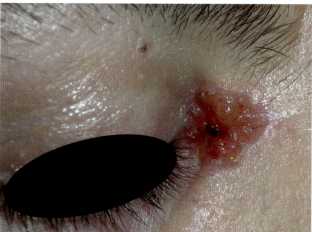

Fig. 11.5 Basal cell carcinoma on the medial canthus of the eye. Surprisingly this minimally sun-exposed area is frequently involved

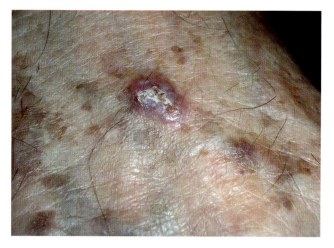

Fig. 11.4 Basal cell carcinoma on the dorsal aspect of the hand, an unusual location. Note the actinic lentigines on the same area

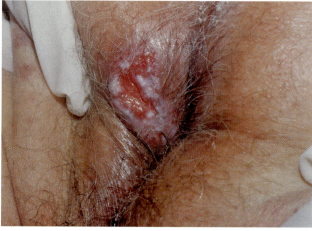

Fig. 11.6 Perianal basal cell carcinoma, a very rare presentation of the tumor

the medial canthus of the eye (*see* Fig. 11.5) and the retroauricular area. Therefore, basal cell carcinoma should not only be considered in the differential diagnosis of tumors located on sun-exposed areas. Basal cell carcinoma is rarely found on the penis, vulva, and perianal skin (*see* Fig. 11.6). It also does not arise primarily on mucosal sites or the nails. However, tumors around the mouth may invade the lips secondarily (*see* Figs. 11.7 and 11.8). Lesions of the eyelid may masquerade as ectropion (*see* Figs. 11.9 and 11.10).

Basal cell carcinoma occurs mostly on normal skin. Unlike squamous cell carcinoma, it does not develop on precursor lesions such as actinic keratosis, but it may arise on nevus sebaceus (*see* Figs. 11.11 and 11.12).

Basal cell carcinoma may also arise on scars after thermal burns (*see* Fig. 11.13) or on scars of some dermatoses such as lupus vulgaris (*see* Fig. 11.14) and discoid lupus erythematosus. Chronic arsenic exposure is another rare cause of basal cell carcinoma. Patients previously exposed to irradiation for many years have an increased risk of developing basal cell carcinoma, especially on the border areas of chronic radiodermatitis (*see* Fig. 11.15). Multiple lesions may be seen concurrently in these patients (*see* Figs. 11.16 and 11.17).

Immunosuppression is another well-known etiologic factor for basal cell carcinoma. Transplant recipients and immunosuppressed patients with systemic lymphoma are at increased risk. The course of the tumor may be more aggressive in this group, and even visceral metastasis may be seen in patients infected with Human immunodeficiency virus.

Patients who have had one basal cell carcinoma are at increased risk of developing another one (*see* Fig. 11.18) and squamous cell carcinoma as well. Most patients have solitary lesions but some, such as those living in sunny climates, immunosuppressed patients, and patients with a history of

11.1 Basal Cell Carcinoma

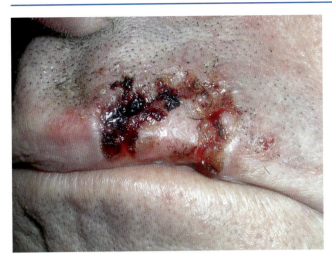

Fig. 11.7 Secondary invasion of the upper lip caused by basal cell carcinoma, which occurred as a late complication of the tumor

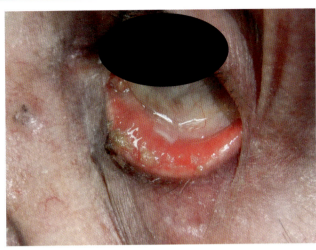

Fig. 11.10 Basal cell carcinoma of the lower eyelid which masquerades as an ectropion

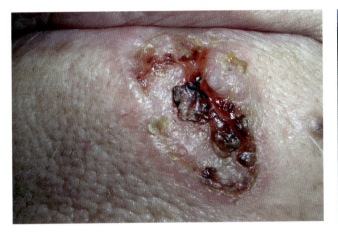

Fig. 11.8 Secondary invasion of the vermilion border of the lower lip due to basal cell carcinoma

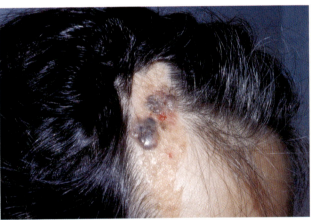

Fig. 11.11 Pigmented basal cell carcinoma developing in nevus sebaceus on the forehead and scalp. Multiple nodules are seen

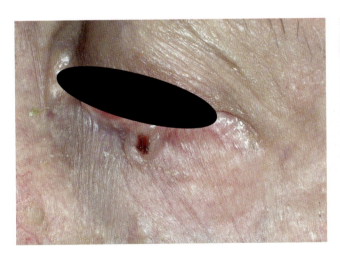

Fig. 11.9 Basal cell carcinoma on the lower eyelid. Note the associated ectropion

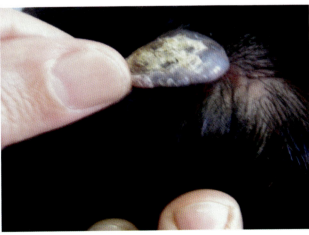

Fig. 11.12 Polypoid basal cell carcinoma, a rare clinical appearance, arising on nevus sebaceus in this case

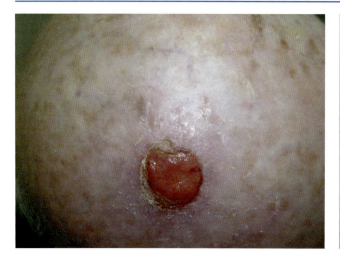

Fig. 11.13 Basal cell carcinoma developing in a thermal burn scar on the scalp

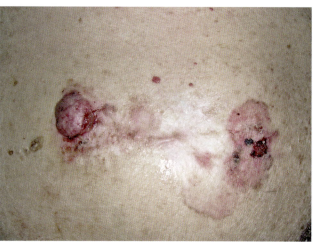

Fig. 11.16 Multiple basal cell carcinomas of superficial and noduloulcerative types developing in the setting of chronic radiodermatitis

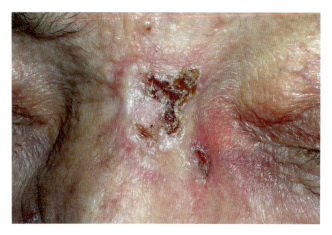

Fig. 11.14 Basal cell carcinoma developing in the scar of lupus vulgaris

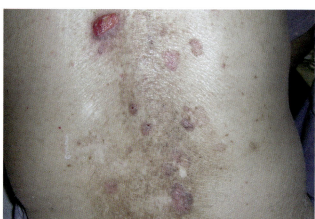

Fig. 11.17 Multiple basal cell carcinomas developing in an area treated with radiotherapy many years previously. Most tumors seen in the figure are of the superficial type

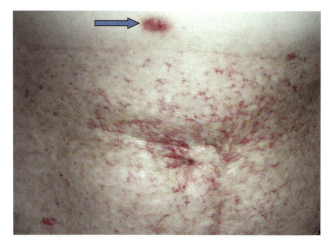

Fig. 11.15 Basal cell carcinoma developing on the border of chronic radiodermatitis. The tumor is visible on the upper part of the figure

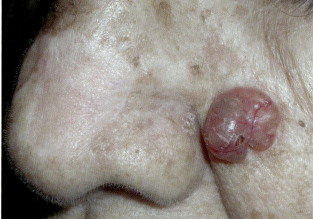

Fig. 11.18 Patients with one basal cell carcinoma are at increased risk of developing another. Note the scar of tumor excision on the nose and a second basal cell carcinoma on the cheek

11.1 Basal Cell Carcinoma

irradiation (*see* Fig. 11.17) or chronic arsenic exposure, may develop more than one lesion. However, some patients with multiple basal cell carcinomas do not have any detectable risk factors (*see* Figs. 11.18 and 11.19). Multiple basal cell carcinomas may also occur as a prominent feature in patients with hereditary tumor syndromes, including Gorlin syndrome, Bazex-Dupré-Christol syndrome, Rombo syndrome, and xeroderma pigmentosum (*see* Figs. 11.20 and 11.21). These are discussed in detail in this chapter. Moreover, the incidence of basal cell carcinomas is increased in those with other genodermatoses with different etiopathogenesis, including albinism (*see* Fig. 11.22), Werner syndrome, Muir-Torre syndrome, Brooke-Spiegler syndrome, and Schöpf-Schulz-Passarge syndrome.

Basal cell carcinoma does not metastasize through blood vessels or lymphatics in the great majority of cases. However, it progresses slowly in the absence of treatment and causes an irregular outgrowth toward adjacent tissue. Direct invasion of the tumor may be detected on fasciae, periosteum, perichondrium, and nerve sheaths. In neglected cases it may even penetrate bone.

Five major clinical types of basal cell carcinoma have been described. Noduloulcerative, superficial, and morphoeic types have different clinical and histopathologic features and different biological behaviors. The pigmented type may show clinical features similar to those of noduloulcerative or superficial types, but it presents as dark-colored lesions, since histopathologically it is rich in melanin. However, this has no prognostic significance. The fibroepithelial type of basal cell carcinoma has distinct clinical and histopathologic features but is very rare compared with the above-mentioned types. The main clinical types and some variants of the tumor will be discussed.

11.1.1 Noduloulcerative (Nodular) Type

More than half of the patients with basal cell carcinoma present with the noduloulcerative type. It is more common on the head but may also occur on the trunk, extremities, and rarely in the anogenital area. The nose (*see* Fig. 11.1), inner canthus of the eye (*see* Fig. 11.5), and the forehead (*see* Fig. 11.19) are the most typical locations. It arises as an elevated, smooth, shiny translucent papule (*see* Fig. 11.23). At this stage it can be confused with an intradermal melanocytic nevus (*see* Fig. 3.122), a palisaded encapsulated neuroma (*see* Fig. 7.41), a fibrous papule of the nose (*see* Fig. 8.16), and benign adnexal tumors such as trichoepithelioma (*see* Fig. 5.38). Because the tumor grows slowly, patients do not usually seek medical advice in the early phase. The center becomes umbilicated in time (*see* Fig. 11.24). Some lesions have a yellowish hue mimicking senile sebaceous hyperplasia (*see* Fig. 5.57). The tumor extends peripherally and vertically. Even papules or

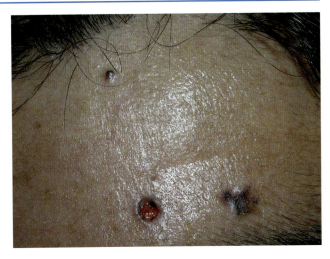

Fig. 11.19 Multiple basal cell carcinomas on the forehead of an otherwise healthy man. Note that all of them are of the pigmented type

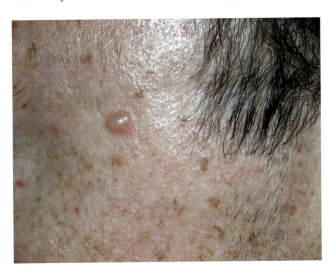

Fig. 11.20 Basal cell carcinoma presenting as a skin-colored papule on the face of a patient with xeroderma pigmentosum

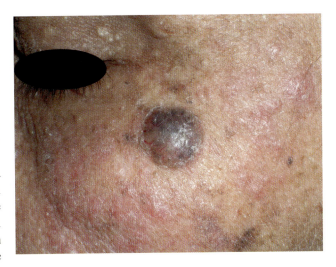

Fig. 11.21 Basal cell carcinoma seen as a pigmented nodule in a patient with xeroderma pigmentosum

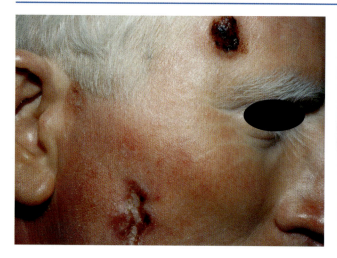

Fig. 11.22 Multiple basal cell carcinomas in a patient with albinism

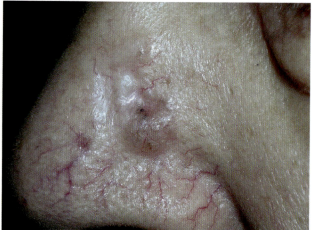

Fig. 11.25 A translucent (pearly) plaque of basal cell carcinoma

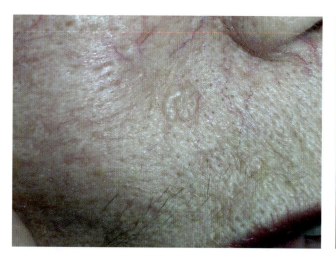

Fig. 11.23 The early lesion of basal cell carcinoma. The tumor has started as a shiny translucent papule in this case

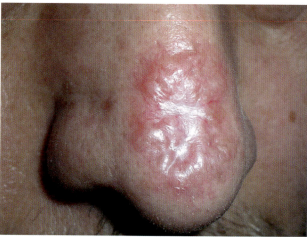

Fig. 11.26 A translucent, irregular plaque of basal cell carcinoma

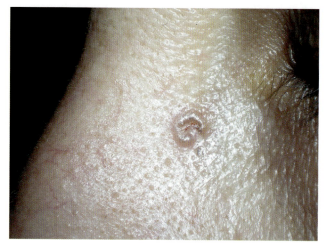

Fig. 11.24 The center of on early papular basal cell carcinoma may become umbilicated in time, as seen in the figure

nodules that are 0.5 to 1 cm in size may be ignored by the patients, mostly because of the absence of pain. The papules may gradually transform into pearly, dome-shaped, well-defined nodules or plaques with a grey or pink hue (*see* Figs. 11.25, 11.26 and 11.27). Some lesions may appear reddish (*see* Fig. 11.28). Fine telangiectasia traversing the whole surface of the lesion is a typical feature (*see* Fig. 11.29). Small foci of brown pigmentation (*see* Fig. 11.30) may be seen owing to the presence of dermal melanin.

The umbilicated center of most lesions becomes ulcerated (*see* Figs. 11.31, 11.32 and 11.33) in a period of 1 to 2 years. However, ulceration may either develop earlier (*see* Figs. 11.34 and 11.35) or never occur (*see* Fig. 11.27). Spontaneous bleeding is a common symptom in ulcerative basal cell carcinoma. The centrally located superficial ulceration is called "rodent ulcer." Scales and crusts mostly develop on the site of ulceration (*see* Figs. 11.36, 11.37, 11.38 and 11.39). Squamous cell carcinoma (*see* Fig. 11.119),

11.1 Basal Cell Carcinoma

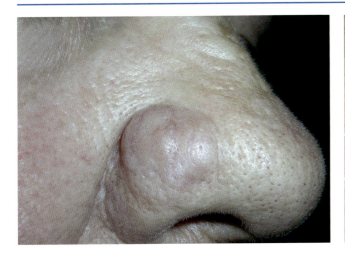

Fig. 11.27 A well-defined, skin-colored nodule of basal cell carcinoma

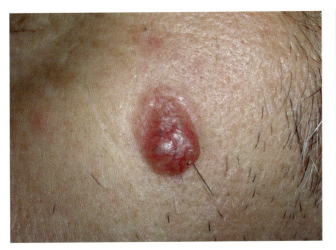

Fig. 11.28 Reddish nodular basal cell carcinoma. Tumor may sometimes appear red in relation to pronounced telangiectases

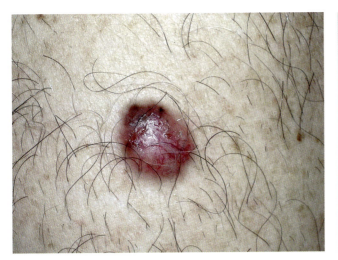

Fig. 11.29 Fine telangiectases on the surface of a translucent nodular basal cell carcinoma on the trunk

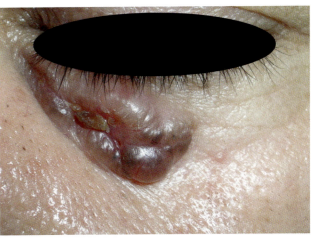

Fig. 11.30 A translucent nodule of basal cell carcinoma with brown foci of pigmentation due to dermal melanin; a typical appearance

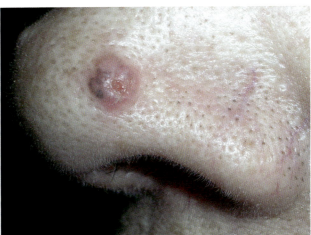

Fig. 11.31 A very small focus of ulceration is remarkable on the umbilicated center of a basal cell carcinoma

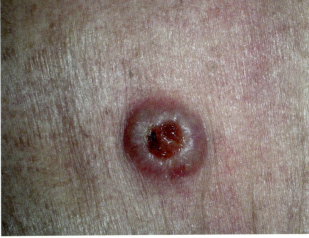

Fig. 11.32 The umbilicated center of basal cell carcinoma may become ulcerated in time as seen in the figure

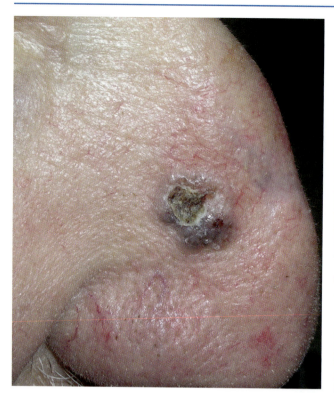

Fig. 11.33 Basal cell carcinoma with a crusted ulceration on the upper part

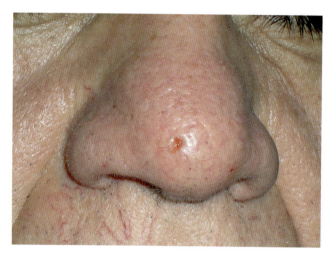

Fig. 11.34 Small superficial ulceration on a flat papule; an early diagnosed basal cell carcinoma

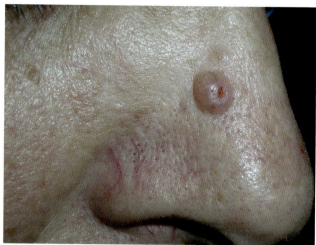

Fig. 11.35 An ulceration that has newly occurred on a nodule of basal cell carcinoma

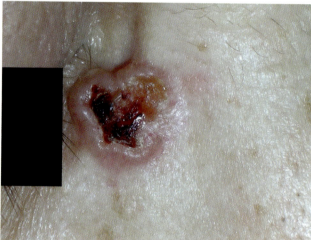

Fig. 11.36 Centrally located deep ulceration on a basal cell carcinoma; rodent ulcer

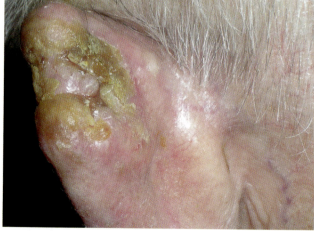

Fig. 11.37 Crusting on the ulceration site of an indurated plaque of basal cell carcinoma

atypical fibroxanthoma (see Fig. 13.63), Merkel cell carcinoma (see Fig. 11.167), and amelanotic malignant melanoma (see Fig. 12.59) may be considered in the differential diagnosis of ulcerated lesions. The presence of a translucent, rolled border, even in ulcerated lesions, is a distinctive clinical feature of basal cell carcinoma (see Fig. 11.40). Although not as frequently as on the head and neck, noduloulcerative basal cell carcinoma may occur on the trunk (see Figs. 11.29, 11.32 and 11.41), extremities (see Fig. 11.42), and rarely on

11.1 Basal Cell Carcinoma

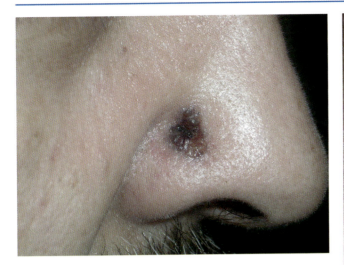

Fig. 11.38 Noduloulcerative basal cell carcinoma; central ulceration is covered with crusts

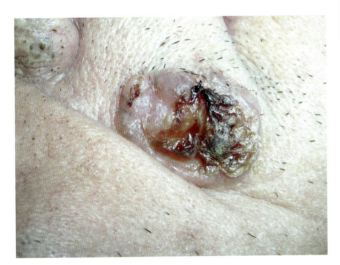

Fig. 11.39 Crusting on the ulceration site of a large noduloulcerative basal cell carcinoma

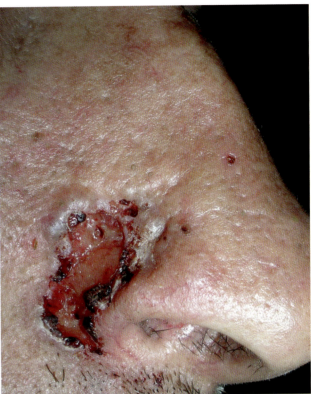

Fig. 11.40 Translucent, rolled, infiltrated border may be noticed even in an ulcerated basal cell carcinoma, as seen here. It is a distinctive sign

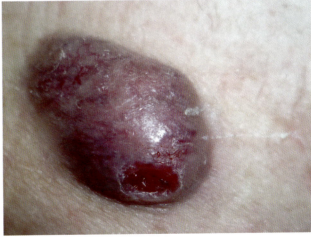

Fig. 11.41 Noduloulcerative basal cell carcinoma on the trunk. The typical rolled border is not always present as in this case

the fingers (see Fig. 11.43). The diagnosis may be delayed in such infrequent locations.

Noduloulcerative basal cell carcinoma may sometimes lack typical clinical clues and be noticed by different clinical features such as a flat indurated endophytic plaque (see Fig. 11.44), a cluster of several elevated nodules (see Fig. 11.30), an exophytic lobulated nodule (see Fig. 11.45), or a hyperkeratotic plaque. Sometimes a large mass or a protracted nonspecific ulcer (see Fig. 11.46), even in an atypical location, may be the presentation of basal cell carcinoma. Untreated tumors may penetrate subcutaneous tissue, causing large deeply ulcerated lesions (see Fig. 11.47). These disfiguring or even mutilating lesions are particularly troublesome when located on the midfacial area and ears. Lesions may penetrate more deeply, destroy cartilage (see Figs. 11.47 and 11.48), and even invade bone. Eye involvement may cause diplopia and ophthalmoplegia. In extreme cases, penetration to the brain has been documented.

Histologically basal cell carcinoma is characterized by tumoral lobules in the superficial dermis that consist of basophilic-staining small basaloid cells resembling the basal layer cells of the epidermis. Cells on the periphery of tumor islands are distinctively arranged in a palisade. Tumor islands and the surrounding mucinous inflammatory stroma may

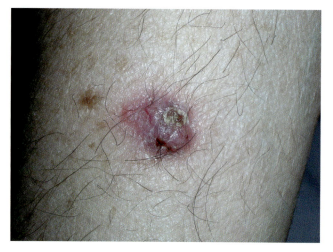

Fig. 11.42 Noduloulcerative basal cell carcinoma located on the arm, not a common location for this type

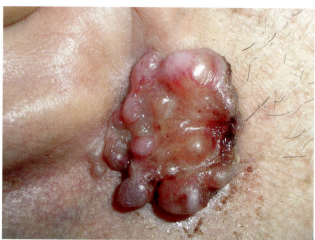

Fig. 11.45 Basal cell carcinoma appearing as an exophytic lobulated nodule

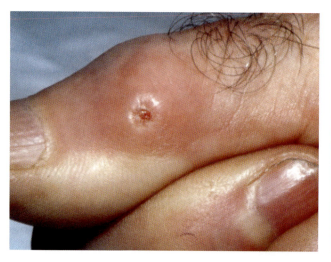

Fig. 11.43 Noduloulcerative basal cell carcinoma on the finger, a very rare location

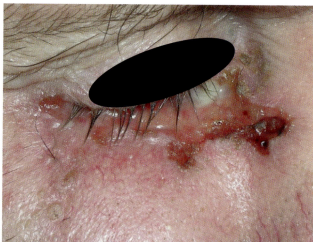

Fig. 11.46 Basal cell carcinoma presenting as a protracted nonspecific ulcer on the lower eyelid

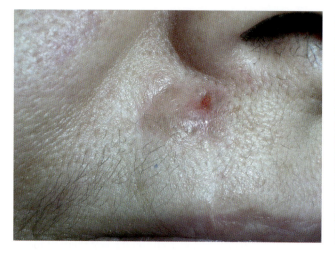

Fig. 11.44 Noduloulcerative basal cell carcinoma presenting as a flat, indurated plaque (endophytic growth)

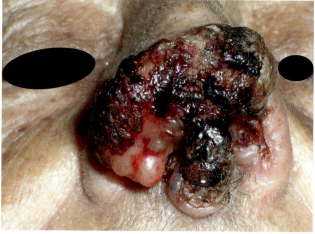

Fig. 11.47 A deeply ulcerated, large basal cell carcinoma, which is destroying the cartilage of the nose. Note the typical translucent, rolled border of the tumor

11.1 Basal Cell Carcinoma

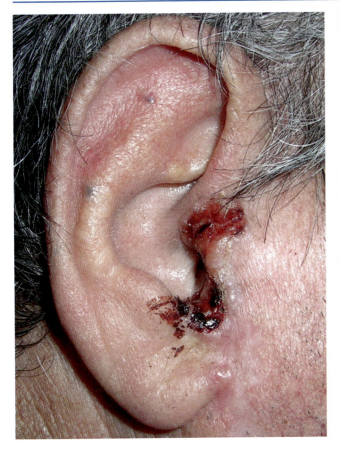

Fig. 11.48 Basal cell carcinoma on the tragus that is destroying the cartilage of the ear

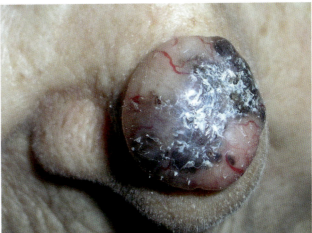

Fig. 11.49 Cystic basal cell carcinoma with fine telangiectases on the surface

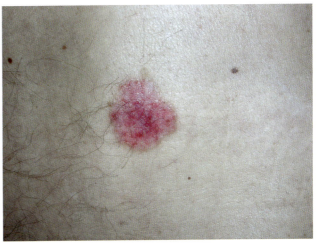

Fig. 11.50 Early small patchy lesion of superficial basal cell carcinoma on the trunk, the most typical location

invade the reticular dermis or subcutis in advanced cases. This typical histologic appearance is characteristic of noduloulcerative basal cell carcinoma. Other types of the tumor show some additional histopathologic features.

Cystic basal cell carcinoma is a variant of the noduloulcerative type. It presents as a well-defined, bluish-gray, translucent nodule with a smooth surface. Fine telangiectases may be present on the surface (see Fig. 11.49). The clinical appearance mimics benign cysts, particularly apocrine hidrocystoma (see Fig. 5.36). It may be ulcerated in the late period. Histologically the cystic variant is characterized by a tumoral cell mass with a large central cystic area devoid of cells, sometimes containing cellular debris or mucin. Tumor cells at the periphery of the nodule are usually small basaloid cells.

Basal cell carcinomas developing on nevus sebaceus are mostly of the noduloulcerative or pigmented type but may also appear as protruding polypoid lesions (see Fig. 11.12). They arise mostly after puberty.

11.1.2 Superficial Type

Superficial basal cell carcinoma is the least aggressive type of the tumor. It is the second most common type and occurs on the average, at a later age than the nodular type. Sun damage is possibly not a major etiologic factor, as the tumor is mostly localized on the trunk (see Fig. 11.50), although it can sometimes be seen on the extremities and face (see Fig. 11.51). Superficial basal cell carcinoma may present as a solitary lesion or a few lesions. It arises as a slightly erythematous, flat patch (see Figs. 11.50 and 11.52). Lesions are asymptomatic and may be ignored for a long time as the tumor grows slowly. Sometimes tumors may reach several centimeters before diagnosis (see Fig. 11.53). The tumor may be misinterpreted as nummular eczema or psoriasis.

Advanced superficial basal cell carcinoma may appear as a sharply demarcated reddish plaque with a typical minimally raised, thin, pearly border (see Fig. 11.54). The central part of the lesion may be atrophic (see Figs. 11.55 and 11.56). Foci of adherent scales (see Fig. 11.56), crusted shallow ulcers (see Fig. 11.53), or hyperpigmentation (see Fig. 11.57) may cause a variegated appearance. Lesions may become thicker after years as a result of deep invasion. Papulonodular

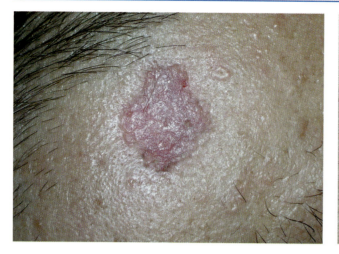

Fig. 11.51 Superficial basal cell carcinoma presenting as a flat patch on the face

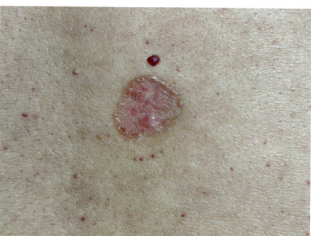

Fig. 11.54 Superficial basal cell carcinoma with a distinctive, slightly raised, thin, pearly border

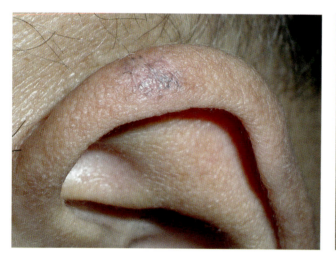

Fig. 11.52 Superficial basal cell carcinoma presenting as a flat, slightly hyperpigmented patch on the ear

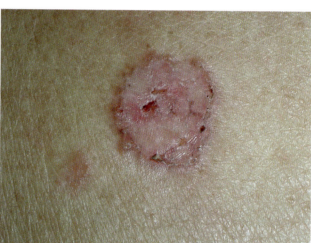

Fig. 11.55 Superficial basal cell carcinoma with slight central atrophy and foci of scales

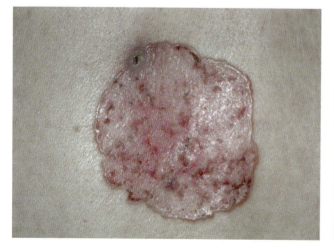

Fig. 11.53 A large thin plaque of superficial basal cell carcinoma. Crusted shallow small ulcers are seen on the surface

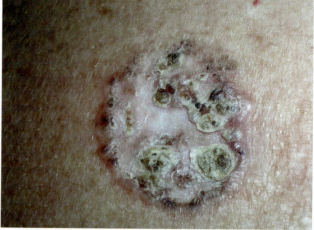

Fig. 11.56 Superficial basal cell carcinoma with prominent central atrophy. Note also the overlying scales and crusts

11.1 Basal Cell Carcinoma

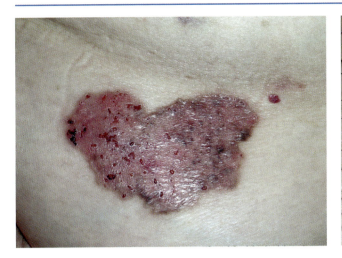

Fig. 11.57 Partially hyperpigmented, sharply demarcated flat plaque of superficial basal cell carcinoma

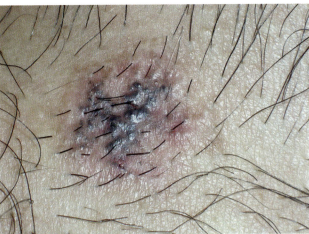

Fig. 11.58 Papulonodular areas may develop on the flat patch of superficial basal cell carcinoma over a period of years. Note the overlying pigmented papules

areas (*see* Fig. 11.58) or elevated masses (*see* Fig. 11.59) overlying a flat lesion may develop as the tumor enlarges. These large lesions may show foci of superficial (*see* Fig. 11.60) or deep ulceration (*see* Fig. 11.61). Some lesions are completely hyperpigmented (*see* Fig. 11.62). Bowen disease (*see* Fig. 2.20), extramammary Paget disease (*see* Fig. 2.80), and superficial spreading melanoma (*see* Fig. 12.20) may be considered in the differential diagnosis of these lesions. Histologically, superficial basal cell carcinoma is characterized only by superficial multifocal buds of basaloid cells extending from the epidermis and invading the papillary dermis.

11.1.3 Morphoeic (Sclerosing) Type

Morphoeic basal cell carcinoma is a relatively rare type with increased potential for deep invasion. It may occur at a relatively younger age than the other main types. This type is more commonly seen on the upper trunk and face. It is mostly larger than the noduloulcerative type of tumor and may reach 1 to 3 cm before the diagnosis (*see* Figs. 11.63 and 11.64). Pale, poorly-defined, flat or sometimes depressed solitary lesions (*see* Fig. 11.63) may look like a small plaque type of morphea or a scar. The tumor is firm on palpation. Raised and rolled borders typical of basal cell carcinoma may be noticed in some parts on the periphery (*see* Figs. 11.65 and 11.66). Pearly appearance, overlying telangiectases, and foci of ulceration (*see* Fig. 11.67) may be seen in some lesions, supporting the clinical diagnosis. Larger lesions on the face may cause retraction (*see* Fig. 11.68). Scleroderma-like cutaneous metastasis manifesting as indurated plaques (*see* Fig. 16.32) may also be considered in the differential diagnosis, but this tumoral infiltration usually has a more acute onset. Microcystic adnexal carcinoma and early lesions

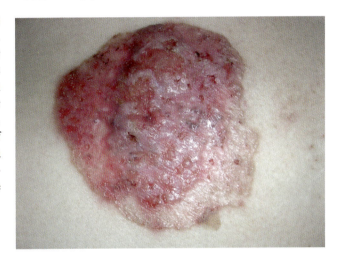

Fig. 11.59 Nodularity may arise on the flat patch of superficial basal cell carcinoma. In the illustrated case the nodular component has developed many years later than the flat component

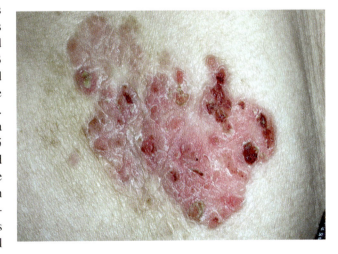

Fig. 11.60 A giant superficial basal cell carcinoma. Note the crusts covering foci of superficial ulcerations

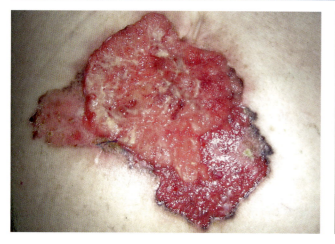

Fig. 11.61 Deep ulceration on the nodular component of a giant superficial basal cell carcinoma

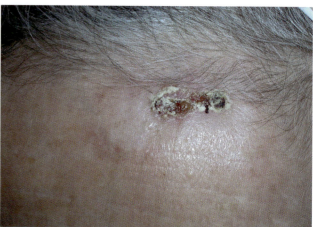

Fig. 11.64 Ill-defined, large, pale plaque of morphoeic basal cell carcinoma. Note the crusted ulceration on one site of the tumor

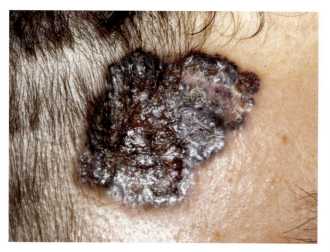

Fig. 11.62 Hyperpigmented superficial basal cell carcinoma

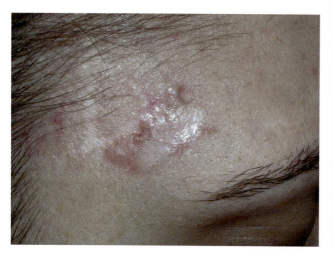

Fig. 11.63 Morphoeic basal cell carcinoma presenting as a solitary depressed lesion on the face. These lesions are firm on palpation

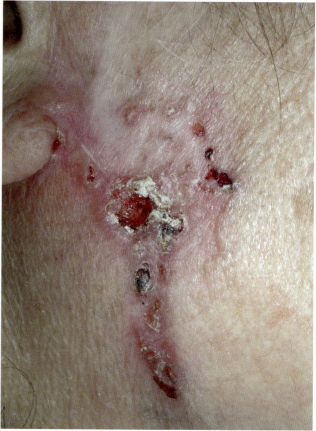

Fig. 11.65 A large morphoeic basal cell carcinoma. Note the raised rolled border, which is helpful for diagnosis

11.1 Basal Cell Carcinoma

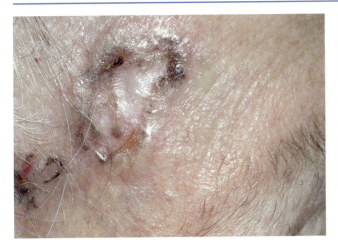

Fig. 11.66 Morphoeic basal cell carcinoma. Note the central depression and the raised border of the plaque

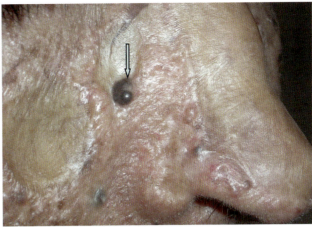

Fig. 11.69 Pigmented basal cell carcinoma (*arrow*) in a patient with xeroderma pigmentosum. Note also the surgical scars of previously performed skin cancer operations

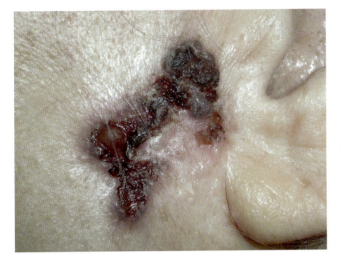

Fig. 11.67 Morphoeic basal cell carcinoma with foci of ulceration and crusting

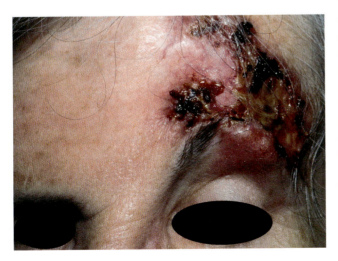

Fig. 11.68 A large morphoeic basal cell carcinoma causing retraction

of dermatofibrosarcoma protuberans (*see* Fig. 13.59) are other diagnostic challenges. Histologically, tumoral islands seen in morphoeic basal cell carcinoma are strands or thin cords of neoplastic cells embedded in a fibrous or desmoplastic stroma. Peripheral palisading is usually not noticeable. This picture is different from other histologic types of the tumor.

Invasion of the underlying tissue occurs more commonly than in the other clinical types of the tumor. Early lesions are asymptomatic, but perineural infiltration may occur in advanced cases of morphoeic type tumors causing paresthesia and sensory loss. The treatment of this type of basal cell carcinoma is a challenge because extension beyond clinical borders is frequently present.

11.1.4 Pigmented Type

The lesions of pigmented basal cell carcinoma are similar to those of other types but also have brown, black, or blue pigmentation. The color is attributable to melanin pigment present in the tumor cells and the stroma. Pigmented tumors may also be associated with tumor syndromes such as xeroderma pigmentosum (*see* Fig. 11.69). Some patients have more than one pigmented basal cell carcinoma (*see* Fig. 11.70). Lesions similar to the noduloulcerative type are more common on the face (*see* Fig. 11.71), and those similar to the superficial type are more common on the trunk (*see* Fig. 11.58). Pigmentation of the basal cell carcinoma may be homogeneous (*see* Fig. 11.72) or speckled (*see* Fig. 11.71). The presence of a pearly component (*see* Fig. 11.71) or of the typical rolled border supports the diagnosis. However, it can clinically be misdiagnosed as a melanocytic nevus, particularly a blue nevus (*see* Fig. 3.63), a pigmented seborrheic keratosis (*see* Fig. 1.38), or a malignant melanoma

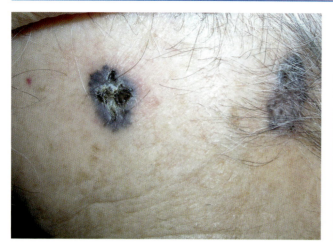

Fig. 11.70 Multiple pigmented basal cell carcinomas

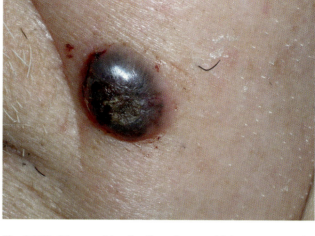

Fig. 11.72 Pigmented basal cell carcinoma with homogeneous pigmentation. Clinically it can be mistaken for malignant melanoma

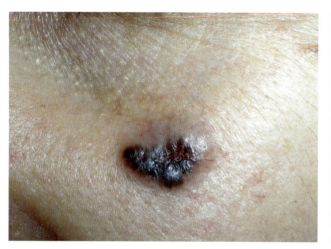

Fig. 11.71 Pigmented basal cell carcinoma on the face with a speckled pattern. Note the similarity to the noduloulcerative type except for the hyperpigmentation

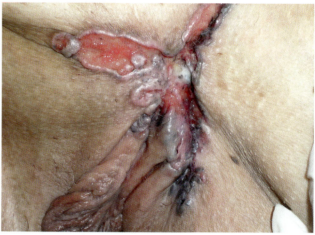

Fig. 11.73 Basosquamous carcinoma on the genital area of a woman. The lesion was very extensive which is unusual for classic basal cell carcinoma

(*see* Fig. 12.42). Dermoscopy may be helpful in diagnosing these tumors, but in most cases histopathologic confirmation is needed. Pigmentation of the tumor does not affect its biological behavior.

11.1.5 Fibroepithelial Type (Pinkus Tumor)

Fibroepithelial basal cell carcinoma is the rarest type and has distinct clinicopathologic features. Tumors mostly locate on the trunk, especially on the lower back, and are sometimes multiple. The lesion is a pink or skin-colored, sessile or pedunculated papule or nodule resembling acrochordon or seborrheic keratosis. Histologically it is characterized by thin, anastomosing cords of basaloid cells extending downward from the epidermis and embedded in a loose stroma.

11.1.6 Basosquamous Carcinoma (Metatypical Carcinoma)

Basosquamous carcinoma is a rare tumor showing histopathologic features of both basal cell carcinoma and squamous cell carcinoma. Although it may show the classic clinical features of basal cell carcinoma, it may also present as a nonspecific tumor, thereby causing delay in diagnosis. It is more common on the head and neck but may be seen anywhere, including the genital area (*see* Fig. 11.73). Its biological behavior is more aggressive, with a higher metastatic rate compared with the main types of basal cell carcinoma. The diagnosis is only made upon biopsy. Histologically, in addition to tumor islands of basaloid cells, squamous cells with abundant eosinophilic cytoplasm and keratinization and a transition zone with intermediate cells are seen. Immunohistochemically this tumor bears

11.1 Basal Cell Carcinoma

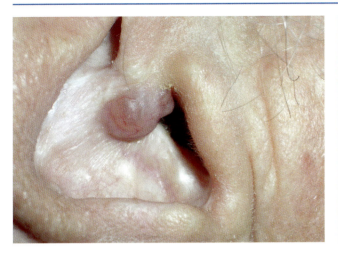

Fig. 11.74 Recurrent basal cell carcinoma on the concha of the ear. Note the absence of the typical raised border

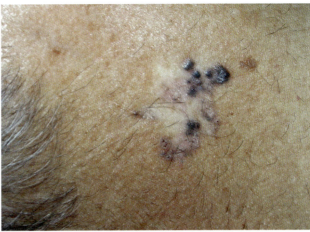

Fig. 11.75 Recurrent basal cell carcinoma overlying the scar tissue of the primary tumor

positive areas with markers of basal cell carcinoma, such as Ber-EP4 stain, which is negative in a standard squamous cell carcinoma.

11.1.7 Recurrent Basal Cell Carcinoma

Patients with one basal cell carcinoma are at increased risk of developing another. On the other hand, although low, there is also a risk of recurrence of the treated tumors. Recurrence occurs for the most part in the first 5 years but may be later. The clinical presentation of the recurrent tumor may be different from that of the primary lesion. Recurrent tumors are associated with increased morbidity and are more difficult to treat.

Inadequate treatment is the main cause of recurrence. On the other hand, recurrence is relatively more common in some conditions. The morphoeic type of the tumor, an infiltrative histopathologic pattern, basosquamous carcinoma, and large lesions are considered to have a higher risk of recurrence. Lesions located on the nose and ears, where subcutaneous tissue is thin, may show invasion of the underlying cartilage, which is further associated with an increased risk of recurrence.

Typical clinical features of basal cell carcinoma such as a rolled border are usually absent on recurrent lesions (*see* Fig. 11.74), and thus the diagnosis is more difficult. Recurrence may be found overlying the scar tissue (*see* Figs. 11.75 and 11.76), on graft areas (*see* Fig. 11.74) or just on their borders (*see* Fig. 11.77), mostly as one or more superficial papules, elevated nodules, and infiltrated plaques that may be pearly or hyperpigmented. Sometimes recurrences may present as erosions, ulcerations, or deeply located masses (*see* Fig. 11.78). Recurrent tumors located in the subcutis may mimic an epidermoid cyst (*see* Fig. 4.16).

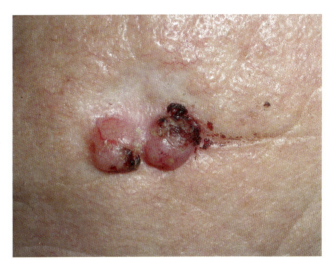

Fig. 11.76 Recurrent basal cell carcinoma occurring as two nodules on the scar site. Inadequate surgical margins are the main cause of recurrence

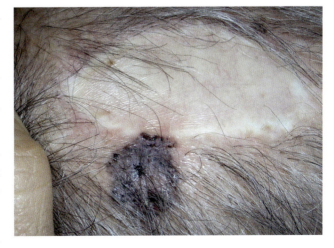

Fig. 11.77 Recurrent basal cell carcinoma on the border of the skin graft area

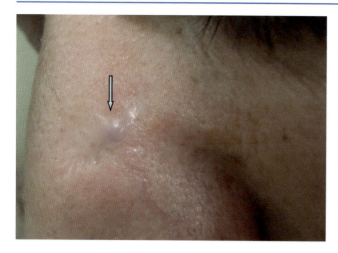

Fig. 11.78 Recurrent basal cell carcinoma presenting as a deeply located nodule (*arrow*) on the surgery site; diagnosis may be difficult in such tumors

Recurrence of morphoeic basal cell carcinoma may be difficult to distinguish from the scar tissue of an excised primary tumor. If there is any doubt of recurrence, a biopsy should be performed.

Recurrent tumors show a tendency to involvement of deeper tissue and perineural invasion. Sometimes recurrence of basal cell carcinoma is associated with neuropathic pain, muscle weakness, paresthesia, or paralysis.

11.1.8 Metastatic Basal Cell Carcinoma

Untreated basal cell carcinomas may eventually invade underlying structures, and in extremely rare cases may also metastasize via the lymphatics to the lymph nodes and hematogenously to the lungs, bones, and other visceral organs. However, in most cases no further routine evaluation of patients after diagnosis is necessary. Neglected cases with very large ulcerated lesions, basosquamous carcinoma, morphoeic type, therapy-resistant or recurrent tumors, and lesions with perineural invasion or blood vessel infiltration have a relatively higher risk of metastasis. After the occurrence of metastasis, the prognosis is poor.

Management. Basal cell carcinoma is a slow growing but destructive tumor and may cause mutilation and disfigurement. In addition to the age and general health of the patient, other factors such as the clinical type, location, size, and growth pattern of the tumor and the presence of ulceration should be considered when deciding on the method of therapy. Additionally, patients with multiple lesions should be evaluated specially. The cosmetic concern of the patients is usually greater for tumors on the face. However, complete removal or destruction of the tumor is necessary because inadequate or superficial interventions applied for better cosmetic results increase the risk of invasion to deeper tissues.

Topical agents, destructive modalities, photodynamic therapy, radiotherapy, surgery and even chemotherapy may be used for basal cell carcinoma. In general, excisional surgery is associated with a lower recurrence rate and is considered prior to other therapies. However, it may be contraindicated because of the age or systemic problems of the patient or the possibility of undesirable scars. Furthermore, superficial or smaller lesions may also initially be treated with other methods. Topical options (5 percent imiquimod, 5-fluorouracil) may be used, especially in superficial basal cell carcinoma. Imiquimod cream may be a practical modality in multiple superficial lesions. This immunomodulator drug may also be helpful in reducing the size of the tumor before surgery (*see* Fig. 11.79a–d). However, the duration of therapy is long and control biopsy is necessary. Photodynamic therapy may be utilized in the superficial type of the tumor even in lesions with a large size. Small papulonodular lesions on the trunk and extremities that do not show deep invasion can be treated with cryotherapy or curettage combined with electrocautery. The main advantage of cryotherapy is that it can be used in patients in poor general health and in those using anticoagulant therapy. However, any of these destructive methods should not be chosen in high-risk lesions.

Noduloulcerative type basal cell carcinoma located on the eyelids, ears, nose, nasolabial folds, and scalp are preferentially removed, and Mohs micrographic surgery is the first-line therapy in these areas. In cases with free surgical margins, the recurrence rate is low. Radiotherapy may also be used on these areas, especially in larger lesions and when surgery is contraindicated. Because the cosmetic results of radiotherapy are not always satisfactory, it is not preferred in young patients.

Pigmented basal cell carcinomas are mostly treated with surgery. Radiotherapy may result in hyperpigmentation and is not a primary option. Morphoeic type of basal cell carcinoma deserves special therapeutic consideration. It should always be treated with surgery, as other methods are not effective. This type of tumor, with high risk of subclinical extension, should be removed leaving large margins. Therefore, surgery can be debilitating and disfiguring. If Mohs micrographic surgery is used, the recurrence rate is lower.

Mohs micrographic surgery is the ideal choice for recurrent basal cell carcinoma. Radiotherapy is another option for these lesions, but the results are not always good. Lymph node metastasis may be managed by lymphadenectomy combined with radiotherapy. Classic chemotherapy and radiotherapy are not very effective in systemic metastasis of basal cell carcinoma. Vismodegib, a hedgehog signaling pathway targeting systemic agent, is a new option in recurrent or large unresectable tumors and metastatic cases. It may show a dramatic effect. Close follow-up of all patients for five years is recommended for prompt diagnosis of recurrences and possible second cutaneous malignancies with solar etiology.

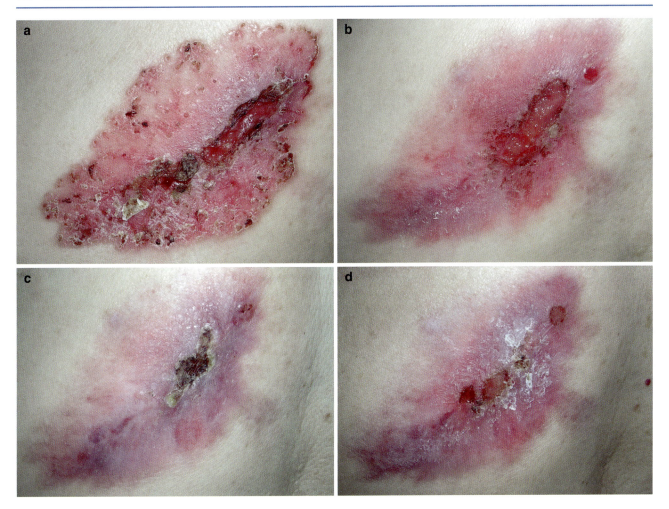

Fig. 11.79 (**a**) A giant, focally ulcerated superficial basal cell carcinoma on the trunk. (**b–d**) The response to therapy with topical imiquimod was observed as prominent reduction in the lesion size

11.1.9 Hereditary Tumor Syndromes

Basal cell carcinoma usually occurs sporadically. However, especially multiple lesions may be associated with some genodermatoses that are also referred to as tumor syndromes. Basal cell carcinomas occurring in the setting of these syndromes may develop at a younger age and at unusual locations. Gorlin syndrome, Bazex-Dupré-Christol syndrome, Rombo syndrome, and xeroderma pigmentosum are the main tumor syndromes related to basal cell carcinomas that are accompanied by other skin manifestations or involvement of visceral organs. Except for xeroderma pigmentosum, these syndromes are associated only with basal cell carcinomas and do not show any relationship with squamous cell carcinoma and other malignant skin neoplasms. In contrast, the risk of all cutaneous neoplasms associated with solar etiology, including squamous cell carcinoma and malignant melanoma, is increased in patients with xeroderma pigmentosum.

11.1.9.1 Gorlin Syndrome (Nevoid Basal Cell Carcinoma)

Gorlin syndrome is an autosomal dominant genodermatosis caused by germline mutation of the *PTCH1* gene, a tumor-suppressor gene. Patients are predisposed to multiple basal cell carcinomas over a lifetime and may develop multiorgan abnormalities. They typically have a positive family history. In family members different manifestations of the disease may be dominant.

Basal cell carcinomas are not present at birth and usually begin in early childhood. The number of tumors is variable, but most patients have numerous lesions (*see* Fig. 11.80). In addition to the face (*see* Figs. 11.80 and 11.81) and neck, areas not densely exposed to sunlight such as the trunk (*see* Fig. 11.82), intertriginous areas (*see* Fig. 11.83), and the extremities (*see* Fig. 11.84) are commonly involved. This type of basal cell carcinoma may have an unusual clinical appearance when compared with the classic types, especially in children. Involvement of the eyelids is typical (*see*

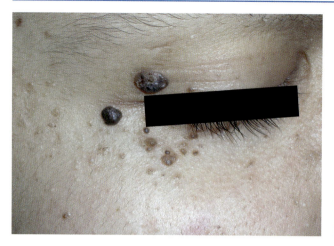

Fig. 11.80 Numerous papular lesions of basal cell carcinoma in a child with Gorlin syndrome. Involvement of the eyelids is typical

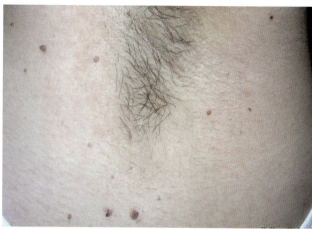

Fig. 11.83 Multiple papular lesions of basal cell carcinomas on the axilla of a patient with Gorlin syndrome

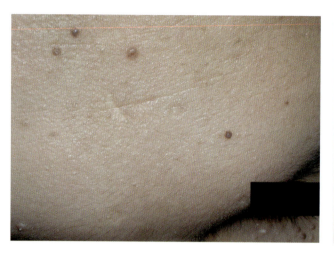

Fig. 11.81 Multiple facial basal cell carcinomas presenting as small papules in Gorlin syndrome. These lesions grow very slowly

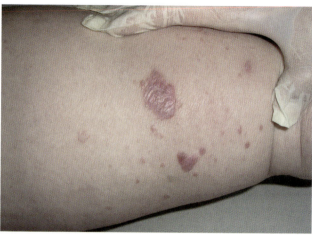

Fig. 11.84 Multiple basal cell carcinomas on the lower leg of a patient with Gorlin syndrome

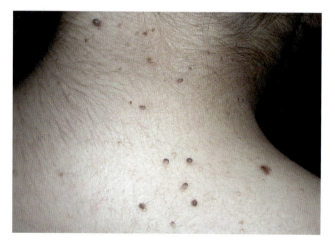

Fig. 11.82 Multiple acrochordon-like basal cell carcinomas on the neck and trunk of a patient with Gorlin syndrome

Figs. 11.80 and 11.85). The lesions are flesh- or pale brown-colored, dome-shaped or pedunculated papules measuring 2 to 3 mm in diameter (see Figs. 11.80, 11.81, 11.82 and 11.83). Tiny papular lesions (see Fig. 11.85) look like milia (see Fig. 4.32), and pedunculated lesions (see Fig. 11.86) are similar to acrochordons (see Fig. 8.69). Some patients have tens to thousands of lesions distributed nearly over the whole body (see Figs. 11.82 and 11.84). Lesions may be stable for decades but some transform into aggressive tumors after puberty. Small papular lesions of Gorlin syndrome may also show the typical histopathologic features of basal cell carcinoma. Noduloulcerative (see Fig. 11.87) and superficial types (see Fig. 11.88) are more common, but pigmented and morphoeic types may also be seen.

Gorlin syndrome has additional dermatologic features. Small pits on palmoplantar skin (see Figs. 11.89 and 11.90)

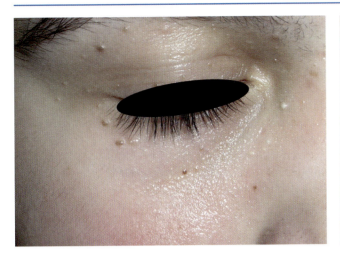

Fig. 11.85 Multiple tiny basal cell carcinomas around the eye of a child with Gorlin syndrome

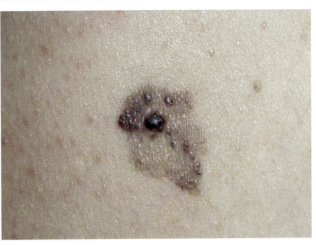

Fig. 11.88 Superficial basal cell carcinoma with overlying pigmented small papules in Gorlin syndrome

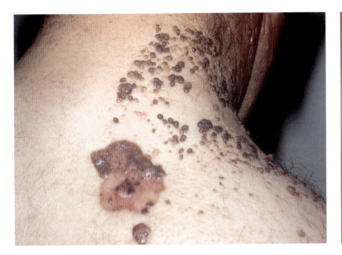

Fig. 11.86 Multiple basal cell carcinomas in Gorlin syndrome. In addition to a typical large plaque of the hyperpigmented type tumor, multiple pedunculated lesions similar to acrochordons are seen

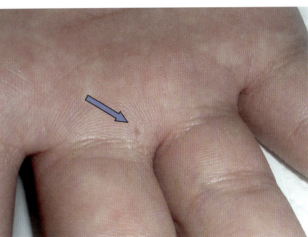

Fig. 11.89 Tiny pits on palmar area, a distinctive feature of Gorlin syndrome

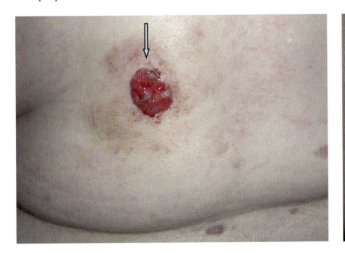

Fig. 11.87 Noduloulcerative type of basal cell carcinoma located on the trunk of an adult with Gorlin syndrome

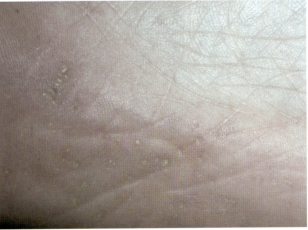

Fig. 11.90 Multiple tiny pits on the sole of the foot in a patient with Gorlin syndrome. They are not seen in all patients

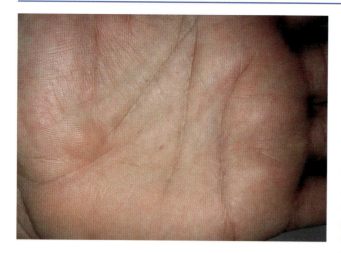

Fig. 11.91 Epidermoid cyst on the palmar area. Atypically located cysts may be seen in Gorlin syndrome

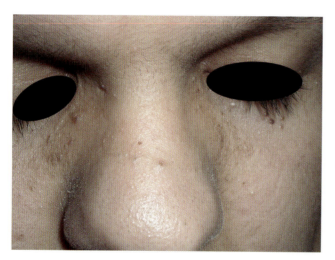

Fig. 11.92 Typical appearance of the face with frontal bossing in a patient with Gorlin syndrome. Note also the milia and small basal cell carcinomas on the face

are typical signs of the disease occurring in early childhood but are not seen in all patients. A few or sometimes numerous pits measuring 1 to 3 mm size are asymmetrically distributed on the palmar area (see Fig. 11.89). The plantar area may be involved less frequently (see Fig. 11.90). These pits only show local absence in the stratum corneum and are not basal cell carcinomas. Epidermoid cysts in unusual locations may be seen in the course of the syndrome. The typical ones are acral epidermoid cysts (see Fig. 11.91). Milia are found in some patients (see Fig. 11.92).

The phenotypical appearance of the patients may be helpful for diagnosis. Most have the typical phenotype with hypertelorism, coarse facies, and frontal bossing (see Fig. 11.92). Head circumference is usually enlarged. Congenital blindness, colobomas, cataract and strabismus are major ocular anomalies seen in this syndrome.

Bony cysts of the jaw are common and distinctive features of the disease. Patients may be diagnosed first by dentists. Odontogenic keratocysts of the mandible are typically multiple and may be associated with malaligned dentition and cause secondary swelling and pain. New cysts may occur throughout the patient's life. Abnormalities of the ribs (bifid or fused ribs) and a short fourth metacarpal bone are other typical but rare bone findings.

Neurologic changes such as intracranial calcification (calcified dural folds), mental retardation, and increased risk of medulloblastoma may also be seen. Moreover, fetal rhabdomyoma and lymphomesenteric cysts may develop in some patients. Ovarian fibromas are common and may cause infertility. Fibrosarcomas of the ovary and the jaw and ameloblastoma are rare malignancies seen in patients with Gorlin syndrome. It is uncommon for all these manifestations to be seen in the same patient.

Differential diagnosis of Gorlin syndrome consists of mainly Bazex-Dupré-Christol syndrome and other syndromes with numerous basal cell carcinomas. In addition to basal cell carcinomas, milia are also common in both syndromes. However in Bazex-Dupré-Christol syndrome, follicular atrophoderma and hypotrichosis may also be present. Milia and hypotrichosis may also be seen in Rombo syndrome, but trichoepitheliomas, atrophoderma vermiculata, and cyanosis may be present as well. Patients with xeroderma pigmentosum may develop multiple classic basal cell carcinomas on sun-exposed areas in early childhood, but these patients also have an increased risk of developing squamous cell carcinoma, malignant melanoma, and fibrosarcoma. Profuse ephelides and lentigines on sun-exposed areas are typically found in xeroderma pigmentosum, which are not expected in Gorlin syndrome. Although basal cell carcinomas seen in Gorlin syndrome may have distinctive clinical features, its diagnosis can be established in the presence of other dermatologic and extracutaneous findings. Patients with multiple papular and acrochordon-like lesions may be confused with patients with Birt-Hogg-Dubé syndrome (see Fig. 8.44).

Management. If Gorlin syndrome is diagnosed early and adequately managed, the morbidity of basal cell carcinomas can be minimized, and patients who do not develop rare sarcomatous tumors may have a normal life span. Vigilant sun protection throughout life is obligatory to reduce the occurrence of aggressive skin tumors. Systemic retinoids may also be used to prevent the development of new basal cell carcinomas. However, it is difficult to tolerate this therapy for prolonged periods.

Smaller basal cell carcinomas arising in childhood may be treated with electrodesiccation and curettage, cryotherapy, photodynamic therapy, or topical imiquimod. Early removal of basal cell carcinomas may prevent disfiguring scars and the need for more aggressive therapies. Radiotherapy should be avoided because it may accelerate the occurrence of basal

11.2 Squamous Cell Carcinoma

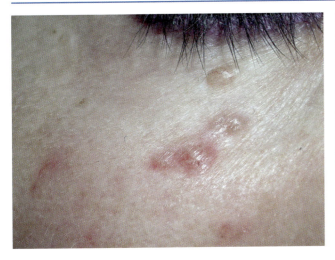

Fig. 11.93 A few basal cell carcinomas on the face of a patient with Bazex-Dupré-Christol syndrome

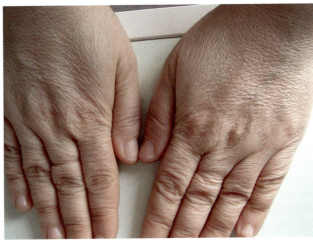

Fig. 11.94 Follicular atrophoderma on the dorsum of the hands; a typical feature of Bazex-Dupré-Christol syndrome

cell carcinomas and additional aggressive tumors. Careful ongoing surveillance of the patients is crucial.

11.1.9.2 Bazex-Dupré-Christol Syndrome

Bazex-Dupré-Christol syndrome is a rare disease characterized by multiple basal cell carcinomas and other dermatologic manifestations. It is inherited in an X-dominant fashion. Patients usually have a family history, but the phenotype is variable among family members. Basal cell carcinomas start at early ages and are not clinically different from the sporadic ones (see Fig. 11.93). Follicular atrophoderma is among the frequent clinical findings of the syndrome, involving the dorsum of the hands (see Fig. 11.94) and feet or extensor surfaces of the elbows (see Fig. 11.95) and knees. It is seen as grouped lesions showing depression of the epidermis. Other frequent clinical features are hair abnormalities (see Fig. 11.96) including hypotrichosis and profuse milia (see Figs. 11.96 and 11.97), which all begin at early ages. Epidermoid cysts, hyperpigmentation of the face, hypohidrosis, and trichoepitheliomas can also be seen in patients with Bazex-Dupré-Christol syndrome. It should be distinguished from other syndromes manifesting with multiple basal cell carcinomas such as Gorlin syndrome (see Fig. 11.80) and xeroderma pigmentosum (see Fig. 11.103). Hypohidrotic ectodermal dysplasia may also be confused with Bazex-Dupré-Christol syndrome, since hypotrichosis and hypohidrosis can be seen in both syndromes but basal cell carcinoma is not expected in the former syndrome.

Management. Patients and their families should be screened regularly for the development of basal cell carcinomas starting from childhood. Lifelong photoprotection should be recommended. Basal cell carcinomas should be treated in the early period. Systemic retinoids may be tried to suppress the development of these carcinomas.

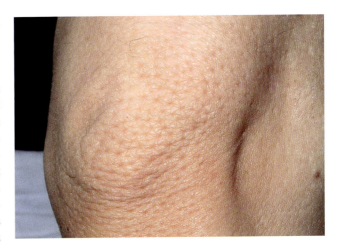

Fig. 11.95 Follicular atrophoderma on the extensor surface of the elbow in a patient with Bazex-Dupré-Christol syndrome

11.2 Squamous Cell Carcinoma

Squamous cell carcinoma is a malignancy deriving from the epidermal keratinocytes of the skin and mucous membranes. It is the second most common skin cancer in humans following basal cell carcinoma, another non–melanoma skin cancer. The potential of metastatic spread increases its importance. Various etiologic factors are suggested, but the most significant one is overexposure to ultraviolet radiation. Accordingly, the tumor is more common in light-complexioned individuals, and the highest incidence rates are reported in Australia. Its incidence is lower in the black population, as expected. On the other hand, patients receiving long-term PUVA therapy are also at increased risk of developing squamous cell carcinoma. The tumor may arise on sun-damaged but otherwise normal skin or progress from in situ carcinomas such as actinic keratosis (see Fig. 11.98), Bowen disease

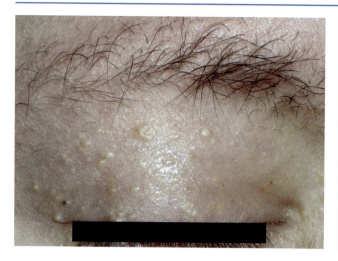

Fig. 11.96 A patient with Bazex-Dupré-Christol syndrome. Note the hair abnormality on the eyebrow and milia on the eyelid

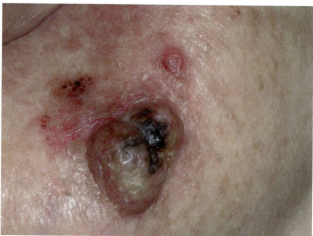

Fig. 11.98 Squamous cell carcinoma progressing from actinic keratosis; other actinic keratoses are also noticeable in the vicinity of the large tumor

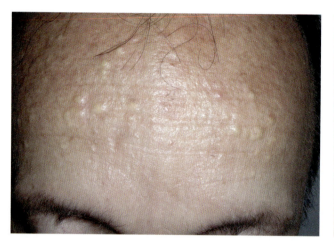

Fig. 11.97 Profuse milia on the face of a patient with Bazex-Dupré-Christol syndrome

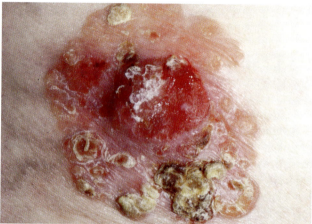

Fig. 11.99 Squamous cell carcinoma evolving from Bowen disease. Note the central nodule representing malignant transformation (dermal invasion) of the large flat plaque

(*see* Fig. 11.99), actinic cheilitis (*see* Fig. 11.100), leukoplakia (*see* Fig. 11.101), and erythroplasia of Queyrat.

Furthermore, the incidence of squamous cell carcinoma is markedly increased in some genodermatoses such as xeroderma pigmentosum (*see* Fig. 11.102), which is characterized by deficient repair of DNA damage induced by ultraviolet radiation; or albinism, this in turn is associated with the absence of photo-protective melanin. In patients with xeroderma pigmentosum other skin malignancies, particularly basal cell carcinoma (*see* Fig. 11.103) and malignant melanoma, may also be found. Squamous cell carcinoma may also develop on precancerous lesions such as the scars of some chronic infectious diseases like lupus vulgaris (*see* Fig. 11.104), inflammatory dermatoses like discoid lupus erythematosus (*see* Fig. 11.105), chronic radiodermatitis (*see* Fig. 11.106), long-standing ulcers, and draining sinuses or fistula (*see* Fig. 11.107). Hypertrophic lichen planus may also be rarely a precancerous lesion of squamous cell carci-

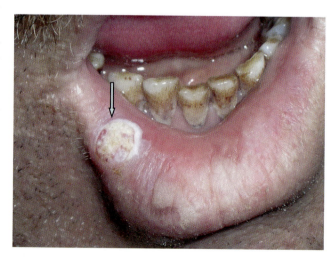

Fig. 11.100 Squamous cell carcinoma (*arrow*) arising from actinic cheilitis on the lower lip. A raised nodule should be alarming for malignant transformation

11.2 Squamous Cell Carcinoma

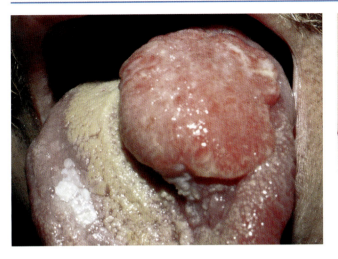

Fig. 11.101 Intraoral squamous cell carcinoma developing on leukoplakia. Note the white patch of leukoplakia (*left side*) in addition to the tumoral mass (*right side*)

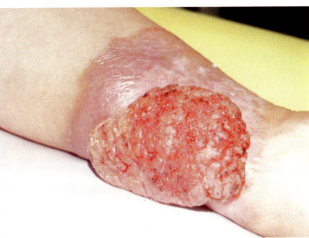

Fig. 11.104 Large squamous cell carcinoma arising on the scar of lupus vulgaris

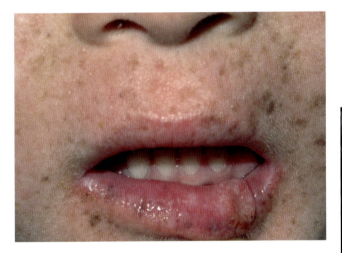

Fig. 11.102 Squamous cell carcinoma on the lower lip of a patient with xeroderma pigmentosum

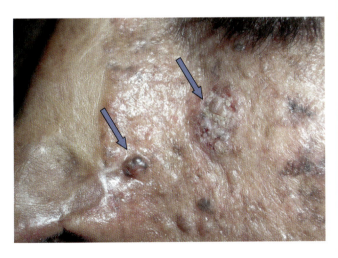

Fig. 11.103 A pigmented basal cell carcinoma on the nose (*left arrow*) and a squamous cell carcinoma with a hyperkeratotic surface on the cheek (*right arrow*) in a patient with xeroderma pigmentosum

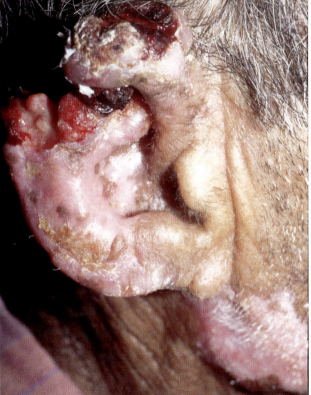

Fig. 11.105 Squamous cell carcinoma developing on the scar of discoid lupus erythematosus. The tumor caused serious cartilage destruction in this case. (With kind permission from Springer Science+Business Media: Baykal C, Yazganoğlu KD. Dermatological diseases of the nose and ears; 2010)

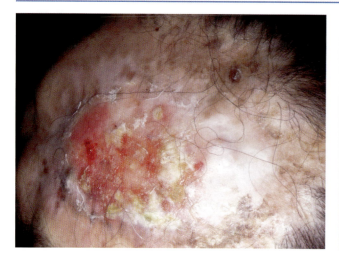

Fig. 11.106 Squamous cell carcinoma occurring on the site of chronic radiodermatitis. Note the ill-defined ulceration

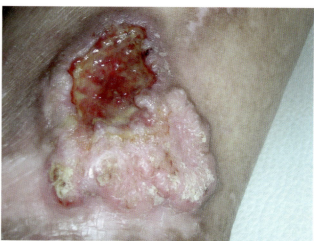

Fig. 11.108 A large ulcerated squamous cell carcinoma arising on the scar of hypertrophic lichen planus on the leg

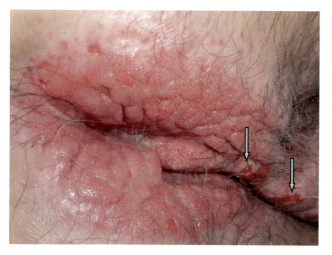

Fig. 11.107 Squamous cell carcinoma (*arrows*) arising on a chronic perianal fistula

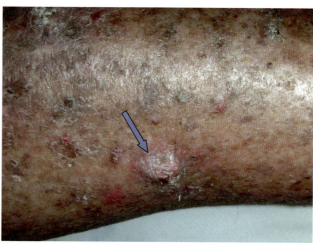

Fig. 11.109 Squamous cell carcinoma in an organ transplant recipient (*arrow*). Note also the many verrucal keratoses on the legs

noma (*see* Fig. 11.108). Drug-induced immunosuppression, especially seen after organ transplantation, is another major risk factor for this carcinoma (*see* Figs. 11.109 and 11.110). In metastatic melanoma patients treated with vemurafenib, squamous cell carcinoma may arise in a short time.

Squamous cell carcinoma mostly occurs in middle-aged or elderly patients. Since cumulative ultraviolet exposure plays a major role in the etiology, the incidence increases with age. It is more common in men than women. Most squamous cell carcinomas arise on sun-exposed sites. Thus, the head and neck, the dorsum of the hands (*see* Fig. 11.111) and forearms (*see* Fig. 11.112) are the preferred sites. The cheeks, forehead (*see* Fig. 11.113), and nose (*see* Fig. 11.114) are the predominant locations on the face. Lesions may be located on the scalp, especially in males with androgenetic alopecia. On the other hand, squamous cell carcinoma may occur anywhere on the skin and also on some unexpected sites

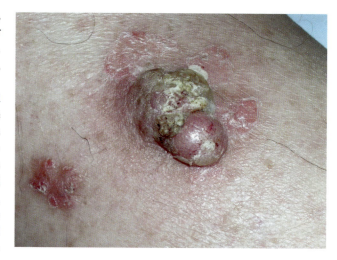

Fig. 11.110 Squamous cell carcinoma presenting as an irregular nodularity on the leg of an immunosuppressed patient

11.2 Squamous Cell Carcinoma

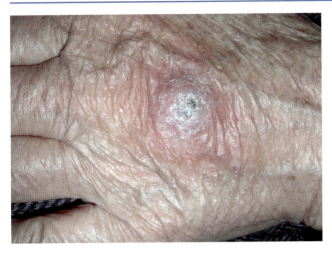

Fig. 11.111 Squamous cell carcinoma on the dorsum of the hand, a typical sun-exposed site

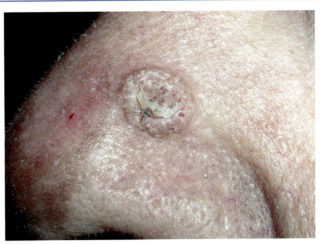

Fig. 11.114 Squamous cell carcinoma on the nose. Note the hyperkeratotic surface of an early lesion

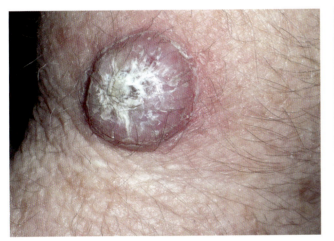

Fig. 11.112 Squamous cell carcinoma presenting as a dome-shaped nodule on the forearm

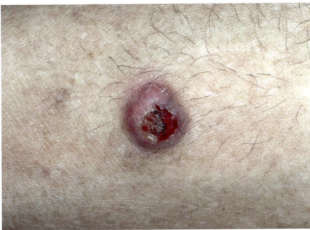

Fig. 11.115 Dome-shaped (round) squamous cell carcinoma with a superficial ulceration. This lesion had a short history of onset

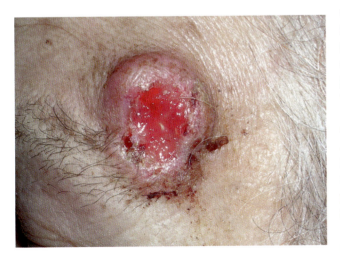

Fig. 11.113 Squamous cell carcinoma on the forehead. Face is a typical location

such as the genitalia and oral mucosa. In patients exposed to prolonged PUVA therapy tumors may be seen on body sites normally covered on the daily life. The tumor is usually solitary, but multiple lesions may be observed in organ transplant recipients, in melanoma patients under therapy with vemurafenib, and in patients with xeroderma pigmentosum.

The lesion begins as an erythematous papule or nodule (*see* Figs. 11.111 and 11.115). The size of the tumor is usually 0.5 to 1.5 cm at the time of diagnosis (*see* Fig. 11.116). It usually grows in a few months but rarely expands as rapidly as a keratoacanthoma. Furthermore, tumors occurring in patients under therapy with vemurafenib may also show rapid tumor enlargement. A skin-colored to dull red, mildly scaly, dome-shaped nodule (*see* Fig. 11.112) or indurated plaque is a typical presentation. The outline of the tumor may be round (*see* Fig. 11.112), oval (*see* Fig. 11.116), or irregular (*see* Fig. 11.110). The surface of the asymptomatic

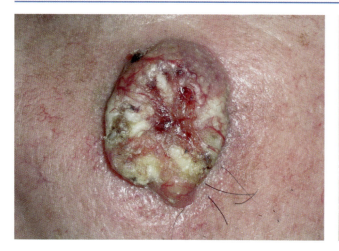

Fig. 11.116 Squamous cell carcinoma presenting as an oval-shaped nodule 1.5 cm in diameter

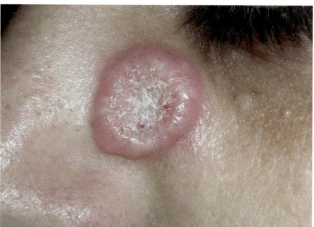

Fig. 11.118 Centrally depressed lesion of squamous cell carcinoma

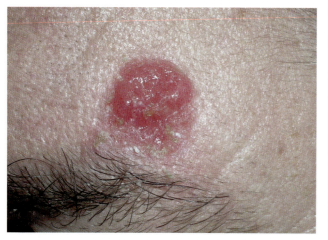

Fig. 11.117 A nodule of squamous cell carcinoma with a raw eroded surface

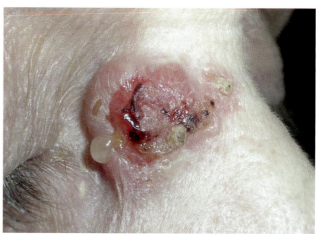

Fig. 11.119 Shallow ulceration on squamous cell carcinoma

tumor may be smooth, hyperkeratotic (*see* Figs. 11.103 and 11.114), papillomatous or eroded (*see* Fig. 11.117). Some lesions are centrally depressed (*see* Fig. 11.118), similar to those in keratoacanthoma (*see* Fig. 2.65). A central shallow ulceration occurs mostly in the early period (*see* Fig. 11.119). In time the entire surface of the lesions may become ulcerated (*see* Figs. 11.120 and 11.121) and covered by hemorrhagic crusts (*see* Fig. 11.122). Weeping, purulation, and malodorous scent may be additional findings in these cases.

In neglected cases the tumor may present as a large mass (*see* Figs. 11.123 and 11.124) and may also show invasion beyond the skin. It is generally more elevated than basal cell carcinoma, and the typical pearly rolled border of the latter tumor (*see* Fig. 11.36) is not seen. Contrary to keratoacanthoma, there is no tendency to spontaneous healing. Another clinical diagnostic challenge is atypical fibroxanthoma (*see* Fig. 13.64). Adequate tissue of the epidermis and dermis should be obtained

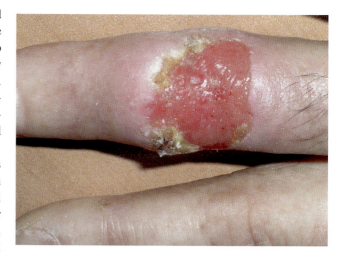

Fig. 11.120 The entire surface of the squamous cell carcinoma may become ulcerated as seen in the figure on a finger lesion

11.2 Squamous Cell Carcinoma

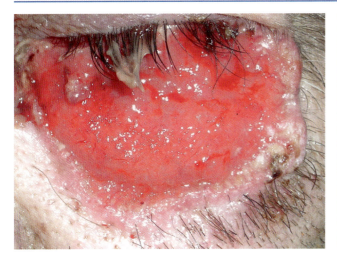

Fig. 11.121 Ulcerated squamous cell carcinoma on the face

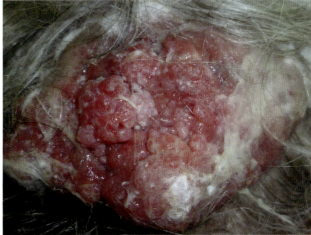

Fig. 11.124 A large ulcerated mass of squamous cell carcinoma

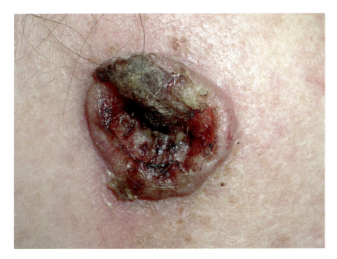

Fig. 11.122 Hemorrhagic crusts on ulcerated squamous cell carcinoma

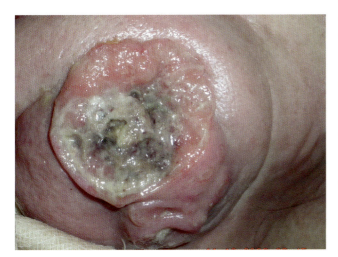

Fig. 11.123 A neglected lesion of squamous cell carcinoma presenting as a large mass on the chin

by a biopsy to confirm the diagnosis. Islands of atypical keratinocytes with abundant eosinophilic cytoplasm and large nuclei extending from the epidermis into the deeper dermis, dyskeratotic cells, and keratin pearls are histopathologic hallmarks of well-differentiated squamous cell carcinomas. In poorly differentiated tumors, anaplasia becomes prominent, and differential diagnosis from other cutaneous malignant tumors may be a challenge. Immunohistochemical markers such as high molecular weight keratins are helpful in such cases.

The course of squamous cell carcinoma is quite variable. Underlying immunosuppression, location of the tumor, and associated precursor or precancerous conditions are the predictive features of the prognosis. In immunosuppressed individuals, squamous cell carcinoma occurs at a younger age and has a relatively aggressive course. It is considered among the important causes of mortality in organ transplant recipients.

As mentioned above, more than half of the squamous cell carcinomas are located on sun-exposed areas. There is usually actinic damage on the surrounding skin. Lesions occurring on normal skin but in the setting of sun damage or arising from actinic keratoses have a relatively good prognosis with a very low metastatic rate. However, invasive squamous cell carcinoma progressing from Bowen disease has a relatively higher risk of metastasis. Squamous cell carcinoma may locate anywhere on the ear, especially on the helix (*see* Fig. 11.125). The metastatic rate of the ear lesions is higher than that of the lesions of the face. Invasive lesions of the external ear may result in destruction of cartilage (*see* Fig. 11.126) and, rarely, hearing loss.

The lower lip is directly exposed to sunlight and therefore is the most common location of squamous cell carcinoma. Nearly 90 percent of lip lesions are located on the lower lip (*see* Fig. 11.127), and they are seen mostly in patients with a history of chronic solar exposure. It may be associated with actinic cheilitis in some cases (*see* Fig. 11.100) and appears

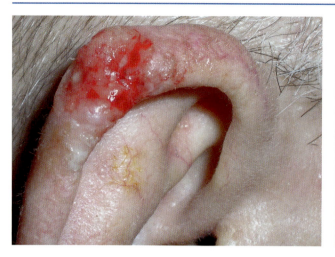

Fig. 11.125 Squamous cell carcinoma on the helix of the ear, a frequently affected area

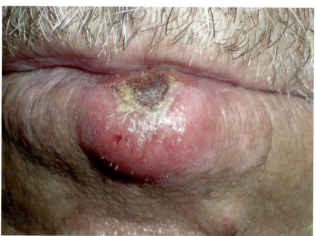

Fig. 11.127 Squamous cell carcinoma on the lower lip, the most common location of this tumor

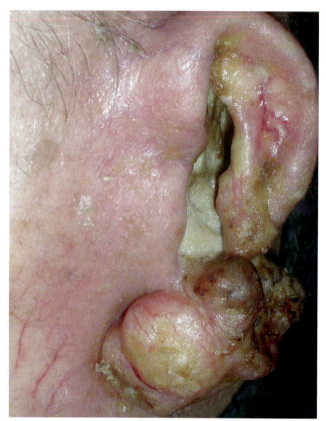

Fig. 11.126 Invasive squamous cell carcinoma seen as destroying the cartilage of the ear

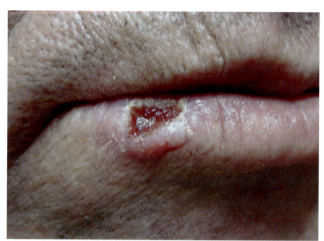

Fig. 11.128 Squamous cell carcinoma on the lateral side of the lower lip. The tumor is firm on palpation

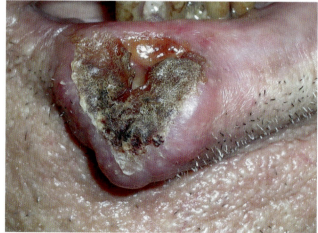

Fig. 11.129 Squamous cell carcinoma located on the lower lip. The tumor has everted margins and a central ulceration with crusting

mostly on the middle (*see* Fig. 11.127) or slightly lateral areas (*see* Figs. 11.128 and 11.129) of the lower lip. The tumor usually begins with a local thickening, and erosion or crusting may also be early findings (*see* Fig. 11.128). It grows progressively inward, outward, and laterally (*see* Figs. 11.130, 11.131 and 11.132). The lesions are usually elevated and indurated at the time of diagnosis (*see*

11.2 Squamous Cell Carcinoma

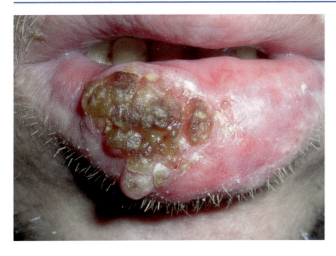

Fig. 11.130 Squamous cell carcinoma on the lower lip growing outward

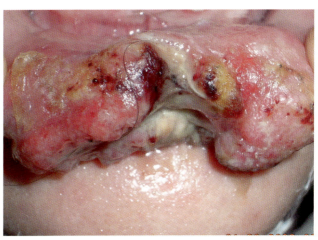

Fig. 11.133 A large irregular tumoral mass of a neglected squamous cell carcinoma destroying the lower lip

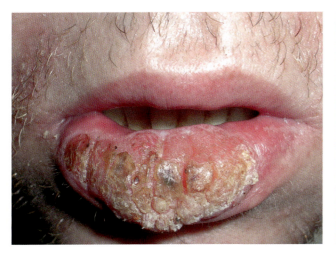

Fig. 11.131 A large squamous cell carcinoma on the lower lip growing both inward and outward

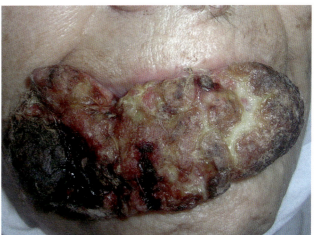

Fig. 11.134 A neglected squamous cell carcinoma presenting as a large exophytic mass on the lower lip with crusting on the surface

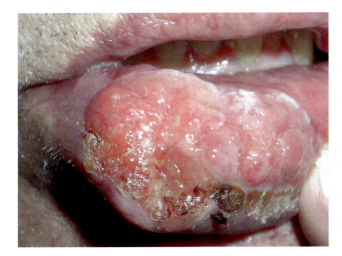

Fig. 11.132 Squamous cell carcinoma presenting as an elevated mass on the lower lip. Note the lateral growth of the lesion

Figs. 11.127 and 11.132). Secondary inflammation may also occur, and ulceration may be hidden by adherent crusts (*see* Figs. 11.129 and 11.131). The tumor bleeds easily. If neglected, large masses may also be seen on the lips (*see* Figs. 11.133 and 11.134). Squamous cell carcinoma on the lower lip is more aggressive than other lesions on the face. It may infiltrate the underlying musculature. Larger, thicker, and undifferentiated lesions tend to be more aggressive and to metastasize earlier. Furthermore the biological behavior of tumors located on the oral commissure are also usually more aggressive. Squamous cell carcinoma metastasizes primarily through the lymphatics in 5 to 20 percent of patients with lower lip involvement. Ipsilateral submandibular and submental node involvement is typical.

Squamous cell carcinoma may also be located intraorally (*see* Fig. 11.101) and is considered the most common malignant tumor of the oral cavity. Intraoral tumors are more

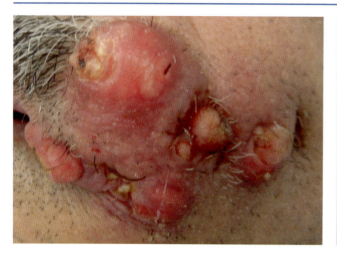

Fig. 11.135 Intraoral squamous cell carcinoma located on the buccal mucosa spreading through the facial muscles to the skin

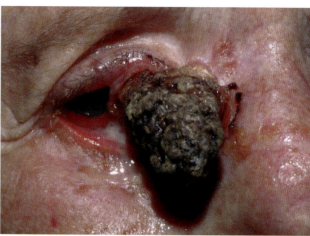

Fig. 11.137 Squamous cell carcinoma on the conjunctivae. Note the associated cutaneous horn

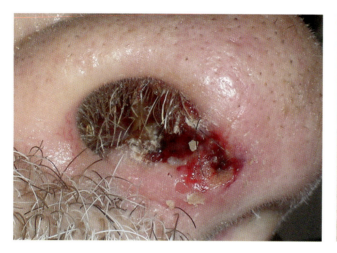

Fig. 11.136 Squamous cell carcinoma in the nasal vestibule

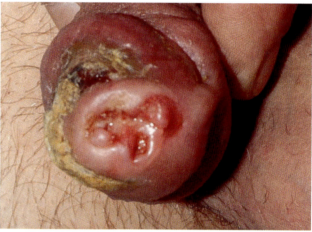

Fig. 11.138 Penile squamous cell carcinoma presenting as an irregular ulcerated mass with everted margins in a circumcised male

common in older men. Smoking and tobacco chewing are risk factors. The anterior floor of the mouth and anterior part of the tongue (see Fig. 11.101) are the most common locations. Tumors may also be located on the palate, tonsilla, gingivae, and buccal mucosa, especially on the oral commissure. They may occur de novo on normal mucosa or develop from precancerous lesions such as leukoplakia (see Figs. 2.40 and 11.101) and rarely erosive lichen planus. The tumor manifests mostly as an infiltrated or exophytic nodule or as a persistent erosion or ulceration. Initial lesions are asymptomatic and thus cannot be discovered early. If left untreated, the tumor may invade deep structures and may spread through muscles (see Fig. 11.135). The metastatic rate of intraoral squamous cell carcinoma is high.

Squamous cell carcinoma rarely begins in the nasal vestibule (see Fig. 11.136). In the case of diagnostic delay, it may be disseminated to the adjacent skin of the nose. Conjunctival squamous cell carcinoma is mostly seen in elderly and fair-skinned individuals. It is more common in the interpalpebral area of the perilimbal conjunctiva. It begins as a flesh-colored nodule (see Fig. 11.137), grows rapidly, and may be locally invasive. Symptoms of chronic conjunctivitis, decreased vision, and diplopia may be helpful in the diagnosis. There is a risk of metastasis to regional lymph nodes.

Anogenital region is a rare location for squamous cell carcinoma. Human papilloma virus is suggested to play a role in the development of lesions in this sun-protected area. If the genital region is not adequately protected during PUVA therapy, the risk of development of squamous cell carcinoma increases. HIV-infected patients have increased risk for anogenital carcinoma. Tumors at this site are more aggressive and have high metastatic potential. Penile lesions mostly occur on the glans of uncircumcised individuals. Erythroplasia of Queyrat and balanitis xerotica obliterans are the main precancerous lesions of male genitalia. The

11.2 Squamous Cell Carcinoma

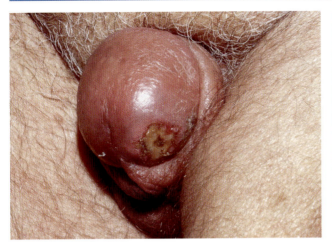

Fig. 11.139 Penile squamous cell carcinoma seen as a large mass with focal ulceration on the glans of a circumcised male

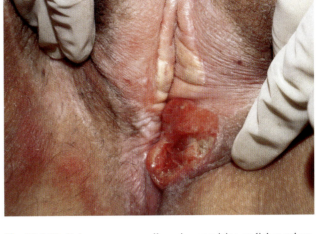

Fig. 11.141 Vulvar squamous cell carcinoma arising on lichen sclerosus et atrophicus

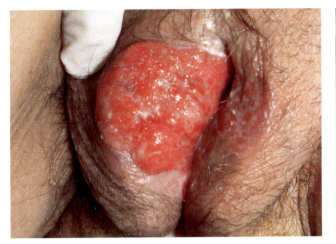

Fig. 11.140 Vulvar squamous cell carcinoma in an older woman

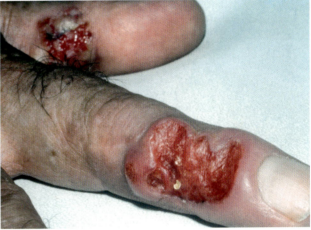

Fig. 11.142 Two squamous cell carcinomas on the fingers. The one on the index finger has progressed from Bowen disease

tumor has also rarely been observed in circumcised men (*see* Figs. 11.138 and 11.139), occasionally on the circumcision scar. Dorsal parts of the glans penis and sulcus coronarius are more commonly involved. The tumor may later invade deeper tissue and the urethra. Kaposi sarcoma (*see* Fig. 13.9) should be considered in the differential diagnosis of penile lesions. Squamous cell carcinoma of the vulva (*see* Figs. 11.140 and 11.141) occurs mostly in elderly patients. It may occur de novo (*see* Fig. 11.140) or on lichen sclerosus et atrophicus (*see* Fig. 11.141). It presents as a nodule or an infiltrated plaque, generally with an eroded or ulcerated surface, and may cause pruritus, pain, and bleeding. Perianal carcinomas begin as an indurated mass and may become protuberant in time. Diagnosis is mostly delayed in this location.

Squamous cell carcinoma may rarely present as acral tumors involving the fingers (*see* Figs. 11.120 and 11.142) and nail unit (*see* Fig. 11.143). Subungual tumors are mostly located on the nailfolds. Early symptoms of the tumor such as erythema, swelling, and pain are similar to those of paronychia,

and in the advanced cases the tumor may lead to nail destruction. It may be associated with HPV 16. Bowen disease located on the periungual area or on the fingers (*see* Fig. 11.142) may be the precursor lesion of the carcinoma. Dentists who have used their terminal phalanx during x-ray films in the past are also at increased risk of developing squamous cell carcinoma on the exposed fingers. Huriez syndrome is a rare autosomal dominant palmoplantar keratoderma syndrome associated with scleroatrophy and sclerodactyly on the hands (*see* Fig. 11.144), hypoplastic nail changes, and an increased risk of squamous cell carcinoma development in the scleroatrophic areas (*see* Figs. 11.144 and 11.145). Carcinoma may occur at early age and may metastasize.

Ulcerating squamous cell carcinoma arising on the scars of chronically inflamed skin lesions such as thermal burn scars (*see* Figs. 11.146 and 11.147), chronic venous ulcers, draining sinuses, and fistulous tracts (as in hidradenitis suppurativa) (*see* Fig. 11.148) are called Marjolin ulcer. It is

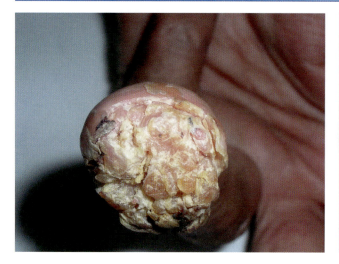

Fig. 11.143 Subungual squamous cell carcinoma causing a large mass on the fingertip extending to the subungual area

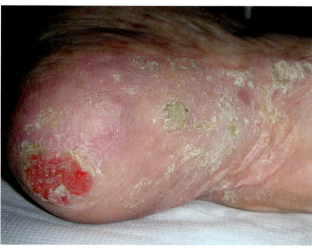

Fig. 11.146 Ulcerating squamous cell carcinoma on the heel arising on the scar of a thermal burn (Marjolin ulcer)

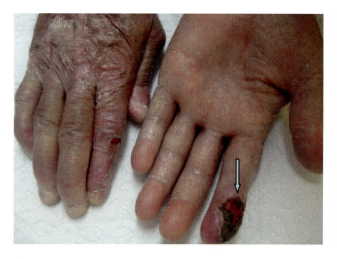

Fig. 11.144 Squamous cell carcinoma (*arrow*) located on the volar aspect of the finger with sclerodactyly in patient with Huriez syndrome

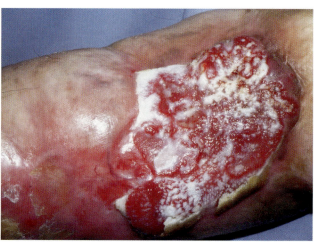

Fig. 11.147 Squamous cell carcinoma shown presenting as a large ulcerated mass arising on the scar of a thermal burn

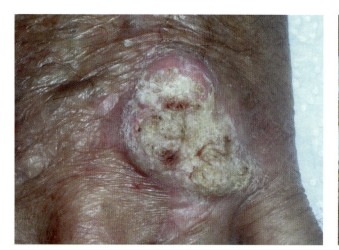

Fig. 11.145 Squamous cell carcinoma developing on scleroatrophic skin of the dorsum of the hand in a patient with Huriez syndrome

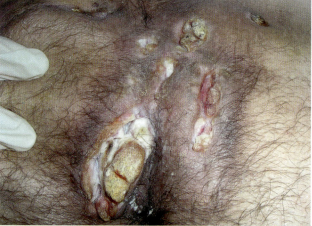

Fig. 11.148 Ulcerating squamous cell carcinoma arising on the chronic fistulous tract of hidradenitis suppurativa. Note the multifocal hyperkeratotic lesions

11.2 Squamous Cell Carcinoma

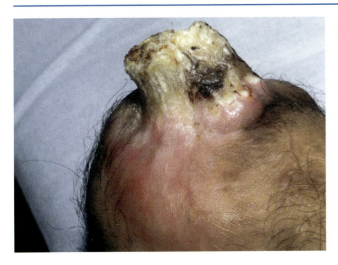

Fig. 11.149 Squamous cell carcinoma with overlying cornu cutaneum arising on the scar of the amputation stump

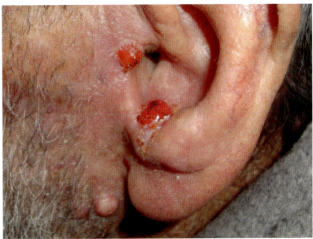

Fig. 11.151 A subcutaneous nodule near the earlobe representing the in-transit metastasis of ulcerated squamous cell carcinoma on the ear

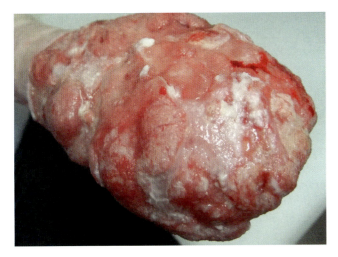

Fig. 11.150 Squamous cell carcinoma arising on the chronic ulceration of epidermolysis bullosa. Note multiple hyperkeratotic nodules

more common on the lower limbs. A recently developing induration, persistent nodule, or ulceration on the above-mentioned lesions should arouse suspicion for this subtype of squamous cell carcinoma. The tumor grows slowly but has an aggressive course. Chronic radiodermatitis (*see* Fig. 11.106), atrophic scars of discoid lupus erythematosus (*see* Fig. 11.105), scars of lupus vulgaris (*see* Fig. 11.104), amputation stump scars (*see* Fig. 11.149), porokeratosis Mibelli, and erythema ab igne are also among precancerous lesions of squamous cell carcinoma. Furthermore, squamous cell carcinoma is a major cause of mortality in severe forms of epidermolysis bullosa (*see* Fig. 11.150) and can occur at a younger age. The carcinoma diagnosis may be delayed owing to the presence of multiple erosions, chronic ulcers, and scars concomitantly occurring in the course of this chronic bullous dermatosis. The risk of metastasis is high in these patients.

Immunosuppressed patients are at a high risk of developing squamous cell carcinoma. Organ transplantation such as of the heart, kidney, and liver increases the risk of tumor development significantly in the following decades. Tumors located on the trunk and extremities are common in these patients (*see* Figs. 11.109 and 11.110).

11.2.1 Metastatic Squamous Cell Carcinoma

In general, squamous cell carcinoma has a low metastatic potential. But as described earlier, the risk of metastasis may be relatively higher depending on the etiologic factors, size and location of the tumors, level of infiltration, and poor differentiation in histopathologic examination. Tumors developing from actinic keratoses are not frequently associated with metastasis. The incidence of metastasis is also low for squamous cell carcinomas arising on normal skin sites with chronic sun damage, but it is higher on the lower lip. Patients with lesions of the oral cavity and anogenital area are also at a high risk of developing metastases. Regardless of location, tumors developing in immunosuppressed patients and lesions occurring in scars all carry a high risk of metastasis. Histopathologic features such as undifferentiated tumor and perineural involvement are also in that category.

Squamous cell carcinoma usually metastasizes first to the regional lymph nodes. Therefore careful palpation of the regional lymph nodes and additional radiologic examinations such as ultrasonography are especially helpful in determining the lymph node involvement. Dermal in-transit metastases appearing with papules or nodules may rarely occur (*see* Fig. 11.151). Distant metastases to visceral organs such as the lungs, liver, bones, and brain may also be found in long-standing or high-risk lesions. After the occurrence of metastasis, squamous cell carcinoma has a poor prognosis with a high mortality rate.

Management. Squamous cell carcinoma is a malignant tumor with a variable metastatic potential influenced by multiple factors that affect the choice of the therapeutic modality. Therefore, determining the risk of the tumor can be an initial step in patient management. The location and size of the tumor, the underlying condition, and the existence of metastasis all play a prominent role when deciding on the therapeutic modality. In general, all tumors should be treated as early as possible to achieve good cosmetic results and minimal dysfunction. Excisional surgery is usually the therapy of choice. Simple removal, including subcutaneous fat tissue, results in the cure of early small lesions. Mohs micrographic surgery is generally used for larger lesions, for tumors on high-risk sites, and those arising on scars. Reconstructive surgery may also be indicated in some cases with large lesions. Extensive lesions on the acral sites of the limbs or involvement of bones may be an indication for amputation.

The risk of local recurrence is increased in the first years of the follow-up period. It is associated significantly with the size of the tumor, and the risk is higher in tumors that are excised especially with narrow surgical margins. Recurrence may be confined to deep tissues and rarely may initially cause neurologic symptoms. Recurrent tumors have a high risk of metastasis.

If surgery is contraindicated, radiotherapy may be the main treatment option. However, it is difficult to identify the tumor margins accurately with this method. It is more commonly preferred in old patients. Adjuvant radiotherapy may also be applied after surgery in high-risk tumors.

Destructive methods such as curettage and electrodesiccation or cryotherapy followed by the use of topical imiquimod cream may be used infrequently in cases in which surgery cannot be performed or in selected low-risk lesions such as small tumors evolving from actinic keratosis. However, these methods are not efficacious in deeper lesions.

In cases with lymph node involvement, regional nodal dissection followed by adjuvant radiotherapy or systemic chemotherapy is indicated. Chemotherapy may also be used for inoperable tumors and visceral metastasis. However, the results are not always satisfactory.

In addition to therapy, prevention is also essential for this type of skin carcinoma. Patients diagnosed with squamous cell carcinoma carry a lifetime risk of developing a second non–melanoma skin cancer anywhere on the body. Therefore regular sun protection, including extra protection of the lower lip, should be advised. Strict sun avoidance may decrease the incidence of skin carcinoma development in patients with xeroderma pigmentosum, albinism, and organ transplant recipients. Administration of systemic retinoids as prophylaxis can be effective in organ transplant recipients with multiple cutaneous carcinomas and in xeroderma pigmentosum patients.

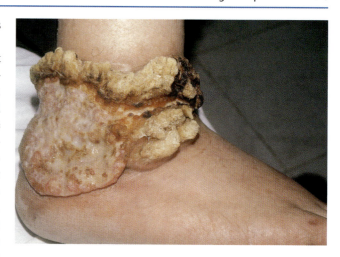

Fig. 11.152 Cutaneous verrucous carcinoma manifesting as a large vegetating mass on the leg

Precancerous lesions should be treated early. In patients with oral cancer, use of tobacco and alcohol should be prohibited. Patients with epidermolysis bullosa or with high-risk precursor lesions such as scars should be warned against the risk of developing new nodules or ulcerations on these areas. These patients need a careful and close follow-up for early detection of squamous cell carcinoma.

After the treatment of squamous cell carcinoma, patients require close surveillance. While the lesion site should be monitored for recurrence, other parts of the body should be examined for another primary non–melanoma skin cancer. In addition, regional lymph nodes should be placed under periodic surveillance.

11.3 Verrucous Carcinoma

Verrucous carcinoma is a distinct type of squamous cell carcinoma characterized by a slow growing, locally invasive course and has low metastatic potential. As opposed to classic squamous cell carcinoma, sun damage is not viewed as an etiologic factor. Three variants related to the anatomic site have been described: oral florid papillomatosis in the mouth, Buschke-Löwenstein tumor on the anogenital area, and carcinoma cuniculatum on the palmoplantar area. Moreover, it may rarely be seen on other areas of the skin such as the leg (cutaneous verrucous carcinoma) (*see* Fig. 11.152).

11.3.1 Oral Florid Papillomatosis (Aerodigestive Verrucous Carcinoma)

Oral florid papillomatosis presents as a grayish or white, soft verrucous lesion (*see* Figs. 11.153 and 11.154) that may be exophytic (cauliflower-like) and extensive. It may be

11.3 Verrucous Carcinoma

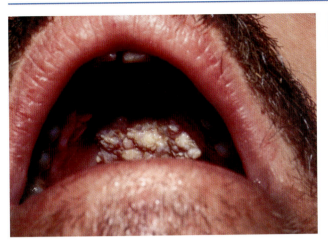

Fig. 11.153 Oral florid papillomatosis (aerodigestive verrucous carcinoma) presenting as a white verrucous lesion on the palate

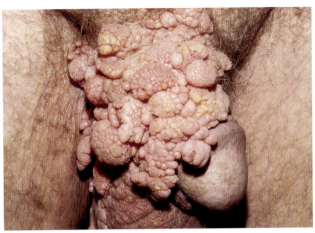

Fig. 11.155 Buschke-Löwenstein tumor (anogenital verrucous carcinoma) presenting as a condyloma acuminata-like vegetating mass

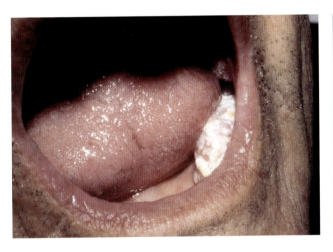

Fig. 11.154 Oral florid papillomatosis shown as a white verrucous lesion on the floor of the mouth

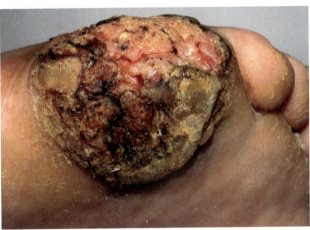

Fig. 11.156 A sharply demarcated, slightly elevated large plaque on the sole representing carcinoma cuniculatum

localized anywhere in the oral cavity, but involvement of the buccal mucosa is most common. Verrucous leukoplakia (*see* Fig. 2.48) and white sponge nevus (*see* Fig. 1.136) are the main differential diagnostic challenges but the latter appears at a younger age. The tumor may be ulcerated in the advanced stages. Invasion of the underlying soft tissue and bone may be seen in neglected cases.

11.3.2 Buschke-Löwenstein Tumor (Anogenital Verrucous Carcinoma)

Buschke-Löwenstein tumor is a verrucous carcinoma presenting as a condyloma acuminata-like vegetating lesion (*see* Fig. 11.155). It is more common on the glans and prepuce of the penis in uncircumcised middle-aged men. The anus, vulva, vagina, and scrotum may also rarely be involved. Ulceration and fistulae may be seen on the advanced lesions.

11.3.3 Carcinoma Cuniculatum

Carcinoma cuniculatum is the most common form of verrucous carcinoma and is usually found on the plantar surface of the feet and rarely on the palms. It is more common in older men. The initial solitary papular lesion with a hyperkeratotic surface is clinically similar to verruca plantaris and therefore the diagnosis might be delayed. The lesion becomes larger (*see* Fig. 11.156) and exophytic in time (*see* Fig. 11.157). Ulceration may also be observed. This tumor also has a tendency to endophytic growth, invading underlying tissues, including tendons, muscles, and bones in the late stage. It then becomes indurated and painful. Sinus formation associated with discharge is also possible. Acral lentiginous melanoma (*see* Fig. 12.32) and Kaposi sarcoma (*see* Fig. 13.21) may be considered in the differential diagnosis of ulcerated lesions. Radiologic examinations such as MRI and CT may be helpful to show the depth of the invasion of the tumor.

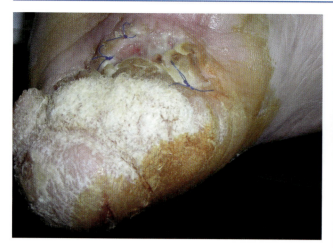

Fig. 11.157 Carcinoma cuniculatum manifesting as a hyperkeratotic exophytic lesion on the heel. In this case multiple biopsies were performed to confirm the diagnosis

Histopathologically, exophytic and endophytic epidermal thickening and hyperkeratosis are the main findings of verrucous carcinoma, and keratinocyte atypia is minimal. At the dermoepidermal junction the rete ridges are broad and have a "pushing" border toward the underlying dermis. Because the keratin layer and epidermis are considerably thickened, a deep and large incisional biopsy is needed to confirm the diagnosis. Multiple biopsies may be required, especially in carcinoma cuniculatum. It is well known that anogenital verrucous carcinoma can only be differentiated from condyloma acuminata by its histopathologic features.

Management. Although verrucous carcinoma is considered a low-grade malignancy, it is difficult to eradicate the primary tumor. Mohs micrographic surgery is the therapy of choice. Radiotherapy is not a first option as the tumor may sometimes become more aggressive (anaplastic transformation). This method is only used if surgery is amenable. Patients should be followed up carefully because of the risk of local recurrence (*see* Fig. 11.158). Prognosis of recurrent lesions is considered to be poor.

11.4 Malignant Adnexal Tumors

Malignant adnexal tumors can be categorized according to their origin and differentiation into follicular, sebaceous, eccrine, and apocrine structures. Malignant adnexal tumors, particularly carcinomas with differentiation to sweat glands, are difficult to classify as eccrine or apocrine.

11.4.1 Sebaceous Carcinoma

Sebaceous carcinoma is a malignant tumor that originates from the sebaceous glands and shows an aggressive biological behavior. It is more commonly seen on the eyelid (ocu-

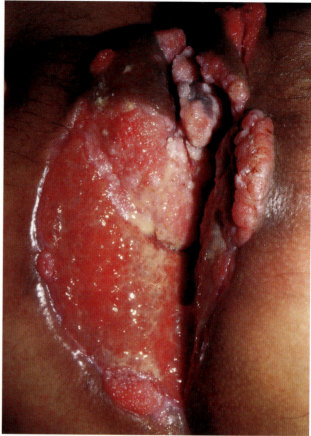

Fig. 11.158 Local recurrence of anogenital verrucous carcinoma on the excision site

lar type), scalp, and face, where sebaceous glands are numerous. However, it may be seen anywhere on the skin where sebaceous glands are present. Ocular sebaceous carcinoma is derived from the modified sebaceous glands (Meibomian and Zeis glands). It rarely arises on nevus sebaceus. Most sebaceous carcinomas are sporadic, but like some benign sebaceous tumors they may be the sign of Muir-Torre syndrome, which is associated with visceral malignancies.

Sebaceous carcinoma is more common in older patients. Involvement of the lower eyelid is more common than the upper one. It begins as a slightly erythematous painless nodule (*see* Fig. 11.159). Because it has clinical similarities to chronic conjunctivitis or chalazion, the proper diagnosis is often delayed at this location.

Extraocular sebaceous carcinoma may arise as yellow or pinkish papule or nodule with telangiectatic vessels. Involvement of head and neck is more common, but it may occur anywhere on the skin. The tumor grows slowly and may develop into a large mass with ulcerated surface (*see* Fig. 11.160). Lesions tend to bleed easily. Clinically many benign and malignant skin tumors, including basal cell carcinoma, squamous cell carcinoma and other malignant adnexal tumors may be considered in the differential diagnosis. Histopathologic examination reveals large masses of

11.4 Malignant Adnexal Tumors

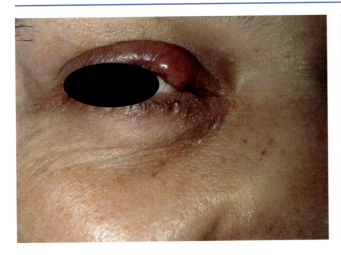

Fig. 11.159 Ocular sebaceous carcinoma presenting as an erythematous nodule of the upper eyelid

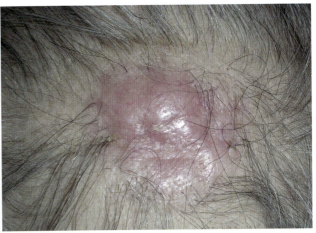

Fig. 11.161 Secondary infiltration of adenoid cystic parotid gland carcinoma. Note the indurated alopecic plaque on the scalp

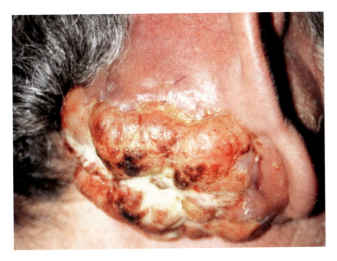

Fig. 11.160 A large ulcerated tumor of extraocular sebaceous carcinoma

pleomorphic cells with centrally located hyperchromatic nuclei. The cytoplasm occasionally shows a microvacuolated appearance reminiscent of sebaceous differentiation. This has to be confirmed either by immunohistochemistry as epithelial membrane antigen (EMA) or androgen receptor positivity, by lipid stains on fresh frozen tissue, or by electron microscopic examination. Prompt diagnosis is essential for a better prognosis.

This tumor first metastasizes to draining lymph nodes and later visceral metastasis may occur.

Management. Patients diagnosed with either ocular or extraocular sebaceous carcinoma and their family members should be checked for visceral cancers commonly occurring in the setting of Muir-Torre syndrome. Treatment of the skin tumor generally includes excision with wide margins or Mohs micrographic surgery. Adjuvant regional radiotherapy may also be used. However, local recurrence is possible. Regional lymph node dissection should be planned for nodal metastasis. In cases with visceral metastasis, systemic chemotherapy should be considered. Cases associated with Muir-Torre syndrome have a better prognosis.

11.4.2 Primary Cutaneous Adenoid Cystic Carcinoma

Primary adenoid cystic carcinoma of the skin is a rare eccrine gland carcinoma characterized by a slowly invasive course and a risk of visceral metastasis. It is mostly seen in middle-aged or older patients showing female predominance. It usually appears on the scalp and face as a pink- to skin-colored, poorly defined, firm intradermal or subcutaneous nodule measuring 0.5 to 8 cm in diameter. It may also be seen on the trunk and extremities. The lesion may be associated with regional alopecia. Clinical features are not distinguishing, and the diagnosis is based on histopathology. The histologic hallmarks are the cribriform pattern seen in large nests of small basaloid cells and the very infiltrative pattern. Basophilic-staining mucinous material fills the cribriform spaces. Basal cell carcinoma of the adenoid histologic type may be confused with this malignancy.

The tumor grows slowly, but if neglected, it may become a large mass. Lung and lymph node metastases are seen in nearly 20 percent of the patients. A detailed radiologic investigation for metastasis should be performed after diagnostic confirmation. On the other hand, adenoid cystic parotid gland carcinoma may also rarely spread to the skin (*see* Fig. 11.161) causing a similar histologic appearance.

Management. Wide excision with large margins or Mohs micrographic surgery is the therapy of choice. However, local recurrence is frequent, possibly due to the perineural invasion of the tumor. Chemotherapy is indicated in the treatment of metastatic disease. Close follow-up of the patients is mandatory.

11.4.3 Microcystic Adnexal Carcinoma (Sclerosing Sweat Duct Carcinoma)

Microcystic adnexal carcinoma is a rare, locally aggressive tumor with a disputed histogenesis. It has been previously believed that the tumor showed pure eccrine differentiation, but recently, a combination of eccrine, apocrine, sebaceous and follicular differentiation, namely mixed adnexal lineage of the tumor has been shown. Most patients are middle-aged adults. Nasolabial folds, periorbital areas and the lips are typical locations on the face. Rarely, other body sites can be involved. As the tumor grows very slowly, it may be misdiagnosed as a benign tumor. It presents as a nodule or an indurated plaque with indistinct borders. Morphoeic basal cell carcinoma (see Fig. 11.63) is a common clinical pitfall in the differential diagnosis. A deep biopsy including the base of the tumor is required for a proper diagnosis. Histopathology reveals ducts and nests of small epithelial cells without prominent atypia and islands and chords of squamous epithelial cells and horn cysts in the dermis and subcutaneous tissue. Perineural and intraneural invasion is typical, and infiltration of the deep underlying tissues, extending through muscles, may occur in time. However metastasis to distant sites is not expected.

Management. Mohs micrographic surgery is the best therapeutic approach, since delineation of tumor margins is difficult. Local recurrence is frequent because of the invasion of deep tissue and perineural spreading of the advanced tumors (see Fig. 11.162).

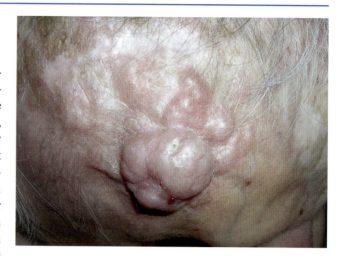

Fig. 11.162 Recurrent microcystic adnexal carcinoma presenting as multiple indurated nodules close to the excision site

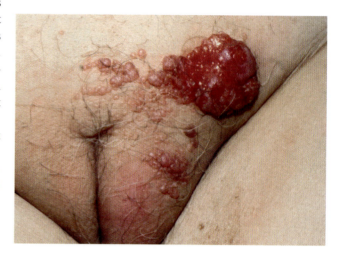

Fig. 11.163 Multiple skin-colored and reddish nodules of hidradenocarcinoma located on the pubic area

11.4.4 Hidradenocarcinoma

Hidradenocarcinoma is a very rare tumor with metastatic potential. It is accepted as the malignant counterpart of hidradenoma and may be of eccrine or apocrine origin. It may arise on normal skin but may also originate from a pre-existing hidradenoma. It is more common in older patients. It may be located anywhere on the skin. A typical clinical feature has not been described, but most tumors appear as reddish nodules and poorly defined margins (see Fig. 11.163). Histologically a dermal tumor with solid sheets or nodules of clear cells with intracytoplasmic vacuoles is seen. Cytoplasmic membranes are distinct. Cellular pleomorphism is prominent. Evidence of benign hidradenoma remnants may be detected. Regional lymph node metastasis may occur in 1 to 2 years, and involvement of distant lymph nodes and visceral metastasis worsen the prognosis.

Management. Surgical excision, regional lymph node dissection, and chemotherapy are the main therapeutic modalities. However, there may be local recurrence (see Fig. 11.164) and metastases may cause death.

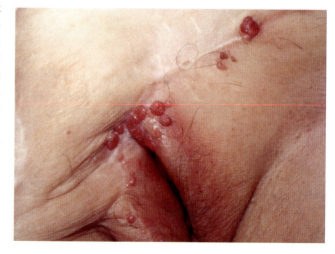

Fig. 11.164 Local recurrence of hidradenocarcinoma. Note the multiple papules and nodules around the excision scar

11.4.5 Porocarcinoma (Malignant Eccrine Poroma)

Porocarcinoma is the malignant counterpart of poroma. It is the most common eccrine carcinoma. This adnexal tumor may occur de novo or may be associated with pre-existing poroma. It may rarely arise on nevus sebaceus. The lower extremities, especially the feet, face, and buttocks, are the most common locations but it may occur anywhere.

A reddish verrucous plaque or a polypoid mass with ulceration may be the clinical presentation (*see* Fig. 11.165). The differentiation from seborrheic keratosis, squamous cell carcinoma, Merkel cell carcinoma, and amelanotic melanoma can be determined by skin biopsy. It may completely be intraepidermal or may invade into the dermis. Poroid small cells sharply demarcated from the adjacent epidermis, solid broad cords and columns of cells extending from the epidermis toward the deep dermis, and sometimes ductal lumina and cyst formation are the main histopathologic features.

The tumor may show an aggressive course. There is a risk of regional lymph node and visceral metastases. We have observed a cutaneous metastasis of porocarcinoma presenting as carcinoma erysipeloides (*see* Fig. 11.166).

Management. Wide surgical excision is the mainstay of the therapy. However, the tumor may recur on the excision site. Regional lymph node dissection and chemotherapy are used in metastatic cases.

11.5 Merkel Cell Carcinoma

Merkel cell carcinoma, also called neuroendocrine carcinoma of the skin, is a rare and highly aggressive neoplasm derived from Merkel cells that locate in the epidermis and have mechanoreceptor function. Merkel cell polyoma virus (MCV) is suggested to contribute to the pathogenesis of this neoplasm. It is more common in the older population and its incidence is also increased in immunocompromised individuals such as solid organ transplant recipients and HIV-infected patients. It is mainly located on sun-exposed skin sites such as the face, scalp, neck, and upper extremities but may also be seen on the trunk, buttocks, and lower extremities and on the mucosal surfaces. It manifests as a rapidly growing solitary tumor. A reddish, violet, or flesh-colored, raised, painless nodule with a mostly intact surface is clinically not distinctive (*see* Fig. 11.167). Larger tumors may be ulcerated. The differentiation from squamous cell carcinoma (*see* Fig. 11.110), angiosarcoma (*see* Fig. 13.48), and cutaneous lymphomas is possible after biopsy. Histologically, there is a dense infiltration of small cells in the dermis and invasion of subcutaneous tissue. The tumor cells may be arranged in a trabecular pattern and they frequently show nuclear molding. The cytoplasm is inconspic-

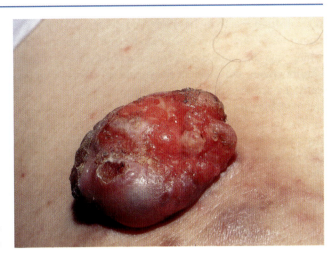

Fig. 11.165 A red polypoid mass of porocarcinoma (malignant eccrine poroma). Foci of ulceration are noticeable

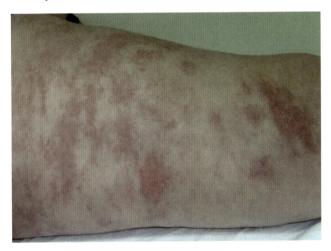

Fig. 11.166 Cutaneous metastasis of eccrine porocarcinoma manifesting as carcinoma erysipeloides on the leg. This is an exceptional presentation of this tumor

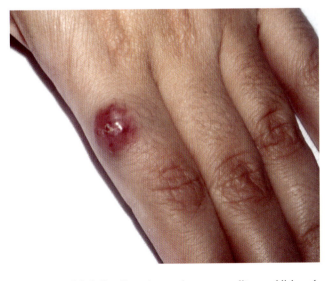

Fig. 11.167 Merkell cell carcinoma shown as a solitary reddish nodule on the finger

uous. Mitotic activity is high and apoptotic cells are numerous. They show neuroendocrine differentiation, which can be demonstrated immunohistochemically by chromogranin and other neuropeptide positivity. Tumoral cells characteristically show dot-like paranuclear cytoplasmic positivity for cytokeratin 20.

The tumor is highly aggressive and may invade underlying tissue in a relatively short time. Rarely, satellite skin lesions may also be seen. Regional lymph node metastasis is the first route of dissemination of the tumor, which may be followed by distant lymph node metastasis and visceral metastasis to the liver, brain, bone, and lungs.

Management. Early diagnosis and appropriate management are critical to decrease the mortality rate of Merkel cell carcinoma. Surgical excision with wide margins should be performed in all cases. Mohs micrographic surgery may be preferred and adjuvant radiotherapy may be administered. The recurrence rate is higher in larger tumors, and recurrent lesions may be multiple. Sentinel lymph node mapping and biopsy are indicated for all cases. Regional lymph node dissection combined with adjuvant regional radiotherapy to draining lymph nodes may improve survival in cases with nodal involvement. Chemotherapy may be used simultaneously with radiotherapy for nodal metastasis and additionally for systemic involvement. The efficacy of the therapy in cases with systemic metastases is limited. Immunosuppressed patients have the worst prognosis. Close follow-up is mandatory for all patients.

Suggested Reading

Ang JM, Alai NN, Ritter KR, Machtinger LA. Muir-Torre syndrome: case report and review of the literature. Cutis. 2011;87:125–8.

Attili SK, Evans A, Fleming CJ. Recurrent pigmented eccrine porocarcinoma presenting as carcinoma erysipeloides. Clin Exp Dermatol. 2009;30;e493–5.

Brantsch KD, Meisner C, Schoenfisch B, et al. Analysis of risk factors determining prognosis of cutaneous squamous-cell carcinoma: a prospective study. Lancet Oncol. 2008;9:713–20.

Burgdorf WHC, Plewig G, Wolff HH, Landthaler M. Braun-Falco's dermatology, edn 3. Italy: Springer-Verlag; 2009.

Calonje JE, Brenn T, Lazar AJ, McKee PH. McKee's pathology of the skin, edn 4. China: Elsevier; 2012.

Caputo R, Tadini G. Atlas of genodermatoses. Spain: Taylor and Francis; 2006.

Castori M, Morrone A, Kanitakis J, Grammatico P. Genetic skin diseases predisposing to basal cell carcinoma. Eur J Dermatol. 2012;22:299–309.

Ceilley RI, Del Rosso JQ. Current modalities and new advances in the treatment of basal cell carcinoma. Int J Dermatol. 2006;45:489–98.

Chu EY, Wanat KA, Miller CJ, et al. Diverse cutaneous side effects associated with BRAF inhibitor therapy: a clinicopathologic study. J Am Acad Dermatol. 2012;67:1265–72.

Gollnick H, Barona CG, Frank RG, et al. Recurrence rate of superficial basal cell carcinoma following treatment with imiquimod 5% cream: conclusion of a 5-year long-term follow-up study in Europe. Eur J Dermatol. 2008;18:677–82.

James WD, Berger T, Elston D. Andrew's diseases of the skin: Clinical Dermatology, edn 11. China: Saunders Elsevier; 2011.

Liu LS, Colegio OR. Molecularly targeted therapies for nonmelanoma skin cancers. Int J Dermatol. 2013;52:654–65.

Lortscher DN, Sengelmann RD, Allen SB. Acrochordon-like basal cell carcinomas in patients with basal cell nevus syndrome. Dermatol Online J. 2007;13:21.

Madan V, Lear JT, Szeimies R-M. Non-melanoma skin cancer. Lancet. 2010;375:673–85.

Mougel F, Kanitakis J, Faure M, Euvrard S. Basosquamous cell carcinoma in organ transplant patients: a clinicopathologic study. J Am Acad Dermatol. 2012;66:e151–7.

Nehal KS, Levine VJ, Ashinof R. Basal cell carcinoma of the genitalia. Dermatol Surg. 1998;24:1361–3.

Obaidat NA, Alsaad KO, Ghazarian D. Skin adnexal neoplasms–part 2: an approach to tumours of cutaneous sweat glands. J Clin Pathol. 2007;60:145–59.

Otley CC, Stasko T, Tope WD, Lebwohl M. Chemoprevention of nonmelanoma skin cancer with systemic retinoids: practical dosing and management of adverse effects. Dermatol Surg. 2006; 32:562–8.

Renzi C, Mastroeni S, Passarelli F, et al. Factors associated with large cutaneous squamous cell carcinomas. J Am Acad Dermatol. 2010;63:404–11.

Rigel DS, Robinson JK, Ross M, Friedman RJ, Corkerell CJ, Lim HW, Stockfleth HW, Kirkwood JM. Cancer of the skin, edn 2. China: Saunders Elsevier; 2011.

Robson A, Greene J, Ansari N, et al. Eccrine porocarcinoma (malignant eccrine poroma): a clinicopathologic study of 69 cases. Am J Surg Pathol. 2001;25:710–20.

Roewert-Huber J, Lange-Asschenfeldt B, Stockfleth E, Kerl H. Epidemiology and aetiology of basal cell carcinoma. Br J Dermatol. 2007;157:47–51.

Röwert-Huber J, Patel MJ, Forschner T, et al. Actinic keratosis is an early squamous cell carcinoma: a proposal for reclassification. Br J Dermatol. 2007;156:8–12.

Schwartz RA. Skin cancer: recognition and management, edn 2. Singapore: Blackwell Publishing; 2008.

Sekulic A, Migden MR, Oro AE, et al. Efficacy and safety of vismodegib in advanced basal-cell carcinoma. N Engl J Med. 2012;366:2171–9.

Shiohara J, Koga H, Uhara H, et al. Eccrine porocarcinoma: clinical and pathological studies of 12 cases. J Dermatol. 2007; 34:516–22.

Tang JY, Mackay-Wiggan JM, Aszterbaum M, et al. Inhibiting the hedgehog pathway in patients with the basal-cell nevus syndrome. N Engl J Med. 2012;366:2180–8.

Telfer NR, Colver GB, Morton CA; British Association of Dermatologists. Guidelines for the management of basal cell carcinoma. Br J Dermatol. 2008;159:35–48.

Vidal D, Matias-Guiu X, Alomar A. Fifty-five basal cell carcinomas treated with topical imiquimod: outcome at 5-year follow-up. Arch Dermatol. 2007;143:264–8.

Weedon D. Weedon's skin pathology, edn 3. China: Elsevier; 2010.

Wong CS, Strange RC, Lear JT. Basal cell carcinoma. BMJ. 2003;327:794–8.

Malignant Melanoma 12

Malignant melanoma is a tumor that arises from melanocytes and nevus cells. Skin is the most important site of malignant melanoma. However, rarely the oral mucosa, genital mucosae, eyes, leptomeninges, and other visceral organs may be the initial sites. It is the most common cause of death among skin diseases. It originates from the melanocytes of normal skin or from melanocytic nevi. Individuals with more than 100 melanocytic nevi are three to ten times more likely to develop malignant melanoma than others with fewer melanocytic nevi (*see* Fig. 12.1). Most melanoma patients present with a history of a newly developing lesion on normal skin. However, although the exact number is not definite, it is estimated that approximately 20 to 25 percent of melanoma patients have a pigmented lesion of long duration, namely, a precursor melanocytic nevus that has changed recently (*see* Fig. 12.2). Moreover, some types of melanoma develop very slowly, and therefore patients may not remember the prior lesion exactly. Sometimes only histopathologic examination may determine the origin of a melanoma arising from a melanocytic nevus. Malignant melanoma is mostly seen in adults. However, it may rarely be seen in childhood, especially in individuals with large congenital melanocytic nevi.

Genetic and environmental factors play role in the etiology of melanoma. Familial melanoma represent a small percentage of all cases. However, in last years, various genes involved in melanoma susceptibility, such as *CDKN2A* and *NC1R* have been identified, showing high or low risk. Excessive sun exposure is the major environmental risk factor of the melanoma causing neoplastic change in melanocytes. However, it is not related with all types of this heterogeneous tumor. BRAF mutation is common in lesions related with intermittent sun exposure and c-kit mutation in lesions without relation with sun damage, namely acral lentiginous melanoma. The clinical appearance of the primary tumor and the risk of metastasis are mainly related to the location of atypical melanocytes. The risk of metastasis increases as the tumor reaches deep tissues (dermis, subcutis), which are rich in blood and lymph vessels. Malignant melanoma can metastasize to neighboring skin, lymph nodes, and eventually to visceral organs as well as distant skin regions.

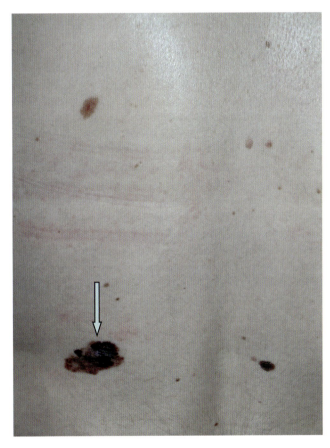

Fig. 12.1 Superficial spreading melanoma (*arrow*) in a patient with multiple dysplastic melanocytic nevi

Primary and metastatic melanomas of the skin have different clinical features. Both of them are discussed in this chapter.

12.1 Primary Cutaneous Malignant Melanoma

Most patients with melanoma have a solitary lesion and are usually otherwise healthy at diagnosis. The tumor may be located on any site of the skin or mucosae. Therefore, a

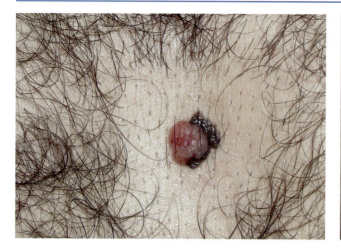

Fig. 12.2 Melanoma arising in a congenital melanocytic nevus

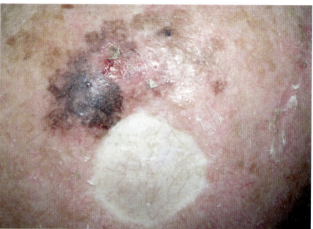

Fig. 12.3 Melanoma on the scalp of a bald male with severe sun damage. Note the adjacent excision scar of a squamous cell carcinoma

thorough dermatologic examination, including the scalp, intertriginous areas, and oral and genital mucosa is advised in melanoma screening. Four main types of primary cutaneous melanoma are described. Racial predisposition, location of the tumor, age of onset, biological behavior, and histopathologic features may differ according to the type. Apart from the nodular type, which shows dermal invasion from the onset, the other three main types of the tumor, namely, lentigo maligna melanoma, acral lentiginous melanoma, and superficial spreading melanoma, show biphasic development. Initially proliferating neoplastic cells stay confined to the epidermis, which is called the radial growth (in situ or microinvasive) phase. Subsequently they penetrate the dermoepidermal junction extending vertically to the dermis, which is the vertical growth phase. Lesions in the radial growth phase are flat, and tumors in the vertical growth phase have a more or less raised component. While the location of the tumors in these clinical types is usually different, their basic clinical features are common. Nodular malignant melanoma, which lacks the radial growth phase, has a clinical appearance different from that of the other types of the tumor; it presents as a raised papule or nodule from the onset and has the worst prognosis. In addition to the four types of melanoma, there are some variants.

12.1.1 Lentigo Maligna Melanoma

Lentigo maligna melanoma is nearly always seen in fair-skinned individuals who are prone to actinic damage. Patients usually have a history of chronic sun exposure and sometimes a non–melanoma skin cancer (*see* Fig. 12.3). Individuals with outdoor occupations such as sailors or farmers are in the high risk group. Most patients are older than 60 years, but middle-aged people may also be affected. It is extremely rare in childhood. Lentigo maligna melanoma is two times more common in females than in males. It is usually not related to prior melanocytic nevi. It may rarely be

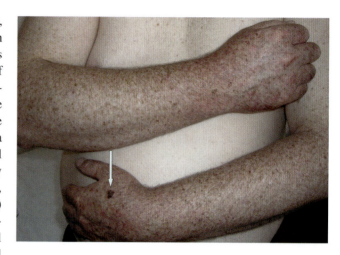

Fig. 12.4 Lentigo maligna melanoma on the dorsum of the hand (*arrow*) in a patient with xeroderma pigmentosum. The presence of profuse ephelides and benign lentigines in these patients can make an early diagnosis more difficult

associated with desmoplastic melanoma. In patients with xeroderma pigmentosum, different types of malignant melanoma, including lentigo maligna melanoma, can be seen on sun-exposed areas with onset at young ages (*see* Fig. 12.4).

Lentigo maligna melanoma favors the head and neck regions (*see* Figs. 12.3 and 12.5) and on occasion occurs on other skin sites such as the dorsum of the hands (*see* Fig. 12.4) and the forearms (*see* Fig. 12.6), which are also exposed to dense sunlight. The nose, temple (*see* Fig. 12.7), and cheeks (*see* Figs. 12.8 and 12.9) in both sexes and the ears (*see* Fig. 12.10) in men are typically involved. The scalp may be another common site of the tumor in bald men (*see* Fig. 12.3). The lesion appears as a light brown macule; it may darken (*see* Figs. 12.7) and spread out slowly to the surrounding skin (*see* Fig. 12.8). The border of the tumor is usually irregular and not sharply defined (*see* Figs. 12.6 and 12.9). Wood lamp examination may be useful for determining the borders of the lesion. In time, the color of the lesion changes, acquiring a mottled

12.1 Primary Cutaneous Malignant Melanoma

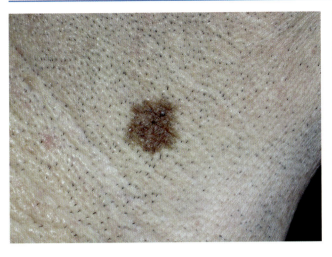

Fig. 12.5 Lentigo maligna on the neck

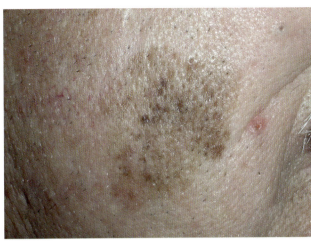

Fig. 12.8 Lentigo maligna presenting as a mottled macular lesion with ill-defined borders located on the cheek

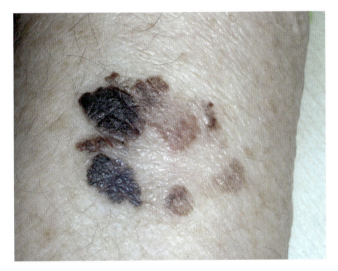

Fig. 12.6 Lentigo maligna melanoma on the forearm with features of regression. Note the light-colored depressed areas

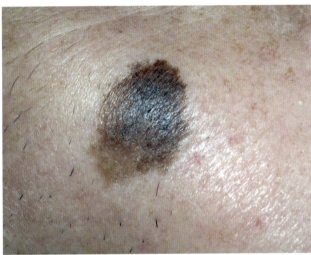

Fig. 12.9 Slightly raised lentigo maligna with uneven pigmentation on the cheek

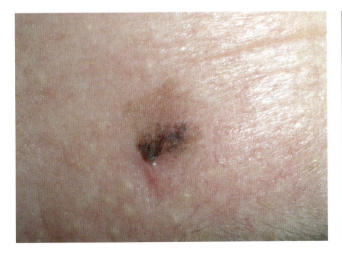

Fig. 12.7 Lentigo maligna presenting as a flat hyperpigmented lesion with irregular borders located on the forehead

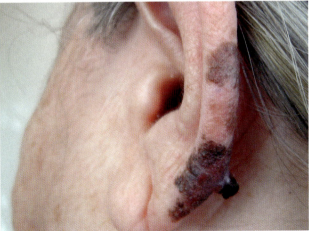

Fig. 12.10 Lentigo maligna melanoma located on the ear helix, a heavily sun-exposed area. The raised black papule has appeared years after the enlargement of the flat component

appearance with various shades of brown and black areas (*see* Figs. 12.8 and 12.10). The pigmentation may sometimes show a reticular pattern. These thin lesions are on the skin level and nonpalpable or sometimes mildly elevated. They are compatible with the radial growth phase of the tumor. Lentigo maligna may also be used as a synonym for a lesion in the radial growth phase representing early in situ melanoma, indicating that the abnormal melanoncytes are confined to the epidermis and show a lentiginous pattern. Solar elastosis is another standard histopathologic feature of lentigo maligna.

While some in situ lesions do not evolve and stay nearly unchanged throughout life, some may evolve slowly into the vertical growth phase if not treated. Lentigo maligna melanoma is the term for these lesions invading the dermis. The borders of the growing lesion may be notched. While some parts of the lesion become thickened, others show features of regression, such as a pale or shallow depression caused by destruction of atypical melanocytes related to an immune response (*see* Figs. 12.6 and 12.11). Furthermore, one or more raised papules (*see* Fig. 12.8) or nodules (*see* Figs. 12.11 and 12.12) may be seen on the flat patch or plaque. These parts of the lesions reflecting the vertical growth phase may be brown, black (*see* Fig. 12.10), blue, or sometimes light-colored (*see* Fig. 12.11). Papulonodular lesions have a tendency to rapid growth and may be eroded or ulcerated in a short time.

Because the tumor does not cause subjective symptoms and grows slowly in the early period, some patients with numerous benign and especially facial lesions such as pigmented actinic keratoses (*see* Fig. 2.13), or flat seborrheic keratoses (*see* Fig. 1.39) may ignore the lesion of lentigo maligna melanoma, thereby delaying medical attention. Some lesions may reach 10 to 15 cm (*see* Fig. 12.13). On the other hand, if destructive methods like cryotherapy or

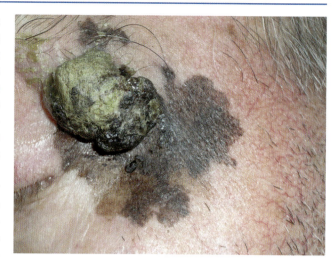

Fig. 12.12 A raised nodule on an irregularly pigmented lesion on the face. This kind of lesion should always arouse a suspicion of melanoma; when found on the face a lentigo maligna melanoma should be suspected

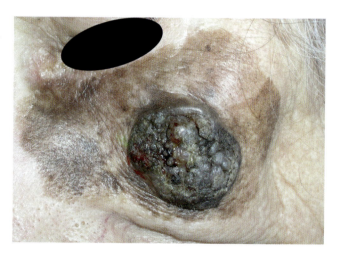

Fig. 12.13 A neglected case of lentigo maligna melanoma with an extensive lesion. The large ulcerated nodule in the center represents the vertical growth phase of the tumor and has occurred after a very long radial growth phase (more than 10 years)

electrocautery are applied on a misdiagnosed lesion, the clinical features of melanoma may change, causing further delay in diagnosis. These tumors may sometimes be initially diagnosed only in the invasive phase.

Lentigo maligna melanoma has the longest radial growth phase (5 to 20 years) among all types of melanoma, and therefore it is considered to be the type with the best prognosis. However, the prognosis of malignant melanoma is actually determined by Breslow thickness (vertical tumor thickness), which is measured on histopathologic examination. The vertical distance between the granular layer of epidermis or the ulcer base in ulcerated tumors and the deepest tumor cells in the dermis or subcutis equal the Breslow thickness. Once melanoma has evolved in the vertical growth phase, the different histologic types have no significant

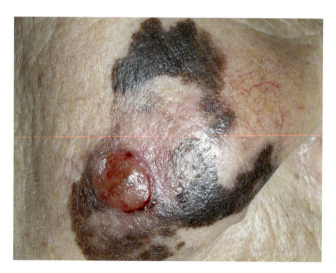

Fig. 12.11 A broad lesion of lentigo maligna melanoma showing a depressed hypopigmented area representing regression and an eroded nodule indicating the invasive stage

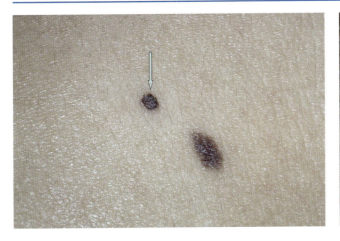

Fig. 12.14 Early diagnosed small (4 to 5 mm) malignant melanoma with a relatively symmetric appearance (*arrow*). The patient also had a benign melanocytic nevus close to the melanoma (the lower one)

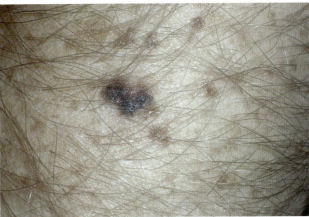

Fig. 12.15 Superficial spreading melanoma in the radial growth phase in a patient with xeroderma pigmentosum. Lesion approximately 1 cm in size is just palpable

influence on survival, and the prognosis is worsened. In addition to Breslow thickness, ulceration and high mitotic count are other histopathologic prognostic markers.

12.1.2 Superficial Spreading Melanoma

This is the most common type of malignant melanoma in Caucasians. It is most commonly seen in individuals between the ages of 30 and 50 with a slight predominance in females. It is also the common type in childhood. Fair-skinned individuals who do not tan after sun exposure (skin types I and II), people with many ephelides or actinic lentigo, and patients who have a history of intermittent intense sun exposure in childhood or puberty are more prone to develop superficial spreading melanoma. It is rare in black people. The relationship with preexisting melanocytic nevi is more prominent than in other types of melanoma. It is more commonly found in individuals with dysplastic nevi (*see* Fig. 12.1). The risk is especially increased in individuals with familial dysplastic nevi. On the other hand, an early lesion of superficial spreading melanoma may not be easily distinguished from a dysplastic nevus, causing a diagnostic challenge, especially in individuals with multiple nevi.

Superficial spreading melanoma is more commonly found on the back in both sexes and on the legs of females. However, it may occur anywhere on the body. When the lesion is smaller than 5 mm, the diagnosis can be difficult because of its uniform color and regular appearance (*see* Fig. 12.14). The tumor has a predominant radial growth phase. In situ superficial spreading melanoma is generally 1 cm in size at diagnosis and is observed as sharply defined, slightly elevated, palpable lesions with oval, round, or irregular shapes (*see* Figs. 12.15 and 12.16). Asymmetry and mild color variegation may also be observed (Fig 12.17). The tumor

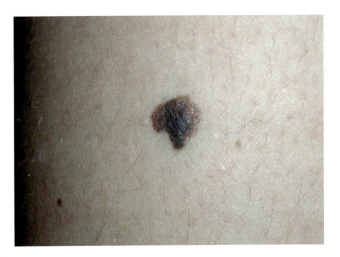

Fig. 12.16 Superficial spreading melanoma in situ presenting as a sharply defined, unevenly pigmented, slightly elevated lesion

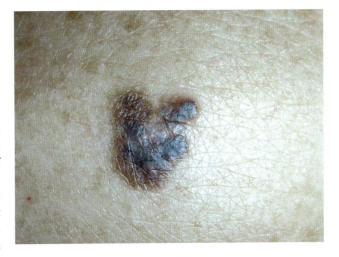

Fig. 12.17 Superficial spreading melanoma in situ. Note the mild color variegation

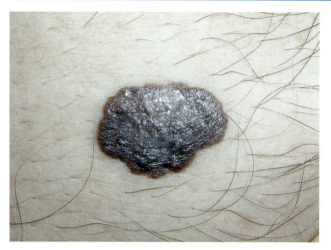

Fig. 12.18 Superficial spreading melanoma manifesting as a slightly raised black plaque nearly 2 cm in diameter

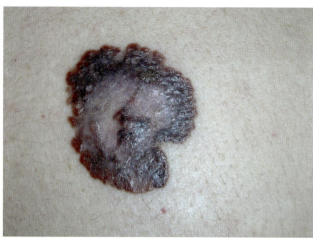

Fig. 12.20 Prominent asymmetry caused particularly by incomplete regression in superficial spreading melanoma. The borders are notched

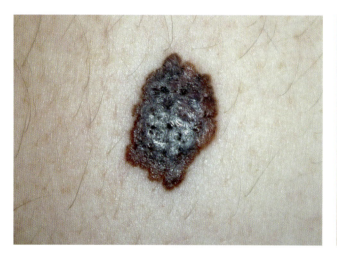

Fig. 12.19 Superficial spreading melanoma with typical notched borders

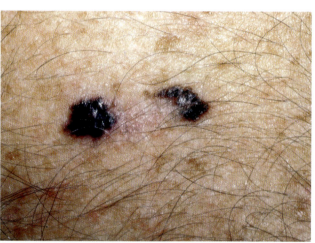

Fig. 12.21 Centrally regressed superficial spreading melanoma causing an appearance of split islands of tumors

spreads out to the peripheral skin gradually (see Fig. 12.18). The borders of the enlarged plaque may be notched (see Figs. 12.19 and 12.20). Skin creases may not be noticed on the surface of the tumor.

While a part of the lesion elevates and extends peripherally, another part may regress, causing an asymmetric appearance (see Fig. 12.20). One or more parts of the irregular plaque may be depressed (see Fig. 12.21). Furthermore, papulonodular parts may be noticed on tumors and indicate the vertical growth phase (see Figs. 12.22 and 12.23). Papules or nodules overlying the flat plaque may be dark like other parts of the melanoma (see Fig. 12.22) or light-colored, especially pink or red (see Figs. 12.24 and 12.25). Plaques that have grown a few centimeters in diameter usually show prominent variegation of color (see Figs. 12.26 and 12.27). Brown and black hues related to melanin in the epidermis and superficial dermis mostly dominate, but foci of blue, red, pink, yellow, gray, and white colors may also be

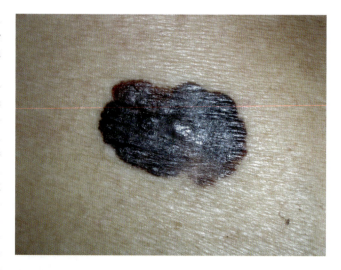

Fig. 12.22 Small central papule on a flat hyperpigmented plaque indicating the vertical growth phase (invasive stage) of superficial spreading melanoma

12.1 Primary Cutaneous Malignant Melanoma

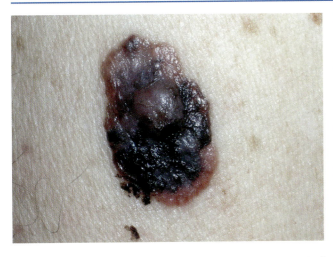

Fig. 12.23 A nodule overlying a flat hyperpigmented plaque with notched borders, typical of superficial spreading melanoma in the invasive stage

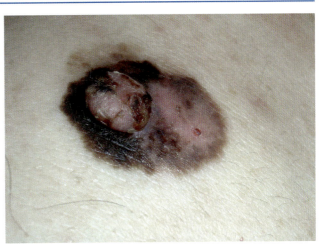

Fig. 12.26 Superficial spreading melanoma in the invasive stage showing prominent color variegation related with partial regression

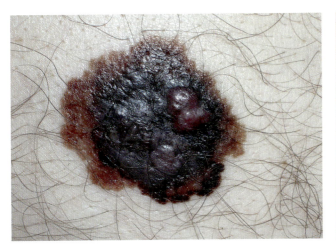

Fig. 12.24 Superficial spreading melanoma in the invasive stage; several nodules with reddish and black color are remarkable on an asymmetric lesion

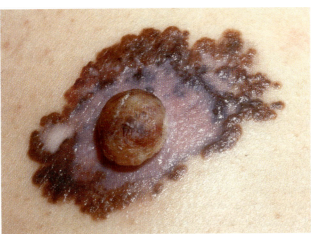

Fig. 12.27 Superficial spreading melanoma in the invasive stage. ABCDE criteria including asymmetry, border irregularity, and variegations of color are prominent in this rapidly growing large lesion

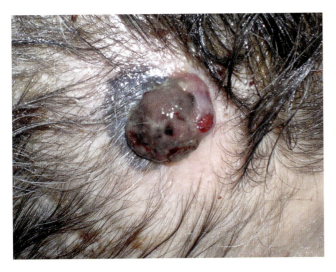

Fig. 12.25 Large eroded nodule on a flat plaque representing the invasive stage of superficial spreading melanoma

noticed. Blue color corresponds to dense melanin pigment deposition in the deep dermis. Pink and red colors may be related to inflammation or erosion and ulceration on the surface. A yellow color may be seen in crusted parts. Gray and white colors occur as a result of regression, an immune response to the tumor. Sometimes the brown or black colors remain only as small foci on the regressed tumor (*see* Fig. 12.28). Regression of large areas may result in an appearance of split islands of tumors (*see* Fig. 12.21). Apart from the depigmented parts within the lesion, another sign of regression may be an irregular depigmented halo at the periphery. Neglected tumors may reach 5 to 6 cm in diameter. Pruritus may accompany some cases in the invasive phase.

The so-called ABCDE criteria (asymmetry, border irregularity, color variegation, diameter, and evolution) may be found in lesions of superficial spreading melanoma, lentigo

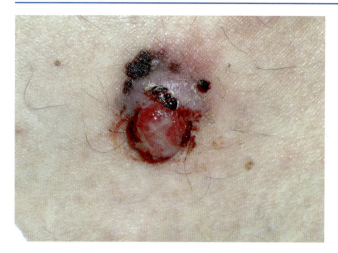

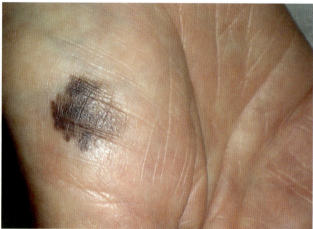

Fig. 12.28 Superficial spreading melanoma in the invasive stage. Note that a great part of the lesion is depigmented, but the presence of small dark foci of pigmentation on the periphery is helpful for clinical diagnosis

Fig. 12.29 In situ acral lentiginous melanoma on the palm

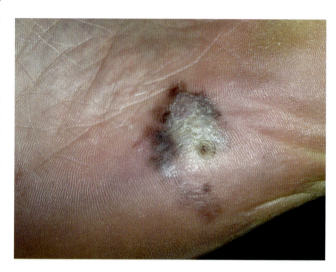

Fig. 12.30 Acral lentiginous melanoma in situ presenting as a poorly defined pigmented lesion on the sole

maligna melanoma, and acral lentiginous melanoma. Although not specific, the existence of these criteria may be helpful in distinguishing malignant melanoma from benign melanocytic nevi. On the other hand, most of these criteria may not be present in the evaluation of in situ stage lesions. Dysplastic nevus (*see* Fig. 3.199) and pigmented superficial basal cell carcinoma (*see* Fig. 11.62) are the main differential diagnostic challenges in early lesions of superficial spreading melanoma. Dermoscopy and confocal microscopy may support the diagnosis. Histology of an in situ superficial spreading melanoma reveals abnormal melanocytes generally clustered in nests at the dermoepidermal junction. Intraepidermal "pagetoid" spread of atypical melanocytes toward the surface is another important clue to the diagnosis.

Sometimes melanoma may disappear, reflecting complete regression. This is more commonly seen in the superficial spreading type. Poorly defined, white, gray or pinkish patches without pigmentation can sometimes be detected only during the screening examination following the diagnosis of metastasis. Many melanophages in the dermis, edematous loosely arranged collagen fibers, neovascularization, an inflammatory infiltrate containing lymphocytes and plasma cells are the histopathologic clues for regression areas that are devoid of atypical melanocytes. These features vary in intensity among individual cases.

In terms of good prognosis, for tumors at the radial growth phase, superficial spreading melanoma is the second most common type after lentigo maligna melanoma. Lesions on the legs and arms have a better prognosis than lesions on the head, especially scalp, and trunk, probably because they can be seen more easily and earlier by the patients or their relatives, thus patients can seek medical advice earlier.

12.1.3 Acral Lentiginous Melanoma

This is the type of malignant melanoma that is mainly located on the palms, soles, and nails. Ultraviolet rays are not considered to be an etiologic factor in acral lentiginous melanoma. It is relatively rare in Caucasians. However, in the black population, among all types of malignant melanoma, acral lentiginous type is seen in nearly half of the cases. It is also common in Asians. It appears most frequently at between 50 and 70 years of age. The lesion arises de novo from normal skin and is usually not associated with the common acquired junctional nevi of the palmoplantar area.

Acral lentiginous melanoma is more common on the plantar than the palmar area. The tumor can also be located on lateral sides of the feet, heels, and on interdigital sites. It appears as a brown, bluish-black, or black-colored macular lesion (*see* Figs. 12.29 and 12.30) and extends slowly.

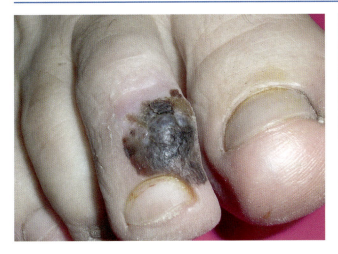

Fig. 12.31 Acral lentiginous melanoma in the invasive stage around the toenail. Note the prominent nodular component

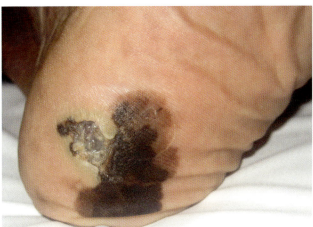

Fig. 12.33 Acral lentiginous melanoma in the invasive stage on the sole. In addition to a large hyperpigmented area, an ulceration is seen

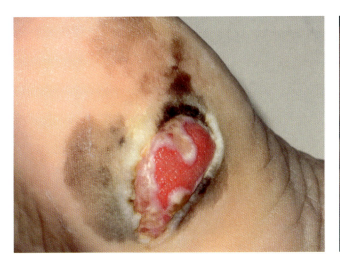

Fig. 12.32 Varying shades of brown pigmentation and hypopigmented areas related to partial regression are remarkable on an acral lentiginous melanoma. Note the associated ulcerated nodule representing the invasive stage

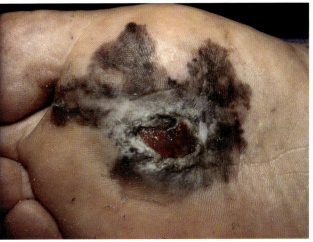

Fig. 12.34 A broad lesion of acral lentiginous melanoma with irregular margins. Note the eroded red nodule arising within the flat dark in situ component

Contrary to benign melanocytic nevi of the palmoplantar area, in situ lesions of melanoma are larger, poorly defined, and irregularly shaped (*see* Fig. 12.30). As opposed to lentigo maligna melanoma and superficial spreading melanoma, even flat nonpalpable palmoplantar lesions may show invasion to deep tissue. Elevated parts like papules or nodules, sometimes with a verrucous surface, may be noticed over time within the growing pigmented lesions (*see* Fig. 12.31). Different colors, including white and gray reflecting partial regression, can also be present (*see* Fig. 12.32). Partial or complete ulceration may develop on some lesions. Ulceration may occur overlying raised nodules (*see* Fig. 12.32) or as a depressed area (*see* Fig. 12.33). Some patients have large tumors measuring 5 to 10 cm on diagnosis (*see* Fig. 12.34), which mostly fulfill the ABCDE criteria.

The radial growth phase of acral lentiginous melanoma is slightly shorter than that of superficial spreading melanoma. Additionally, diagnosis is usually delayed because of its location. Therefore axillary or epitrochlear lymph node involvement may be present at diagnosis. In conjunction with these features, the prognosis is worse than that of lentigo maligna melanoma and superficial spreading melanoma. Pyogenic granuloma (*see* Fig. 6.57), Kaposi sarcoma (*see* Fig. 13.24), poroma (*see* Fig. 5.15), verruca plantaris, callus, and carcinoma cuniculatum (*see* Fig. 11.156) can be considered in the differential diagnosis of invasive stage lesions. On histopathologic examination the epidermis is irregularly acanthotic, and atypical spindle-shaped and dendritic melanocytes proliferate along the junction and later invade the dermis. Perineural extension can be a feature of invasive tumors, occurring relatively more frequently than in other types of melanoma.

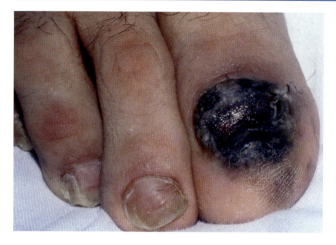

Fig. 12.35 Nail melanoma on the big toe causing nail destruction and hyperpigmentation on the nail bed. Pigmentation extending to the pulpa is a typical additional feature

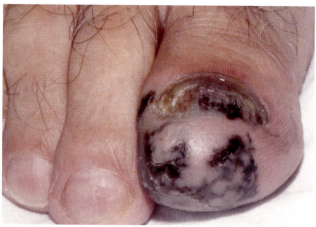

Fig. 12.37 Nail melanoma presenting as nail destruction and irregular pigmentation around the nail caused by incomplete regression

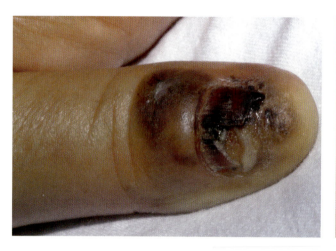

Fig. 12.36 Nail melanoma on the thumb with darkening and destruction of the nail plate and hyperpigmentation on the proximal nail fold (Hutchinson melanocytic whitlow)

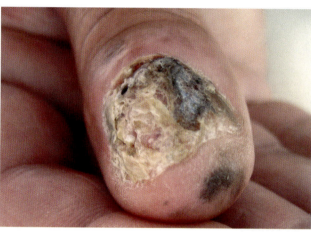

Fig. 12.38 The diagnosis of a nail melanoma may be delayed because nail dystrophy similar to onychomycosis or psoriatic nail may sometimes be the prominent feature. Irregular pigmentation on the pulpa accompanying nonspecific nail dystrophy was diagnostic in this case

Nail melanoma is mostly located on the big toe (*see* Fig. 12.35) and sometimes on the thumb (*see* Fig. 12.36). Other fingers and toes are more rarely affected. It commonly starts on the nail matrix, sometimes on the nail bed or nailfolds, and extends peripherally. A part or whole nail plate can be black or brown in matrix melanomas (*see* Fig. 12.36). Some melanomas can present as melanonychia striata. Contrary to melanonychia striata caused by benign melanocytic nevi, the longitudinal pigmented bands of malignant melanoma are thicker, irregular, and variegated in colour. Pigmentation increases in width in time and can also spread to the cuticle. Irregular pigmentation of the nail can spread out to adjacent proximal or lateral nailfolds (Hutchinson melanotic whitlow) (*see* Fig. 12.36) or pulpa (*see* Fig. 12.35) in the radial growth phase. Splitting of the nail may also occur (*see* Fig. 12.36), especially as the tumor thickens at the vertical growth phase. Irregular pigmentation caused by incomplete regression may be observed (*see* Fig. 12.37). Malignant melanoma arising on the nail bed appears mostly as a papule or nodule. The whole nail plate may be destroyed (*see* Fig. 12.38), and an ulcerated and sometimes nonpigmented nodule with crusting (*see* Fig. 12.39) can be seen on the nail bed. The existence of periungual foci of pigmentation is helpful for the diagnosis (*see* Fig. 12.38).

Some nail melanomas can be amelanotic (*see* Fig. 12.39) and mimic pyogenic granuloma (*see* Fig. 6.61a) or hypertrophic granulation tissue caused by an ingrown toenail. Therefore histopathologic confirmation and close follow-up of periungual tumors are mandatory. Matrix biopsy is required in patients with melanonychia striata only if there is any suspicion of melanoma. Nail melanoma has a poor prognosis, possibly owing to an increased rate of delay in diagnosis. Metastasis may occur as a consequence of late diagnosis (*see* Fig. 12.40a and b). On the other hand, as malignant

12.1 Primary Cutaneous Malignant Melanoma

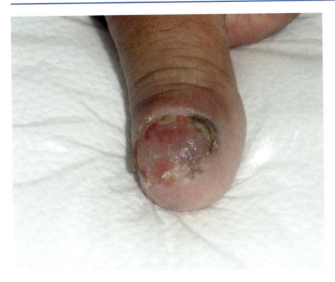

Fig. 12.39 Ulcerated amelanotic nodule on the nail bed. The periungual foci of pigmentation are supportive of the diagnosis of nail melanoma

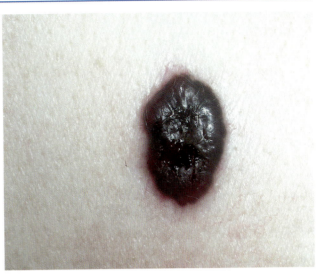

Fig. 12.41 Nodular malignant melanoma on the neck showing a small focus of erosion. Note that a flat component is absent in this lesion

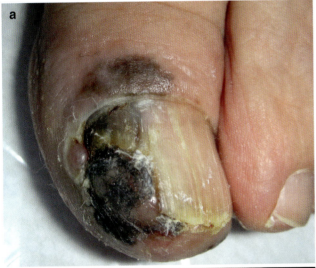

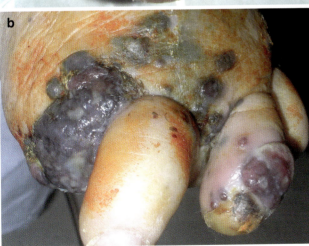

Fig. 12.40 (a) Nail melanoma associated with regional nail destruction, hyperpigmentation on the proximal nailfold and a skin-colored papule (macrosatellite) on the lateral nailfold. (b) Despite the amputation of the great toe, followed by immunotherapy and chemotherapy, melanoma has spread to the other toes and foot

melanoma is very rare in children, routine biopsy of thin and regular pigmented bands caused by benign melanocytic nevi (*see* Fig. 3.88) is mostly unnecessary in young children.

12.1.4 Nodular Malignant Melanoma

This type of melanoma is different from the other three main types of the tumor as the transition to the vertical growth phase is direct bypassing the radial growth phase; this is associated with a poor prognosis. It appears as a raised dark papule or nodule without peripheral pigmentation or a flat component (*see* Fig. 12.41). It is more commonly seen between the ages of 40 and 60 with a slight male preponderance. It may rarely be seen in childhood. The tumor usually starts de novo from the normal skin. Like superficial spreading melanoma, acute sunburn and intermittent sun exposure in childhood seem to be the main risk factors.

Sometimes nodular lesions arise in a preexisting congenital melanocytic nevus (*see* Fig. 12.2). Melanoma occurring within small or medium-sized congenital nevi is usually seen after puberty. On the other hand, the ones arising within large congenital nevi can be seen in the first 10 years of life. Melanoma that arises on melanocytic nevi may also be accepted as a distinct variant. The typical presentation is rapidly growing, dark or flesh-colored, raised asymmetric papules or nodules. Subcutaneous nodules may rarely be observed.

The head (*see* Fig. 12.42), neck (*see* Fig. 12.41), and trunk are common locations of nodular melanoma. However, it may arise at any skin site. Nodular melanoma may appear as dome-shaped (*see* Fig. 12.43), exophytic, or irregular (*see* Fig. 12.44) papules or nodules. Rarely, pedunculated or polypoid (*see* Fig. 12.45) or plaque-like (*see* Fig. 12.46) lesions may be found. It grows rapidly in comparison to other types

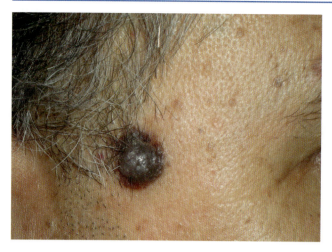

Fig. 12.42 Nodular malignant melanoma on the face. There is no apparent flat component or peripheral pigmentation

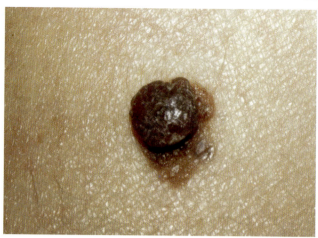

Fig. 12.45 A polypoid nodular malignant melanoma; a rare presentation

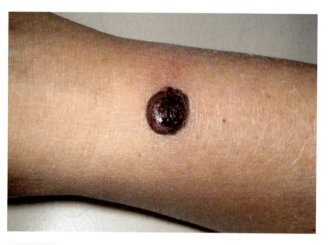

Fig. 12.43 Nodular malignant melanoma presenting as a dome-shaped nodule with crusted surface

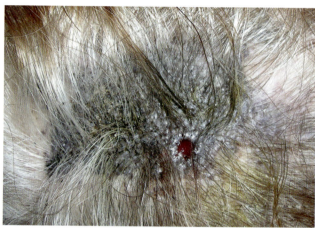

Fig. 12.46 A plaque-like nodular malignant melanoma on the scalp. In this location the diagnosis is often delayed

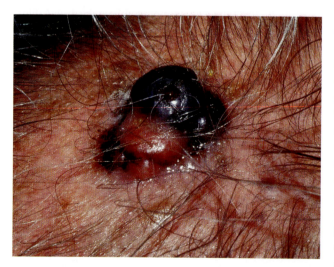

Fig. 12.44 Nodular malignant melanoma with an irregular appearance. History of rapid-growth is usually present

of melanoma. Most lesions are black or brown, but gray, bluish-black, purple, or bluish-red tumors may also be seen. This type of melanoma may sometimes be difficult to differentiate clinically from other dark-colored skin tumors such as pigmented basal cell carcinoma (*see* Fig. 11.71), dermatofibroma (*see* Fig. 8.10), seborrheic keratosis (melanoacanthoma) (*see* Fig. 1.38), Reed nevus (*see* Fig. 3.223), or cellular blue nevus (*see* Fig. 3.79). Apart from the other three main types of primary cutaneous melanoma, the lesion may be relatively uniform; thus ABCDE criteria may not be completely fulfilled. However, it has a rapid progressive course. In other words, only criteria "D" and "E" are usually present at diagnosis. Erosion (*see* Fig. 12.41) or ulceration (*see* Fig. 12.47) on the surface of the tumor is a common finding and associated with a poor prognosis. Sometimes the whole surface of the tumor is ulcerated or covered with hemorrhagic crusts (*see*

12.1 Primary Cutaneous Malignant Melanoma

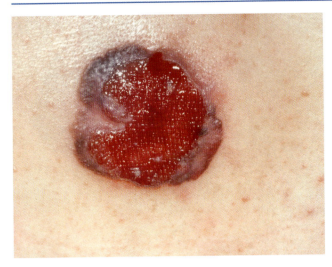

Fig. 12.47 Nodular malignant melanoma with ulceration involving nearly the whole surface of the tumor

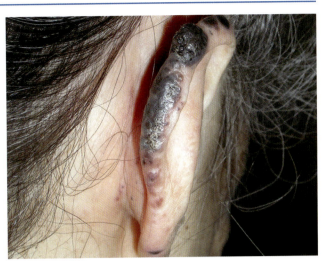

Fig. 12.49 Macrosatellites in different sizes around a nodular malignant melanoma on the ear

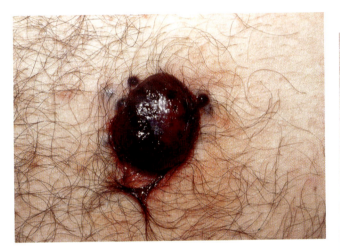

Fig. 12.48 Small pigmented papules in the vicinity (*upper part*) of a large nodular malignant melanoma representing macrosatellites, a form of lymphatic metastasis

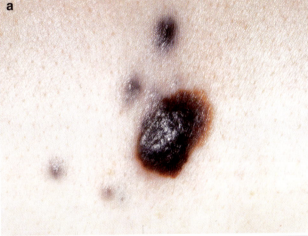

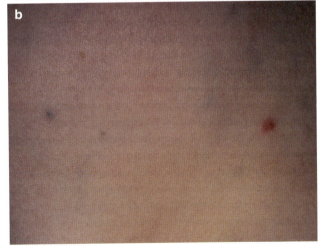

Fig. 12.50 (**a**) Macrosatellites manifesting as pigmented macules around a nodular malignant melanoma. These macules had malignant blue nevus-like histopathologic features. (**b**) Distant skin metastasis as pigmented macules occurred one year later after the excision of the primary tumor

Fig. 12.43). Bleeding may occur on these sites. Lesions may be asymptomatic or sometimes pruritic, tender, and painful. Tumors in the late stage may expand laterally. Histologically large, cluster-forming pleomorphic melanocytes distributed asymmetrically in the junctional area and dermis are observed.

Nodular melanoma is considered to have the worst prognosis among the main types of primary cutaneous melanoma because Breslow thickness is usually high at the time of diagnosis. On some locations like the scalp, the tumor may not be easily detected, and thus it may be enlarged and thickened until diagnosed. The thickness of melanoma developing within a large congenital melanocytic nevus is also usually high because it mostly derives from the deep part of the nevus.

Small pigmented papules (*see* Figs. 12.48 and 12.49) or macules (*see* Fig. 12.50a) at the periphery of melanoma called macrosatellites are not rare in nodular melanomas.

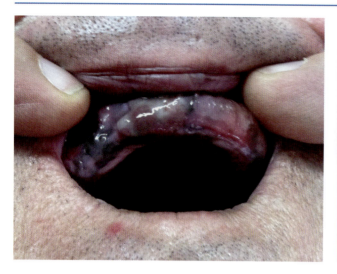

Fig. 12.51 Mucosal melanoma on the gingivae seen as irregular diffuse hyperpigmentation

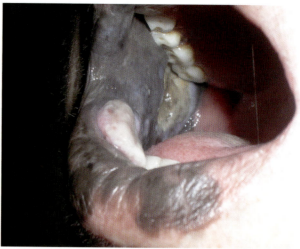

Fig. 12.52 Mucosal melanoma covering a large area as an irregular hyperpigmented patch. The light-colored, eroded nodule on the labial mucosa represents the vertical growth phase of the tumor

Satellite lesions (macrosatellites) may be the first presentation of metastasis and are indicators of a poor prognosis. Metastasis is usually present in large nodular melanomas. However, even small lesions may metastasize. Many patients have regional lymph node metastasis by the time of presentation.

12.1.5 Mucosal Melanoma

Apart from skin, melanoma may also develop on oral, nasal, nasopharyngeal, laryngeal, anorectal, and urinary mucosae. Oral melanoma is more commonly located on the hard palate, but it may be seen anywhere in the oral mucosa. It shows mostly a biphasic growth pattern similar to that of the three main types of melanoma. The tumor appears as an irregularly shaped, dark macule and enlarges gradually, developing into flat or slightly elevated lesions with indistinct borders (*see* Figs. 12.51 and 12.52). It may later be infiltrated and ulcerated. Advanced lesions may cause bleeding and pain.

Polypoid lesions may be noticed on nasal mucosa. These may present with epistaxis. Melanoma of the vulva is seen in the older population, mostly on the labia majora and minora. Irregular dark macules evolve into nodules, plaques, or ulcers. Bleeding may be a late symptom. Penile melanoma is mostly located on the glans as an irregular hyperpigmented patch or plaque that enlarges gradually (*see* Fig. 12.53). Involvement of scrotum is very rare (*see* Fig. 12.54). Anorectal melanoma is usually diagnosed after bleeding of the ulcerated lesions. The prognosis of mucosal melanoma is not good because it is usually detected late. Metastases may be found in many patients, and local recurrence after excision is a common problem. The risk of distant metastasis is also increased.

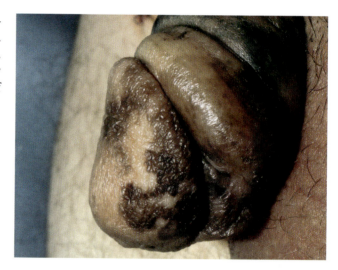

Fig. 12.53 Early malignant melanoma on the glans penis shown as an irregular hyperpigmented patch

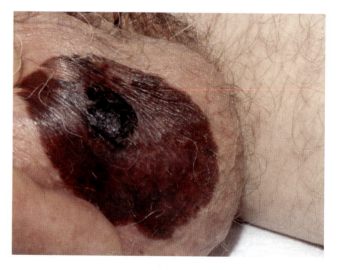

Fig. 12.54 Scrotal melanoma in the invasive stage. This is an extremely rare location for the tumor

12.1 Primary Cutaneous Malignant Melanoma

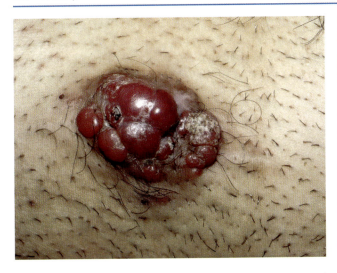

Fig. 12.55 Amelanotic melanoma presenting as a homogeneous red lobulated tumor

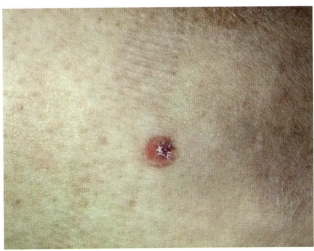

Fig. 12.57 Amelanotic melanoma in situ on the trunk. This entirely amelanotic small flat lesion is similar to in situ superficial spreading melanoma except for the color

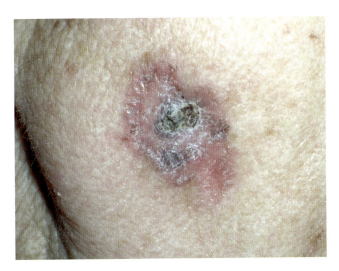

Fig. 12.56 Amelanotic melanoma on the face. Apart from the color, this lesion looks like lentigo maligna melanoma

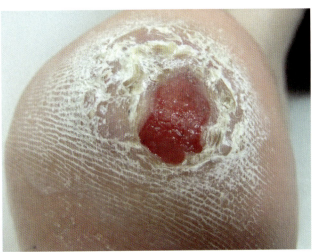

Fig. 12.58 Amelanotic melanoma on the heel. This lesion has clinical features similar to those of acral lentiginous melanoma other than the colour

12.1.6 Amelanotic Melanoma

Amelanotic lesions represent a distinct variant of malignant melanoma that is generally devoid of melanin pigment. Pink or red colors are predominantly found in this type of melanoma (Fig 12.55). Since the characteristic dark color is absent, clinical diagnosis is much more difficult. Amelanotic lesions are seen in nearly 5 percent of all melanomas and may occur anywhere on the body. Other than the color, the clinical findings are similar to the main types of malignant melanoma (*see* Figs. 12.56, 12.57, 12.58, and 12.59). The entire lesion may be amelanotic (*see* Figs. 12.55, 12.56, 12.57, 12.58, and 12.59). Sometimes only a small focus of brown or black color within the tumor or at its periphery may be a clue to diagnosis (*see* Figs. 12.28 and 12.39). Flat lesions may be clinically similar to Bowen disease (*see* Fig. 2.20). Merkel cell

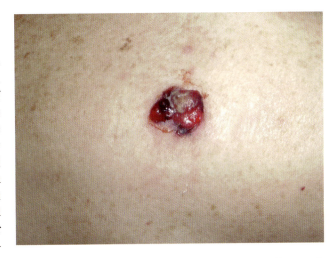

Fig. 12.59 Amelanotic melanoma on the trunk looking similar to nodular malignant melanoma except for its colour

carcinoma (*see* Fig. 11.167), squamous cell carcinoma (*see* Fig. 1.117), basal cell carcinoma (*see* Fig. 11.13) and epithelioid sarcoma can be considered in the differential diagnosis of amelanotic nodular lesions. Erosions covering the entire surface of the reddish tumor (*see* Fig. 12.59) may mislead the examiner to a diagnosis of pyogenic granuloma (*see* Fig. 6.49) or other vascular tumors. Early nodular lesions may be confused with verruca vulgaris or seborrheic keratosis (*see* Fig. 1.51). In these cases, application of destructive modalities such as electrocautery and cryotherapy can cause further delay in diagnosis. In some of these cases the correct diagnosis can only be made after the tumor metastasizes. Therefore amelanotic melanoma has a poor prognosis. Even metastatic lesions can be amelanotic.

Histologically, amelanotic melanoma has features similar to other types. However, melanin pigment may either be totally absent or present only in small amounts. Special techniques like Masson-Fontana stain may help to disclose small amounts of melanin. Immunohistochemical methods using melanocytic markers such as S100, Mart-1/Melan-A, and HMB45 are very helpful for diagnostic confirmation.

12.1.7 Desmoplastic Melanoma

Desmoplastic melanoma is a rare variant of melanoma with light-colored papulonodular lesions or plaques and distinct histopathologic features. It is predominantly seen in men and patients over 60 years old. Sun-exposed skin areas such as the face, scalp, and neck are most commonly involved. It arises de novo on normal skin or from lentigo maligna. Most lesions are skin-colored and nonulcerated (*see* Fig 12.60). Desmoplastic melanoma may mimic scars, benign connective tissue tumors, or cutaneous sarcomas due to sclerosis or induration. Therefore the diagnosis is usually delayed. Amelanotic spindle cells in a fibrotic stroma are the main histopathologic features, and a junctional component is usually absent. As it spreads through cutaneous nerves (neurotropism), it may cause severe pain. Its metastatic potential is not high. On the other hand, the tumor may particularly infiltrate the deep tissue, including periosteum and bone; therefore excision with wide surgical margins is required. Otherwise there may be local recurrence, which is relatively more common than in other types of malignant melanoma.

12.1.8 Spitzoid Melanoma

Spitzoid melanoma is a rare variant of melanoma mostly seen in children. It is more common on the head and extremities but may occur anywhere. It is not well known whether spitzoid melanoma may occur as a result of transformation from Spitz nevus and atypical spitzoid melanocytic neoplasm. It presents as a pinkish round nodule clinically similar to its benign counterpart, Spitz nevus (*see* Fig. 3.218) or angiomatous tumors such as pyogenic granuloma (*see* Fig. 6.43). It changes rapidly, may darken (*see* Fig. 12.61) or remain amelanotic, and a mildly asymmetric appearance may occur. However, ABCDE criteria are not completely positive. These tumors are mostly excised in order to exclude malignancy. The distinction of spitzoid melanoma from Spitz nevus may be also difficult from a histopathologic point of view. Cytologic atypia may be more prominent in spitzoid melanoma, but this is not a unique reliable criterion, as many more, such as asymmetry, deep penetration, and spontaneous ulceration are important in the differentiation. The biological behavior of spitzoid melanoma is not well known, but possibly it does not have a different prognosis from other types of melanoma.

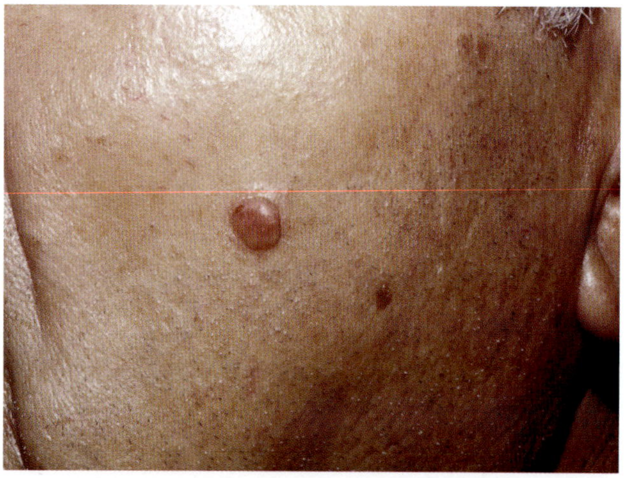

Fig. 12.60 Desmoplastic melanoma on the face presenting as a smooth-surfaced, skin-colored nodule

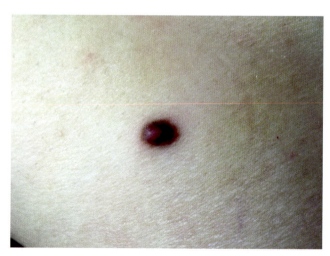

Fig. 12.61 Spitzoid malignant melanoma presenting as a round pigmented nodule

12.2 Metastatic Malignant Melanoma

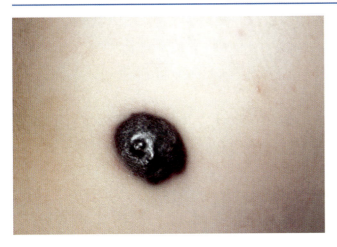

Fig. 12.62 Malignant blue nevus shown as a bluish-black nodule in a child

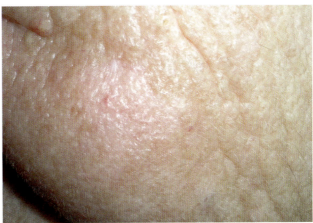

Fig. 12.63 Hypopigmented, slightly atrophic lesion on the face representing complete regression of melanoma. The depicted patient had associated regional lymph node metastasis

12.1.9 Malignant Blue Nevus

Malignant blue nevus arises from normal skin or within a pre-existing blue nevus, especially the cellular type, and rarely within other types of dermal melanocytoses. The deep dermis is commonly involved during diagnosis, and detection of this uncommon variant of melanoma is usually delayed. It is a slow-growing tumor. The head is the most common involved site, followed by the buttocks. Lesions may exceed 2 to 3 cm. Blue or black nodules are typically found (*see* Fig. 12.62). Histologically this tumor generally shows features of cellular blue nevus and malignancy criteria such as prominent cellular atypia, a high number of mitoses, and necrosis. There is no intraepidermal component. Recurrence rate and metastatic potential, including visceral metastasis, are considered high.

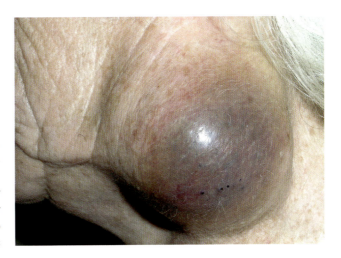

Fig. 12.64 Soft-tissue metastasis of melanoma presenting as a large bluish black-colored mass on the neck

12.2 Metastatic Malignant Melanoma

Untreated cutaneous melanomas eventually invade deeper parts of the skin. The possibility of metastasis also increases in parallel to the depth of the tumor. Thanks to better public education about melanoma in the last years, more patients can be diagnosed earlier, and metastasis, which is a marker of a poor prognosis, is found in approximately 20 percent of the patients. Owing to lymphatic spread, the sentinel lymph node (the first draining node) is usually the primary site of metastasis. In time, the tumor spreads hematogenously and can metastasize to almost all organs. On the other hand, some patients with metastatic melanoma may have the primary tumor on extracutaneous sites or sometimes melanoma on the skin may have completely regressed at the time of detection of metastasis. A slightly atrophic, irregular, white area (*see* Fig. 12.63) may be the evidence of regression of a primary melanoma, especially if supported by the history of the patient.

Skin and soft tissues (*see* Fig. 12.64) are among the common sites of metastasis. Different types of cutaneous metastasis of malignant melanoma are described according to their distance from the primary tumor. Dissemination of neoplastic cells through local lymphatic channels causes locoregional metastases called macrosatellites and in-transit metastases. Skin metastases found within a 2 cm distance around the primary tumor are called macrosatellites (*see* Figs. 12.48, 12.49 and 12.50a). They may be solitary or multiple, presenting as papules or nodules. Macrosatellites on the palmoplantar area may be clinically similar to acral lentiginous melanoma (*see* Fig. 12.65).

Skin metastasis between the primary tumor and the sentinel lymph node is called in-transit metastasis (*see* Fig. 12.66). The number of the lesions is variable. Macrosatellites and in-transit metastases may be hyperpigmented (*see* Fig. 12.65) or amelanotic (*see* Fig. 12.66). They generally have an intact

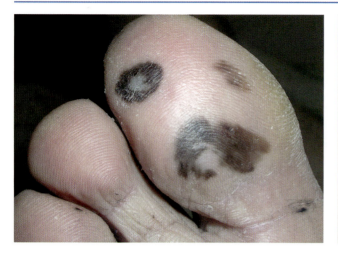

Fig. 12.65 In-transit metastases of nail melanoma shown as pigmented macules on the toe

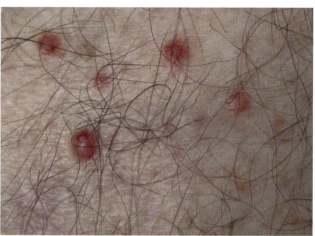

Fig. 12.67 Multiple in-transit metastases of melanoma on the leg. The flesh-colored papules have smooth surface

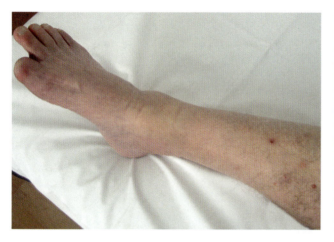

Fig. 12.66 Skin-colored papules on the shin representing in-transit metastasis which occurred despite the amputation of the phalanx with nail melanoma

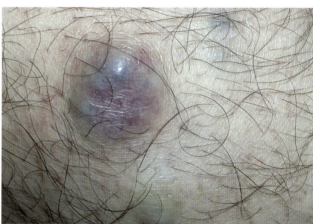

Fig. 12.68 In-transit metastasis of melanoma presenting as a large smooth-surfaced amelanotic nodule

surface (*see* Figs. 12.67 and 12.68). The presence of macrosatellites or in-transit metastases is associated with a worse prognosis.

Distant skin metastasis beyond the regional nodes occurs via hematogenous spread. It is a late feature, and on rare occasions patients may seek a physician only after this stage. Brown or black papules or nodules are the most common presentation (*see* Fig. 12.69). Sometimes multiple grouped (*see* Fig. 12.70) or scattered (*see* Figs. 12.71 and 12.72) lesions are observed. Even hundreds of metastatic skin lesions are possible (*see* Figs. 12.70, 12.71 and 12.72). Firm, asymptomatic, elevated dermal papules or nodules are typical (*see* Figs. 12.70 and 12.72), but pigmented patches (*see* Fig. 12.50b) may also be found. In general, they have a uniform appearance. Besides hyperpigmented lesions, pinkish red (amelanotic) lesions are not rare. Cutaneous metastasis of a hyperpigmented primary melanoma may also be amelanotic. Some patients have disseminated papulonodular lesions. Pinkish or

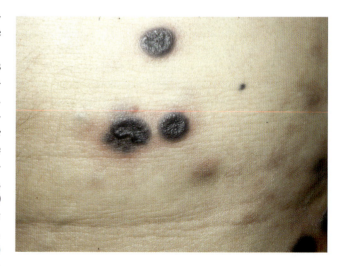

Fig. 12.69 Cutaneous metastasis of melanoma via hematogenous spread typically presenting as hyperpigmented papules and nodules devoid of a surrounding flat component

12.2 Metastatic Malignant Melanoma

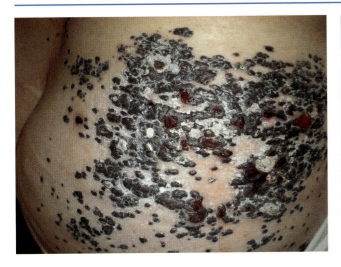

Fig 12.70 Cutaneous metastasis of melanoma. The number of lesions may be in the hundreds and some lesions may be grouped as seen here, and the surface of some lesions may be eroded or ulcerated

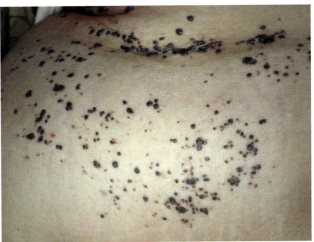

Fig. 12.72 Disseminated pigmented metastatic papules in the late stage of melanoma

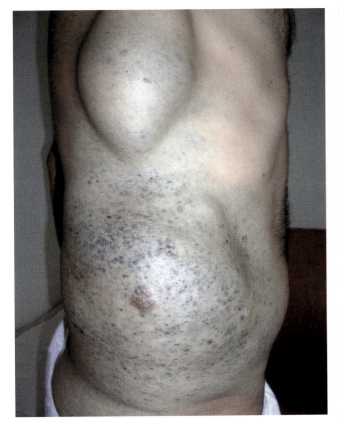

Fig. 12.71 Disseminated cutaneous metastasis, soft tissue metastasis (large masses), and bluish pigmentation owing to generalized melanosis are seen concomitantly on the trunk of this melanoma patient

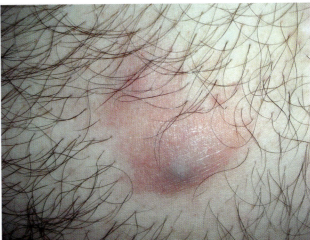

Fig. 12.73 The pinkish subcutaneous nodule seen in the figure may rarely be a presentation of metastatic melanoma

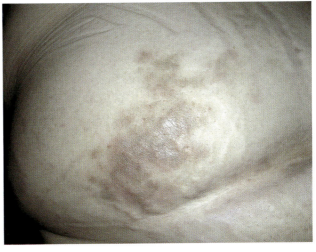

Fig. 12.74 Metastatic melanoma presenting as a large, indurated, skin-colored plaque

skin-colored subcutaneous nodules or large masses may be other presentations of melanoma metastasis (*see* Figs. 12.73 and 12.74). Erosion and ulceration are uncommon in early metastatic lesions, since atypical melanocytes are mostly present in the dermis and are not found in the epidermis.

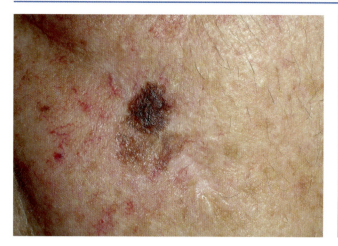

Fig. 12.75 Lentigo maligna on the cheek that has relapsed on the excision site. Inadequate excision is a common cause of recurrence

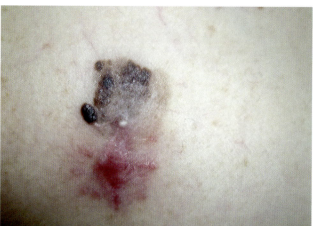

Fig. 12.76 Superficial spreading melanoma that has relapsed on the excision site

However, they may occur in the late, stage (*see* Fig. 12.70). Histopathologic features of metastatic lesions are also different from those of primary melanomas. In the vast majority of cases, the tumor lacks connection with the epidermis, except for the rare "epidermotropic" melanoma metastases. Dense atypical melanocytes may be seen in the reticular dermis and subcutis. Metastatic skin lesions may occasionally be similar to blue nevus clinically and histopathologically.

Sometimes diffuse brown or bluish discoloration (generalized melanosis) may be found on the whole body skin and mucous membranes as a result of dense melanin deposition in the dermis (*see* Fig. 12.71). Systemic symptoms like fatigue and weight loss may be seen in patients with metastatic melanoma. The prognosis is relatively good in patients with cutaneous metastases lacking systemic parenchymatous organ metastasis.

Other than systemic metastasis on the skin, recurrence at the primary lesion site and development of another primary melanoma may also be seen. A second primary cutaneous melanoma is mostly found in patients with many dysplastic nevi. A second melanoma can be diagnosed relatively earlier if the awareness of such patients is increased. Recurrence is more common in thicker melanomas and is usually seen within 5 years after removal. These lesions are found on the excision site (*see* Figs. 12.75 and 12.76), on the sides of the graft area (*see* Fig. 12.77), or around it (*see* Fig. 12.78). Recurrent tumors may show typical clinical features of the excised primary tumor (*see* Figs. 12.75 and 12.76) or clinical features of metastatic melanoma. There may be solitary (*see* Fig 12.79) or multiple (*see* Fig. 12.80) papules or nodules adjacent to the site of surgery. Recurrent lesions are mostly hyperpigmented (*see* Fig. 12.78) but may rarely be amelanotic (*see* Figs. 12.81 and 12.82). Local recurrence is usually related to incomplete excision of the primary tumor or clinically inapparent microsatellites or macrosatellites that have

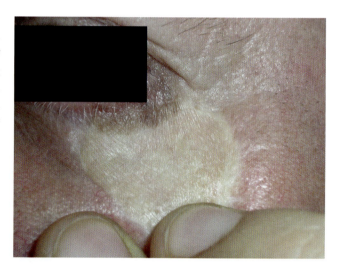

Fig. 12.77 Relapse of melanoma on one side of the skin graft area. Note the brownish hyperpigmentation close to the lower eyelid

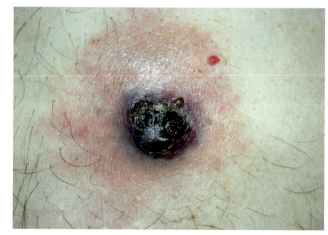

Fig. 12.78 Relapse of melanoma as an eroded pigmented nodule

12.2 Metastatic Malignant Melanoma

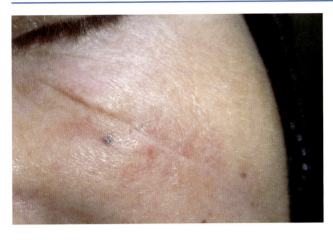

Fig. 12.79 Nonspecific small pigmented solitary papule near the excision site representing metastatic melanoma

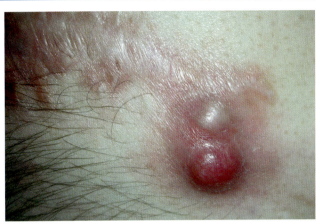

Fig. 12.82 Metastatic melanoma showing as amelanotic subcutaneous nodules adjacent to the excision site

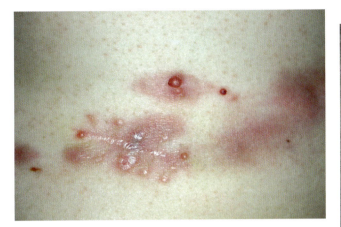

Fig. 12.80 Metastatic melanoma presenting as multiple erythematous nodules around an inadequate excision site

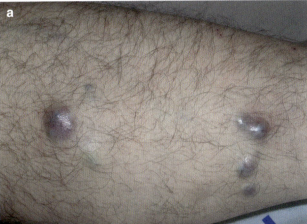

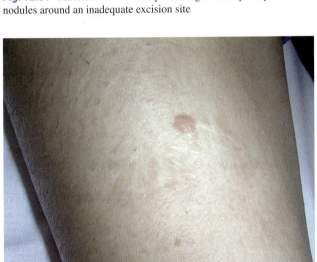

Fig. 12.81 Metastatic melanoma occurring as a solitary skin-colored papule on the site of an excision scar

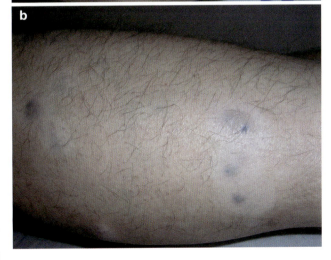

Fig. 12.83 (a) Multiple in-transit metastases on the leg. (b) Partial involution of the lesions during chemotherapy with temozolamide

not been excised. However, in advanced melanoma recurrence is possible even after wide excision. There may be multiple papulonodular metastatic lesions around the amputation site (*see* Fig. 12.40). After the excision of the primary tumor, the excision site must be regularly checked in the follow-up period.

Management (Primary and Metastatic Melanoma). Early detection of malignant melanoma is of vital importance because surgery performed for in situ melanomas is generally curative. Diagnosis in advanced stages may be related to the patient's lack of awareness of the tumor or sometimes is the consequence of misdiagnosis. Differential diagnosis of malignant melanoma includes a rich spectrum of skin tumors. As the clinical findings of melanoma extend over a wide spectrum, the clinical diagnosis may sometimes be difficult even for an experienced physician. Therefore, any changing tumoral skin lesion that cannot be diagnosed accurately should also be evaluated as suspicious for melanoma and if possible biopsied. Destructive therapy modalities should not be used in these cases before the confirmation of diagnosis.

Follow-up of high-risk benign melanocytic lesions is also critical for early recognition of malignant melanoma. Photographic and dermoscopic records of the congenital melanocytic nevi, dysplastic nevi, and other atypical nevi are important in the follow-up of the patients. However, when malignant melanoma is suspected, histopathologic confirmation is essential. Total excision of the tumor, including subcutaneous fat, is the ideal approach. As the thickness of the tumor is the most important prognostic parameter, an incisional or punch biopsy may not be adequate. However if the differential diagnosis of a large tumor includes other tumors such as seborrheic keratosis, total excision for histopathologic evaluation may not always be appropriate. In these cases, a biopsy must be taken from the thickest or the most elevated part of the tumor. Sometimes multiple biopsies from different parts of a large tumor may be required. Shave excision should not be performed. According to the current concept, the risk of local recurrence or metastasis is not related to biopsy trauma.

After the confirmation of the diagnosis, the patient should be examined dermatologically to search for macrosatellites, in-transit metastases, and distant metastases. In addition to physical examination of the lymph nodes, basic blood tests, and simple imaging stuies such as lymph node ultrasonograhy and chest radiography may be done in patients with thin melanomas. Patients with thick melanomas or with lymph node metastasis should be investigated for systemic metastasis with laboratory examinations such as serum lactate dehydrogenase (LDH), S100-B levels, and radiologic examinations such as computed tomography, magnetic resonance imaging or positron-emission tomography. A routine genetic testing is not indicated.

Surgery is the therapy of choice in all types of primary melanoma. The tumor should be excised with margins established according to its thickness. Surgical margins are the lowest (0.5 cm) for in situ melanomas. Lentigo maligna has a higher tendency to subclinical invasion of the surrounding skin; hence recurrence is common after removal with standard margins (*see* Figs. 12.75 and 12.77). Mohs micrographic surgery may be preferred in this type. Wide excision (1-2 cm) and grafting are performed for thicker lesions of all types of melanoma. Conventional surgery is efficacious in great majority of the cases. Amputation of the phalanx (proximal interphalangeal joint) may be indicated for some nail melanomas in the vertical growth phase (*see* Fig. 12.40a and b).

If a solitary or a few macrosatellites or in-transit metastases are detected clinically or radiologically, they may also be resected. However, surgery may not be feasible for multiple lesions.

Intraoperative lymphatic mapping followed by sentinel node biopsy is performed in patients with intermediate and thick melanomas to determine the stage of the tumor. Regional node dissection should be performed if nodal micrometastasis (positive sentinel lymph node) is detected.

While there is generally no need for adjuvant therapy for thin melanomas, an adjuvant therapy is usually combined with surgery for the treatment of patients in the vertical growth phase and with regional lymph node metastasis. Systemic high-dose interferon alpha is the main choice of therapy and is also used for subsequent maintenance therapy.

Radiotherapy is not routinely used for malignant melanoma. It can be administered in lentigo maligna if surgery cannot be performed and in desmoplastic melanoma or sometimes as an adjuvant treatment modality after lymphadenectomy. Another adjuvant therapeutic modality is isolated limb perfusion, which is sometimes used in high-risk melanomas and in-transit metastases of the extremities.

Once systemic metastasis occurs, the prognosis of melanoma is very negative. Various therapeutic options can be tried in metastatic or unresectable melanomas, but none of them is curative (*see* Fig. 12.83a and b). Dacarbazine and temozolomide are the most commonly used classic chemotherapeutic agents. Temozolomide is more effective for brain metastasis. Immunotherapies or targeted medications used in metastatic melanoma include ipilimumab (human cytotoxic T-lymphocyte antigen 4-blocking antibody), BRAF inhibitors like vemurafenib and dabrafenib, a MEK inhibitor trametinib and PD-1 receptor targeting drugs like lambrolizumab and nivolumab. BRAF inhibitors can be chosen in patients with metastatic melanoma who are positive for BRAF V600E mutation. The results are good in cases with visceral metastases, but severe side effects, including eruptive non–melanoma skin cancers, may occur, and duration of remission is usually not very long.

Various combinations of the targeted therapeutic options may prolong remission duration or reduce some adverse effects. In general, overall survival of metastatic melanoma has improved after the development of these agents. On the other hand, metastasectomy may be used in patients with solitary or localized metastatic lesions of various visceral organs and skin. Long term remissions may be achieved if complete excision can be performed.

All patients with malignant melanoma should be followed up carefully for local recurrence, in-transit metastasis and systemic metastasis. Physical, laboratory, and radiologic examinations for surveillance of malignant melanoma in the follow-up period should be more frequent for thicker melanomas than thin ones. It should be kept in mind that local recurrence and even metastasis may occur years later. Sun protection including using sunscreen creams, protective clothes, sunglasses and hat is lifelong necessary.

Suggested Reading

Abbasi NR, Show HM, Rigel DS, et al. Early diagnosis of cutanesus melanoma: revisiting the ABCD criteria. JAMA. 2004;292:2771–6.

Barnhill RL, Fitzpatrick TB, Fandrey K, Kenet RO, Mihm MC, Sober AJ. Color atlas and synopsis of pigmented lesions. New York: McGraw-Hill; 1995.

Baumert J, Plewing G, Volkenandt M, Schmid-Wendtner MH. Factors associated with a high tumor thickness in patients with melanoma. Br J Dermatol. 2007;156:938–44.

Betti R, Vergani R, Tolomio E, et al. Factors of delay in the diagnosis of melanoma. Eur J Dermatol. 2003;13:183–8.

Bevona C, Goggins W, Quinn T, Fullerton J, Tsao H. Cutaneous melanomas associated with nevi. Arch Dermatol. 2003;139:1620–4.

Briggs JC, Ibrahim NB. Late recurrence of cutaneous melanoma. J Am Acad Dermatol. 1988;18:147–9.

Calonje JE, Brenn T, Lazar AJ, McKee PH. McKee's pathology of the skin, edn 4. China: Elsevier; 2012.

Cascinelli N, Belli F, MacKie RM, et al. Effect of long-term adjuvant therapy with interferon alpha-2a in patients with regional node metastases from cutaneous melanoma: a randomised trial. Lancet. 2001;358:866–9.

Chamberlain AJ, Fritschi L, Giles GG. Nodular type and older age as the most significant associations of thick melanoma in Victoria, Australia. Arch Dermatol. 2003;138:609–14.

Chamberlain AJ, Fritschil, Kelly JW. Nodular melanoma: patients perceptions of presenting features for earlier detection. J Am Acad Dermatol. 2003;48:694–701.

Chapman PB, Hauschild A, Robert C, et al. BRIM-3 Study Group. Improved survival with vemurafenib in melanoma with BRAF V600E mutation. N Engl J Med. 2011;364:2507–16.

Clark WH Jr, Elder DE, van Horn M. The biologic forms of malignant melanoma. Hum Pathol. 1986;17:443–50.

Connelly J, Smith JL Jr. Malignant blue nevus. Cancer. 1991;67:2653–7.

Cox NH, Artchison TC, MacKie RM. Extrafacial lentigo maligna melanoma: analysis of 71 cases and comparison with lentigo maligna melanoma of the head and neck. Br J Dermatol. 1998;139:439–43.

de Sa BC, Reze GG, Seramin AP, et al. Cutaneous melanoma in adolescence: retrospective study of 32 patients. Melanoma Res. 2004;14:487–92.

Demierre MF, Chung C, Miller DR, Geller AC. Early datection of thick melanoma in the United States: beware of the nodular type. Arch Dermatol. 2005;141:745–50.

Garbe C, Büttner P, Bertz J, et al. Primary cutaneous melanoma. Prognostic classification of anatomic location. Cancer. 1995;75:2492–8.

Garbe C, Peris K, Hauschild A, et al. Diagnosis and treatment of melanoma. European consensus-based interdisciplinary guideline-Update 2012. Eur J Cancer. 2012;48:2375–90.

Gershenwald JE, Thompson W, Mansfield PF, et al. Multi-institutional melanoma lymphatic mapping experience: the prognostic value of sentinel lymph node status in 612 stage I or II melanoma patients. J Clin Oncol 1999;17:976–83.

Hill SJ, Delman KA. Pediatric melanomas and the atypical spitzoid melanocytic neoplasms. Am J Surg. 2012;203:761–7.

Hodi FS, O'Day SJ, McDermott DF, et al. Improved survival with ipilimumab in patients with metastatic melanoma. N Eng J Med. 2010;363:711–23.

Kanzler MH, Swetter SM. Malignant melanoma. J Am Acad Dermatol. 2003;48:780–3.

Kanzler MH, Mraz-Gernhard S. Primary cutaneous malignant melanoma and its precursor lesions: diagnostic and therapeutic overview. J Am Acad Dermatol. 2001;45:260–76.

Koch H, Zelger B, Cerroni L. Malignant blue nevus: malignant melanoma in association with blue nevus. Eur J Dermatol. 1996;6:335–8.

Kuchelmeister C, Schaumburg-Lever G, Garbe C. Acral cutaneous melanoma in caucasions: clinical features, histopathology and prognosis in 112 patients. Br J Dermatol. 2000;143:275–80.

Kunishige JH, Brodland DG, Zitelli JA. Surgical margins for melanoma in situ. J Am Acad Dermatol 2012;66:438–44.

Lack KE, Karagiannis SN, Nestle FO. Advances in the treatment of melanoma. Clin Med. 2012;12:168–71.

LeBoit PE, Burg G, Weedon D, Sarasin A. Pathology and genetics of skin tumours. World Health Organization Classification of Tumours. France: IARC Press; 2006.

Ledermon J, Sober A. Does biopsy influence survival in clinical stage I melanoma? J Am Acad Dermatol. 1985;13:983–7.

Lens MB, Newton-Bishop JA, Boon AP. Desmoplastic malignant melanoma: a systematic review. Br J Dermatol. 2005;152:673–8.

Marghoob AA, Schoenbach SP, Kopf AW, et al. Large congenital melanocytic nevi: a prospective study. Pediatr Dermatol. 1996;132:170–5.

Martin RC 2nd, Scoggins CR, Ross MF, et al. Is incisional biopsy of melanoma harmful? Am J Surg. 2005;190:913–7.

McKenna JK, Florell SR, Goldman GD, Bowen GM. Lentigo maligna/lentigo maligna melanoma: current state of diagnosis and treatment. Dermatologic Surg. 2006;32:493–504.

Meleti M, Leemons CR, Mooi WJ, van der Waal I. Oral malignant melanoma: the Amsterdam experience. J Oral Maxillofac Surg. 2007;65:2181–6.

Patrick RJ, Fenske NA, Messina JL. Primary mucosal melanoma. J Am Acad Dermatol. 2007;56:828–34.

Posther KE, Selim MA, Mosca PJ, et al. Histopathologic characteristics, recurrence patterns, and survival of 129 patients with desmoplastic melanoma. Ann Surg Oncol. 2006;13;728–39.

Rigel DS, Robinson JK, Ross M, Friedman RJ, Corkerell CJ, Lim HW, Stockfleth HW, Kirkwood JM. Cancer of the skin, edn 2. China: Saunders Elsevier; 2011.

Ruocco E, Argenziano G, Pellaconi G, Seidenori S. Noninvasive imaging of skin tumors. Dermatol Surg. 2004;30:301–10.

Schwartz RA. Skin cancer: recognition and management, edn 2. Singapore: Blackwell Publishing; 2008.

Skender-Kalneas TM, English DR, Heenan PJ. Benign melanocytic lesions: risk marker or precursors of cutaneous melanoma? J Am Acad Dermatol. 1995;33:1000–7.

Soyer HP, Argenziano G, Hofmann-Welenhof R, Johr R . Color atlas of melanocytic lesions of the skin. Germany: Springer-Verlag; 2010.

Stevenson O, Ahmed I. Lentigo maligna: prognosis and treatment options. Am J Clin Dermatol. 2005;6:151–64.

Temple-Camp CR, Saxe N, King H. Benign and malignant blue nevus: a clinicopathological study of 30 cases. Am J Dermatopothol. 1988;10:289–96.

Toung W, Cheng LS, Armstrong AW. Melanoma: epidemiology, diagnosis, treatment and outcomes. Dermatol Clin. 2012;30:113–24.

Weedon D. Weedon's skin pathology, edn 3. China: Elsevier; 2010.

Wolf IH, Richtig E, Kopera D, Kerl H. Locoregional cutaneous metastases of malignant melanoma and their management. Dermatol Surg. 2004;30:244–7.

Cutaneous Sarcomas

Malignant tumors of mesenchymal tissue (sarcomas) originating from the dermis and subcutis are discussed in this chapter. In addition, some sarcomas locate in deeper soft tissue (subfascial sarcomas), and the skin may be involved secondarily by the extension of the tumor. These sarcomas are mainly diagnosed and treated by orthopedic surgeons. Sarcomas are classified according to the cell of origin. All cutaneous sarcomas of vascular, fibrous, fatty tissue, nerve sheath, and smooth muscle origin are rare. Cutaneous sarcomas with vascular differentiation are localized on relatively superficial parts of the skin and have typical clinical features, but most other sarcomas present with nonspecific nodules or poorly defined deep masses that may only be diagnosed by histopathologic examination. Cutaneous sarcomas are generally not transformed from benign skin or soft tissue tumors. While some of these cutaneous sarcomas are low grade and have a better prognosis than their counterparts in deeper tissue, many have an aggressive course with a potential for systemic metastasis. Early diagnosis is essential to decrease the morbidity and mortality of these tumors.

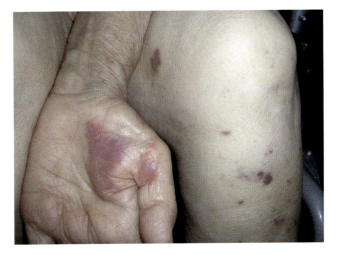

Fig. 13.1 Classic Kaposi sarcoma involving the hand and leg concomitantly

13.1 Kaposi Sarcoma

Kaposi sarcoma is a malignant neoplasm characterized by multicentric skin and mucous membrane lesions that may be associated with visceral involvement. It is the most common skin sarcoma. Endothelial cells of lymphatics, smooth muscle cells of vessel walls, and dermal dendrocytes are the suggested cellular origins of the tumor. Human herpes virus type-8 (HHV-8) plays an important role in the etiopathogenesis but is possibly not the single factor. This virus originally was named Kaposi sarcoma herpes virus (KSHV). The tumor may be seen in different clinical presentations and varying frequencies throughout the world. Familial occurrence is very unusual. Clinical and epidemiologic subtypes of the tumor have been described. The number and extension of skin lesions, favored sites, possibility of mucosal involvement the severity of visceral involvement, and the course and prognosis of the disease are variable in these subtypes. On the other hand, the histopathologic features of all subtypes of Kaposi sarcoma are common.

13.1.1 Classic Kaposi Sarcoma

Classic Kaposi sarcoma is the most common form of the disease in many countries, excluding those where the endemic form is frequently seen. It is more common in people of Mediterranean and Eastern European Jewish origin. It occurs primarily in the elderly population and sometimes in the middle-aged group, with a clear male predominance. Patients having the classic subtype of the tumor nearly always have only dermatologic manifestations. One or more body sites may be involved (*see* Fig. 13.1). Lesions occur predominantly on the feet (*see* Fig. 13.2), followed by the lower legs (mostly around the ankles) (*see* Fig. 13.3) and hands. Both dorsal and volar surfaces of the hands (*see* Fig. 13.4) and feet (*see* Fig. 13.5), including the digits (*see* Figs. 13.1 and 13.6), may be affected. The periungual area may also be involved

C. Baykal, K.D. Yazganoğlu, *Clinical Atlas of Skin Tumors*,
DOI 10.1007/978-3-642-40938-7_13, © Springer-Verlag Berlin Heidelberg 2014

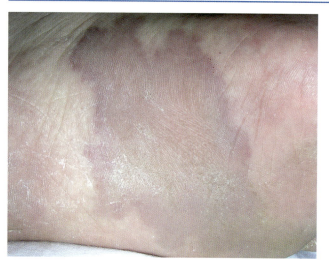

Fig. 13.2 Classic Kaposi sarcoma appearing as a purplish patch on the sole of the foot

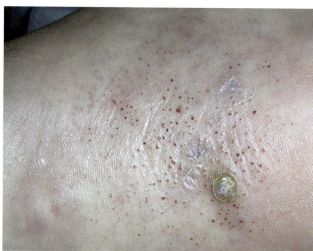

Fig. 13.5 Classic Kaposi sarcoma seen as multiple tiny papules and a small nodule on the sole

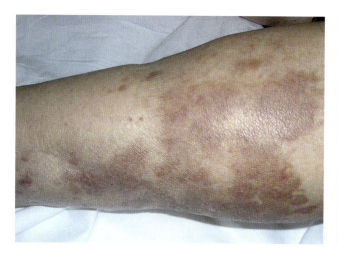

Fig. 13.3 Classic Kaposi sarcoma as brownish patches on the lower leg

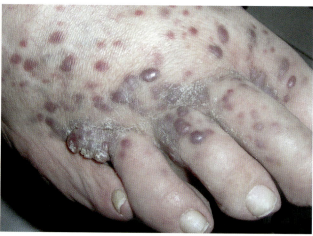

Fig. 13.6 Classic Kaposi sarcoma presenting as multiple purple papules on the toes and dorsum of the foot

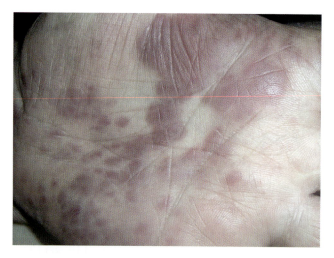

Fig. 13.4 Classic Kaposi sarcoma on the palm

(see Fig. 13.7). Lesions on the head and neck are seen in a small percentage of patients (see Fig. 13.8). Mucosal involvement, including the genital mucosae may also be seen but is rare in classic Kaposi sarcoma (see Fig. 13.9). Most patients have a few lesions, but solitary or multiple cutaneous lesions are also possible. In patients with multiple lesions, bilateral and partially symmetric involvement may be seen (see Fig. 13.10).

The clinical presentation of Kaposi sarcoma is variable. Lesions may start as small patches that may be purple (see Fig. 13.11), reddish-blue, brown (see Fig. 13.3), or flesh-colored. They slowly enlarge, becoming large indurated plaques (see Figs. 13.12, 13.13 and 13.14), sometimes with overlying papules and raised nodules (see Fig. 13.15). However, the tumor also may appear as an isolated papule or nodule from the onset (see Figs. 13.16, 13.17, 13.18 and 13.19). The lesions may be smooth-surfaced but are sometimes

13.1 Kaposi Sarcoma

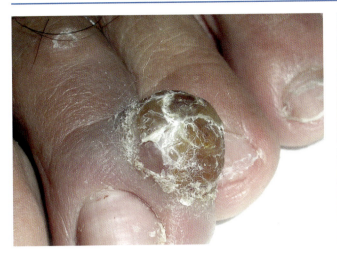

Fig. 13.7 A solitary crusted nodule on the periungual area representing classic Kaposi sarcoma

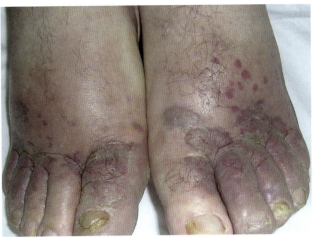

Fig. 13.10 Typical bilateral involvement of Kaposi sarcoma on the feet

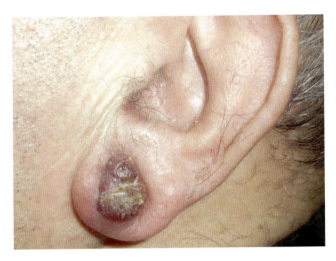

Fig. 13.8 Kaposi sarcoma on the earlobe in an otherwise healthy patient. This is a rare location for the classic subtype

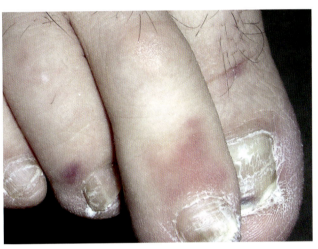

Fig. 13.11 Purplish macules on the toes. A typical presentation of the early stage of classic Kaposi sarcoma

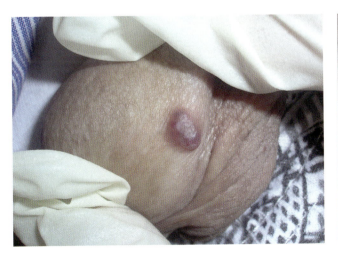

Fig. 13.9 A solitary lesion on the urethral meatus in an otherwise healthy patient; a rare site of involvement of classic Kaposi sarcoma

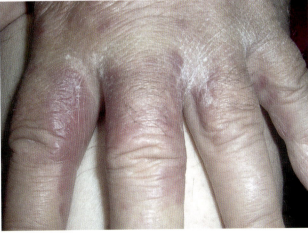

Fig. 13.12 Plaque lesions on the fingers of a patient with classic Kaposi sarcoma

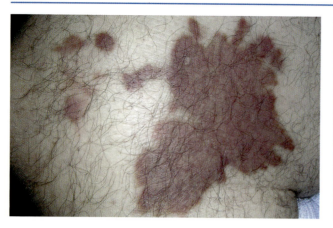

Fig. 13.13 Sharply demarcated irregular plaque on the leg of a patient with classic Kaposi sarcoma

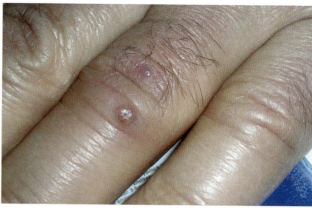

Fig. 13.16 A small papule on the hand. Initial presentation of classic Kaposi sarcoma

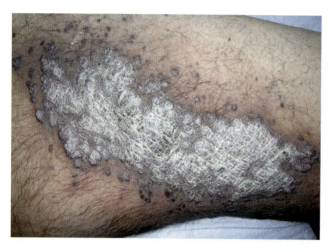

Fig. 13.14 Large hyperkeratotic plaque of classic Kaposi sarcoma that existed for a long time period

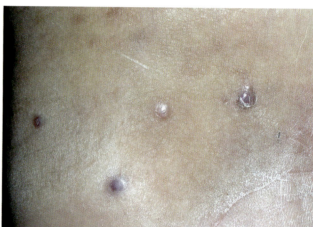

Fig. 13.17 Scattered purple papules on the foot representing classic Kaposi sarcoma

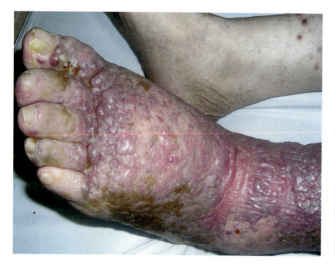

Fig. 13.15 Classic Kaposi sarcoma presenting as a plaque covering a large area with overlying papules. Note the enlargement of the same extremity owing to lymphedema

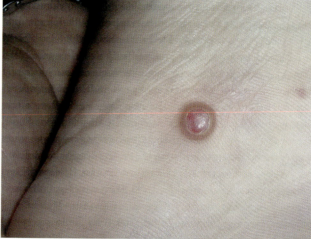

Fig. 13.18 Red solitary nodule on the sole of a patient with classic Kaposi sarcoma

13.1 Kaposi Sarcoma

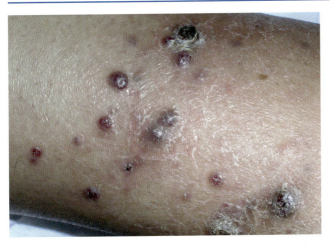

Fig. 13.19 Multiple papules and nodules on the leg of a patient with Kaposi sarcoma

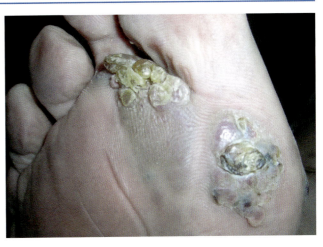

Fig. 13.21 Kaposi sarcoma on the sole, causing a verrucous appearance

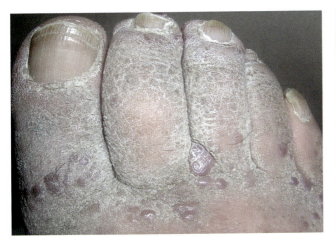

Fig. 13.20 Confluent plaques of Kaposi sarcoma with hyperkeratotic surface on the dorsum of the toes

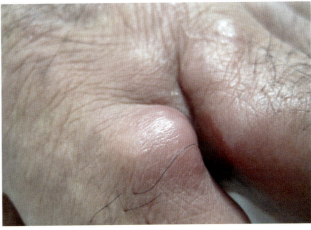

Fig. 13.22 Kaposi sarcoma appearing as subcutaneous nodules on the fingers. Diagnosis is more challenging in such cases

hyperkeratotic (*see* Figs. 13.14 and 13.20) or verrucous (*see* Fig. 13.21). Rarely, they may appear as subcutaneous firm nodules (*see* Fig. 13.22). Telangiectasia on the surface is uncommonly observed. The classic type of the tumor usually has a very slow progression. Older lesions may be eroded or ulcerated and covered with crusts (*see* Fig. 13.23). Large tumors may cause bleeding and pain. As related to the rich spectrum of clinical presentation, a large number of diseases may be considered in the differential diagnosis. Macular lesions should be differentiated from pseudo-Kaposi sarcoma and early lesions of cutaneous angiosarcoma (*see* Fig. 13.48), but the latter is mostly located on the head and neck. Papulonodular lesions have similarities with pseudolymphoma (*see* Fig. 14.193), dermatofibroma (*see* Fig. 8.1), sarcoidosis, angiolymphoid hyperplasia with eosinophilia (*see* Fig. 6.76), and many other vascular tumors. Exophytic lesions with an eroded surface (*see* Figs. 13.24 and 13.25)

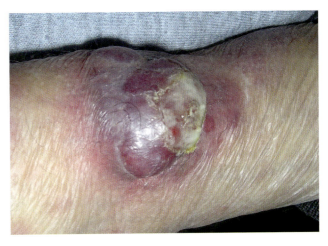

Fig. 13.23 Advanced classic Kaposi sarcoma presenting as a large ulcerated tumor on the forearm

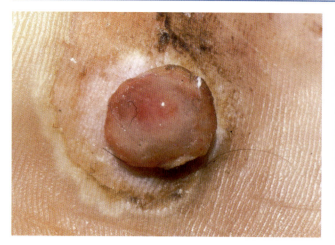

Fig. 13.24 A pyogenic granuloma-like exophytic Kaposi sarcoma with eroded surface on the sole of the foot

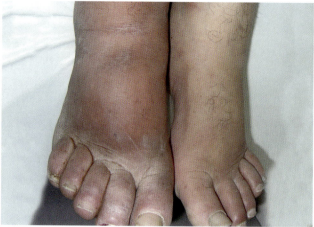

Fig. 13.26 Prominent lymphedema and diffuse skin infiltration on one foot (*left*) caused by Kaposi sarcoma

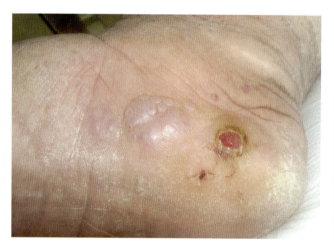

Fig. 13.25 Multiple lesions of Kaposi sarcoma on a lymphedematous foot. Note the erosion on the surface of the large nodule

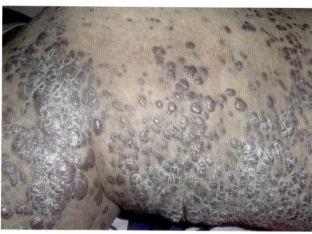

Fig. 13.27 Numerous papulonodular lesions with a tendency to confluence and covering a large area of the leg in a patient with Kaposi sarcoma

look like pyogenic granuloma (*see* Fig. 6.49). Histologically early patch and plaque type lesions may show only subtle changes such as slit-like abnormal vascular channels, a few spindle cells, and a reactive inflammatory infiltrate containing plasma cells and hemosiderin deposition related with erythrocyte extravasation. In early macular lesions the correct diagnosis may be missed. Papulonodular or tumoral lesions are characterized by spindle cells forming sheets and nodules in the dermis. In relation to the tumor's etiology, anti-HHV8 staining is always positive.

Lymphedema, especially on the lower legs and genitalia, may accompany some lesions of Kaposi sarcoma. Involved limbs are typically enlarged (*see* Fig. 13.26). This chronic condition has been attributed to secondary lymphatic obstruction caused by the tumor.

Skin lesions seen in the classic subtype of the tumor generally have an indolent course. Although they gradually increase in size and number over many years, lesions covering large areas (*see* Fig. 13.27) and infiltration of underlying deep tissue rarely occur (*see* Fig. 13.28). Lymphadenopathy and symptomatic visceral involvement are rare in this subtype of Kaposi sarcoma. The usual site of visceral involvement is the gastrointestinal tract, which may be detected by endoscopic examination. However, routine use of endoscopy is not indicated unless the patient is symptomatic. The lung and very rarely other visceral organs may also be involved.

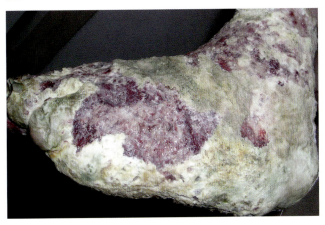

Fig. 13.28 Kaposi sarcoma with deep tissue involvement, causing diffuse ulcerations that are secondarily infected. This otherwise healthy patient had a long duration of disease

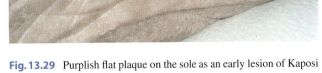

Fig. 13.29 Purplish flat plaque on the sole as an early lesion of Kaposi sarcoma in an HIV-infected patient

13.1.2 Acquired Immunodeficiency Syndrome (AIDS)–Related (Epidemic) Kaposi Sarcoma

Contrary to the classic subtype, Kaposi sarcoma seen in patients with untreated Human immunodeficiency virus (HIV) infection has an aggressive course and has been described as a special subtype. On the other hand, the incidence and morbidity of this malignant tumor are seriously reduced after the use of highly activated antiretroviral therapy (HAART). This subtype is more commonly seen in homosexual or bisexual men and appears at a younger age than the classic Kaposi sarcoma. The lesions are mostly seen in the later stages of HIV infection, when the CD4+ cell count is decreased. However, sometimes the diagnosis of HIV infection can be made after the development of Kaposi sarcoma. In addition to the classic location on the distal extremities (*see* Figs. 13.29 and 13.30), the head (especially the nose and ears), neck, upper trunk (*see* Fig 13.31), and genitalia are commonly involved in this subtype of Kaposi sarcoma. Lesions have a rapid progressive course, and many patients have disseminated skin lesions with oval or elongated, reddish or purple nodules and plaques (*see* Fig 13.32). A symmetric distribution of lesions may be observed (*see* Figs. 13.30 and 13.32). Ulceration of the tumors may occur. Mucosal involvement is very often seen in patients, especially those who are not treated with HAART. The hard palate is a typical location, but any areas of the oral mucosa may be involved. Difficulty during eating may occur. Bacillary angiomatosis is a Bartonella infection manifesting with multiple angiomatous nodules occurring eruptively and may be a differential diagnostic challenge of Kaposi sarcoma in HIV-infected patients. The differentiation is critical because

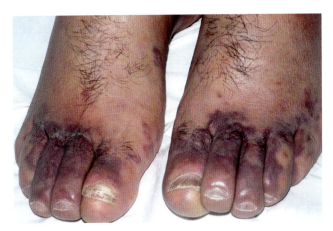

Fig. 13.30 AIDS-related Kaposi sarcoma with bilateral feet involvement occurring in a short period of time. Associated white superficial onycomycosis is also noticeable

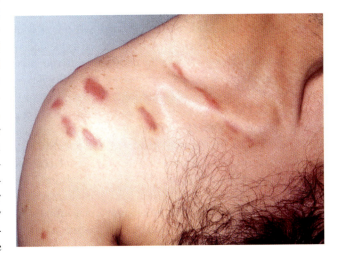

Fig. 13.31 Disseminated oval plaques of Kaposi sarcoma on the shoulders of an HIV-infected patient

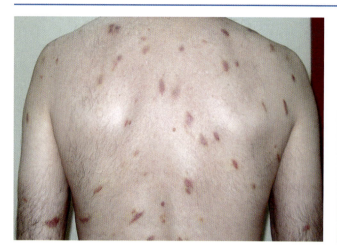

Fig. 13.32 Multiple oval plaques on the trunk with symmetric distribution; typical presentation of the tumor in HIV-infected patients

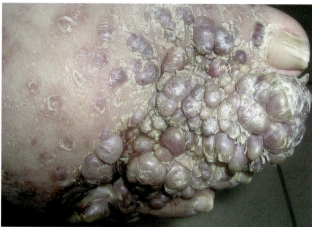

Fig. 13.33 Confluent papules of Kaposi sarcoma causing a verrucous plaque on the foot of an immunosuppressed patient. Lesions may be exaggerated in the iatrogenic subtype of Kaposi sarcoma

this life-threatening bacterial disease should be treated with antibiotics.

Lymph node and visceral involvement are more frequent and widespread than in the classic form and may also occur in the absence of skin lesions. AIDS-related Kaposi sarcoma may cause gastrointestinal involvement, pulmonary parenchymal disease, pleural effusion, and involvement of other organs, causing dysfunction. Therefore, it should be treated as early as possible.

13.1.3 Iatrogenic Kaposi Sarcoma

The incidence of Kaposi sarcoma is increased significantly in patients with weakened immune systems as a result of organ transplantation, systemic lymphomas, or long-term systemic corticosteroid administration. In rare cases, long-term use of potent topical corticosteroids may also be associated with Kaposi sarcoma. The course is typically related to the underlying condition. It may occur in the early period of immunosuppression or up to ten years later. Patients with this subtype of the tumor usually have multiple lesions. Lesions are primarily located on the distal extremities (*see* Fig. 13.33), but also on other areas of the skin, including the proximal extremities (*see* Figs. 13.34), the trunk (*see* Figs. 13.35 and 13.36), and face (*see* Fig 13.37). In addition, mucous membranes such as the conjunctival (*see* Fig 13.38), intraoral (*see* Figs 13.39, 13.40, and 13.41), nasal, and genital areas may also be involved in most cases. Nodules and plaques may be observed anywhere on the oral mucosa. The inferior fornix of the conjunctiva is the most commonly involved site of the eye. Lagophthalmia, ectropion, and trichiasis are complications of eye involvement. Lesions have a progressive course (*see* Fig. 13.42a and b), and ulceration, dissemination, or confluence (*see* Fig. 13.34) of cutaneous lesions may be observed in patients with immunosuppression of long duration.

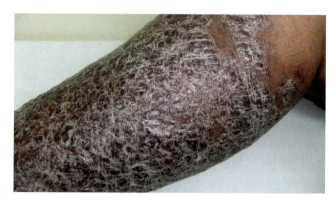

Fig. 13.34 Kaposi sarcoma appearing during a prolonged course of high-dose systemic corticosteroid therapy. Note the confluent papules covering a large part of the shin

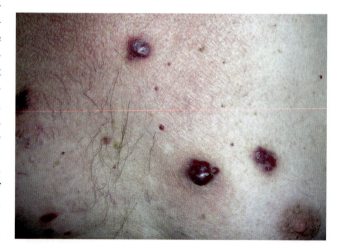

Fig. 13.35 Multiple reddish nodular lesions on the trunk of an immunosuppressed patient. Kaposi sarcoma is not rare in atypical locations in the iatrogenic subtype

13.1 Kaposi Sarcoma

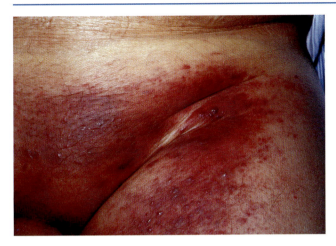

Fig. 13.36 Kaposi sarcoma presenting as a large plaque on the pubic area and groin of a patient with systemic lymphoma

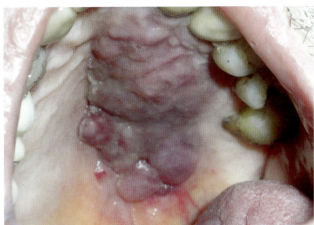

Fig. 13.39 Mucosal involvement in iatrogenic Kaposi sarcoma. Raised purplish plaque is seen on the hard palate, a very typical location

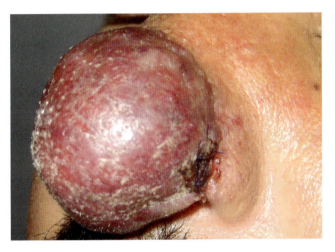

Fig. 13.37 Kaposi sarcoma manifesting as a large mass on the tip of the nose in a renal transplant recipient. Involvement of the nose is also common in AIDS-related Kaposi sarcoma (With kind permission from Springer Science+Business Media: Baykal C, Yazganoğlu KD. Dermatological diseases of the nose and ears; 2010.)

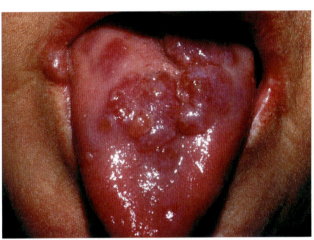

Fig. 13.40 Mucosal involvement in iatrogenic Kaposi sarcoma. Red nodules on the tongue and oral commissure are seen

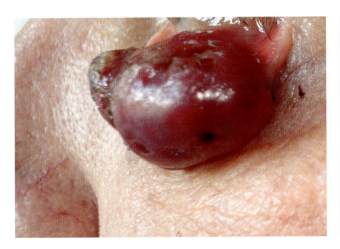

Fig. 13.38 Mucosal involvement in iatrogenic Kaposi sarcoma. A large red nodule arising from the conjunctiva is seen

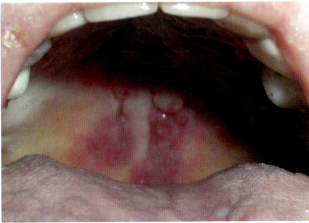

Fig. 13.41 Iatrogenic Kaposi sarcoma presenting as purplish macules on the soft palate

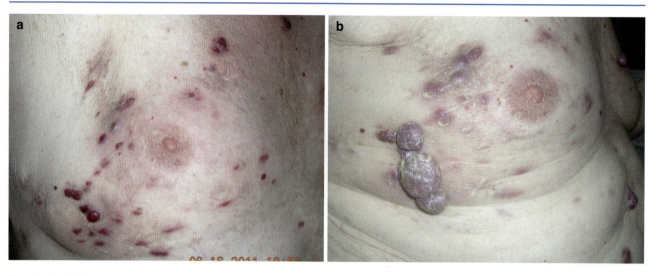

Fig. 13.42 (a) Iatrogenic Kaposi sarcoma presenting as multiple papular lesions on the trunk. (b) Lesions enlarged to nodules and tumors as the immunosuppressive therapy could not be stopped

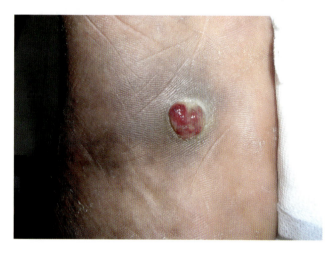

Fig. 13.43 Kaposi sarcoma presenting as an ulcerated exophytic nodule surrounded by macular component on the sole of an African American patient

Visceral involvement may be seen in some patients and may cause numerous symptoms. Life-threatening hemorrhages, intussusception, perforation, protein-loosing enteropathy, pulmonary obstruction, and cardiac tamponade are rare complications, especially if withdrawal of immunosuppressive agents is not possible. Gastrointestinal symptoms such as nausea, abdominal pain, odynophagia, hematemesis, or melena seen in patients with skin lesions of Kaposi sarcoma should be of great concern for gastrointestinal tract involvement and necessitate further investigation, including endoscopy. Pulmonary involvement may also rarely cause symptoms such as cough, hemoptysis, or dyspnea. It is mostly detected by radiologic examination and bronchoscopy.

13.1.4 Endemic (African) Kaposi Sarcoma

Kaposi sarcoma is more common in the African black population and is endemic in some countries near the equator in Africa. This represents a subtype that may be seen in middle-aged adult men and also in children with no gender difference. However, clinical features varies due to age of the patient. In adults, involvement of the distal extremities is more common (*see* Fig. 13.43). As in the classic subtype of the tumor, systemic involvement is rare in adults. However, the endemic subtype is locally more aggressive. It may show an aggressive course with lymphadenopathy and visceral involvement in children. Skin lesions may be absent in this age group.

Management. The clinical course of Kaposi sarcoma is unpredictable. The management decision depends on the individual condition of each patient. Identifying the subtype of Kaposi sarcoma is the first step to determine the ideal therapeutic approach. In patients with HIV infection, even the disseminated skin lesions of Kaposi sarcoma may regress after using antiretroviral therapy. However, in some cases other modalities should be added. Similarly, if possible, withdrawal of immunosuppression is the main step in the management of the iatrogenic subtype of Kaposi sarcoma. Cessation of systemic corticosteroid therapy may result in complete healing (*see* Fig. 13.44a and b). Sirolimus (rapamycin), a tumor growth inhibitor, may be preferred as an immunosuppressive drug in patients with iatrogenic Kaposi sarcoma associated with transplantation, and after switching to this drug the mucocutaneous lesions may disappear in some cases (*see* Fig. 13.45a and b). Other therapeutic modalities can be used if this drug change is not efficient.

The age of the patient as well as the number and extension of mucocutaneous lesions, their anatomic distribution, and the cosmetic concerns are important factors in determining

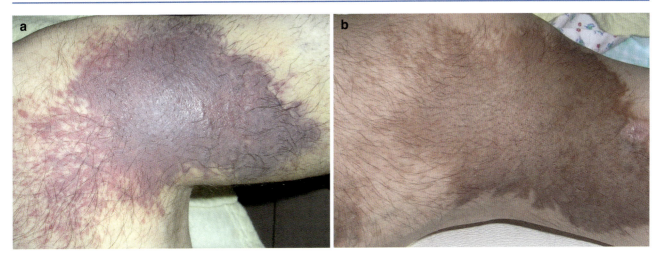

Fig. 13.44 (a) A large patch of Kaposi sarcoma on the leg occurring during systemic corticosteroid therapy. (b) Healing of the lesion after discontinuation of corticosteroid therapy (postinflammatory pigmentation in the figure resolved later)

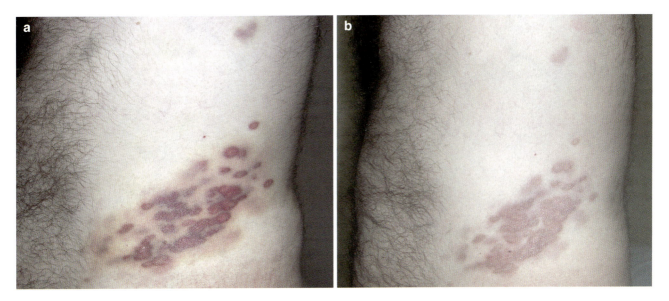

Fig. 13.45 (a) Kaposi sarcoma seen as confluent purple papules forming a large plaque on the trunk of a transplant recipient. (b) Regression of the lesions after switching the immunosuppressive therapy

the therapy of classic Kaposi sarcoma. Elderly without a rapid progressive course and symptomatic systemic involvement can only be followed up without therapy.

Various local therapeutic modalities are used in all subtypes of Kaposi sarcoma. Solitary or only a few lesions can be excised surgically (*see* Fig. 13.46a–c) or destroyed with lasers or cryotherapy. However new lesions and recurrence may occur on the same site (*see* Fig. 13.47). Therefore multiple minor surgical interventions may be required for many years in classic Kaposi sarcoma. Mucosal lesions of Kaposi sarcoma are more difficult to treat with surgery. Radiotherapy is generally used for larger skin lesions, and complete regression can be obtained with this method. Intralesional vinca alkaloids (vinblastine, vincristine) and interferon alpha are other options for limited lesions and for some mucosal lesions.

A topical retinoid, alitretinoin (0.1 percent gel), has also been shown to be effective in Kaposi sarcoma. However, development of new lesions cannot be avoided with local therapies.

Lesions refractory to other therapies, rapidly progressive or disseminated lesions, and tumors associated with lymphedema or symptomatic visceral involvement need to be treated with systemic chemotherapy. Low-dose vinblastine is generally preferred. Other chemotherapeutic medications such as liposomal doxorubicin, liposomal daunorubicin, paclitaxel, and etoposide may be used in rapidly progressive skin lesions and visceral involvement seen in AIDS-related Kaposi sarcoma, iatrogenic Kaposi sarcoma, and endemic Kaposi sarcoma. Recurrent lesions may be re-treated with the same modalities. Systemic and local therapies can be combined in some cases. Amputation

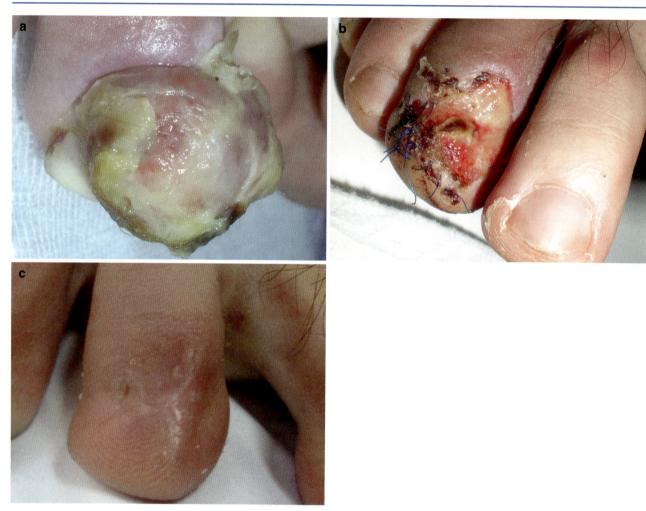

Fig. 13.46 (a) Kaposi sarcoma manifesting as a solitary eroded nodule on the nailfold. (b) Tumor is removed surgically. (c) Healing with the formation of scar tissue

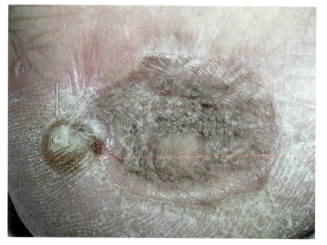

Fig. 13.47 Recurrence of Kaposi sarcoma as a nodule (*arrow*) around the excision scar on the foot

may be indicated in deep acral lesions with ulceration and secondary infection which are refractory to aggressive medical therapy.

13.2 Cutaneous Angiosarcoma

Angiosarcoma is a neoplasm of endothelial cell origin that may be seen in visceral organs, soft tissue, and skin. Cutaneous angiosarcoma is a very rare tumor with a highly aggressive course. It may appear in relation to several clinical conditions. It may develop spontaneously in the older population on normal skin, may appear rarely at the site of previous radiotherapy as a late complication, or sometimes may occur in the setting of chronic lymphedema (Stewart-Treves syndrome). Moreover, patients with Maffucci syndrome have an increased risk of developing angiosarcoma.

The scalp, face, and neck are the favored sites of cutaneous angiosarcoma that occurs in older men on normal skin, but it may also be seen on the lower extremities. It begins typically as a bruise-like, bluish-black patch that is not well-defined (*see* Fig. 13.48) and may be multicentric (*see* Fig. 13.49). In the early stage, ecchymosis, nevus flammeus (*see* Fig. 6.92), and macular lesions of Kaposi sarcoma (*see* Fig. 13.2) may be considered in the differential diagnosis.

13.2 Cutaneous Angiosarcoma

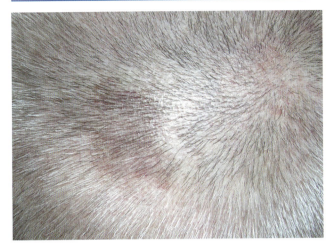

Fig. 13.48 An ill-defined, bruise-like patch on the scalp representing an early lesion of cutaneous angiosarcoma

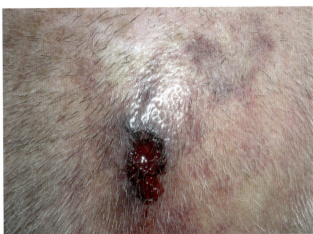

Fig. 13.50 Cutaneous angiosarcoma shown as multiple ill-defined, reddish patches resembling ecchymosis and a bluish-black raised nodule

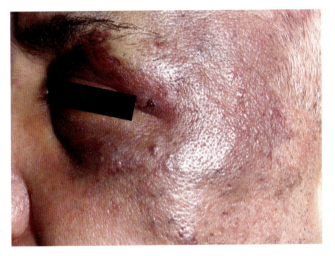

Fig. 13.49 Multifocal lesions of cutaneous angiosarcoma involving a large part of the face; an advanced case is seen

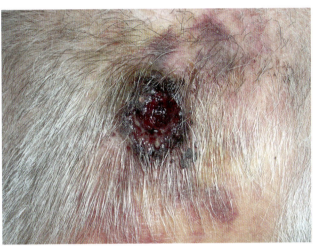

Fig. 13.51 Ulcerated nodule of cutaneous angiosarcoma seen concomitantly with patchy lesions

The diagnosis may be delayed, especially if the lesions are limited to the scalp (see Fig. 13.48). Histologically, anastomosing irregular vascular channels lined by pleomorphic endothelial cells, dissecting dermal collagen, and infiltrating subcutaneous tissue represent the well-differentiated tumor. Less differentiated areas without vascular channels but with a proliferation of spindle-shaped or epithelioid cells may also be seen.

Macular lesions spread rapidly to the near vicinity and infiltrate deeper tissue, causing raised nodules (see Fig. 13.50) and large plaques. They may be eroded or ulcerated (see Fig. 13.51) in a short time and may be painful. They bleed easily and may be covered with necrotic crusts (see Figs. 13.52 and 13.53). Satellite skin lesions may also occur. Metastases to regional lymph nodes and hematogenous metastases to the lungs, liver, spleen, and bones worsen the prognosis of the tumor.

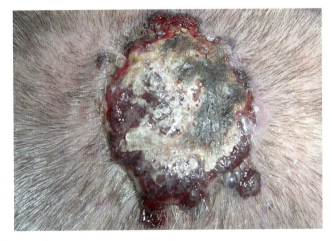

Fig. 13.52 Cutaneous angiosarcoma presenting as a large nodule covered with crusts on the scalp. This lesion has shown rapid growth

Stewart-Treves syndrome is a special type of cutaneous angiosarcoma occurring in the setting of chronic

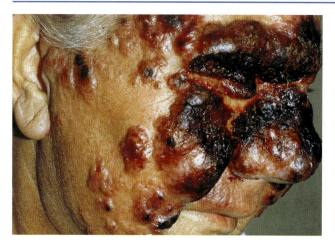

Fig. 13.53 Infiltrated lesions of angiosarcoma covered with necrotic crusts. The tumor may involve large areas in advanced stage (With kind permission from Springer Science+Business Media: Baykal C, Yazganoğlu KD. Dermatological diseases of the nose and ears; 2010.)

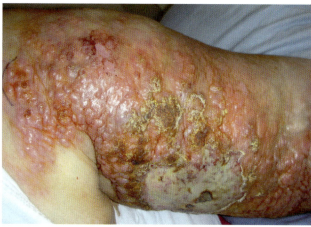

Fig. 13.55 Confluent papules and nodules on edematous tissue of the upper arm in Stewart-Treves syndrome

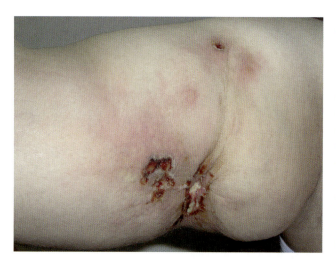

Fig. 13.54 Ulcerative nodules on edematous upper arm representing Stewart-Treves syndrome in a patient who has undergone radical mastectomy

lymphedema. It is especially seen on the upper extremities, which become lymphedematous after mastectomy, but it may also rarely arise in congenital lymphedema. The interval between mastectomy and the appearance of angiosarcoma may be 10 to 20 years. The medial aspect of an edematous upper arm ipsilateral to the mastectomy is the typical site of onset in these patients, and lesions may invade the periphery later (*see* Fig. 13.54). Multiple purplish hemorrhagic infiltrating papules or nodules with a tendency to confluence are typical (*see* Fig. 13.55). Erosions and ulcerations may develop on a diffusely indurated area. They should be distinguished from skin metastases of breast carcinoma (*see* Fig. 16.16). The histopathology is similar to that of angiosarcoma occurring on normal skin. The prognosis is poor.

Management. The main therapeutic option of cutaneous angiosarcoma is wide excision laterally and in depth. However, lesions may be multiple and extensive at the time of diagnosis, and thus excision is not always possible. Furthermore, clinically visible margins are not reliable. Amputation of the affected arm may be required in Stewart-Treves syndrome. Palliative radiotherapy can be done in unresectable lesions (*see* Fig. 13.56a and b), but local recurrence or new lesions on the vicinity (*see* Fig. 13.56c and d) mostly occur in a short time. Chemotherapy is preferred in unresectable advanced tumors, in recurrent tumors, and for visceral metastases but its effect is limited.

13.3 Epithelioid Hemangioendothelioma

Epithelioid hemangioendothelioma is a rare tumor of soft tissue arising from the vascular endothelium. It may be seen on visceral organs such as the liver, lung, and bone and extremely rarely on the dermis or subcutis of the skin. It is a well-differentiated tumor considered a borderline malignancy. It is more common in young adults and may be seen in children. Skin lesions may be associated with other visceral lesions as part of multifocal involvement or may be isolated. Its form is mostly solitary or rarely with multiple erythematous papules, nodules (*see* Fig. 13.57), plaques, or ulcerations. The lesion may be painful. Differentiation from other vascular tumors such as pyogenic granuloma, Kaposi sarcoma, and cutaneous angiosarcoma is possible on histopathologic examination. Polygonal epithelioid endothelial cells forming cords and strands in the dermis are typical features.

Management. All patients diagnosed with skin lesions should be evaluated for systemic involvement. If the tumor is located only on the skin, surgery with wide margins is usually most effective. The clinical course of the visceral tumors is unpredictable. Although not very often, lymphogenous and hematogenous metastasis may occur.

13.4 Dermatofibrosarcoma Protuberans

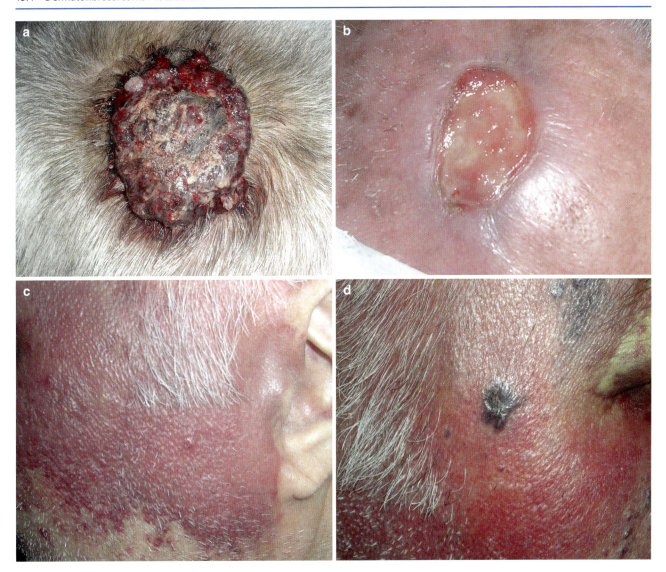

Fig. 13.56 (**a**) A large nodule and bruise-like patches on the scalp histologically diagnosed as angiosarcoma. (**b**) Good response to radiotherapy. (**c-d**) New lesions occurred extensively on the face in a short time after cessation of radiotherapy

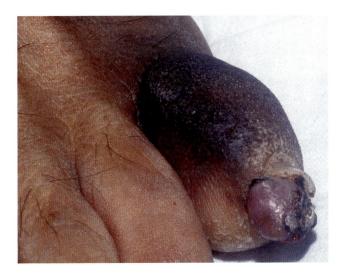

Fig. 13.57 Epithelioid hemangioendothelioma manifesting as a pyogenic granuloma-like nodule around the nail

13.4 Dermatofibrosarcoma Protuberans

Dermatofibrosarcoma protuberans is a low-grade and slowly growing malignancy originating from dermal fibroblasts. It is mostly seen in young and middle-aged adults but is occasionally congenital (*see* Fig. 13.58). The chest, back, buttocks, and thighs are the preferred sites. Head and neck involvement may rarely be seen. The confluence of skin-colored, pinkish, or brown nodules form irregularly shaped raised plaques (*see* Figs. 13.59 and 13.60). Protuberant or pedunculated nodules may overlie firm plaques, which are fixed to the underlying subcutaneous tissue (*see* Fig. 13.61). Tumors are usually smaller than 5 cm at the time of diagnosis but may become larger if ignored (*see* Fig. 13.62). Keloid (*see* Fig. 8.97), plaque type morphea, desmoplastic malignant melanoma (*see* Fig. 12.60), morphoeic basal

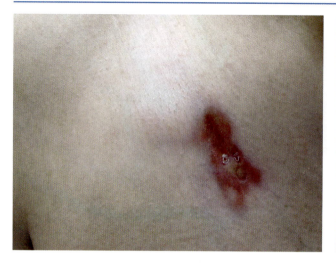

Fig. 13.58 Dermatofibrosarcoma protuberans. In this patient the lesion had been present since birth

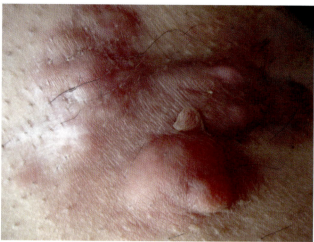

Fig. 13.60 Pedunculated nodules overlying an indurated plaque representing dermatofibrosarcoma protuberans

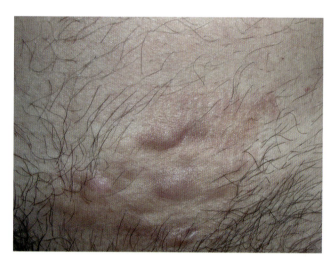

Fig. 13.59 Dermatofibrosarcoma protuberans shown as a flesh-colored solitary, slightly elevated irregular plaque

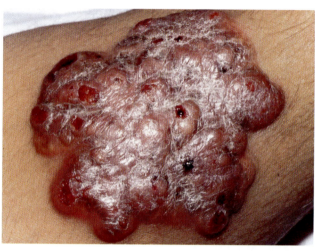

Fig. 13.61 Large elevated plaque of dermatofibrosarcoma protuberans. In neglected cases, lesions may enlarge as seen in this figure

cell carcinoma (*see* Fig. 11.64), and dermatofibroma (*see* Fig. 8.7) may be clinically considered in the differential diagnosis.

The tumor is usually asymptomatic. A rare presentation of dermatofibrosarcoma protuberans is atrophic plaques resembling lipoatrophy. The diagnosis of the sarcoma is established after biopsy. Dermal proliferation of spindle cells with a low degree of atypia extending to the subcutis are the hallmarks. Spindle cells proliferate in a "storiform" pattern, which means extending centrifugally from a virtual central point. They infiltrate the fat tissue, leaving small islands and even single lipocytes in between, which is called the "honeycomb" pattern. Immunohistochemically tumor cells show positivity for CD34.

Dermatofibrosarcoma may slowly invade subcutaneous tissue, fasciae, and muscle. These lesions may be indurated. Although it is rare, lymph node metastasis and hematogenous metastasis to the lungs may be seen.

Management. Early diagnosis and therapy prevent the complications of the tumor. Mohs micrographic surgery or wide local excision is the therapy of choice. Removal of the tumor is more difficult in the head and neck regions. Radiotherapy may be added if there is any concern about the adequacy of the borders of surgery. Local recurrence is a common problem. Imatinib mesylate, a molecular-targeted drug, may be used in inoperable cases to decrease the tumor size and in cases of failed surgery or with visceral metastasis. Careful follow-up of the patients is indicated after therapy.

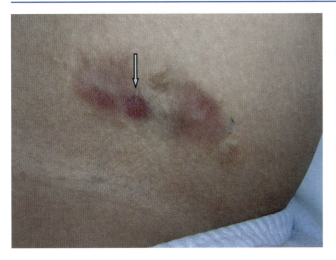

Fig. 13.62 Dermatofibrosarcoma protuberans relapsed after inadequeate excision. Note the erythematous nodule (*arrow*) on the center of surgical scar

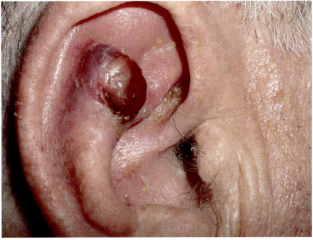

Fig. 13.64 Atypical fibroxanthoma with a crusted surface on the auricle, a typical location

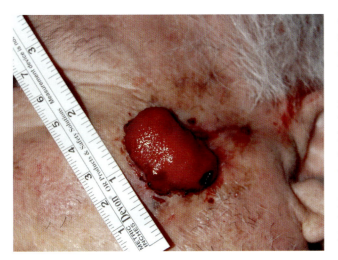

Fig. 13.63 Atypical fibroxanthoma presenting as a reddish nodule with eroded surface on the sun-damaged face of an elder patient

13.5 Atypical Fibroxanthoma

Atypical fibroxanthoma is a low-grade malignancy of soft tissue. It has also been suggested to represent a superficial variant of malignant fibrous histiocytoma. Different from other fibrous tissue sarcomas, it is more common on sun-exposed areas such as the face, ears, scalp, neck, and dorsum of the hands, but it may also develop on the trunk and proximal extremities. It may be seen in the setting of xeroderma pigmentosum, after radiotherapy, or on a thermal burn scar. The tumor occurs mostly in older patients but it may rarely be seen in early childhood, especially in children with xeroderma pigmentosum. The patients may have other dermatologic problems related to sun damage. It presents typically as a solitary, firm, reddish, dome-shaped, asymptomatic nodule measuring 1 to 3 cm. It may be eroded or ulcerated and crusted (*see* Figs. 13.63 and 13.64), resembling a squamous cell carcinoma (*see* Fig. 11.121) or amelanotic melanoma (*see* Fig. 12.55). The diagnosis is mostly established after biopsy. Spindle- or polygonal-shaped atypical tumor cells are seen in the dermis. Cellular pleomorphism, giant cells, and many mitotic figures are important histologic features. Since this is considered an exclusionary diagnosis, a large immunohistochemistry panel to exclude sarcomatoid squamous cell carcinoma, malignant melanoma, and other sarcomas (like cutaneous leiomyosarcoma) is essential. Metastasis is very rare.

Management. Complete excision with wide margins or Mohs micrographic surgery is effective. Contrary to other types of cutaneous sarcomas, the recurrence rate is low. Patients should be instructed about future sun protection.

13.6 Malignant Fibrous Histiocytoma

Malignant fibrous histiocytoma is a rapidly growing fibrous tissue sarcoma mostly seen in the elderly. Undifferentiated pleomorphic sarcoma is a synonym of this tumor. The muscles of the extremities and retroperitoneal areas are common locations of malignant fibrous histiocytoma, but the skin is a rare primary site of involvement. Lesions are more commonly seen on the lower extremities, especially on the thigh, but other areas may also be involved. Skin-colored, painless subcutaneous masses may be multinodular and are clinically not distinctive. Rapid growth of the tumor is typical. The diameter of the tumor may reach to 5 to 10 cm before diagnosis. Retroperitoneal tumors tend to be larger and are usually associated with constitutional symptoms such as fever and weight loss. Similar symptoms may also be seen in advanced tumors of other regions. Malignant fibrous histiocytoma is mostly diagnosed on histopathologic examination. There are spindle-shaped tumor cells with prominent nuclear

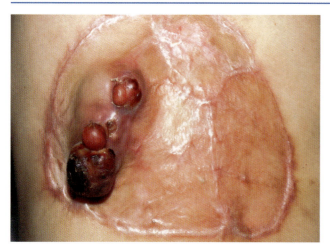

Fig. 13.65 Relapse of malignant fibrous histiocytoma on the graft area

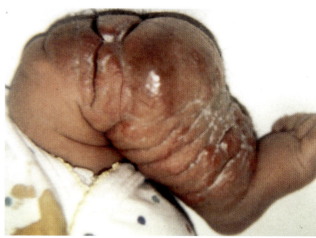

Fig. 13.66 Infantile type fibrosarcoma shown as a very large mass on the leg

pleomorphism and increased atypical mitotic figures. Necrosis may be a feature.

Management. Aggressive surgery is the therapy of choice. While limb-sparing interventions are preferred for the extremity lesions, amputation is sometimes inevitable. Adjuvant radiotherapy may be used after surgery. The rate of local recurrence (*see* Fig. 13.65) is high and systemic metastasis is possible, especially in deeply located lesions. Chemotherapy is used especially in cases with metastasis. If possible, resection of metastases can be performed.

13.7 Fibrosarcoma

Fibrosarcoma is a soft tissue tumor originating from fibroblasts. It arises mostly in deep soft tissue and secondarily involves the overlying skin. Regarding the age of onset, two variants have been described: infantile (congenital) and adult types.

The infantile type may be present at birth or occur in the neonatal period. It presents as an indurated painless mass measuring 1 to 20 cm in diameter (*see* Fig. 13.66). The head, neck, and distal parts of the limbs are most frequently involved. Since it has a vascular appearance, it can be misdiagnosed as a congenital vascular malformation. However, fibrosarcoma tends to grow rapidly. Infantile fibrosarcoma may be locally invasive but metastasis is usually not expected.

Fibrosarcoma in adults usually occurs on the lower extremities followed by the upper extremities as firm nonspecific subcutaneous nodules or masses which may be ulcerated (*see* Fig. 13.67). It can generally be diagnosed after a deep incisional biopsy. Histologically, sheets or uniform solidly packed spindle-shaped cells, arranged in a "herringbone" pattern, are seen. Various histopathologic types of fibrosarcoma exist.

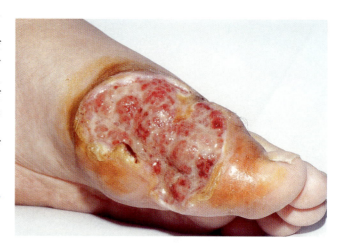

Fig. 13.67 Adult fibrosarcoma presenting as an ulcerated large tumor

Magnetic resonance imaging is useful to show the local extension of the tumor. Early lesions may be asymptomatic. Secondary vascular and neurologic findings may occur in the late stage of the sarcoma due to infiltration of neighboring tissue. Hematogenous metastases to the lungs and bones may be observed. The metastatic rate in adult patients is higher than in infantile cases.

Management. Surgical excision with wide margins is obligatory both in infantile and adult types of fibrosarcoma. However recurrence is possible even in low-grade types (*see* Fig. 13.68). Adjuvant radiotherapy and chemotherapy reduce the risk of recurrence.

13.8 Liposarcoma

Liposarcoma is a malignant tumor of deep soft tissue and is one of the most common ones. It may also arise from intramuscular fasciae, the retroperitoneum, and the mediastinum.

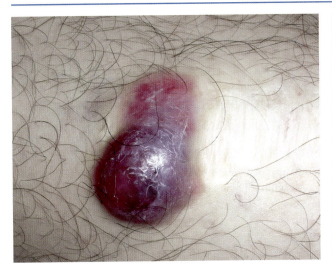

Fig. 13.68 Relapse of low-grade fibromyxoid sarcoma with myxoid type on the excision site in a young adult

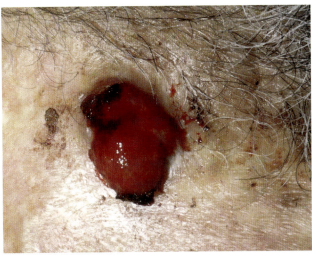

Fig. 13.69 Leiomyosarcoma arising in a thermal burn scar. Note the ulcerated tumor on the temple

Primary cutaneous liposarcomas are very rare. They appear primarily on the upper thigh and buttocks as large masses in adults, mostly in men. Early asymptomatic lesions may clinically be misinterpreted as lipoma. However, liposarcoma does not evolve from lipomas, grows rapidly, and can metastasize hematogenously to the lung and bones, especially in patients who are not diagnosed early or managed appropriately. Several histopathologic subtypes, including well-differentiated (lipoma-like), myxoid, round cell, pleomorphic, and dedifferentiated types exist. The prognosis of liposarcoma is dependent on the histopathologic subtype and the anatomic site.

Management. Complete surgical resection may be curative for lesions of the extremities. Radiotherapy and chemotherapy are used in advanced cases. There is a risk of local recurrence and systemic metastasis. Therefore, careful follow-up is necessary.

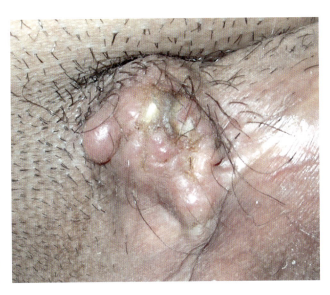

Fig. 13.70 Dermal leiomyosarcoma on the genital area of a male patient

13.9 Leiomyosarcoma

Leiomyosarcoma is a malignant tumor of smooth muscles originating from the uterus, gastrointestinal tract, retroperitoneal tissue, and skin. Leiomyosarcomas of other organs may rarely involve the skin. Two different primary subtypes of the tumor exist in the skin. The superficial (dermal) subtype originates from arrector pili muscles and the deep (subcutaneous) subtype from muscular coats of blood vessels in the subcutaneous tissue. The tumor may occur on normal skin as well as on chronic radiodermatitis and scars (*see* Fig. 13.69). It is more common in the fifth and sixth decades of life. Hair-bearing areas of the lower extremities are more commonly involved, but it may occur anywhere, including the genital area (*see* Fig. 13.70).

Dermal leiomyosarcomas present as irregularly contoured, indurated, single or multiple papules or nodules measuring 1 to 2 cm and may be tender or painful. Some lesions may be ulcerated (*see* Fig. 13.69). Subcutaneous leiomyosarcomas are usually larger nonspecific deep nodules (*see* Fig. 13.71). The differential diagnosis includes benign skin tumors, cysts, and squamous cell carcinoma, occurring especially on scars. It may be diagnosed with biopsy. Leiomyosarcomas are composed of intersecting bundles of spindle cells with eosinophilic cytoplasm and cigar-shaped (blunt-ended) nuclei, reminiscent of smooth muscle cells. Nuclear "palisading" may be a feature and pleomorphism is variable. Cellular areas may be present. Mitosis are seen.

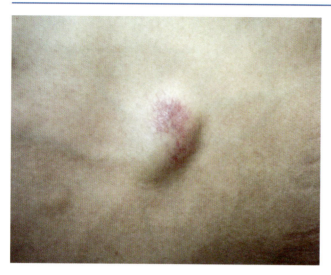

Fig. 13.71 Subcutaneous leiomyosarcoma. The diagnosis can be established with biopsy, since clinical presentation of subcutaneous lesions is nonspecific

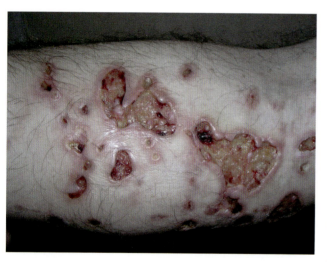

Fig. 13.72 Epithelioid sarcoma presenting with multiple subcutaneous nodules and sharply demarcated, persistent ulcers on the arm

The course of the tumor is unpredictable. Leiomyosarcoma of the skin may metastasize to lymph nodes and visceral organs, especially the lungs, thereby determining the survival time. The metastatic potential of subcutaneous lesions is higher than that of dermal lesions.

Management. Surgical excision with wide margins or Mohs micrographic surgery is the therapy of choice. However, there is a risk of local recurrence, especially if removal is delayed. Adjuvant radiotherapy and chemotherapy have limited effects. Patients should be followed carefully.

13.10 Epithelioid Sarcoma

Epithelioid sarcoma is a rare aggressive type of soft tissue malignancy characterized by large polygonal cells, which can mimic granulomatous inflammation or carcinoma on low-power microscopic examination. It is more common in young males. The typical location is the hands and feet, including the fingers. It may rarely be seen on the proximal extremities and the genital area. Painless, firm, dermal or subcutaneous nodules may be associated with superficial plaques and ulcers (*see* Fig. 13.72). Lesions grow slowly but have a tendency to infiltrate deeper tissue. Multiple lesions in a sporotrichoid pattern may be observed. Early lesions may clinically mimic inflammatory dermatoses such as granuloma annulare, rheumatoid nodule and scar tissue. Palmar lesions can resemble Dupuytren contracture (*see* Fig. 8.64). Finger lesions may resemble giant cell tumor of the tendon sheath (*see* Fig. 8.110). Ulcerative lesions are similar to those of squamous cell carcinoma. Histologically nodules composed of epithelioid and spindle-shaped cells, which contain a central necrobiotic area, are typical. Sometimes tumoral cells may look bland, and this can be the source of a misdiagnosis of granulomatous inflammation. Immunohistochemistry is very helpful in establishing the correct diagnosis. Tumor cells express vimentin, cytokeratin and EMA. The majority of cases are also positive for CD34. The tumor infiltrates underlying structures such as the subcutis, fasciae, and tendons.

Even superficial lesions of this type of sarcoma have a high metastatic rate. They may rapidly spread to distant skin, deep soft tissue, lymph nodes, bones, lungs, pleura, and other visceral organs. Lesions involving underlying large nerves cause paresthesia and pain.

Management. Therapeutic results are not good because most patients are not diagnosed early. Aggressive surgery should be performed as early as possible. Local recurrence is very common. Amputation is indicated in some cases. Adjuvant radiotherapy and chemotherapy can also be used but are not overly efficacious.

13.11 Malignant Peripheral Nerve Sheath Tumor (Malignant Schwannoma, Neurofibrosarcoma)

Malignant peripheral nerve sheath tumor is a rare neoplasm of peripheral nerves that may be associated with benign neural tumors. Up to half of the tumors occur in the setting of neurofibromatosis, usually originating from plexiform neurofibromas. Rarely, schwannomas or other neural tumors may be the origin of this malignant tumor. De novo or sporadic occurrence is also possible. It is more common in middle-aged patients.

It presents as a deep subcutaneous nodule that is clinically not distinctive. Rapid growth of a preexisting neural tumor is suggestive of a malignant degeneration. Histopathologic examination must be performed for a definite diagnosis. It reveals interlacing bundles of spindle cell proliferation with atypia and mitoses. Different patterns of differentiation (mesenchymal, glandular or epithelioid) may be observed.

Management. Aggressive surgery and chemotherapy are indicated but are not effective in all cases, and the prognosis is not good. Sporadic lesions have a relatively higher survival rate than the ones associated with neurofibromatosis.

Suggested Reading

Calonje JE, Brenn T, Lazar AJ, McKee PH. McKee's pathology of the skin, edn 4. China: Elsevier; 2012.

de Morais OO, de Araújo LC, Gomes CM, et al. Congenital dermatofibrosarcoma protuberans. Cutis. 2012;90:285–8.

Hendersen MT, Hollmig ST. Malignant fibrous histiocytoma: changing perceptions and management challanges. J Am Acad Dermatol. 2012;67:1335–41.

Hosseini-Moghaddam SM, Soleimanirahbar A, Mazzuli T, et al. Post renal transplantation Kaposi's sarcoma: a review of its epidemiology, pathogenesis, diagnosis, clinical aspects, and therapy. Transpl Infect Dis. 2012;14:338–45.

Johnson-Jahangir H, Ratner D. Advances in management of dermatofibrosarcoma protuberans. Dermatol Clin. 2011;29:191–200.

Régnier-Rosencher E, Guillot B, Dupin N. Treatments for classic Kaposi sarcoma: a systematic review of the literature. J Am Acad Dermatol. 2013;68:313–31.

Rigel DS, Robinson JK, Ross M, Friedman RJ, Corkerell CJ, Lim HW, Stockfleth HW, Kirkwood JM. Cancer of the skin, edn 2. China: Saunders Elsevier; 2011.

Schwartz RA. Skin cancer: recognition and management, edn 2. Singapore: Blackwell Publishing; 2008.

Sharma A, Schwartz RA. Stewart-Treves syndrome: pathogenesis and management. J Am Acad Dermatol. 2012; 67:1342–8.

Voth H, Landsberg J, Hinz T, et al. Management of dermatofibrosarcoma protuberans with fibrosarcomatous transformation: an evidence-based review of the literature. J Eur Acad Dermatol Venereol. 2011;25:1385–91.

Yaich S, Charfeddine K, Zaghdane S, et al. Sirolimus for the treatment of Kaposi sarcoma after renal transplantation: a series of 10 cases. Transplant Proc. 2012;44:2824–6.

Young RJ, Brown NJ, Reed MW, Hughes D, Woll PJ. Angiosarcoma. Lancet Oncol. 2010;11:983–91.

Ziemer M. Atypical fibroxanthoma. J Dtsch Dermatol Ges. 2012;10: 537–50.

Cutaneous Lymphomas

The skin may be affected by lymphoproliferative diseases either primarily or secondarily. In addition to skin involvement of systemic lymphomas, including Hodgkin disease and non-Hodgkin lymphomas, a heterogeneous group of primary cutaneous lymphomas (extranodal non-Hodgkin lymphomas) originating from B cells, T cells and NK (natural killer) cells, have been described. By definition, these lymphomas are restricted to the skin at the time of diagnosis but may show involvement of lymph nodes, visceral organs, and bone marrow during their course. However, some types of cutaneous lymphomas very rarely involve extracutaneous sites. In the last two decades, many classification systems of these diseases have been proposed. This chapter is mainly organized according to the WHO-EORTC (World Health Organization-European Organization for Research and Treatment of Cancer) classification of cutaneous lymphomas published in 2005 and the WHO classification of lymphomas published in 2008. Most of these primary cutaneous lymphomas included in these classification systems showing different clinical, histopathologic, cytogenetic, and molecular genetic features and prognosis will be discussed. Pseudolymphomas which are clinical and histopathologic imitators of lymphomas, and secondary cutaneous infiltration of systemic hematologic neoplasms are included in this chapter for convenience.

None of the primary cutaneous lymphomas has a high incidence. Many of them cause multifocal skin lesions. The most critical point about cutaneous lymphomas is that they have different biological behavior when compared to nodal lymphomas; thus they require a specialized approach.

14.1 Primary Cutaneous Lymphomas

14.1.1 Cutaneous T-cell Lymphomas

Nearly 70 to 80 percent of primary cutaneous lymphomas are of T-cell origin. These tumors represent a heterogeneous spectrum from indolent lymphomas such as CD30+ lymphoproliferative disorders to highly aggressive tumors such as primary cutaneous CD8+ aggressive epidermotropic cytotoxic T-cell lymphoma. Whereas mycosis fungoides patients present only with patches or thin plaques in the early stages, patients with lymphomatoid papulosis present with papulonecrotic lesions with a tendency to spontaneous regression. Most patients with other types of cutaneous lymphomas commonly present with solitary or multiple, persistent or progressive nodules or tumors which may be ulcerated. On the other hand, erythroderma is the presentation of Sézary syndrome. The diagnosis is usually established with skin lesions, along with histopathologic interpretation. Thereafter, staging examinations regarding systemic involvement should be performed in most but not in all types of cutaneous T-cell lymphomas.

14.1.1.1 Mycosis Fungoides

Mycosis fungoides is the most common type of cutaneous T-cell lymphoma, typically seen in adults in their mid-fifties (*see* Fig. 14.1), although it may appear at any age. Approximately 5 percent of the cases are children (*see* Fig. 14.2). Familial cases are very rare. Men are slightly more frequently affected than women. Mycosis fungoides

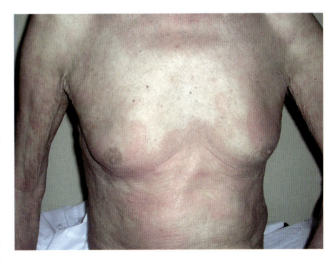

Fig. 14.1 Mycosis fungoides in an adult; patches and plaques are seen

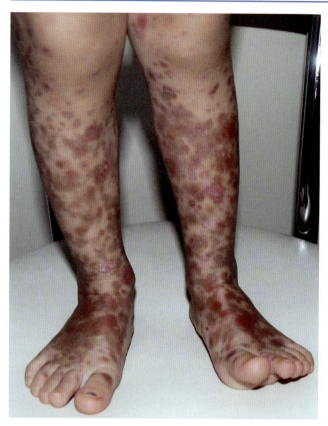

Fig. 14.2 Mycosis fungoides in a two-year-old child. Though rare it can be seen in childhood

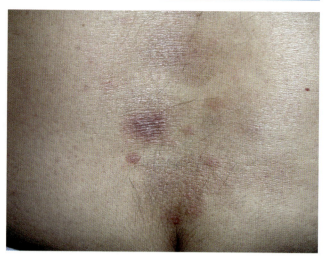

Fig. 14.3 A few nonscaly patches on the trunk representing the premycotic (patch) stage of mycosis fungoides. These lesions are nonspecific and the diagnosis may be delayed

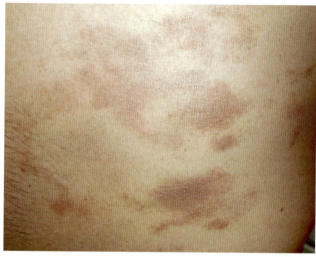

Fig. 14.4 Multiple ill-defined, nonscaly patches of early mycosis fungoides on the trunk

typically begins with skin involvement and may be confined to the skin for a long time — for years or even decades. In a minority of the patients, lymph node, visceral organ, and blood involvement may occur. Even though various clinical presentations of skin involvement have been defined, the classic type is the commonest one.

Classic Mycosis Fungoides

Typical clinical features of "classic mycosis fungoides" include erythematous and mostly scaly patches and plaques, or tumors. Patches and thin plaques represent the initial lesions, whereas tumors are in line with the advanced disease. Especially in early mycosis fungoides, the clinical picture looks like a persistent inflammatory disorder rather than a neoplastic disease. The early lesions, namely, few erythematous, ill-defined, scaly or nonscaly patches (see Figs. 14.3, 14.4 and 14.5) are considered the patch (premycotic) stage of this cutaneous lymphoma. These lesions are commonly clinically misdiagnosed as pityriasis alba, contact dermatitis, atopic dermatitis, or tinea corporis. Therefore, topical corticosteroids may have been administered for various indications before the diagnosis of mycosis fungoides. The patches and plaques may respond well to this treatment, but recurrence after discontinuation of the therapy may occur immediately. Moreover, in the early period, the lesions may resolve with sunlight. Histopathologic misdiagnosis is also not uncommon. The histologic appearance of the patch stage lesions reveals mild or no epidermotropism and mild spongiosis. While the presence of epidermotropism is an important diagnostic finding in mycosis fungoides, spongiosis is rather nonspecific and may result with a misdiagnosis as eczema. Therefore, it is usually difficult to reach a definite diagnosis before the histopathologic findings become more pathognomonic. Several biopsies may be needed to establish a correct diagnosis. Sometimes, it can be hard to convince the patients about the need for multiple biopsies. The punch biopsy is preferred. Close collaboration of clinicians and pathologists is essential at this time. T-cell clonality is also frequently undetectable in early lesions of mycosis fungoides.

14.1 Primary Cutaneous Lymphomas

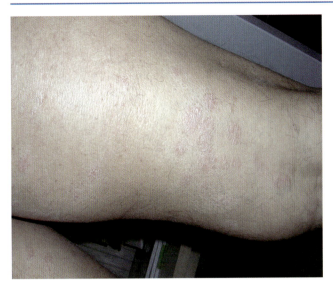

Fig. 14.5 Patches of early mycosis fungoides showing mild scaling

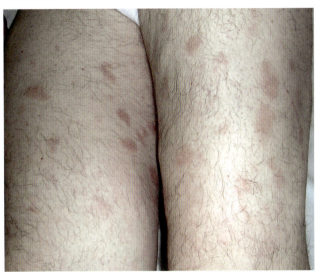

Fig. 14.7 Multiple erythematous patches located on the thighs, a typical presentation of early mycosis fungoides

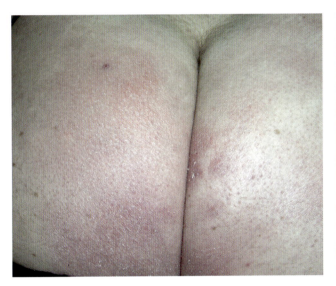

Fig. 14.6 Patches of early mycosis fungoides located on the buttocks. This non-sun exposed area is a typical location

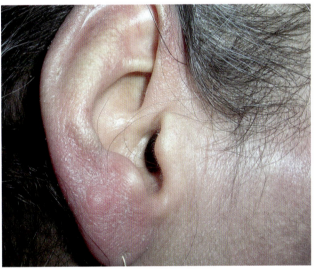

Fig. 14.8 Involvement of the ear, which is mostly seen in advanced stages of mycosis fungoides

The buttocks (see Fig. 14.6) or other non–sun exposed areas of the body like the trunk (see Fig. 14.4) and the proximal parts of the extremities (see Fig. 14.7) are more commonly involved initially. Patch and plaque lesions are generally not expected to occur on the face, possibly because it is highly exposed to the sun. On the other hand, lesions may occur anywhere (see Fig. 14.8). The size, shape, and number of the patches and plaques are variable. Round (see Fig. 14.9), annular (see Fig. 14.10), or polycyclic (see Fig. 14.11) patches or plaques may be seen. Reddish (see Fig. 14.12) and brownish lesions (see Fig. 14.13) are more common but dark yellow, skin-colored (see Fig. 14.14) and black lesions are also possible.

Plaque lesions (plaque stage) may appear de novo or patches may become gradually infiltrated and evolve into plaques. Therefore patches and plaques may be seen concomitantly (see Fig. 14.15). Lesions may become confluent in time (see Fig. 14.16). Fine scales are usually found on both types of the lesions (see Figs. 14.5 and 14.17). Rarely, there can be thicker scales, especially overlying the plaques (see Figs. 14.18 and 14.19). Sometimes, the lesions may be atrophic (see Fig. 14.20) or wrinkled (see Fig. 14.21). More than one clinical form of these lesions may be seen in one individual. Pruritus may accompany the plaques.

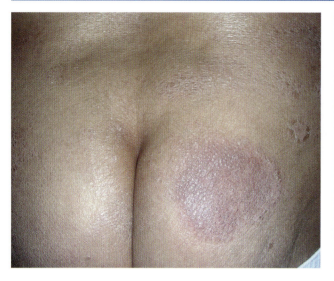

Fig. 14.9 Typical round (nummular) lesions of mycosis fungoides

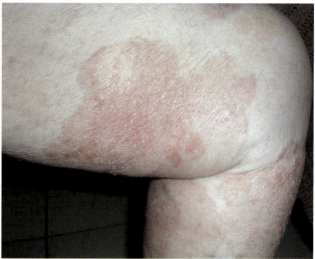

Fig. 14.11 Polycylic patches of mycosis fungoides on the leg

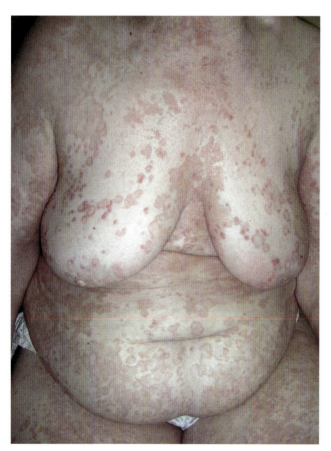

Fig. 14.10 Disseminated erythematous annular lesions, an uncommon presentation of mycosis fungoides

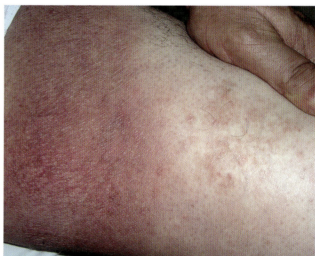

Fig. 14.12 Ill-defined, reddish patches of mycosis fungoides

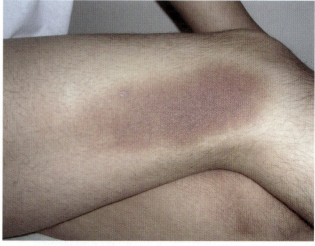

Fig. 14.13 Brownish-colored, sharply demarcated, homogenous plaque of mycosis fungoides in a child

The diagnostic accuracy rate from histopathologic point of view in plaque-type lesions is higher when compared to the patch-type lesions. Histologically, epidermotropism is generally more prominent in plaque stage lesions. Lichenoid infiltration of small to medium-sized lymphocytes, atypia sometimes with cerebriform nuclei, and papillary dermal fibrosis are also seen. Immunohistochemical staining for

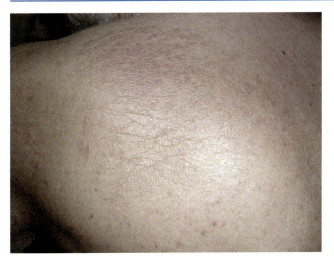

Fig. 14.14 Skin-colored, ill-defined, slightly atrophic patches of mycosis fungoides

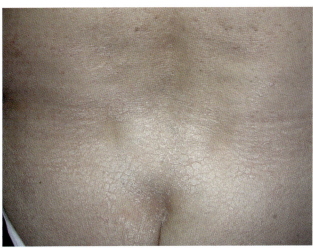

Fig. 14.17 Ill-defined patches covered with fine scales located on the back of a patient with mycosis fungoides

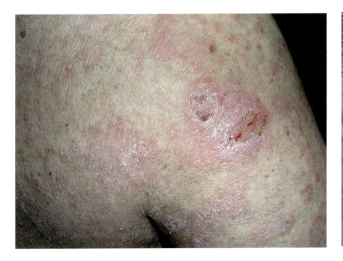

Fig. 14.15 Patches and plaques seen concomitantly in mycosis fungoides

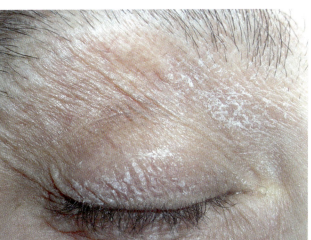

Fig. 14.18 Scaly patches on the eyelids. This rare presentation of mycosis fungoides can easily be misdiagnosed as eczema

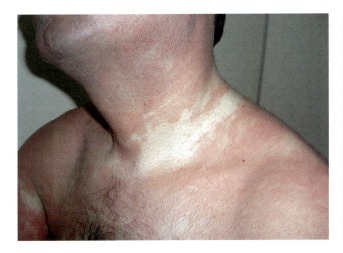

Fig. 14.16 Confluence of erythematous patches that resulted in diffuse involvement of the upper trunk and neck in a patient with mycosis fungoides

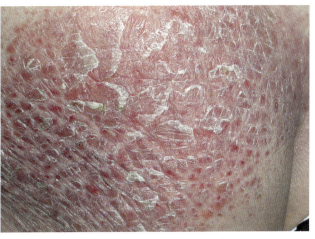

Fig. 14.19 Plaque lesion of mycosis fungoides covered with thick scales

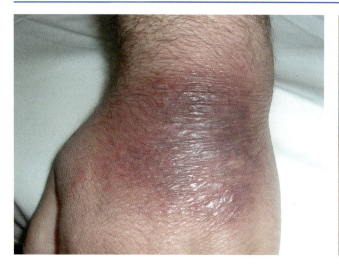

Fig. 14.20 Atrophic, erythematous, well-defined lesion of mycosis fungoides

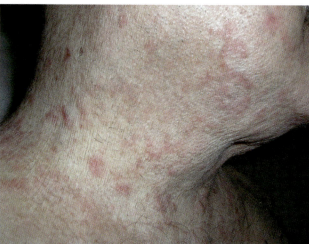

Fig. 14.22 Irregularly distributed plaque lesions of mycosis fungoides on the neck and face

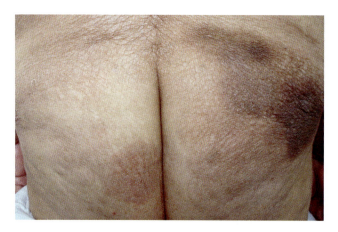

Fig. 14.21 Fine wrinkling on an atrophic lesion of mycosis fungoides

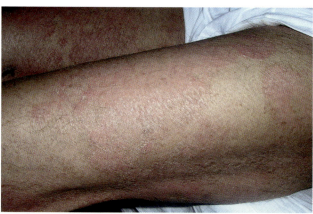

Fig. 14.23 Multiple erythematous plaques of mycosis fungoides located bilaterally on the legs

T-lymphocyte antigens and loss of expression of some of them may contribute to the diagnosis but does not have prognostic significance.

Most patients have multiple irregularly distributed lesions (*see* Figs. 14.22 and 14.23). A subset of patients may have a solitary lesion (*see* Fig. 14.24). Unilesional mycosis fungoides may be observed as an erythematous scaly (*see* Fig. 14.24), psoriasiform (*see* Fig. 14.25), poikilodermatous or hypopigmented patch or plaque. Multiple papular lesions may sometimes be the presentation of mycosis fungoides (*see* Fig. 14.26).

Mycosis fungoides with classic lesions usually remain confined to the skin. Untreated patches or plaques often persist for years and show a slow progressive course. In some patients, generalized involvement of patches and plaques may occur. Clinical evolution from patches to infiltrated

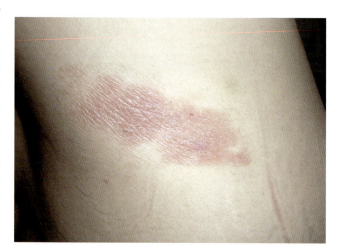

Fig. 14.24 Mycosis fungoides presenting as a solitary scaly plaque

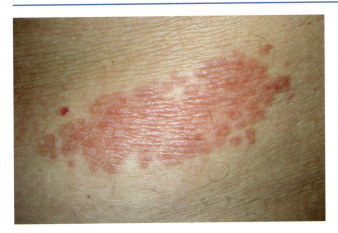

Fig. 14.25 Mycosis fungoides presenting as a solitary psoriasiform plaque

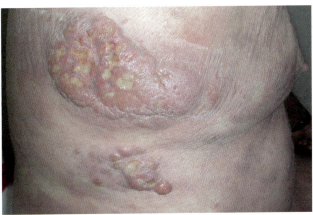

Fig. 14.27 Plaques and tumors of mycosis fungoides are seen concomitantly. Associated patches or plaques are also commonly seen in tumoral stage

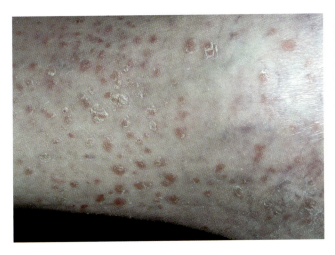

Fig. 14.26 Papular mycosis fungoides. Note multiple discrete erythematous and slightly scaly papules

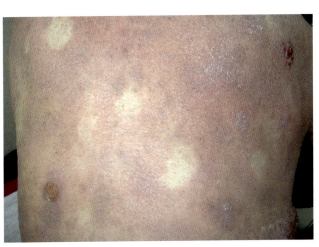

Fig. 14.28 Confluent plaques with a few overlying tumors on the back. Uninvolved areas are also remarkable

plaques and then to tumors may be seen even after decades. However, this kind of evolution is not seen in all patients. Relapse after therapy in the clinical presentation of patches and plaques does not indicate systemic involvement.

The tumoral stage of mycosis fungoides is less commonly seen and it typically evolves from patch or plaque stage disease. There are no known risk factors for the evolution to the tumoral stage. A combination of patches, plaques, and tumors is the typical presentation of this stage (see Fig. 14.27). Tumors may be observed overlying patches and plaques (see Fig. 14.28) or on normal skin (see Fig. 14.29). The presence of associated patches and plaques is helpful in distinguishing tumoral mycosis fungoides from other cutaneous T-cell lymphomas or cutaneous B-cell lymphomas and pseudolymphoma. It is unusual to observe tumors as the initial lesion of mycosis fungoides, especially in the absence of

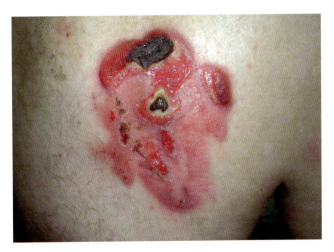

Fig. 14.29 A tumor of mycosis fungoides irregular in shape located on normal skin

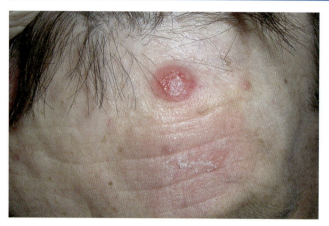

Fig. 14.30 A round tumor of mycosis fungoides located on the forehead. The face is not a rare location for tumors on the contrary to patches or plaques

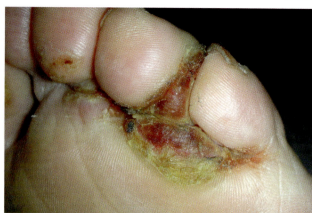

Fig. 14.32 Crusted tumor of mycosis fungoides on the interdigital area

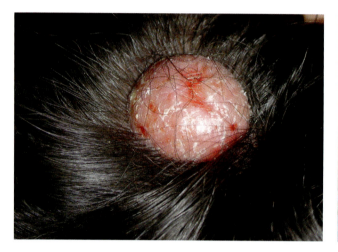

Fig. 14.31 Solitary round tumor of mycosis fungoides located on the scalp

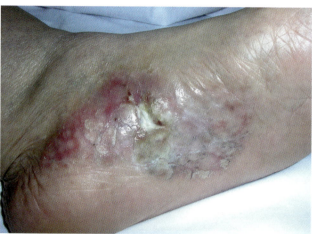

Fig. 14.33 Palmoplantar involvement of mycosis fungoides. These flat but indurated lesions have been evaluated as the tumoral stage of mycosis fungoides on histopathologic examination

patches or plaques. The diagnosis is challenging in these latter cases because the differential diagnosis must also include other types of cutaneous lymphomas.

Unlike patches or plaques, tumors are not rare on the sun-exposed areas. Typical locations of tumors are the face (see Fig. 14.30), scalp (see Fig. 14.31), and intertriginous areas (see Fig. 14.32), although any site, including the palmoplantar area (see Fig. 14.33), can be affected. They may also rarely locate on mucosal sites. Tumoral lesions tend to enlarge rapidly. Their size varies from one or a few centimeters (see Fig. 14.34) to very large lesions (see Fig. 14.35). Tumors may be scattered or may be grouped on one site of the body (see Fig. 14.36). They are typically elevated (see Fig. 14.31), but palmoplantar lesions can be flat (see Fig. 14.33). Lesions may be purple to reddish or brownish in color, and their shapes may be round (see Figs. 14.30 and 14.31) or irregular (see Figs. 14.29 and 14.37). The center of the tumor may be depressed (see Fig. 14.38) and the surface may be intact (see Fig. 14.34), slightly hyperkeratotic (see Fig. 14.39), eroded,

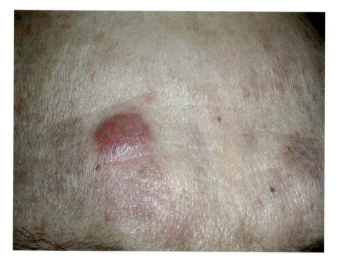

Fig. 14.34 Small nodule on the face with intact surface representing tumoral mycosis fungoides

14.1 Primary Cutaneous Lymphomas

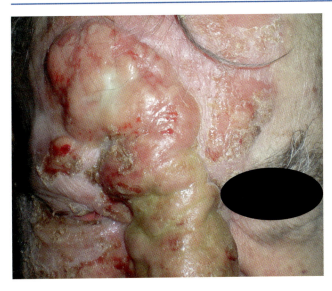

Fig. 14.35 Large ulcerated tumor on the face in a patient with mycosis fungoides

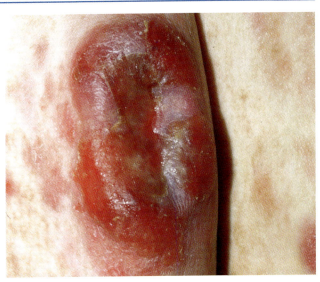

Fig. 14.38 Large tumor of mycosis fungoides with depressed center located on the buttocks

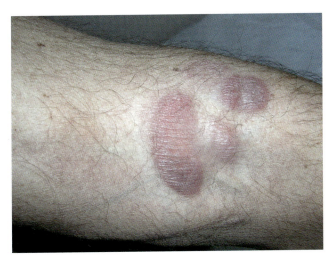

Fig. 14.36 Tumors of mycosis fungoides may be clustered as seen here

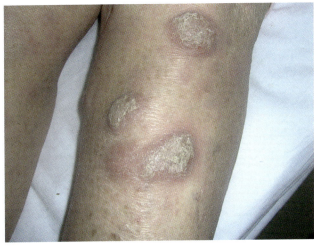

Fig. 14.39 Multiple tumoral lesions of mycosis fungoides with slightly hyperkeratotic surface.

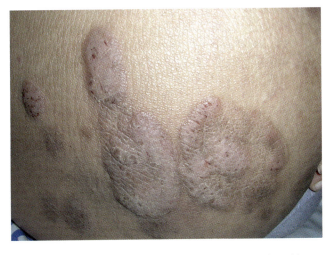

Fig. 14.37 Irregular, slightly elevated tumors of mycosis fungoides on the trunk

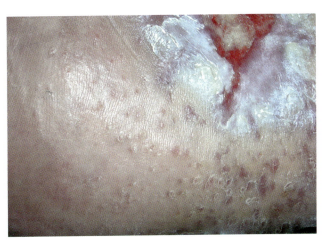

Fig. 14.40 Confluent reddish papulonodular lesions and ulceration on the sole representing the tumoral stage of mycosis fungoides

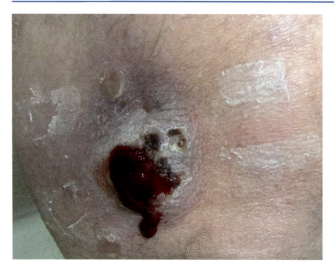

Fig. 14.41 Tumor of mycosis fungoides with ulceration. The bleeding on the surface is noticeable

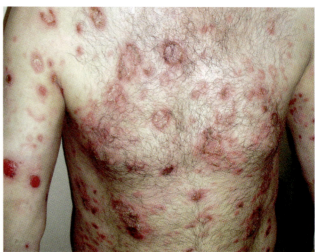

Fig. 14.43 Multiple plaques and ulcerated tumors of mycosis fungoides. Large-cell anaplastic transformation was detected histopathologically in some of them

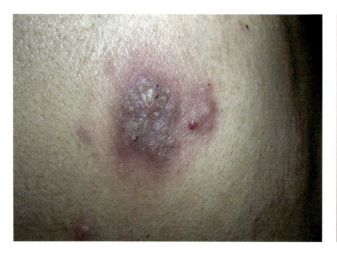

Fig. 14.42 Tumor of mycosis fungoides with superficial bacterial infection. It may be painful

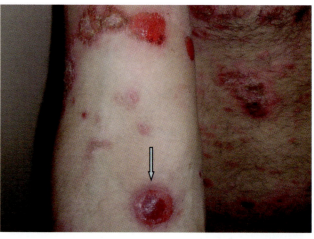

Fig. 14.44 Crusted ulcerated tumor (*arrow*) histologically diagnosed as large-cell anaplastic transformation of mycosis fungoides

crusted, or ulcerated (*see* Figs. 14.38 and 14.40). The tumors bleed easily (*see* Fig. 14.41). Secondary bacterial infections are common, especially on the ulcerated lesions (*see* Fig. 14.42). Chronic septicemia and thrombosis are severe complications of this stage.

The histopathology of the tumors almost always shows confirmatory signs of mycosis fungoides. Different from plaques, epidermotropism is usually absent, whereas diffuse or nodular dermal infiltration of large atypical lymphocytes with cerebriform nuclei is prominent. T-cell clonality is more frequently detected than patch and plaque type lesions. The serum lactate dehydrogenase (LDH) level is mostly elevated in this stage. Tumors are the sign for high risk of systemic involvement.

Transformed mycosis fungoides (anaplastic large-cell transformation) may arise in a minority of patients and present mostly as new papules or nodules within classic patches and plaques, or with enlarging tumors (*see* Figs. 14.43 and 14.44), or it may be seen as an acute eruption of multiple scattered papules or nodules. Histologically, large cells constitute more than 25 percent of the neoplastic population. CD30 may be expressed by these transformed large cells, but not always.

The staging and classification of mycosis fungoides were revised by ISCL (International Society for Cutaneous Lymphomas) and EORTC in 2007. The separation of the morphology of the lesions as patches, plaques, or tumors is important, as the new classification is primarily designated according to the presence and extent of these lesions. Moreover, involvement of lymph nodes and visceral organs is also vital in staging. The prognosis, therapy of choice, and response to therapy differ among stages. Patients in early stages with limited patch or plaque disease have a good prognosis with nearly a similar life expectancy to that of an age-, sex- and race-matched population. Tumors, anaplastic large cell transformation, erythroderma, and extracutaneous involvement are seen in the late stages of mycosis fungoides. The presence of ulceration on plaques or tumors does not affect staging but is usually a sign of poor prognosis. The aggressive clinical course and poor prognosis are associated with extracutaneous involvement and transformation into a large T-cell lymphoma.

Involvement of peripheral lymph nodes is not expected in the patch and plaque stages of mycosis fungoides. A routine biopsy without clinical and radiologic evidence of lymph node involvement is not recommended. In the early stages, dermatopathic lymphadenopathy, representing a reactive process, is usually encountered. This type of lymph node enlargement can also be seen in the course of benign chronic inflammatory dermatoses. Histologically, the paracortical zone of the lymph node is expanded and contains melanin-laden macrophages. Although dermatopathic involvement of the lymph node affects staging, it does not have any prognostic significance and does not alter the choice of treatment. Neoplastic infiltration of the lymph node is histologically characterized by clustered or diffuse infiltration of atypical lymphocytes disrupting the normal nodal architecture. It is more commonly seen in the patients with tumoral lesions or erythroderma and is a marker of a poor prognosis.

Visceral involvement is rarely seen in patients with mycosis fungoides. Various sites such as the liver, spleen, bone marrow, lung, gastrointestinal system, or kidney can be affected. This is the terminal stage of mycosis fungoides, with the worst prognosis. Failure of the involved organs and infections are the common causes of death.

In addition to the classic type, several clinical variants of mycosis fungoides have been described. Because of this great variability in its clinical presentation, the differential diagnosis includes a wide spectrum of diseases. Therefore, dermatologists include mycosis fungoides in the clinical differential diagnosis of many dermatoses or neoplastic diseases especially in uncertain cases, before performing a biopsy for histopathologic examination. These clinical variants mostly show the typical histology of mycosis fungoides in addition to some distinctive histopathologic features. Among these, pagetoid reticulosis, folliculotropic mycosis, fungoides, and granulomatous slack skin are considered as distinct variants of mycosis fungoides in the 2005 WHO-EORTC classification about cutaneous lymphomas. However, other clinicopathologic variants of mycosis fungoides are also present. Some of these variants have prognostic significance, but many of them show a course similar to that of classic mycosis fungoides with patches and plaques. They will be discussed below.

Digitate Parapsoriasis

Digitate parapsoriasis is a term that describes a distinct clinical presentation of early mycosis fungoides. It has been considered as a separate entity in the past. It is typically seen on the trunk, especially on the flanks (see Fig. 14.45), and the proximal parts of extremities. Multiple pinkish or brownish-red, elongated, or finger-shaped lesions measuring 2 to 10 cm in parallel distribution are the hallmarks of digitate parapsoriasis (see Figs. 14.46 and 14.47). This variant of mycosis fungoides may easily be diagnosed clinically. The lesions have fine scales on the surface (see Fig. 14.48) and are asymptomatic. Histologically, slight spongiosis associated with perivascular lymphocytic infiltration without epidermotropism and atypia are the main features but they are not diagnostic.

Digitate parapsoriasis has a stable course, and plaques or tumors are usually not seen in these patients. Digitate parapsoriasis responds well to phototherapy, but it may relapse with similar lesions after cessation of therapy.

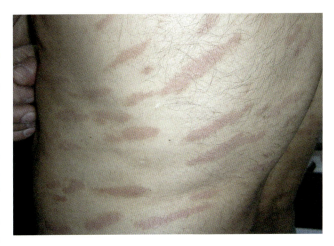

Fig. 14.45 Digitate parapsoriasis located on the flanks

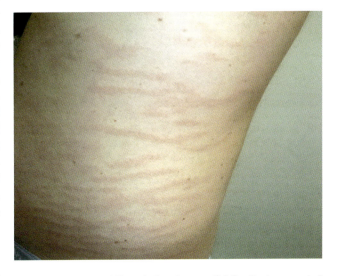

Fig. 14.46 Elongated linear lesions in a parallel distribution, a typical appearance for digitate parapsoriasis

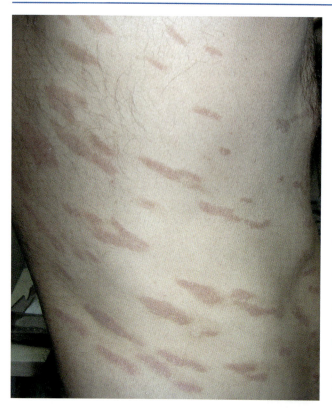

Fig. 14.47 Typical finger-shaped, brownish-red patches of digitate parapsoriasis. These lesions are persistent

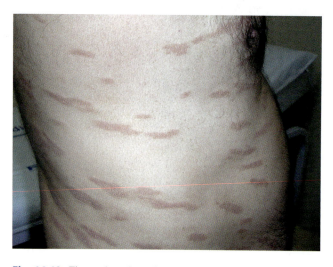

Fig. 14.48 Finger-shaped patches with fine scales scattered on the lower trunk in a patient with digitate parapsoriasis. This clinical presentation is highly suggestive of the diagnosis

Pagetoid Reticulosis

Pagetoid reticulosis is a rare localized type of cutaneous T-cell lymphoma with pathognomonic histopathologic features. It is also called Woringer-Kolopp disease. The usual location is the extremities, especially the soles of the feet. It is observed as a solitary psoriasiform or hyperkeratotic, sharply demarcated, red patch or plaque. The tumor grows slowly. It has histopathologic features distinct from classic unilesional mycosis fungoides, including a hyperplastic epidermis with marked epidermotropism of lymphocytes in a pagetoid pattern. The immune profile is similar to that of mycosis fungoides. The prognosis of this variant of cutaneous T-cell lymphoma is good.

A generalized form of pagetoid reticulosis (Ketron-Goodman disease) has also been described in the past, but it is now considered to be a distinct entity. Primary cutaneous CD8+ aggressive epidermotropic cytotoxic T-cell lymphoma, which has pathognomonic immunohistochemical findings and a totally different prognosis, has also been suggested as a more likely diagnosis for some of the reported cases as Ketron-Goodman disease.

Folliculotropic/Syringotropic Mycosis Fungoides

Neoplastic infiltration of mycosis fungoides rarely involves the hair follicles (folliculotropism, pilotropism) and eccrine glands (syringotropism), resulting in a different clinical picture. The folliculotropic mycosis fungoides (follicular mycosis fungoides, mycosis fungoides-associated follicular mucinosis) is relatively common and syringotropic mycosis fungoides is a very rare presentation. These syringotropic and folliculotropic forms are also designated as a single clinical variant of mycosis fungoides. It is more common in man.

Folliculotropic mycosis fungoides is characterized by neoplastic T-lymphocytes infiltrating the hair follicles but not the epidermis. Mucin may be present or absent.

The diagnosis of folliculotropic mycosis fungoides may be challenging because of the great variability in clinical presentation. Any hair-bearing area, either localized or generalized, may be affected, although the head and neck region, especially the eyebrows (*see* Fig. 14.49), are more commonly involved. Most cases show erythematous scaly, infiltrated, sharply demarcated alopecic plaques in different sizes (*see* Figs. 14.50 and 14.51) with histologic mucinous deposition; hence the term "alopecia mucinosa" is used. Furthermore, folliculotropic mycosis fungoides causes other clinical presentations, including grouped or scattered follicular keratotic papules (*see* Fig. 14.52), milium-like cysts (*see* Fig. 14.53), comedo-like lesions with or without inflammation (*see* Fig. 14.54), acneiform lesions (*see* Fig. 14.55) and rarely tumors. Acneiform lesions may be first misdiagnosed as nodulocystic acne vulgaris or acne conglobata, and follicular papules as lichen spinulosus. Sometimes the lesions are associated with diffuse edema (*see* Fig. 14.56) and mucinorrhea (*see* Fig. 14.56). Elevated, indurated plaques with alopecia may also be seen (*see* Fig. 14.57).

This variant of mycosis fungoides may show a rapid progressive course (*see* Fig. 14.58a and b). In case of generalized involvement on the scalp, eyelids, and eyebrows, the clinical picture may resemble that of alopecia totalis or alopecia universalis (*see* Figs. 14.59 and 14.60). Severe pruritus

14.1 Primary Cutaneous Lymphomas

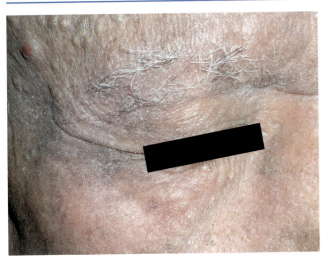

Fig. 14.49 Folliculotropic mycosis fungoides on the face leading to partial loss of the eyebrows (alopecia mucinosa)

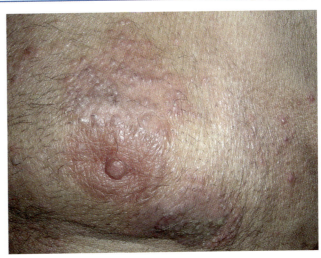

Fig. 14.52 Grouped follicular erythematous papules; a presentation of folliculotropic mycosis fungoides

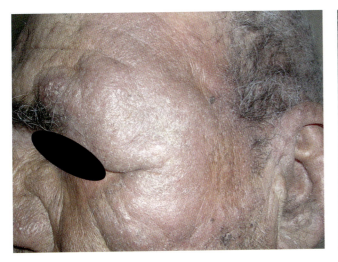

Fig. 14.50 Folliculotropic mycosis fungoides that appear as erythematous infiltrating plaques causing prominent alopecia of the eyebrows

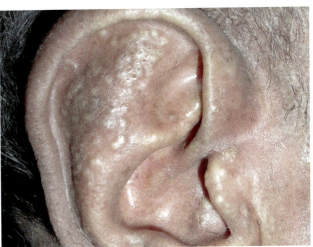

Fig. 14.53 Milium-like cysts; a rare presentation of folliculotropic mycosis fungoides

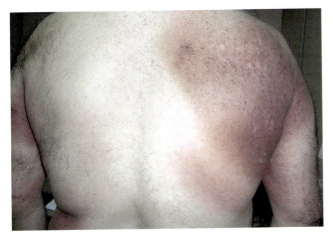

Fig. 14.51 Multiple sharply demarcated erythematous plaques with hair loss on the trunk caused by folliculotropic mycosis fungoides

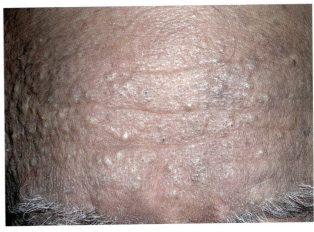

Fig. 14.54 Multiple comedo-like lesions on the face in a patient with folliculotropic mycosis fungoides

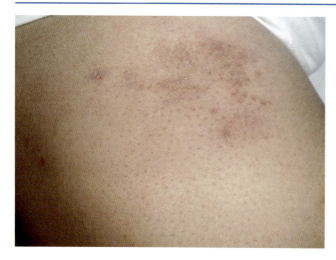

Fig. 14.55 Acneiform and comedo-like lesions grouped on the legs. These were the initial lesions of folliculotropic mycosis fungoides

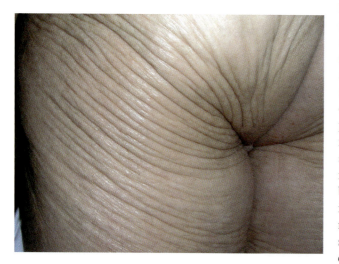

Fig. 14.56 Folliculotropic mycosis fungoides causing diffuse edema in a patient with advanced disease. Edema was associated with mucinorrhea in this patient

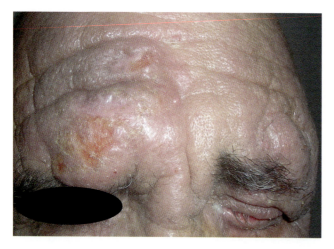

Fig. 14.57 Elevated plaque of folliculotropic mycosis fungoides on the forehead leading to alopecia of the eyebrows

is a major problem of this type of mycosis fungoides and may be an indicator of progressive disease. Secondary bacterial infections are not uncommon.

Generally, because of deep follicular involvement, folliculotropic mycosis fungoides needs to be treated more aggressively than classic mycosis fungoides with patches and plaques. Response to therapy may be delayed in acneiform or cystic lesions. However, regrowth of hairs may also be seen after appropriate treatment. Patients have the risk of relapse and disease progression. The prognosis of folliculotropic mycosis fungoides is poor when compared with that of classic patches or plaques of mycosis fungoides. On rare occasions, folliculotropic mycosis fungoides can progress to Sézary syndrome or may show anaplastic large cell transformation.

Red-brown or skin-colored, sometimes anhydrotic patches, slightly infiltrated plaques, or small papules (*see* Fig. 14.61) are the typical presentations of syringotropic mycosis fungoides. Punctate erythema (*see* Fig. 14.62), accepted as a characteristic feature of eccrine gland involvement, can be seen. Sometimes the lesions are associated with alopecia. The diagnosis can be delayed if the lesions are solitary and if there are no accompanying clinical features of classic mycosis fungoides. Most patients with syringotropism have coexisting folliculotropism, whereas only a small number of patients with folliculotropism have concomitant syringotropism. Therefore, in cases with slight follicular involvement, the presence of eccrine gland involvement can be helpful in diagnosis. Deep and multiple biopsies showing adnexal structures are usually required for accurate diagnosis. Those cases of syringotropic mycosis fungoides with skin involvement only usually have a good prognosis with a chronic course.

Granulomatous Mycosis Fungoides and Granulomatous Slack Skin

Although it is not common, the granulomatous infiltration pattern can be observed histologically in various clinical variants of mycosis fungoides. Granulomatous lesions may occur concomitantly or after the onset of classic mycosis fungoides. However, sometimes they may be the initial presentation and therefore may be misdiagnosed with other diseases causing granulomatous dermatitis. The mechanism of granuloma formation is unknown. The prognosis of this variant is variable; some cases show good prognosis, whereas others follow an aggressive course.

Granulomatous slack skin is a rare presentation of mycosis fungoides with distinctive clinical features. While it may be considered a subgroup of granulomatous mycosis fungoides, it is classified as a separate subtype of mycosis fungoides in the 2005 WHO-EORTC classification. It also demonstrates specific histopathologic features and has a very slow progressive course. Typically,

14.1 Primary Cutaneous Lymphomas

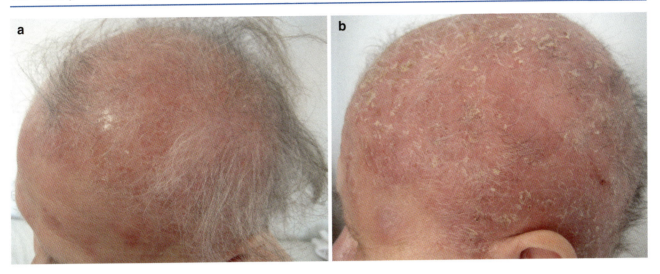

Fig. 14.58 (a) Mild diffuse alopecia due to folliculotropic mycosis fungoides. (b) Infiltration of the whole scalp and severe alopecia affecting nearly all hairs developed in the following two weeks in this patient

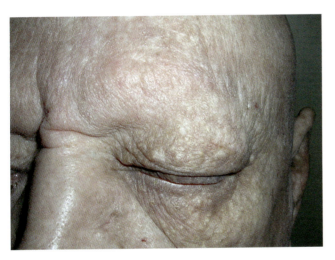

Fig. 14.59 Severe alopecia of the eyelashes and eyebrows in folliculotropic mycosis fungoides. This patient had a history of long-term disease

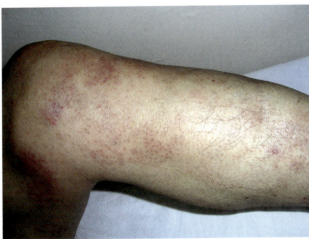

Fig. 14.61 Multiple reddish-brown, tiny papules representing syringotropic mycosis fungoides

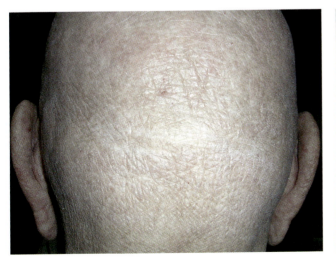

Fig. 14.60 Alopecia universalis-like complete hair loss in a patient with advanced folliculotropic mycosis fungoides

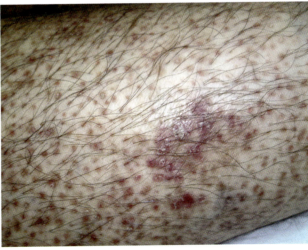

Fig. 14.62 Perifollicular punctuate erythema and papules on the leg. The diagnosis of syringotropic mycosis fungoides was established on histopathologic examination in this case

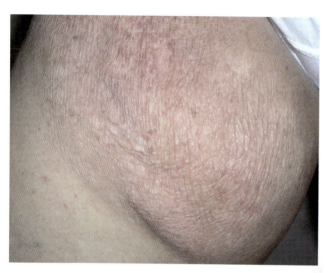

Fig. 14.63 Diffuse involvement of plaque-type mycosis fungoides on the lower abdomen associated with granulomatous slack skin on the groin

Fig. 14.65 Hypopigmented mycosis fungoides on the trunk of a child. Multiple ill-defined patches are seen

Fig. 14.64 Granulomatous slack skin located on the upper thigh. Note the pendulous appearance of the mass

sharply demarcated, atrophic, pendulous, lax plaques are observed which are more common in the axillae and groin (see Figs. 14.63 and 14.64). Lesions may resemble those of cutis laxa. Patients usually have one or only a few granulomatous slack skin lesions, but they may also have associated classic patches and plaques of mycosis fungoides. Histologically interstitial T-cell and histiocyte infiltration in the dermis, forming granulomas with multinucleated giant cells, is accompanied by elastolysis and elastophagocytosis. Loss of the elastic tissue is the cause of slack skin. The prognostic difference from classic mycosis fungoides is not clear.

Hypopigmented Mycosis Fungoides

Hypopigmented mycosis fungoides is an atypical variant of mycosis fungoides rarely seen in adults. However, it is one of the most common types of mycosis fungoides in the pediatric age group (see Fig. 14.65). The reason for this predisposition for children is unknown. Asians and African Americans are more commonly involved than fair or white-skinned patients. Asymptomatic, nonscaly, irregularly scattered small macules (see Fig. 14.66) or large patches (see Fig. 14.67) on the trunk or extremities are the common clinical presentation of this type. However, scaling (see Figs. 14.68 and 14.69) or sometimes purpura (see Fig. 14.70) may be seen on some of the hypopigmented lesions. Solitary hypopigmented lesions may also be observed. Diagnosis is relatively easier when it is found concurrently with other typical lesions of mycosis fungoides. However, it is rather challenging if patients present with only hypopigmented patches. Vitiligo, pityriasis alba, pityriasis versicolor, or postinflammatory hypopigmentation are the typical differential diagnostic challenges. Histopathologic examination shows features of early mycosis fungoides, together with absence or reduced amounts of melanin in the epidermis. The prognosis of this morphologic subtype is good. Repigmentation usually occurs after successful treatment.

14.1 Primary Cutaneous Lymphomas

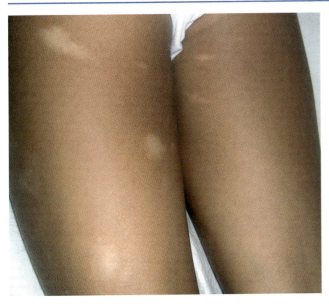

Fig. 14.66 Irregularly distributed, nonscaly white patches representing hypopigmented mycosis fungoides in a child

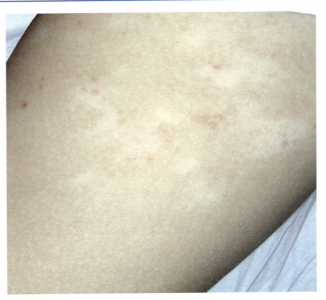

Fig. 14.68 Hypopigmented mycosis fungoides with overlying fine scales on the leg of a child

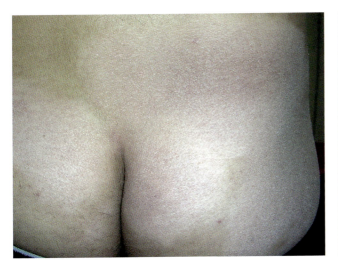

Fig. 14.67 Large well-defined white patch in an adult patient with hypopigmented mycosis fungoides

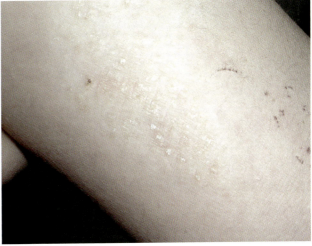

Fig. 14.69 Thick scales overlying hypopigmented mycosis fungoides

Hyperpigmented Mycosis Fungoides

Hyperpigmentation can be seen in different lesions of mycosis fungoides. Sometimes, patches and plaques may be hyperpigmented (see Figs. 14.71 and 14.72). Marked hyperpigmentation causing a reticular appearance can be observed on the lesions of poikilodermatous mycosis fungoides. Moreover, erythroderma of Sézary syndrome may also be hyperpigmented and is called melanoerythroderma. Pigment incontinence seen in the dermis is the reason for hyperpigmentation in mycosis fungoides, which can cause a misdiagnosis of pigmented lichen planus. Mild scaling and infiltration of the dark plaques further support the diagnosis of mycosis fungoides. Treatment can be curative for mycosis fungoides lesions; however, hyperpigmentation, namely melanin in the dermis, can persist for a long time. Therefore, histologic features such as clearance of the neoplastic infiltration are more useful and may be more accurate than the clinical findings in the follow-up period of these cases.

Purpuric Mycosis Fungoides

One of the rare clinicopathologic variants of mycosis fungoides is the purpuric subtype. It is also defined as pigmented purpura-like mycosis fungoides. However, we prefer using the term "purpuric mycosis fungoides." The frequency of this variant is not clear, but we have observed it more commonly in children. Petechiae or ecchymosis on or around the patches and plaques of mycosis fungoides is the typical

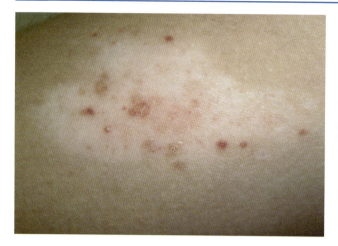

Fig. 14.70 Ill-defined white patch with mild scales and dispersed petechiae; overlap of hypopigmented and purpuric mycosis fungoides in a child

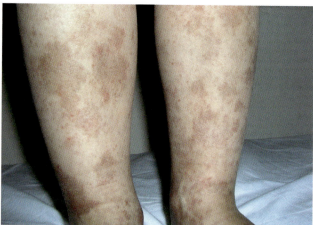

Fig. 14.73 Purpuric mycosis fungoides in a child

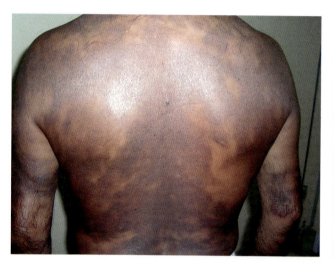

Fig. 14.71 Hyperpigmented mycosis fungoides on the trunk. The existence of mild scaling is helpful in the diagnosis

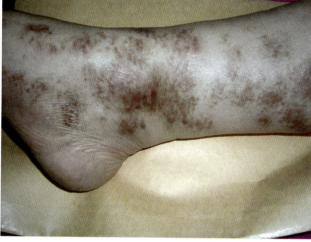

Fig. 14.74 Purpuric mycosis fungoides; mild scaly patches and pigmented purpuric dermatitis-like eruption occurring concomitantly on the foot and leg of an adult

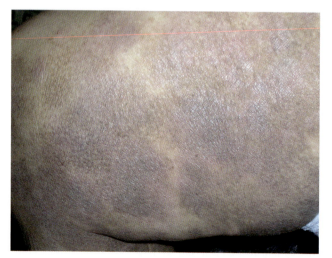

Fig. 14.72 Hyperpigmented mycosis fungoides presenting with confluent patches and plaques

presentation of this variant (see Figs. 14.73 and 14.74). It is stated that mycosis fungoides might mimic pigmented purpuric dermatitis or this benign dermatosis might evolve into mycosis fungoides. Because of the clinical overlap with the purpuric variant of mycosis fungoides, it is suggested that persistent (>1 year) and progressive cases of pigmented purpuric dermatitis should be followed up, and a biopsy may be performed for a suspicion of this cutaneous lymphoma. On the other hand, histopathologic features may be similar in both diseases, leading to a further challenge in diagnosis. The histopathology of purpuric mycosis fungoides usually reveals dense erythrocyte extravasation in the papillary dermis along with other features of classic mycosis fungoides, such as epidermotropism and lymphocyte atypia. Purpura usually resolves with the therapy of mycosis fungoides and does not have any prognostic significance.

14.1 Primary Cutaneous Lymphomas

Poikilodermatous Mycosis Fungoides

Poikilodermatous mycosis fungoides was initially named "poikiloderma vasculare atrophicans" and considered to be a precursor of mycosis fungoides. However, poikilodermatous mycosis fungoides is now considered a distinct clinicopathologic variant. It has also been referred to the lichenoid type of mycosis fungoides. Clinically, it is characterized by patches or plaques with areas of atrophy, telangiectases, and reticulate or mottled hyper- and hypopigmentation. Poikiloderma seen in mycosis fungoides may be reddish-brown (*see* Fig. 14.75) or heavily pigmented (*see* Figs. 14.76 and 14.77), and localized (*see* Fig. 14.78) or diffuse (*see* Fig. 14.79). The flexural areas (*see* Fig. 14.80), trunk (*see* Fig. 14.79), and especially the breasts (*see* Fig. 14.81) and buttocks, are the commonly involved regions. Lesions may also be seen on the arms (*see* Fig. 14.82) and legs. Rarely, face involvement may

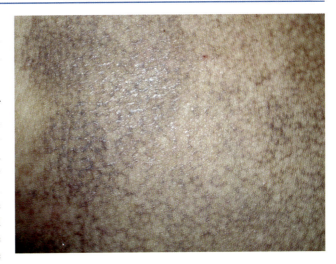

Fig. 14.77 Poikilodermatous mycosis fungoides. Note the typical reticulated hyperpigmentation

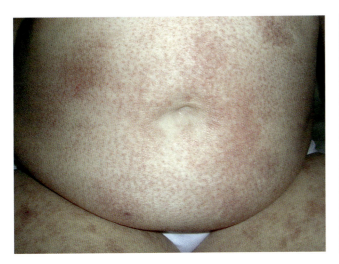

Fig. 14.75 Poikilodermatous mycosis fungoides on the abdomen with reddish-brown color

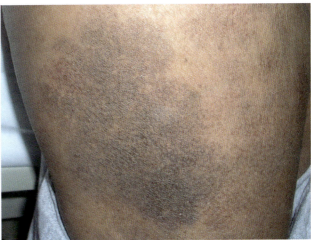

Fig. 14.78 Heavily pigmented poikilodermatous mycosis fungoides on a localized area

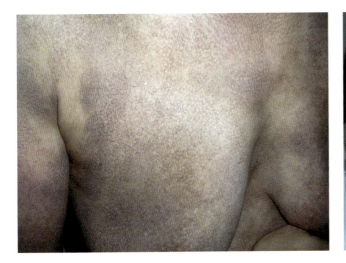

Fig. 14.76 Poikilodermatous mycosis fungoides with pronounced hyperpigmentation

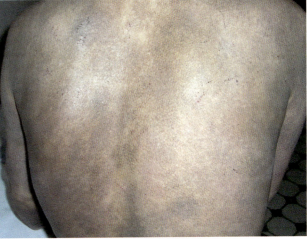

Fig. 14.79 Diffuse involvement of poikilodermatous mycosis fungoides on the trunk

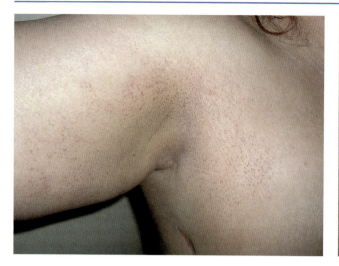

Fig. 14.80 Poikilodermatous mycosis fungoides on the axilla, a typical location

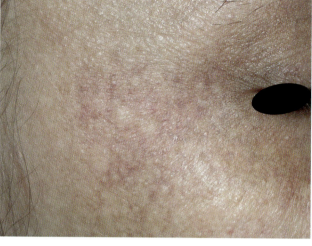

Fig. 14.83 Pigmented poikilodermatous mycosis fungoides on the face, a rare location

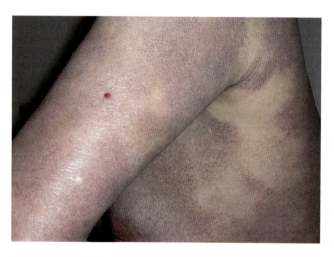

Fig. 14.81 Poikilodermatous mycosis fungoides on the breast, upper trunk and arm

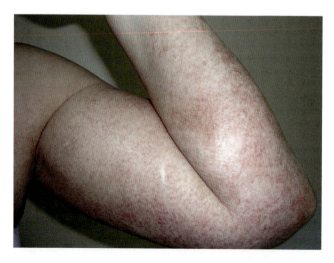

Fig. 14.82 Poikilodermatous mycosis fungoides with reddish-brown color on the arm

be observed (*see* Fig. 14.83). It may be an isolated finding or observed along with other classic patches or plaques of mycosis fungoides. The lesions may be asymptomatic or slightly pruritic.

Multiple biopsies are usually necessary to confirm the diagnosis of poikilodermatous mycosis fungoides. Histopathology reveals typical mycosis fungoides features in conjunction with epidermal atrophy, interface changes, dilated capillaries in the superficial dermis, and numerous melanin-laden macrophages. Clinicopathologic correlation is needed to exclude other poikilodermatous conditions such as poikiloderma of Civatte, connective tissue diseases such as dermatomyositis, topical overuse of corticosteroids, chronic radiodermatitis, graft-versus-host disease, and some genodermatoses. Although the diagnosis of this subtype of mycosis fungoides may be delayed, response to therapy and prognosis is nearly as good as in the early stages of classic mycosis fungoides. However, mild dyspigmentation usually persists and may cause difficulty when evaluating the response to therapy.

Erythrodermic Mycosis Fungoides and Sézary Syndrome

Mycosis fungoides may involve the skin rapidly or slowly to a great extent (*see* Fig. 14.84a and b), and sometimes diffuse erythema with fine scaling involving more than 80 percent of the skin surface (i.e., erythroderma) may occur. Sometimes erythroderma develops as a result of confluence of the infiltrated plaques (*see* Fig. 14.85). The eyelids (*see* Fig. 14.86), ears (*see* Fig. 14.87), and palmoplantar area (*see* Fig. 14.88) may also be involved. Erythrodermic skin may be thin (*see* Fig. 14.89) or infiltrated (*see* Figs. 14.90 and 14.91). Erythrodermic mycosis fungoides and Sézary syndrome may show overlapping skin findings and histologic features

14.1 Primary Cutaneous Lymphomas

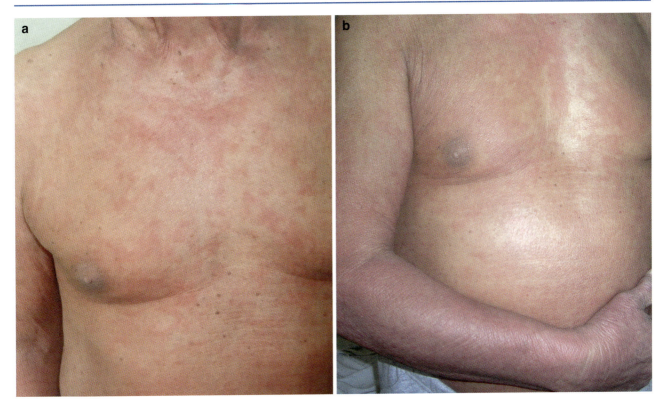

Fig. 14.84 (a) Erythrodermic mycosis fungoides in the early period. (b) The severity of erythroderma increased in 6 months. This patient did not show hematologic involvement over a 5-years follow-up period

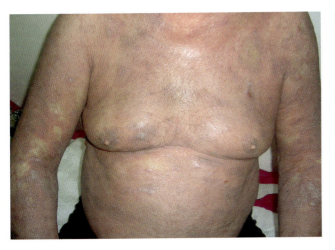

Fig. 14.85 Erythrodermic mycosis fungoides. The confluence of the plaques may lead to erythroderma, as seen this patient. Note the islands of unaffected skin

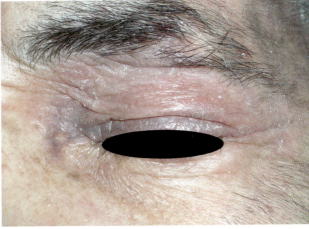

Fig. 14.86 Involvement of the eyelids in a patient with erythrodermic mycosis fungoides

and thereby cause clinical confusion. Erythrodermic mycosis fungoides is defined as erythroderma developing always secondarily in preexisting mycosis fungoides. Desquamation may be prominent in some cases (*see* Fig. 14.88). Islands of unaffected skin may be seen (*see* Fig. 14.85). Eczema-like changes may occur in the course of erythrodermic mycosis fungoides (*see* Fig. 14.92).

Sézary syndrome is described as a separate type of cutaneous T-cell lymphoma with erythroderma and "leukemic" blood involvement, mostly developing without preexisting mycosis fungoides. In rare instances, lesions of mycosis fungoides may precede Sézary syndrome. In an erythrodermic patient with typical histopathologic features of mycosis fungoides or preexisting mycosis fungoides in the history, another differentiating feature between Sézary syndrome

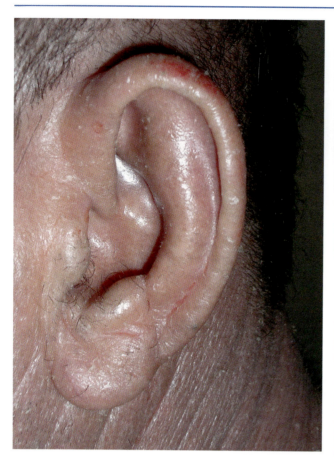

Fig. 14.87 Involvement of the auricle in a patient with erythrodermic mycosis fungoides

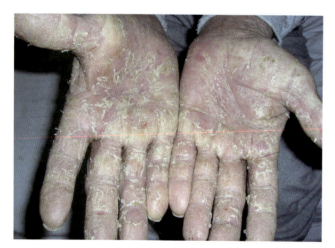

Fig. 14.88 Palmoplantar desquamation, a common feature in erythrodermic mycosis fungoides

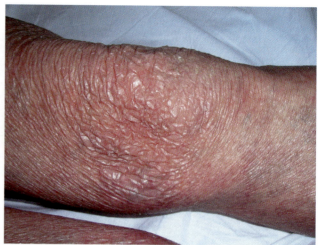

Fig. 14.89 Atrophic skin of a patient with erythrodermic mycosis fungoides

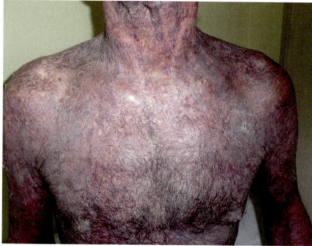

Fig. 14.90 The pigmented and infiltrated skin on the upper trunk in a patient with erythrodermic mycosis fungoides

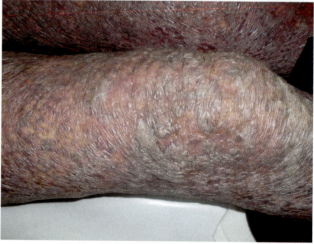

Fig. 14.91 Diffuse infiltration of the skin on the legs in a patient with erythrodermic mycosis fungoides

and erythrodermic mycosis fungoides is the blood findings. Hematologic criteria for Sézary syndrome are defined by the International Society for Cutaneous Lymphomas (ISCL) and these criteria consider mainly the presence of increased circulating Sézary cells, immunophenotypical abnormalities including CD4/CD8 ratio over 10, or the detection of a T-cell clone in the peripheral blood.

Sézary syndrome is more common in elderly men. Apart from the classic acute occurrence of erythroderma, patients with Sézary syndrome may initially manifest with persistent severe pruritus or nonspecific erythematous dermatitis. Erythroderma of mycosis fungoides or Sézary syndrome may be hyperpigmented (melanoerythroderma) (*see* Figs. 14.93 and 14.94). Facial skin of the patients with erythroderma may be infiltrated (*see* Fig. 14.95). Other than erythroderma, skin edema (*see* Fig. 14.96), palmoplantar hyperkeratosis (*see* Fig. 14.97) or desquamation (*see* Fig. 14.98), ectropion (*see* Fig. 14.99), nail dystrophy (*see* Fig. 14.100), and alopecia (*see* Figs. 14.101 and 14.102) may also be found in Sézary syndrome. Follicular mucinosis may sometimes be seen in the course of Sézary syndrome (*see* Fig. 14.103a and b). Palpable lymphadenopathy (*see* Fig. 14.104) and hepatosplenomegaly are other findings of this cutaneous T-cell lymphoma. Lymphadenopathy may be dermatopathic or neoplastic. Some lymph nodes may be very large. The serum LDH level is usually elevated.

The differential diagnosis of erythroderma has to be made against other conditions such as drug eruptions, psoriasis, atopic dermatitis, and adult T-cell leukemia. Dense lichenoid lymphocytic infiltration in the papillary dermis, including Sézary cells with cerebriform nuclei, is typical but cannot always be seen. Even histopathologic examination may sometimes be insufficient to establish the diagnosis of erytrhrodermic mycosis fungoides and Sézary syndrome. Therefore several biopsies may be required.

Erythroderma is important in the staging of mycosis fungoides, and it is related to prognosis. Erythrodermic

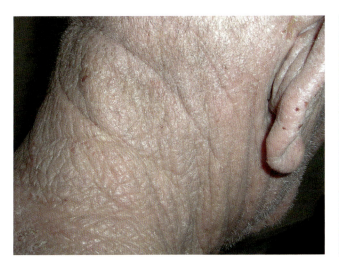

Fig. 14.92 Erythrodermic mycosis fungoides showing eczema-like changes

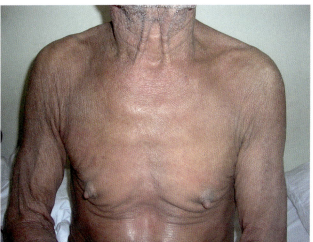

Fig. 14.94 Melanoerythroderma with prominent desquamation in a patient with Sézary syndrome

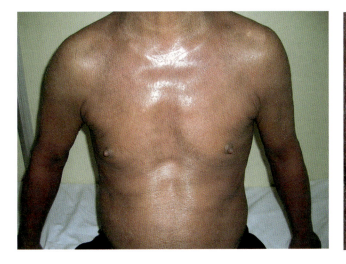

Fig. 14.93 Hyperpigmentation on the background of diffuse erythema and scaling (melanoerythroderma) in Sézary syndrome

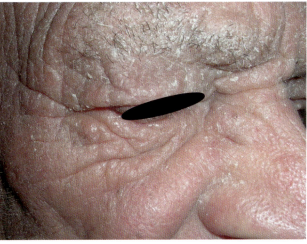

Fig. 14.95 Infiltration of facial skin causing leonine facies in a patient with Sézary syndrome

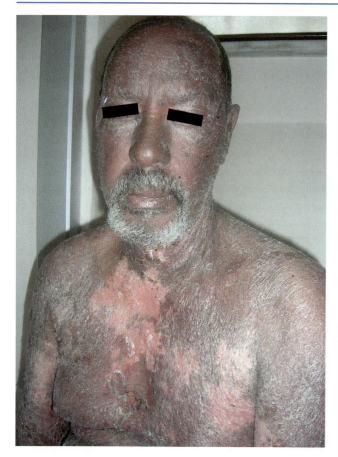

Fig. 14.96 Erythroderma associated with skin edema in a patient with Sézary syndrome

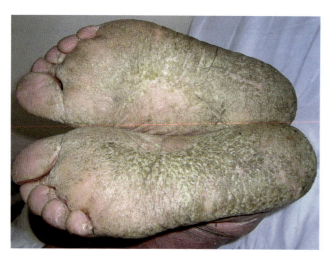

Fig. 14.97 Plantar hyperkeratosis, a frequent feature of Sézary syndrome

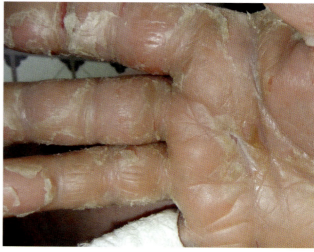

Fig. 14.98 Palmar edema and pronounced desquamation in a patient with Sézary syndrome

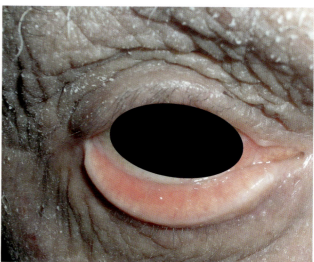

Fig. 14.99 Ectropion: a common complication of longstanding erythroderma in Sézary syndrome

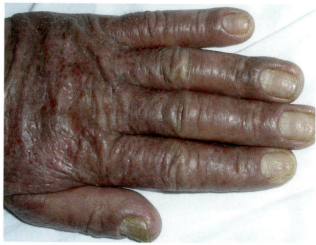

Fig. 14.100 Nonspecific nail dystrophy occurring in the course of Sézary syndrome

mycosis fungoides may sometimes show a chronic stable course effecting only the quality of life. However, in some patients it is rapidly progressive. Tumors may develop over the erythroderma (*see* Fig. 14.105), and the risk of visceral involvement is increased in these patients. In cases misdiagnosed as atopic dermatitis or psoriasis, treatment with cyclosporine makes the prognosis of mycosis fungoides worse.

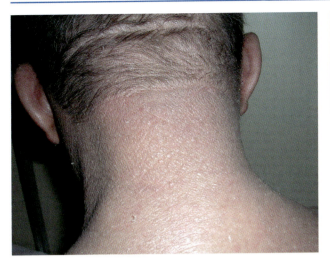

Fig. 14.101 Mild alopecia in a patient with Sézary syndrome

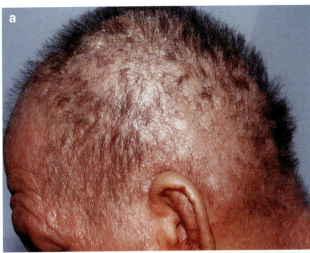

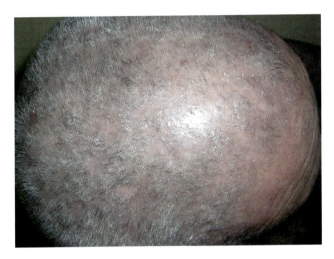

Fig. 14.102 Diffuse involvement of the scalp associated with severe alopecia in a patient with Sézary syndrome

Fig. 14.103 (a) Alopecia resulting from follicular mucinosis in a patient with Sézary syndrome. (b) Severe alopecia and secondary cutis verticis gyrata developed in a short time in the same patient

Secondary cutaneous (see Fig. 14.106) or systemic infections are among the main causes of morbidity and mortality in patients with Sézary syndrome. If the diagnosis of Sézary syndrome is established with extracutaneous findings, it has a poor prognosis.

Other Clinicopathologic Variants of Mycosis Fungoides

These rare variants of mycosis fungoides include anetodermic, bullous (vesiculobullous, dyshydrotic), papular, pustular, isolated palmoplantar, and hyperkeratotic (verrucous) forms. The diagnosis may be delayed in atypical lesions.

Management. The approach to the patient with mycosis fungoides depends mainly on the stage of the disease. However, invasive diagnostic screening protocols should not routinely be used. In early mycosis fungoides, such as in patients with patch/plaque type lesions, detailed radiologic

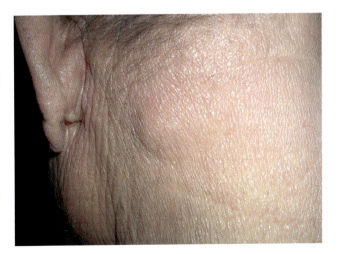

Fig. 14.104 Visible enlarged lymph node in a patient with erythrodermic mycosis fungoides. Histopathologic examination of this lymph node revealed dermatopathic lymphadenopathy

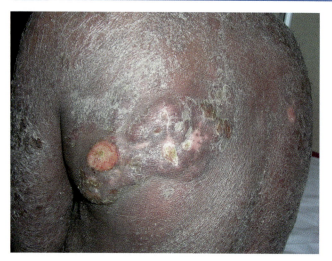

Fig. 14.105 Multiple large tumors arising on erythrodermic mycosis fungoides

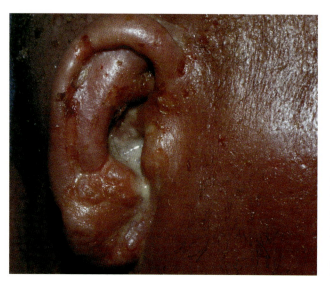

Fig. 14.106 Secondary Pseudomonas infection on the ears (malignant external otitis) in a patient with Sézary syndrome

examination for visceral involvement is not necessary. A complete blood count and routine biochemistry including LDH level and chest x-ray are usually sufficient in these patients. Physical examination of lymph nodes is important. Ultrasound may be used in case of any suspicion. Clinical or radiologic evidence of enlargement of a peripheral lymph node requires excisional biopsy. If dermatopathic lymphadenopathy is detected, further investigations are not necessary. In patients with cutaneous tumors, erythroderma or neoplastic lymphadenopathy detailed investigations for visceral involvement must be performed, such as radiologic examinations (computed tomography, positron emission tomography), peripheral blood smear, and flow-cytometry. Bone marrow biopsy is performed in cases with abnormalities of blood smear or with confirmed lymph node involvement.

Mycosis fungoides has a chronic relapsing course. Recurrence of the disease may be observed in patch and plaque stage patients after a short or long remission period. However many patients stay at early stages of the disease throughout their lives.

There is no proven curative method for mycosis fungoides. Therefore, symptomatic relief and long remission periods are aimed in the management of patients. The choice of the treatment depends mainly on the age and stage of the patient, including the clinical type of the skin lesions, extent of the skin involvement, and lymph node and internal organ involvement. Aggressive methods should not be used in the early stages because they have no proven effect on the prognosis, and the side effects of these therapies may be higher than the morbidity of the disease itself. In general, if the disease is confined to the skin in the form of patches, plaques, or poikiloderma, skin-directed therapies may be efficient.

In patch and plaque stages of mycosis fungoides, highly potent topical corticosteroids or phototherapy are the most commonly used treatment modalities. Topical corticosteroids such as monotherapy are usually the initial choice of treatment in patch stage mycosis fungoides involving less than 10% of the total body surface, whereas they can also be used in the limited recurrent lesions of the disease. Limited lesions seen in childhood, including hypopigmented mycosis fungoides, are mostly treated with topical corticosteroids. Although resolution is usually seen during therapy with topical corticosteroids, occurrence of new patches cannot be prevented. Local side effects on long-term therapy limit their use. Bexarotene, a receptor-specific retinoid, can also be used topically in refractory localized patches and plaques.

If more than 10 percent of the body is involved with patches or plaques, PUVA (psoralen plus ultraviolet A) or narrow band UVB (ultraviolet B) are the preferred treatment modalities. Narrow band UVB has fewer side effects and less carcinogenic potential than PUVA. It is mostly preferred in patch stage disease and digitate parapsoriasis, namely in patients with thinner lesions. On the other hand, PUVA penetrates deeper tissues and is more effective in plaque lesions of mycosis fungoides. These phototherapy or photochemotherapy methods can also be used in combination with topical corticosteroids. Patch and plaque lesions (see Fig. 14.107a–c), and poikiloderma respond well to PUVA (see Fig. 14.108a and b). However, maintenance therapy may be required to prevent the occurrence of new lesions. Therefore, long-term complications of phototherapy such as increased risk for the development of skin cancer can be a problem, especially in young patients treated with PUVA. The duration of maintenance therapy is not clear, and lesions may relapse even after long-term use of PUVA (see Fig. 14.109). Combination of PUVA with systemic interferon alpha or systemic retinoids (bexarotene, rarely acitretine) is an alternative therapy in refractory cases.

14.1 Primary Cutaneous Lymphomas

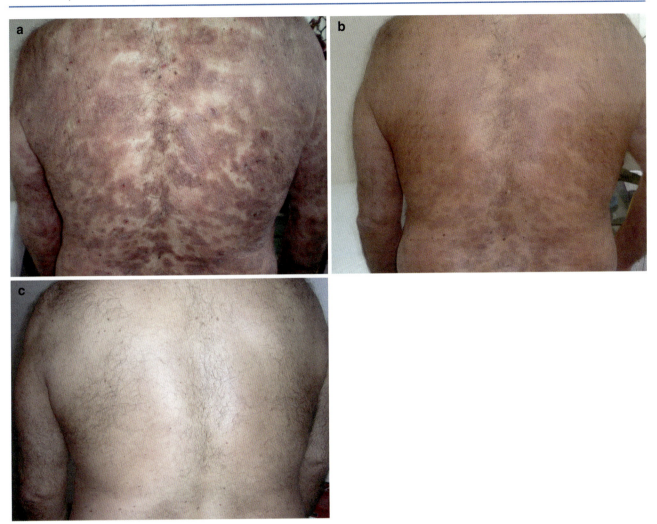

Fig. 14.107 (a) Plaque lesions of mycosis fungoides involving a large portion of the back and arms. (b) Good response to PUVA therapy. (c) Complete clearing at the end of PUVA therapy

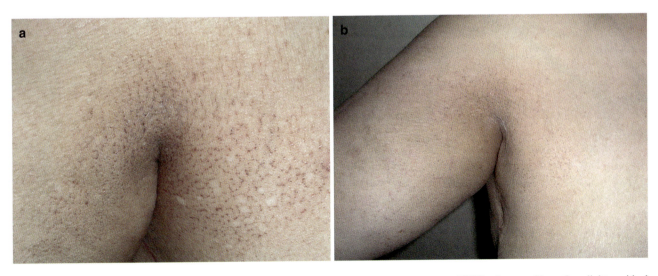

Fig. 14.108 (a) Poikilodermatous mycosis fungoides on the axilla. (b) Good response to PUVA therapy. Note the slight residual hyperpigmentation

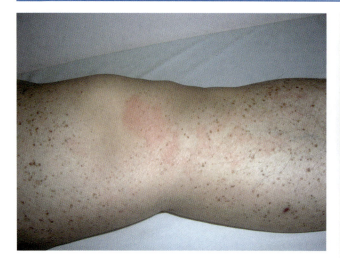

Fig. 14.109 Patchy lesions of mycosis fungoides on the legs that occurred months after PUVA therapy was completed. Note also the associated PUVA lentigines due to long-term use of phototherapy

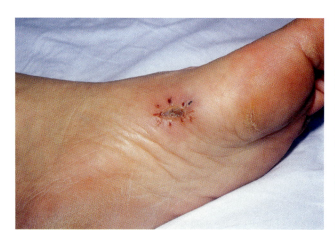

Fig. 14.110 Solitary lesion of pagetoid reticulosis on the sole treated surgically

Topical nitrogen mustard (mechlorethamine) and topical carmustine (BCNU) are other options in the therapy, especially in patients who are refractory to phototherapy. Relapses as patches or plaques that may occur in the early or late period after cessation of the previous therapies are not associated with worsened prognosis and can be treated like the initial lesions.

Local therapies are not effective for some variants of mycosis fungoides. Removal is preferred in solitary lesions of pagetoid reticulosis (*see* Fig. 14.110). If surgery is not feasible, radiotherapy may be used for these lesions. PUVA may be combined with systemic retinoids to treat folliculotropic mycosis fungoides (*see* Figs. 14.111a and b, and 14.112a and b). Total body electron beam therapy may also be preferred in this variant of mycosis fungoides.

In advanced stages of cutaneous disease, including tumors, erythroderma and large-cell transformation systemic interferon alpha, systemic bexarotene, total body

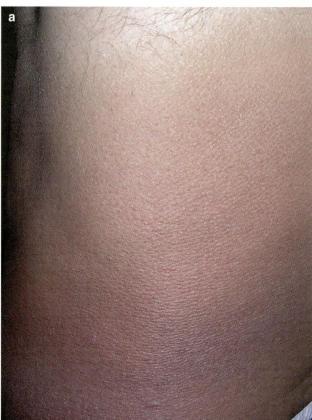

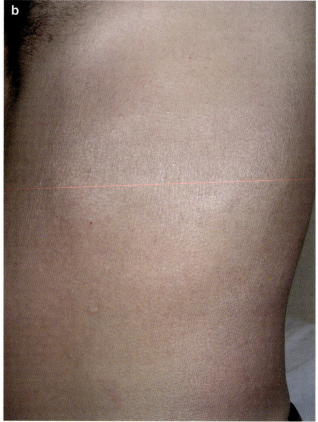

Fig. 14.111 (**a**) A broad plaque of folliculotropic mycosis fungoides on the trunk. (**b**) Improvement of the lesion after PUVA therapy combined with systemic retinoids and interferon alpha

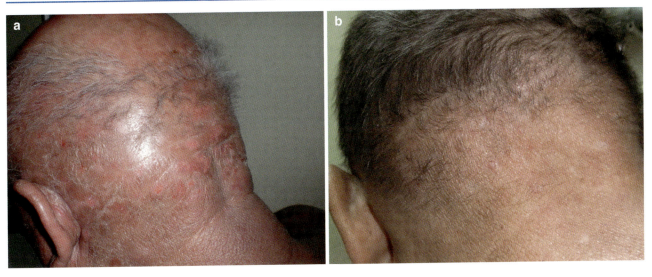

Fig. 14.112 (a) Alopecia caused by folliculotropic mycosis fungoides. (b) Improvement of alopecia after treatment with long-term PUVA and systemic retinoid (acitretine)

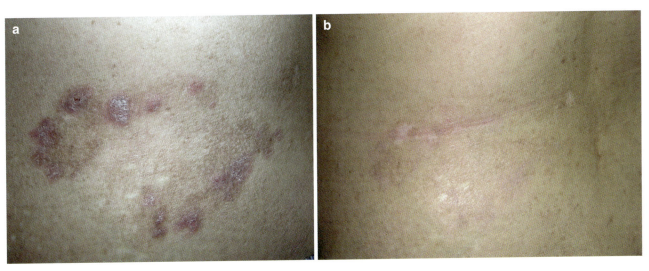

Fig. 14.113 (a) Tumoral mycosis fungoides presenting with an irregular-shaped lesion. The patient had also multiple patches and plaques on other sites. (b) Complete clearance of the tumoral lesion after therapy with PUVA and intralesional interferon alpha

irradiation (electron beam), extracorporeal photopheresis, or a combination of these therapies are the available treatment modalities. They may also be combined with PUVA therapy. In patients with solitary or a few tumors, local radiotherapy or intralesional interferon alpha may be effective, but recurrence is possible (see Fig. 14.113a and b). Systemic bexarotene is effective for multiple tumoral lesions (see Fig. 14.114a –d), but severe side effects such as hyperlipidemia and hypothyroidism limit its long term use. Low-dose methotrexate can also be used. Total body electron beam therapy is mostly preferred in patients with tumoral lesions but in the absence of visceral involvement, and it may be effective in tumors that are refractory to other modalities (see Fig. 14.114a–e). However, duration of remission is not always long. Extracorporeal photochemotherapy (photopheresis) is more commonly used for erythrodermic mycosis fungoides and Sézary syndrome. It may be combined with systemic interferon or systemic bexarotene. Radiotherapy may be added for neoplastic lymph node involvement.

Classic multiagent chemotherapeutic regimens in low doses are able to induce regression of tumors, but almost all patients have serious relapses shortly after cessation of therapy or even during treatment. Therefore these regimens should be avoided unless needed for palliative purposes in systemic involvement.

There are many other drugs that can be used in persistent or recurrent skin lesions and in the advanced stages of mycosis fungoides and Sézary syndrome. Pegylated liposomal doxorubicin, gemcitabine, alemtuzumab (a monoclonal

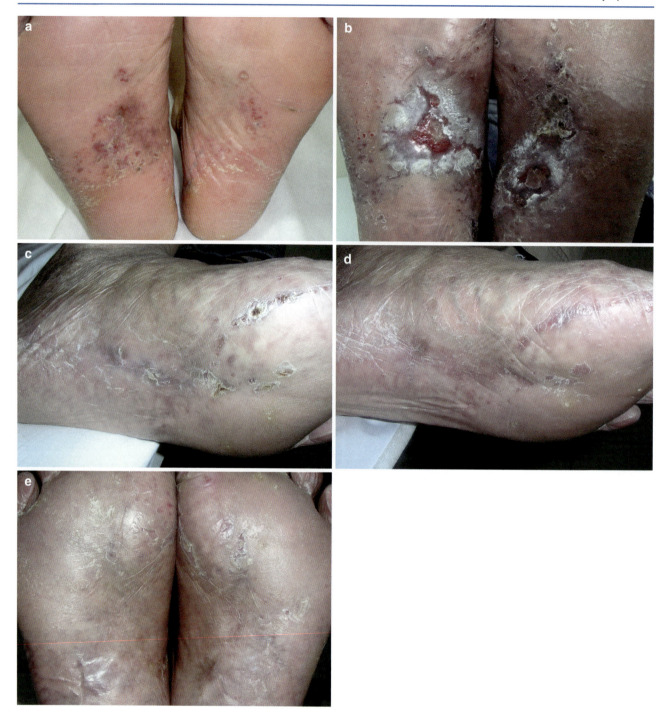

Fig. 14.114 (a) Early lesions of tumoral mycosis fungoides on the soles presenting as multiple erythematous infiltrated papules. (b) PUVA combined with intralesional interferon alpha was not effective; lesions enlarged and ulcerations occurred. (c) Ulceration healed after systemic interferon alpha combined with local radiotherapy, but some papulonodular lesions were refractory. (d) Papulonodular lesions regressed partially after systemic bexarotene therapy. (e) Good response was achieved with total body electron beam therapy

antibody that targets CD52 on lymphocytes), and denileukin diftitox (DAB389-IL2 fusion protein) have been used with variable success. Alemtuzumab may also be effective for blood findings of Sézary syndrome. Zanolimumab (anti-CD4 antibody), romidepsin (histone deacetylase inhibitor), vorinostat (histone deacetylase inhibitor) and bortezomib (proteasome inhibitor) are the new therapeutic alternatives. However, a satisfactory treatment, especially for lymph node and visceral involvement of mycosis fungoides is still lacking. Young patients with advanced stage mycosis fungoides or Sézary

14.1 Primary Cutaneous Lymphomas

syndrome may benefit from allogeneic stem cell transplantation, which may induce remission for a variable duration.

14.1.1.2 Primary Cutaneous CD30+ Lymphoproliferative Disorders

Lymphomatoid papulosis and primary cutaneous anaplastic large cell lymphoma belong to a group of cutaneous T-cell lymphomas called primary cutaneous CD30+ lymphoproliferative disorders. They represent a spectrum and borderline cases have also been described. This group of disorders is the second most common form of cutaneous T-cell lymphoma after mycosis fungoides.

Lymphomatoid Papulosis

Lymphomatoid papulosis is a low-grade cutaneous T-cell lymphoma with a rich spectrum of dermatologic features. This disease, which has an unknown etiology, has a chronic relapsing course: some patients have frequent attacks, whereas others show only a few relapses. It is mostly confined to the skin and has a low rate of morbidity. However, it may sometimes show association with other cutaneous or nodal lymphomas.

Lymphomatoid papulosis affects all age groups but generally is seen in middle-aged adults although onset at childhood (*see* Fig. 14.115) is not uncommon. The clinical presentations of cases in adulthood and childhood are mainly similar. The predominantly affected areas are the limbs (*see* Fig. 14.116), trunk (*see* Fig. 14.117), and the face (*see* Fig. 14.118). Lesions may be seen on the palmoplantar area (*see* Fig. 14.119), fingers (*see* Fig. 14.120), or anywhere on the skin. Recurrent eruption of crops of pink, reddish-brown or purple papules is the typical presentation (*see* Figs. 14.117, 14.121, 14.122, 14.123 and 14.124). Subcutaneous (*see* Fig. 14.125) or raised nodules (*see* Fig. 14.126) may occur. Papulonecrotic lesions (*see* Fig. 14.127) or ulcers covered with hemorrhagic

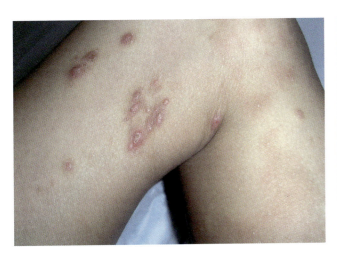

Fig. 14.115 Lymphomatoid papulosis presenting as multiple erythematous papules in a child

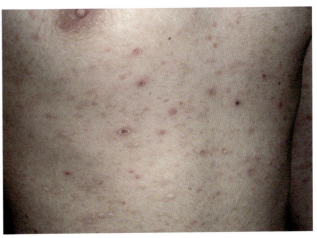

Fig. 14.117 Lymphomatoid papulosis manifesting as generalized papular lesions and atrophic scars on the trunk

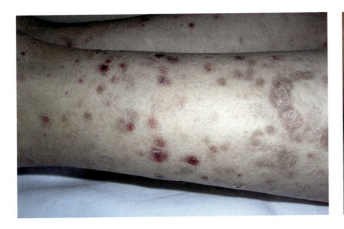

Fig. 14.116 Lymphomatoid papulosis on the legs. Erythematous papules, and nodules and atrophic scars (on the *right*) are seen

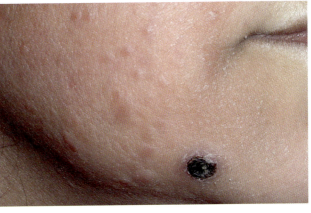

Fig. 14.118 Lymphomatoid papulosis on the face. Multiple erythematous papules and a crusted, ulcerated nodule are seen concomitantly

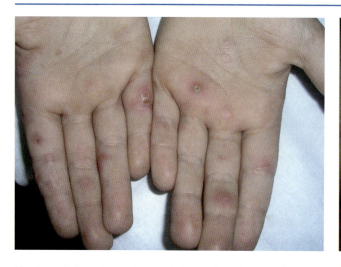

Fig 14.119 Lymphomatoid papulosis on the palms; erythematous papules, nodules and pustules are seen

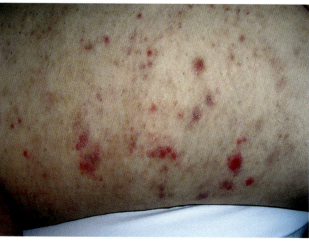

Fig. 14.122 Lymphomatoid papulosis shown as multiple tiny papules. History of a changing eruption is typical

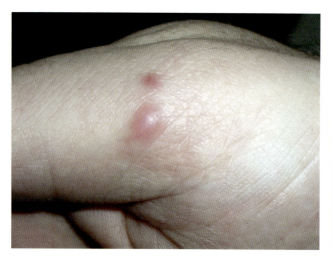

Fig. 14.120 Erythematous papules with smooth surface on the fingers representing lymphomatoid papulosis

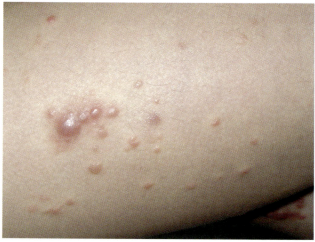

Fig. 14.123 Pinkish, smooth-surfaced papules and nodules in a child with lymphomatoid papulosis

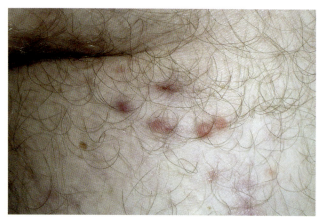

Fig. 14.121 Erythematous small papules of lymphomatoid papulosis; diagnosis may be delayed in such nonspesific lesions

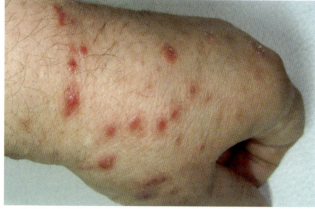

Fig. 14.124 Erythematous papules on the hand. A common presentation of lymphomatoid papulosis

14.1 Primary Cutaneous Lymphomas

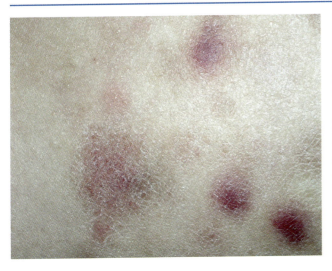

Fig. 14.125 Lymphomatoid papulosis presenting as subcutaneous nodules and purplish papules

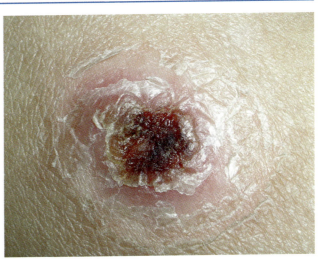

Fig. 14.128 A solitary large erythematous nodule with central ulceration covered with hemorrhagic crust representing lymphomatoid papulosis

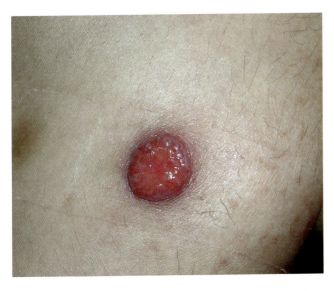

Fig. 14.126 Small erythematous elevated nodule with eroded surface. In such a case differentiation of lymphomatoid papulosis from primary cutaneous anaplastic large cell lymphoma is difficult

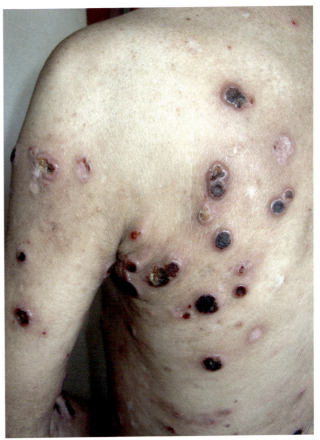

Fig. 14.129 Disseminated ulcerated and crusted nodules which occurred eruptively in a patient with lymphomatoid papulosis. Scars and hypopigmentation related to previous spontaneously healed lesions are also remarkable

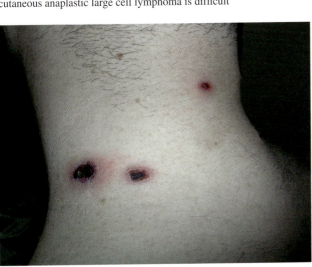

Fig. 14.127 Papulonecrotic lesions of lymphomatoid papulosis, which may be among the polymorphic morphology of the disease

crusts (*see* Figs. 14.128, 14.129 and 14.130) may also be observed. The number of the lesions varies in each episode. The clinical appearance may be highly polymorphic owing to the variety of skin lesions (*see* Fig. 14.131).

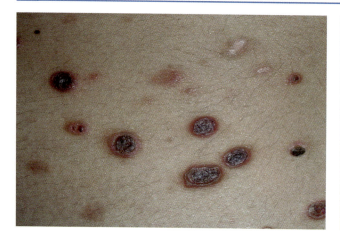

Fig. 14.130 Multiple sharply-demarcated ulcerations with slightly elevated borders. Acute ulcers may rarely be the prominent clinical feature of lymphomatoid papulosis

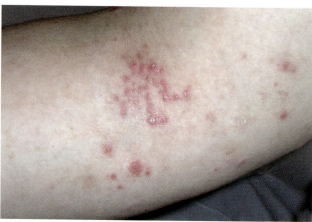

Fig. 14.132 Regional lymphomatoid papulosis. Grouped papular lesions restricted to the antecubital fossa are seen

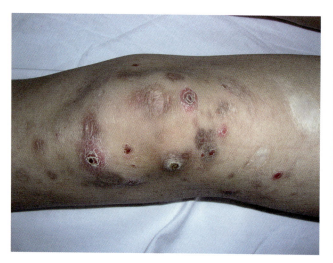

Fig. 14.131 Polymorphic appearance of lymphomatoid papulosis; erythematous papules, necrotic crusts and scars are seen concomitantly

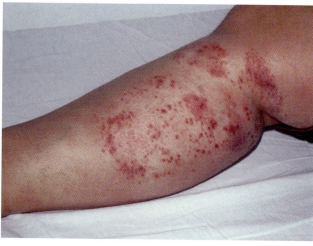

Fig. 14.133 Regional lymphomatoid papulosis. Both the initial and recurrent lesions were restricted to the lower leg in this patient

Most patients have a generalized asymmetrically distributed eruption, but in a subset of patients localized (regional) involvement in one anatomic area (*see* Figs. 14.132 and 14.133) may be the sole clinical presentation. Localized involvement may be more commonly observed in children. Lymphomatoid papulosis is mostly a cutaneous disease, and mucosal surfaces are unusual sites of its involvement. However, lesions on the tongue or other areas of the oral mucosa presenting as raised nodules or ulcerations may rarely be seen (*see* Fig. 14.134). Large tumors or mucosal involvement do not indicate a poor prognosis.

All types of lesions show a tendency to spontaneous regression within 2 to 12 weeks (*see* Fig. 14.135a–e). As some lesions clear new ones may appear on the periphery (*see*

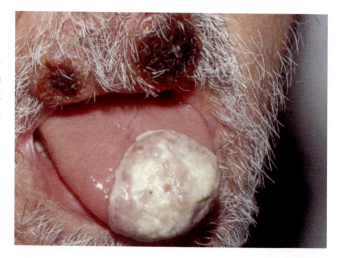

Fig. 14.134 Mucosal lymphomatoid papulosis. Ulcerations on the tongue and upper lip are seen

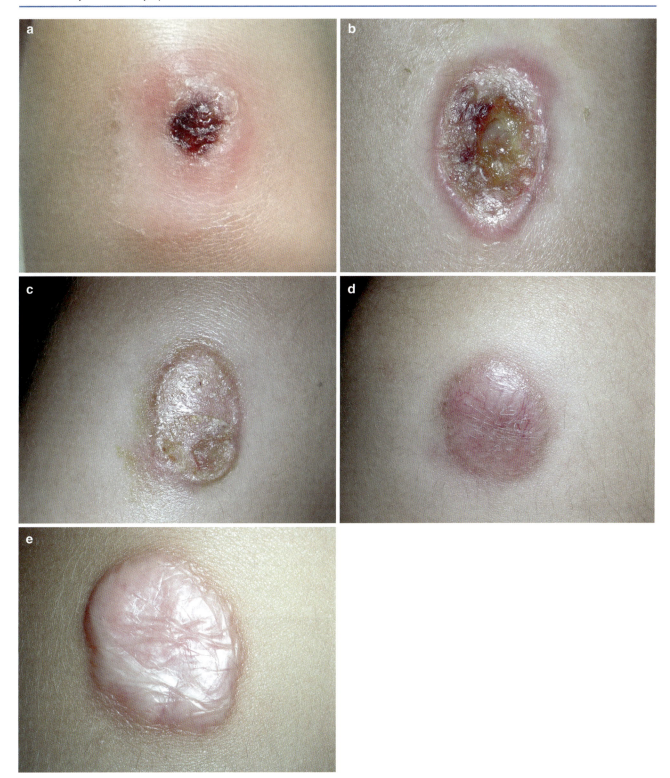

Fig. 14.135 (a) Early lesion of lymphomatoid papulosis presenting as a crusted nodule. (b) The lesion enlarged, and sharply-demarcated ulceration measuring approximately 2 cm in size occurred in a short time. (c) The lesion resolved after one month. (Only symptomatic therapy and topical corticosteroid creams had been administered). (d) An erythematous hypertrophic scar developed in three months on the lesion site. (e) Persistent hypertrophic scar on the lesion site at the end of six months

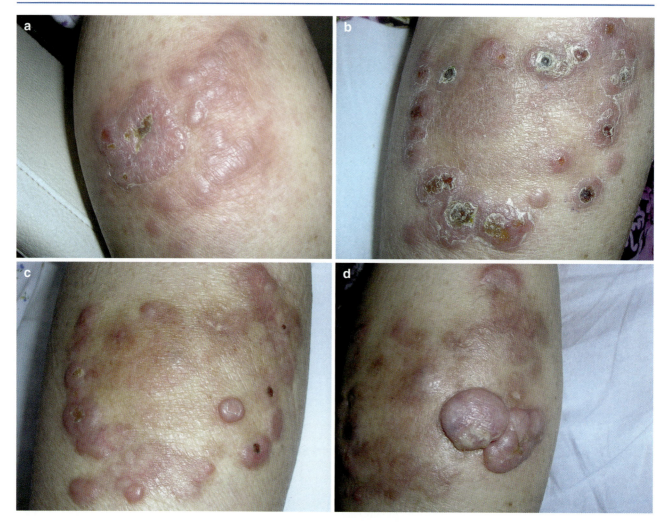

Fig. 14.136 (a) Clustering papules and nodules of lymphomatoid papulosis. (b) Central clearing of the clustering lesions but occurrence of the new nodules at the periphery after 5 weeks. Note most of them are covered with crusts. (c) Healing of peripheral nodules after two weeks. (d) Occurrence of new larger nodules after three weeks (only topical corticosteroids have been used during this period)

Fig. 14.136a–d) or anywhere on the skin. Dyspigmentation (see Fig. 14.129), atrophy (see Figs. 14.117 and 14.137), and hypertrophic scars (see Fig. 14.135e) may be seen, especially after the resolution of large nodules and ulcerations. Smaller papular lesions may heal without scarring.

The self-healing but relapsing course of lymphomatoid papulosis frequently leads to clinical misdiagnosis of inflammatory dermatoses. Ulcerated tumors occurring in a short time may sometimes mimic ecthyma or primary cutaneous CD8+ aggressive epidermotropic cytotoxic T-cell lymphoma. Skin biopsy is usually diagnostic. Although the histopathologic features are quite variable, the main histologic findings of lymphomatoid papulosis are a mixture of reactive inflammatory cells and small groups of large, pleomorphic, CD30+ cells with highly atypical nuclear contours in the dermis. These are features of the so-called "type A" lymphomatoid papulosis, which is the commonest histologic form.

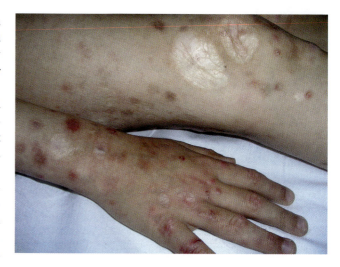

Fig. 14.137 Papulonodular lesions associated with dyspigmentation and large atrophic scars in a child with lymphomatoid papulosis

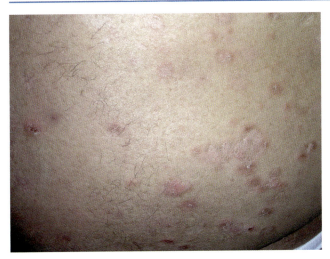

Fig. 14.138 Lesions of mycosis fungoides (patches) and lymphomatoid papulosis (nodules) are seen concomitantly

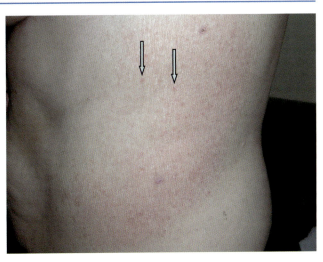

Fig. 14.139 Small papules representing lymphomatoid papulosis (*arrows*) overlying a large plaque of mycosis fungoides

Type C is characterized by sheets or groups of CD30+ large cells, with a few admixed inflammatory elements, a histologic picture close to primary cutaneous anaplastic large cell lymphoma. Type B lymphomatoid papulosis is an extremely rare condition and the histopathology is similar to that of mycosis fungoides. It should be kept in mind, however, that expression of CD30 may also be seen in some other neoplastic (e.g., transformed mycosis fungoides) or inflammatory (e.g., insect bite reaction) conditions. In addition to the classic forms, new histologic variants have been described; type D lymphomatoid papulosis is characterized by CD8 positivity and type E by angioinvasion and necrosis (angiocentric).

The distinction between lymphomatoid papulosis and primary cutaneous anaplastic large cell lymphoma is not always easy to discern. Primary cutaneous anaplastic large cell lymphoma shares most of the clinical and histopathologic features of lymphomatoid papulosis. However, the number of lesions is often fewer, and large tumoral lesions may also occur along with papules and nodules. The tendency to spontaneous healing is also lower and if occurs, it is slower in this type of primary cutaneous anaplastic large cell lymphoma. Typical multiple waxing and waning papular lesions are usually helpful to establish a correct diagnosis of lymphomatoid papulosis. Mycosis fungoides showing anaplastic large cell transformation must also be considered in the differential diagnosis from the clinical, histopathologic, and immunohistochemical points of view. However, these latter patients have typically associated patches or plaques of mycosis fungoides.

Lymphomatoid papulosis may be associated with other cutaneous and nodal T-cell lymphomas, but the incidence of this association and the risk factors related to the development of other lymphomas are not known. The most commonly associated lymphomas are mycosis fungoides (*see* Figs. 14.138 and 14.139) and primary cutaneous anaplastic large cell lymphoma. However, lymphomas like Hodgkin disease and systemic anaplastic large cell lymphoma can also appear. Secondary lymphomas can either precede the diagnosis of lymphomatoid papulosis, occur simultaneously, or even develop after a very long time; therefore lifelong follow-up of these patients is necessary.

Management. Lymphomatoid papulosis is limited to the skin and mucosae. However, after the diagnosis is confirmed, the patient should be checked for an associated systemic lymphoma. The risk of development of a secondary lymphoma remains for the life of the patient, and there is no established protocol to perform repeated aggressive examinations for screening.

The course of lymphomatoid papulosis is unpredictable. Different therapeutic methods mainly produce a partial or temporary response, but the remission cannot be sustained in most cases. Therefore, the adverse effects of a long-term treatment should initially be considered. Furthermore, there is no evidence for any therapy that effectively prevents the development of secondary lymphomas. Reassurance of the patient about the course of this skin disease is important. The existence of secondary lymphomas, the age of the patient, and the extent and type of the lesions determine the choice of treatment. In patients with mild symptoms and limited or localized skin lesions healing without prominent scars, follow-up without any treatment should initially be considered. Topical corticosteroids can be used in these cases. Good results may be achieved with topical imiquimod. However, the effect of topical therapies is only palliative.

In the presence of generalized, persistent, ulcerative, or scarring lesions causing cosmetic disturbance, systemic treatment or phototherapy can be utilized. The most commonly used treatment modalities for these cases include

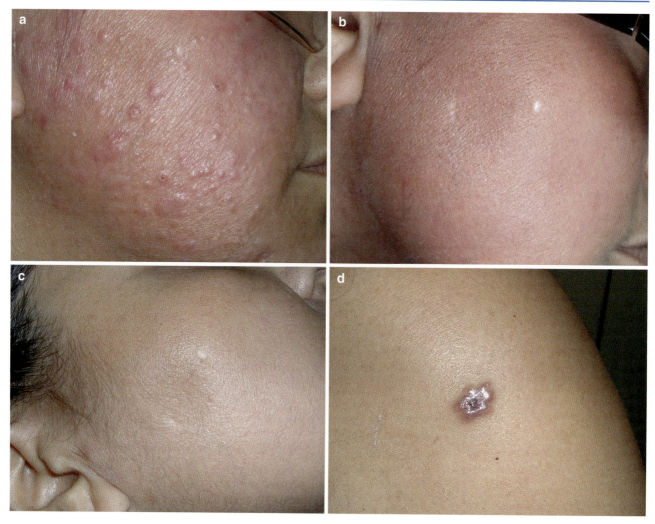

Fig. 14.140 (a) Multiple papular lesions of lymphomatoid papulosis located on the face. (b) Improvement of the lesions during therapy with PUVA. (c) Complete clearance of the lesions at the end of phototherapy. (d) Solitary lesion on the trunk occurred a few months after cessation of the therapy

PUVA and low-dose methotrexate. These methods can also be combined. The occurrence of new lesions may be reduced or even all lesions may be cleared with therapy (see Fig. 14.140a–c). However, after cessation of these therapies, recurrence is frequent on the same site or on other sites (see Fig. 14.140d). Aggressive chemotherapy should be avoided in patients with lymphomatoid papulosis limited to the skin because the disease usually relapses after chemotherapy.

Primary Cutaneous Anaplastic Large Cell Lymphoma
The main histopathologic and immunophenotypic features of primary cutaneous anaplastic large cell lymphoma are similar to those of lymphomatoid papulosis but differ mostly in regard to clinical features and course. This type of primary cutaneous CD30+ lymphoproliferative disorder is more common in adults but may rarely be seen in childhood. It may also be seen in immunosuppressed patients such as organ transplant recipients. The number of lesions is variable. Solitary or multiple red or reddish-brown nodules (see Figs. 14.141 and 14.142) or tumors may be observed anywhere on the skin. In contrast to lymphomatoid papulosis, large tumors (see Fig. 14.143) or thick plaques (see Fig. 14.144) are predominant. As distinct from anaplastic large cell transformation of mycosis fungoides, associated patches and flat plaques are not seen. Multiple lesions have a tendency to be grouped in one anatomic region of the body (see Figs. 14.145, 14.146, and 14.147), but multiple regions may also be involved. Some tumors grow rapidly, but after reaching a certain size they usually have a chronic stable course. Large masses may be observed in some cases (see Fig. 14.148a). Multiple satellite lesions may be located around the initial tumor. The surface of the tumor may be intact (see Fig. 14.142) or ulcerated and crusted (see Fig. 14.147). Nonulcerated tumors clinically resemble cutaneous B-cell lymphomas such as marginal zone lymphoma (see Fig. 14.167) and pseudolymphomas (see Fig. 14.193). Histologically, sheets of large atypical CD30+ cells in the dermis are associated with sparse inflammatory infiltration.

14.1 Primary Cutaneous Lymphomas

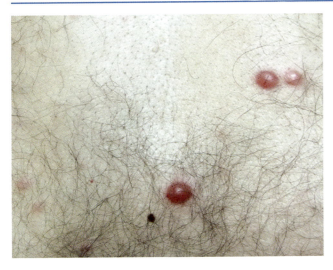

Fig. 14.141 Primary cutaneous anaplastic large cell lymphoma seen as multiple persistent reddish-brown papulonodular lesions on the trunk

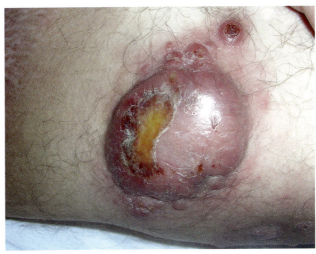

Fig. 14.143 A large red mass and adjacent small nodule in a patient with primary cutaneous anaplastic large cell lymphoma

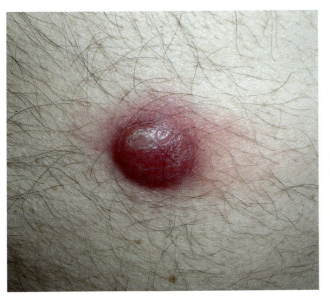

Fig. 14.142 Typical reddish nodular lesion of primary cutaneous anaplastic large cell lymphoma. This lesion has a smooth surface

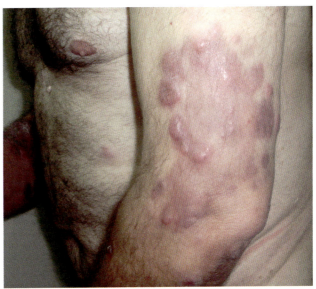

Fig. 14.144 Thick plaque with irregular borders on the arm in a patient with primary cutaneous anaplastic large cell lymphoma

Although self-healing is a prominent feature of lymphomatoid papulosis, partial or complete regression may also be observed spontaneously in patients with primary cutaneous anaplastic large cell lymphoma.

Primary cutaneous anaplastic large cell lymphoma has a chronic relapsing course with a variable prognosis. Extracutaneous involvement is rare, and it is usually in the form of regional lymph node involvement if present. In immunosuppressed patients the course may be aggressive. Primary cutaneous anaplastic large cell lymphoma must be differentiated from systemic anaplastic large cell lymphoma with secondary skin involvement. This differentiation, based on clinical, radiologic, and immunohistochemical findings, is very critical because the nodal counterpart has a high mortality rate. Systemic anaplastic large cell lymphoma typically shows positivity of ALK-1 and epithelial membrane antigen (EMA) in some cases.

Management. The number and extent of the skin lesions are important when determining the choice of therapy. Extensive lesions on the limbs may be more challenging. Surgical excision or local radiotherapy is the initial treatment option in most cases with solitary or localized lesions. Sometimes, both methods can be used concomitantly (*see* Fig. 14.148a and b). Undesirable scars may occur after the removal of large tumors. Moreover, recurrence is possible on the same site or on other body regions (*see* Fig 14.148c and d). Radiotherapy is effective for the treatment of multiple and larger lesions (*see* Fig. 14.149a–d), but relapse is a problem. Even recurrent lesions are generally not associated with systemic involvement.

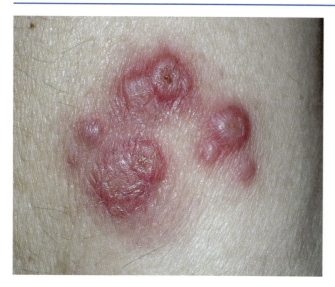

Fig. 14.145 Grouped papulonodular lesions restricted to one region of the body, a typical presentation of primary cutaneous anaplastic large cell lymphoma

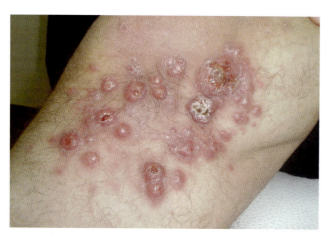

Fig. 14.146 Grouped lesions on one anatomic region in primary cutaneous anaplastic large cell lymphoma

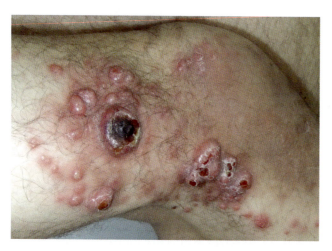

Fig. 14.147 Multiple grouped lesions of primary cutaneous anaplastic large cell lymphoma on the leg. An eroded nodule with crusting on the surface is noticeable

Methotrexate can be used for multiple lesions but may not always be very effective. Moreover, new lesions may occur after cessation of therapy. Brentuximab vedotin (anti CD30 antibody) is a new therapeutic option in refractory cases. Single or multiagent chemotherapy can be considered in disseminated lesions on the limbs or in large masses (*see* Fig. 14.150a and b). Regional lymph node metastasis may be treated with local radiotherapy, brentuximab vedotin or multiagent chemotherapy. Although the initial response to chemotherapy is good, relapse of the skin lesions is not rare (*see* Fig. 14.150c and d).

14.1.1.3 Primary Cutaneous CD8+ Aggressive Epidermotropic Cytotoxic T-cell Lymphoma

Primary cutaneous CD8+ aggressive epidermotropic cytotoxic T-cell lymphoma is a rare type of cutaneous lymphoma with an aggressive course and poor prognosis, as its name implies. CD8+ phenotype may also rarely be seen in mycosis fungoides and is not pathognomonic. However, these two cutaneous T-cell lymphomas have different clinical and histopathologic features. Rapidly evolving scattered lesions, including necrotic and ulcerated tumors (*see* Fig. 14.151), occurs mostly as the initial manifestation of primary cutaneous CD8+ aggressive epidermotropic cytotoxic T-cell lymphoma in contrast to the initiation of mycosis fungoides with patches or plaques. The historical form of mycosis fungoides, called tumeur d'emblée, included cases of this lymphoma. The formerly described generalized form of pagetoid reticulosis (Ketron-Goodman disease) may also overlap with this lymphoma.

Most patients are adults with disseminated eruption on the trunk and limbs. In addition to tumors (*see* Fig. 14.152), irregularly scattered patches, papules, nodules, and plaques (*see* Fig. 14.153) lead to a polymorphic appearance. Lesions may be ulcerated (*see* Figs. 14.154 and 14.155). The face (*see* Fig. 14.156) and palmoplantar areas (*see* Fig. 14.157a) may also be involved. Clinically lymphomatoid papulosis (*see* Fig. 14.29) and pyoderma gangrenosum may be considered in the differential diagnosis. Epidermotropism and diffuse infiltrate of pleomorphic lymphocytes showing CD8 staining are the histopathologic hallmarks of this lymphoma. Many apoptotic/dyskeratotic cells in the epidermis and erosions or ulcers are among the common features. Internal organs, including the central nervous system, lungs, and testes may be involved in a short time. Lymph node involvement is rare.

Management. Primary cutaneous CD8+ aggressive epidermotropic cytotoxic T-cell lymphoma is one of the primary cutaneous lymphomas with the worst prognosis. Multiagent chemotherapy, total body electron beam irradiation, and retinoids used in combination may only be effective for a short time and do not hinder the enlargement of the lesion and the development of ulceration (*see* Figs. 14.157a–e and 14.158a–c). Interferon can exacerbate the disease activity.

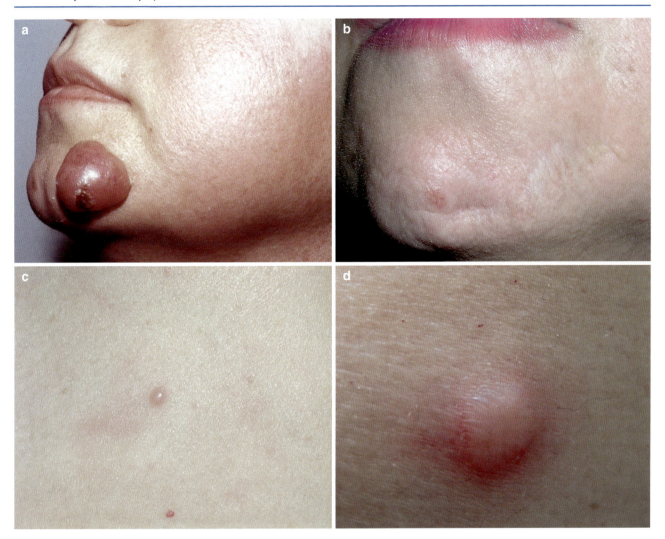

Fig. 14.148 (a) A patient presenting with a solitary large tumor on the face histologically diagnosed as primary cutaneous anaplastic large cell lymphoma. (b) The lesion was excised followed by use of local radiotherapy. (c–d) Relapse as a pink-colored papule and nodules on other sites of the body, one and two years later respectively

14.1.1.4 Extranodal NK/T-cell Lymphoma, Nasal Type

Extranodal NK/T-cell lymphoma, nasal type, formerly known as "lethal midline granuloma," is an aggressive cytotoxic lymphoma. Its pathogenesis is thought to be related to Epstein-Barr virus (EBV). As its name implies, it is located mainly in the nasal cavity. Other areas of the upper respiratory tract may also be involved. The skin may be involved primarily or secondarily. It mostly occurs in adulthood and usually begins with a rapidly growing erythematous and indurated nodule or plaque located on the nose (*see* Fig. 14.159) and cheeks (*see* Fig. 14.160a). This infiltrative lesion may ulcerate in a short time (*see* Fig. 14.160a and b). It may cause epistaxis, destruction of cartilage and bone, and nasal obstruction. There may be accompanying ulcerated tumors of the oral mucosa (*see* Fig. 14.161) and upper respiratory tract. Accompanying systemic symptoms may include weight loss and fever.

Hemophagocytic syndrome as a complication worsens the prognosis markedly. The typical location and highly invasive character of the lesions are helpful in the diagnosis. Visceral involvement may also be seen. Histologically, diffuse infiltration of pleomorphic lymphocytes of various sizes involving the dermis and subcutaneous tissues and angiocentrism are seen. Immunohistochemistry shows a natural killer (NK) or rarely T-cell phenotype. Usually CD2, CD56, and cytotoxic proteins such as TIA-1, granzyme-B, and perforin are expressed. EBV can be demonstrated by in situ hybridization. Rarely, neoplastic cells can be CD3-positive.

On rare occasions, there may be extranasal lesions with localized or generalized erythematous and purpuric plaques (*see* Figs. 14.162 and 14.163) or tumors on the skin. Ulceration is common.

Management. Although systemic polychemotherapy is used, the prognosis is poor. Radiotherapy may be added for solitary lesions.

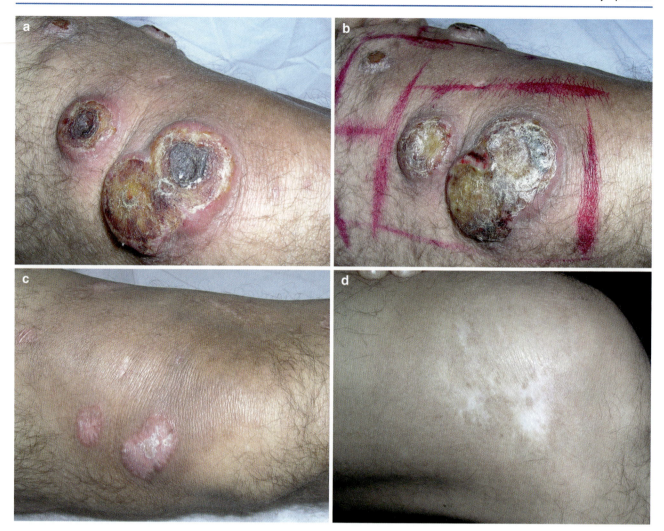

Fig. 14.149 (a) Multiple ulcerated tumors on the legs of a patient with primary cutaneous anaplastic large cell lymphoma with a long-lasting course. (b) Radiotherapy is a preferred option in localized lesions of this type of cutaneous lymphoma. (c) The lesions have regressed during radiotherapy. (d) Complete healing of the lesion with scarring is seen after the end of radiotherapy

14.1.1.5 Primary Cutaneous Gamma/Delta T-cell Lymphoma

Primary cutaneous gamma/delta T-cell lymphoma is a rare cytotoxic lymphoma with a poor prognosis. Most patients are adults. Skin as well as mucosal surfaces may be involved. The disease has a rapid progressive course. The lesions are more common on the extremities, but they may be located anywhere. Concomitant occurrence of erythematous patches or flat plaques similar to mycosis fungoides, panniculitis-like (subcutaneous) lesions (*see* Fig. 14.164), tumoral masses, and ulcerations (*see* Fig. 14.165) may cause a polymorphic appearance. Diagnosis may be delayed in patients with patches. Histologically atypical lymphocytes within the dermis with a pathognomonic phenotype show epidermotropism but also subcutaneous infiltration. It may be associated with visceral involvement, but lymph nodes and bone marrow are usually spared. Hemophagocytic syndrome worsens the prognosis.

Management. There is no effective therapy for this type of cutaneous lymphoma. The mortality rate is high even when multiagent chemotherapy is used.

14.1.1.6 Primary Cutaneous CD4+ Small/Medium (Pleomorphic) T-cell Lymphoma

Primary cutaneous CD4+ small/medium T-cell lymphoma is a rare indolent type of cutaneous lymphoma. The typical clinical presentation is a solitary nodule or tumor on the head and neck, or upper trunk. Sometimes multiple lesions may occur. Ulceration is rare. Extracutaneous involvement is not expected. CD4+ immunoprofile is a shared feature with mycosis fungoides, but patches or plaques are not found in primary cutaneous CD4+ small/medium (pleomorphic) T-cell lymphoma. Pseudolymphoma, especially lymphocytoma cutis (*see* Fig. 14.198), is the main differential diagnostic challenge and can be differentiated only

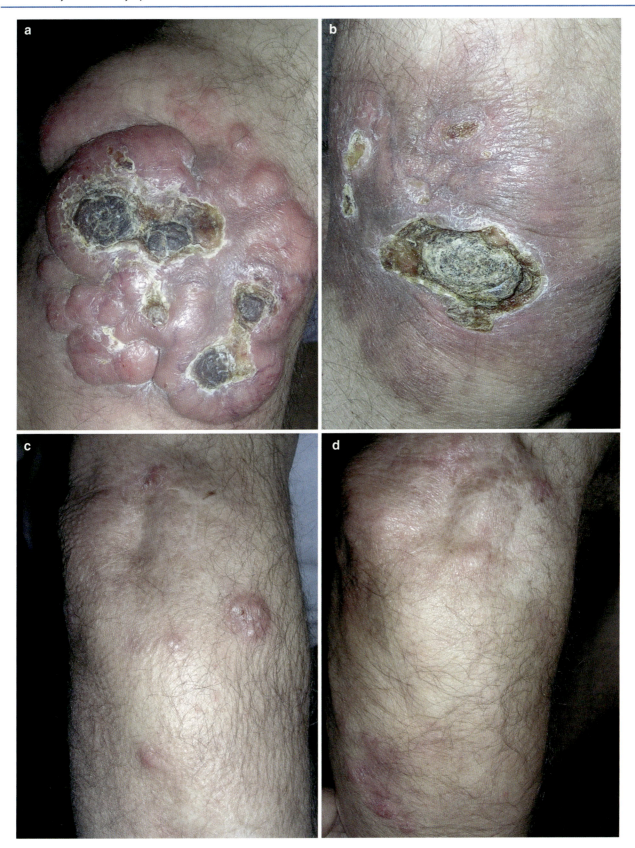

Fig. 14.150 (a) A large reddish lobulated mass on the elbow with eroded and crusted areas in a patient with primary cutaneous anaplastic large cell lymphoma. (b) Good response to multiagent chemotherapy. (c) Relapse of the lymphoma as a solitary nodule on the same site one year after complete healing with chemotherapy. (d) Healing of the relapse lesion with topical corticosteroids

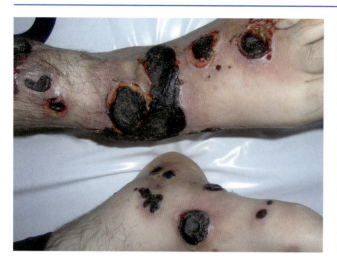

Fig. 14.151 Multiple ulcerated lesions seen in primary cutaneous CD8+ aggressive epidermotropic cytotoxic T-cell lymphoma

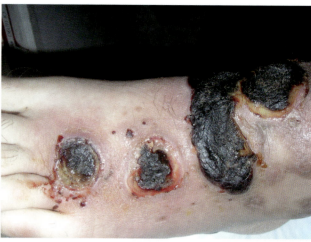

Fig. 14.154 Multiple ulcerated lesions covered with hemorrhagic crusts located on the foot. Lesions may ulcerate in a short time in primary cutaneous CD8+ aggressive epidermotropic T-cell lymphoma

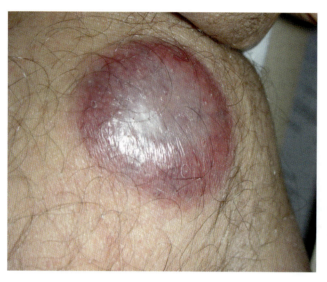

Fig. 14.152 A tumoral mass on the leg; early lesion of primary cutaneous CD8+ aggressive epidermotropic cytotoxic T-cell lymphoma

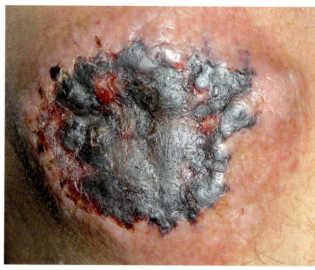

Fig. 14.155 A large tumor with ulceration in a patient with primary cutaneous CD8+ aggressive epidermotropic T-cell lymphoma. These lesions may be clinically misinterpreted as tumors of mycosis fungoides

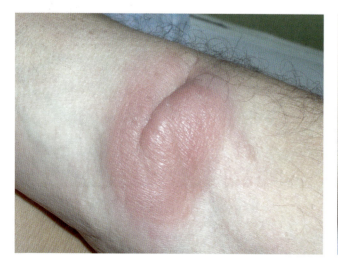

Fig. 14.153 An indurated plaque with a smooth surface representing an early lesion of primary cutaneous CD8+ aggressive epidermotropic T-cell lymphoma

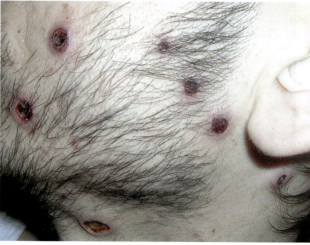

Fig. 14.156 Multiple ulcerated nodules on the face in a patient with primary cutaneous CD8+ aggressive epidermotropic T-cell lymphoma

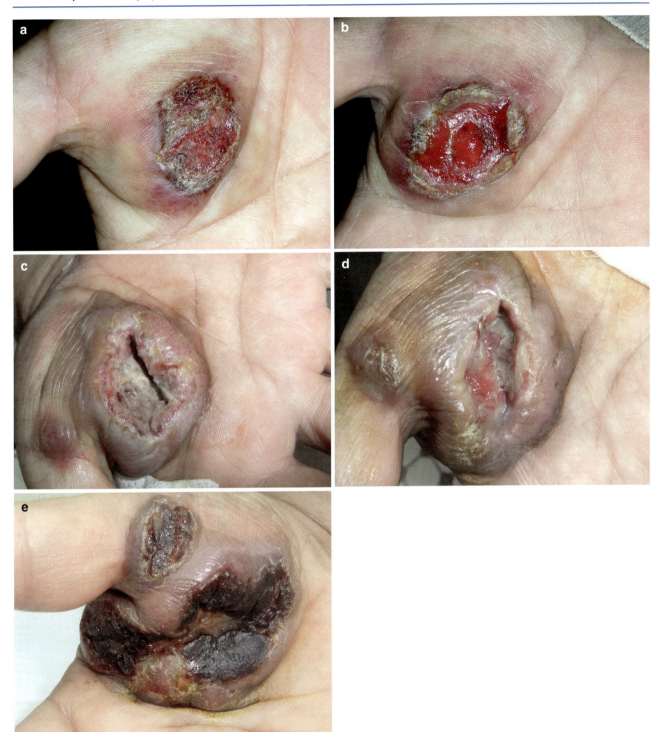

Fig. 14.157 (a) A tumor on the palm; one of the typical locations of primary cutaneous CD8+ aggressive epidermotropic T-cell lymphoma. (b–e) Note the enlargement of the palmar tumor, occurence of a second lesion and development of deep ulcerations in a few months despite the use of systemic chemotherapy

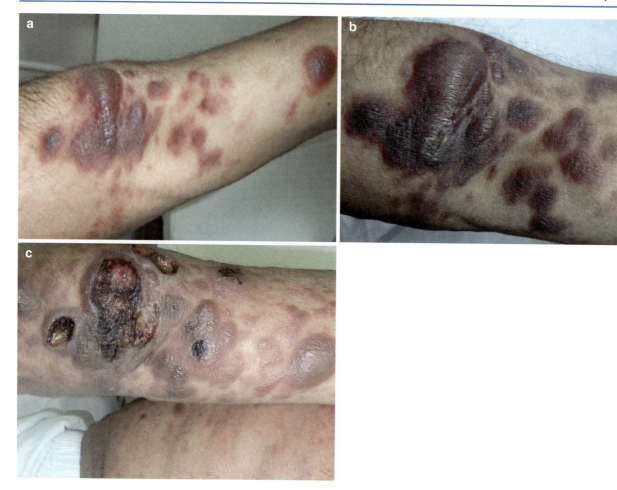

Fig. 14.158 (**a**) Nodular lesions and flat tumors caused by primary cutaneous CD8+ aggressive epidermotropic T-cell lymphoma. (**b**) Increase in size and number of the lesions despite aggressive chemotherapy in the same patient. (**c**) Development of large ulcerations during aggressive chemotherapy. The disease has a poor prognosis

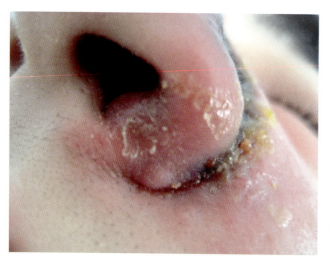

Fig. 14.159 Early lesion of extranodal NK/T-cell lymphoma, nasal type. Note the persistent inflammatory erythema on and around the nose

by histopathologic, immunohistochemical, and molecular biological findings. Histologically, nodular infiltrates of small and medium-sized pleomorphic CD4+ T lymphocytes within the dermis may also invade the subcutis. Marked epidermotropism is not expected.

Management. Aggressive therapies are not preferred. Solitary lesions may be excised sometimes followed by radiotherapy.

14.1.2 Cutaneous B-cell Lymphomas

Following the gastrointestinal tract, the skin is an important extranodal location of B-cell lymphomas. Approximately 20 to 30 percent of skin lymphomas have a B-cell origin. According to the present classifications of cutaneous lymphomas (WHO-EORTC 2005 and WHO 2008), four main

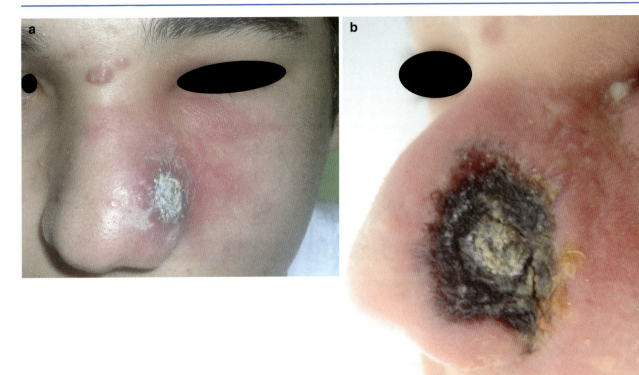

Fig. 14.160 (**a**) Extranodal NK/T-cell lymphoma, nasal type, beginning as an erythematous indurated lesion on one site of the nose and adjacent skin. (**b**) A deep ulceration covered with hemorrhagic crusts developed on the same site of the nose in a short time (With kind permission from Springer Science+Business Media: Baykal C, Yazganoğlu KD. Dermatological diseases of the nose and ears; 2010)

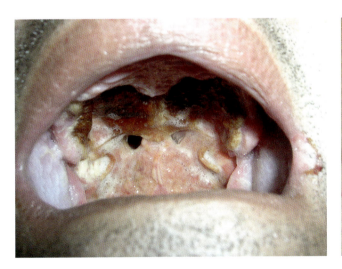

Fig. 14.161 Deep ulceration and crusting on the palate is seen in a patient with extranodal NK/T-cell lymphoma, nasal type

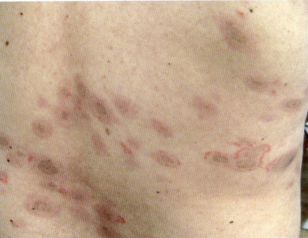

Fig. 14.162 Extranodal NK/T-cell lymphoma, nasal type presenting as multiple erythematous plaques with petecchiae on the trunk

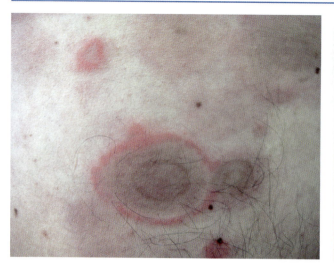

Fig. 14.163 Annular erythematous and purpuric plaque on the trunk of a patient with extranodal NK/T-cell lymphoma, nasal type

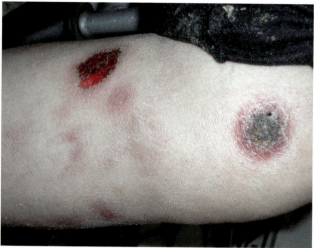

Fig. 14.165 Panniculitis-like subcutaneous lesions and crusted ulcers seen concomitantly in a patient with primary cutaneous gamma/delta T-cell lymphoma

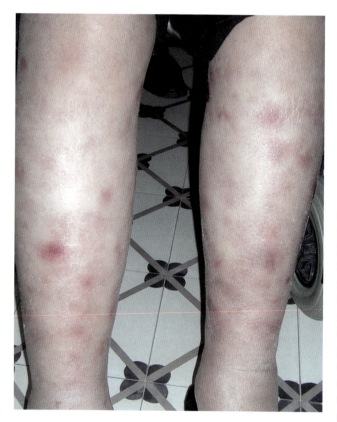

Fig. 14.164 Multiple panniculitis-like lesions in primary cutaneous gamma/delta T-cell lymphoma, typical presentation

types of cutaneous B-cell lymphoma with different clinical and histopathologic features have been described. Although all primary cutaneous B-cell lymphomas originate from B lymphocytes, thus sharing antigenic expression of CD20 or CD79α, they have different architectural and morphologic features, and each one shows some specific antigenic expression. Some of these cutaneous lymphomas have counterparts in the lymph nodes, but the clinical behavior of these nodal lymphomas is completely different. Except for intravascular large B-cell lymphoma, extracutaneous involvement is generally not present at the time of the initial diagnosis of cutaneous B-cell lymphomas. However, lymph node and visceral involvement may be seen during the course of the disease in different types with varying frequency.

14.1.2.1 Primary Cutaneous Marginal Zone Lymphoma

Primary cutaneous marginal zone lymphoma is a low-grade lymphoma composed of mainly centrocyte-like cells and has the best prognosis among cutaneous B-cell lymphomas. It is usually seen in adults and is more common in men. The arms and trunk are mostly involved sites, but it may occur anywhere on the skin. Patients present with solitary or multiple reddish or violaceous papules (*see* Fig. 14.166a), dome-shaped nodules (*see* Fig. 14.167), or plaques. Some papulonodular lesions show a tendency to cluster (*see* Fig. 14.168), whereas others may be irregularly distributed (*see* Fig. 14.169). As the tumor is nonepidermotropic, the surface of the lesion does not show scales, erosion, or ulceration (*see* Fig. 14.170). Even the larger lesions are usually asymptomatic.

Lymphocytoma cutis (*see* Fig. 14.194), primary cutaneous anaplastic large cell lymphoma (*see* Fig. 14.141), Merkel cell carcinoma (*see* Fig. 11.167), leukemia cutis (*see* Fig. 14.213), nodular cutaneous metastasis of solid neoplasms (*see* Fig. 16.12), and cutaneous infiltration of nodal marginal zone lymphoma should be considered in the differential diagnosis. The exact diagnosis of marginal zone lymphoma can only be made after histopathologic

14.1 Primary Cutaneous Lymphomas

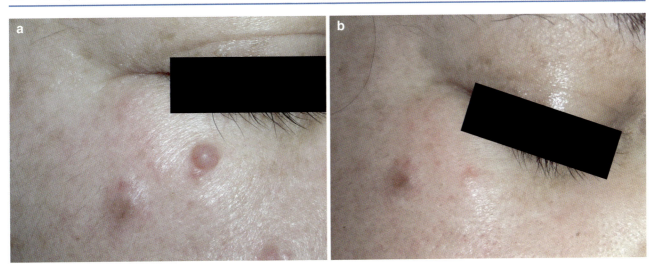

Fig 14.166 (**a**) Dome-shaped reddish solitary papule on the face representing primary cutaneous marginal zone lymphoma. (**b**) Lesion regressed after intralesional corticosteroid therapy

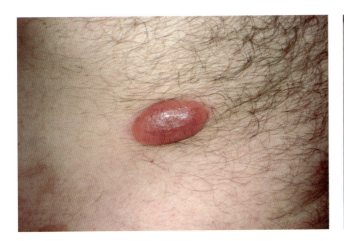

Fig. 14.167 Primary cutaneous marginal zone lymphoma presenting as a solitary erythematous round nodule with a smooth surface on the trunk

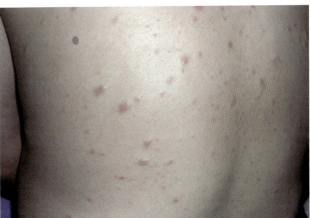

Fig. 14.169 A patient with primary cutaneous marginal zone lymphoma manifesting with multiple scattered lesions on the back

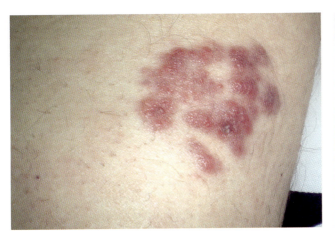

Fig. 14.168 Clustered reddish papules and nodules, a typical presentation of primary cutaneous marginal zone lymphoma

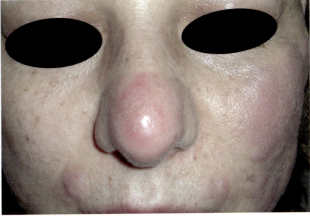

Fig. 14.170 Erythematous nodules with smooth surface on the nose, upper lip and cheeks; pseudolymphoma was also considered in the differential diagnosis, but histopathologic examination revealed primary cutaneous marginal zone lymphoma

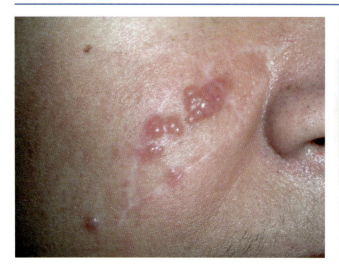

Fig. 14.171 Primary cutaneous marginal zone lymphoma relapsed on the scar of a previous excision

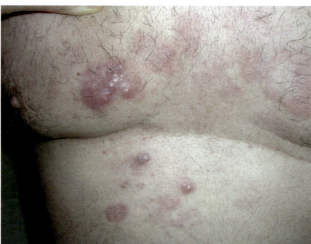

Fig. 14.174 Reddish-brown, infiltrated, raised nodules surrounded by flat erythematous plaques in a patient with primary cutaneous follicle center lymphoma

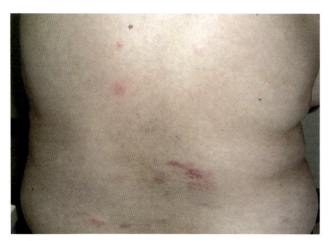

Fig. 14.172 Primary cutaneous follicle center lymphoma seen as irregularly distributed erythematous plaques on the trunk

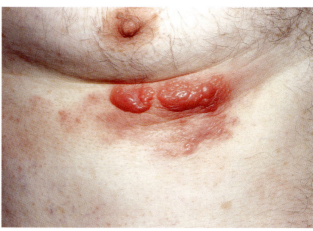

Fig. 14.175 Large tumors and infiltrated erythematous patches on the adjacent skin; this case illustrates a typical presentation for primary cutaneous follicle center lymphoma

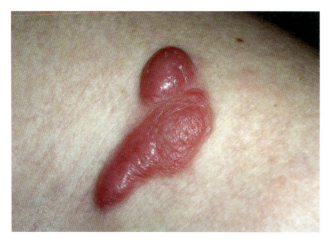

Fig. 14.173 Irregularly shaped solitary tumor representing primary cutaneous follicle center lymphoma

examination supported by immunohistochemical staining or molecular proof of a clonal B cell proliferation. The typical histologic appearance involves infiltration of mainly small to medium-sized atypical lymphocytes showing a nodular or diffuse pattern with a grenz zone below the epidermis. This type of cutaneous lymphoma has a chronic course but remains confined to the skin in the great majority of cases. Visceral involvement is rare.

Management. After the confirmation of the diagnosis with a skin biopsy, peripheral blood examination and radiologic imaging, including MRI and PET, may be performed to eliminate visceral involvement. Lymph node biopsy can be performed in patients with palpable lymph nodes. However, routine bone marrow aspiration and biopsy are not indicated.

Aggressive therapy is not necessary for primary cutaneous marginal zone lymphoma; thus excessive treatment

14.1 Primary Cutaneous Lymphomas

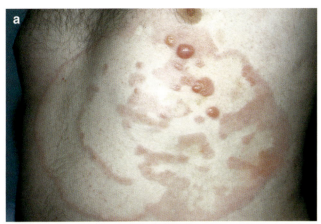

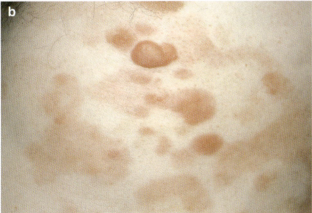

Fig. 14.176 (**a**) A distinctive clinical appearance of primary cutaneous follicle center lymphoma; erythematous nodules located on the center and annular erythematous patches on the periphery. (**b**) Regression of the lesion after two sessions of multiagent chemotherapy (this lesion healed completely at the end of therapy and did not relapse)

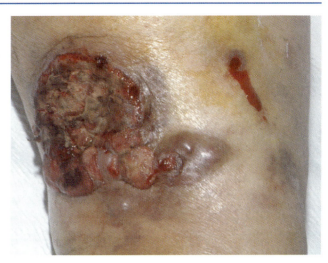

Fig. 14.177 A solitary ulcerated large tumor on the lower extremity. This is a typical presentation of primary cutaneous diffuse large B-cell lymphoma, leg type

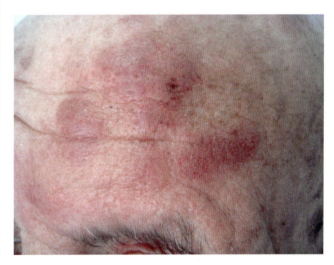

Fig. 14.178 A solitary erythematous infiltrated plaque on the face diagnosed histopathologically as primary cutaneous diffuse large B-cell lymphoma, other type

protocols designed for a systemic lymphoma should be avoided. Although it does not occur very often, spontaneous regression is possible. An isolated lesion can be treated with topical or intralesional corticosteroids (*see* Fig. 14.166a and b). Excision may be an alternative for solitary lesions. Local radiotherapy is another effective modality. Intralesional interferon alpha and rituximab, an anti-CD20 monoclonal antibody, have also been used for localized lesions. Patients with multiple lesions can be treated with systemic rituximab or systemic interferon alpha. However, close follow-up of the patients without therapy may also be preferred. Rarely multiagent systemic chemotherapy may be used in refractory cases. Recurrences are common after all therapeutic interventions and may occur at the same site (*see* Fig. 14.171) or at different areas. Cutaneous relapse does not herald systemic involvement or a poor prognosis.

14.1.2.2 Primary Cutaneous Follicle Center Lymphoma

Primary cutaneous follicle center lymphoma is the most common type of cutaneous B-cell lymphomas. It is characterized by the proliferation of B cells exhibiting a germinal center cell phenotype. It is more commonly seen in adults. The scalp, face, neck, and trunk (*see* Fig. 14.172) are the typical locations, but the lesions may also be seen on the extremities. Lesions are usually localized at one site but on occasion may be dispersed on the body. There may be a solitary (*see* Fig. 14.173) or multiple lesions. Reddish or red-brown firm papules, nodules, and plaques with an intact surface are grouped or irregularly scattered (*see* Fig. 14.174). Infiltrated erythematous patches and plaques surrounding a larger central nodule or tumor is the typical presentation of this type of cutaneous lymphoma (*see* Figs. 14.175a and 14.176). Cutaneous B-cell lymphoma with similar clinical features localized on the back has been named Crosti lymphoma.

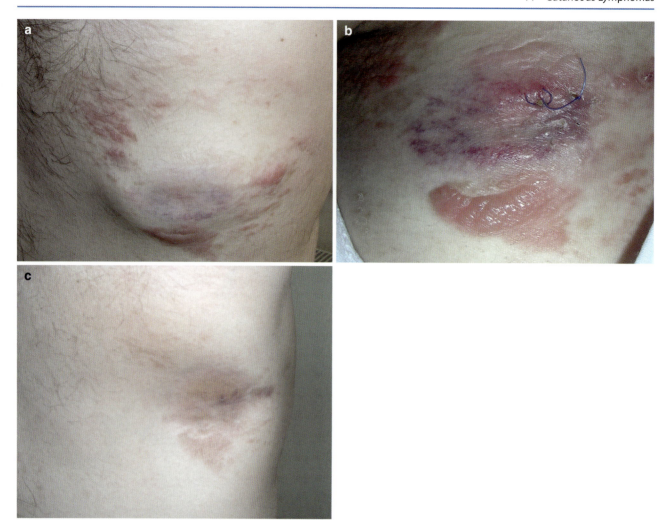

Fig. 14.179 (a) Large subcutaneous mass and adjacent reddish brown nodules histologically diagnosed as primary cutaneous diffuse large B-cell lymphoma, other type. (b) The lesion increased in size in a short time. (c) Complete clearance of lesions after multidrug chemotherapy

Since the typical clinical features are not present in all cases, the condition is generally diagnosed after biopsy. Medium to large centrocytes with a variable number of centroblasts and other inflammatory cells arranged in a follicular or diffuse pattern are the main histopathologic features. Positivity with Bcl-6 is supportive of the diagnosis.

Skin lesions have a chronic lasting course for many years. They grow slowly and increase in number with time. Multifocal lesions do not imply a poor prognosis. Lymph node and visceral involvement is rare in primary cutaneous follicle center lymphoma. However, it may occur in some cases, and the incidence of bone marrow infiltration is relatively higher than in primary cutaneous marginal zone lymphoma. Therefore, all staging investigations, including bone marrow aspiration and biopsy, should be performed in this type of cutaneous B-cell lymphoma.

Management. In general the approach to this indolent lymphoma is similar to the approach to primary cutaneous marginal zone lymphoma. Aggressive methods have no priority. However, because the margins of tumors are not well-defined and are surrounded by patches or papules, surgery and radiotherapy may not be effective. Extensive lesions with a progressive course may be treated systemically with rituximab. Frequent relapses are possible, but the recurrent lesions may be treated with the same options. The response rate of skin lesions to systemic chemotherapy is high, but this option is usually confined to refractory or extensive lesions (*see* Fig. 14.176a and b) or visceral involvement. Patients with bone marrow involvement have a poor prognosis.

14.1.2.3 Primary Cutaneous Diffuse Large B-cell Lymphoma

Primary cutaneous diffuse large B-cell lymphoma, leg type or other, is a rare type of cutaneous lymphoma characterized histologically by large round cells and an aggressive course. It may be located on the leg (leg type) or elsewhere (other). The former variant is usually located unilaterally and on the lower leg (*see* Fig. 14.177). The latter variant may be located on the head (*see* Fig. 14.178), trunk (*see* Fig. 14.179a), and upper extremities. In rare instances, involvement of the leg and other areas may be seen concomitantly. Most patients are elderly and female. Solitary or more commonly multiple lesions are usually restricted to one area of the leg. Contrary to more common, indolent types of cutaneous B-cell lymphoma, large, reddish-brown, firm nodules or tumors grow rapidly and they mostly ulcerate in the advanced stages. Mainly, the location of the tumor determines the prognosis. Patients with lesions located on the leg have an increased risk of lymph node and visceral involvement, including the central nervous system, and thus have a poor prognosis.

If primary cutaneous diffuse large B-cell lymphoma is located solely on areas other than the leg, it shows an indolent course similar to that of primary cutaneous follicle center lymphoma. Histologically lesions on any location show common features. Diffuse dermal infiltration of medium to large centroblasts and immunoblasts may obliterate adnexal structures and invade the subcutis. Immunophenotyping shows positivity for B-cell markers such as CD20, CD79α, and MUM-1. Additionally Bcl-2 is also accurate. Detailed laboratory and radiologic investigations about systemic involvement and aspiration biopsy of bone marrow are indicated in all cases.

Management. In patients with even solitary leg lesions, the risk of mortality is high. If multiple tumors on the legs or associated lesions on other body sites exist, the prognosis is worse. Aggressive multiagent chemotherapy should be considered in all cases and it may be efficacious especially in lesions located outside the leg (*see* Fig. 14.179a–c). Rituximab is another option that can be combined with chemotherapy. Surgery or regional radiotherapy for solitary tumors can be useful and may be combined with medical therapy. However, the recurrence rate is high and may be over a short period.

14.1.2.4 Intravascular Large B-cell Lymphoma

Intravascular large B-cell lymphoma is a rare neoplasm characterized by atypical lymphocytes within the lumina of blood vessels, including capillaries and postcapillary venules. It is considered a subtype of large B-cell lymphoma and carries a poor prognosis. Intravascular lymphocytes are mostly B-cells but rarely they may be lymphocytes of T-cell lineage or NK cells. The reason for the intravascular confinement of these cells is unclear. On occasion they may be localized to the skin, but more commonly skin and visceral organs are concomitantly involved, or visceral organs alone. It shows a predilection for the skin, lungs, and the central nervous system, but the adrenal glands, thyroid, kidneys, and various other organs may also be affected. Occlusion of blood vessels of visceral organs produces a variety of clinical manifestations. Bone marrow involvement is also possible, but lymph node involvement is not present.

This type of lymphoma is more common in adults. Cutaneous lesions are mostly nonspecific, and this causes a delay in the diagnosis. The trunk and lower extremities are more commonly involved but it may occur anywhere. A typical but rare presentation is generalized telangiectasia with relatively thick and large lesions (*see* Figs. 14.180 and 14.181). Other clinical presentations include erythematous or violaceous nodules (*see* Fig. 14.182) or panniculitis-like tender lesions that are irregular in shape (*see* Fig. 14.183), bruise-like plaques (*see* Fig. 14.183), indurated plaques with telangiectases (*see* Fig. 14.184), livedo-like erythema, and nonspecific pitting edema. Fine telangiectasia may overlie these lesions (*see* Fig. 14.182).

The diagnosis is generally established with histopathologic examination of the skin lesions or visceral organs. Large cells with vesicular nuclei are in the lumina of capillaries and postcapillary venules. Immunohistochemical staining is mandatory to determine the lineage of the neo-

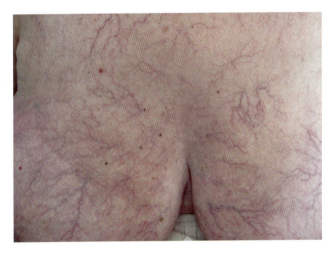

Fig. 14.180 Diffuse telangiectases, a typical feature of intravascular large B-cell lymphoma, are seen on the breast

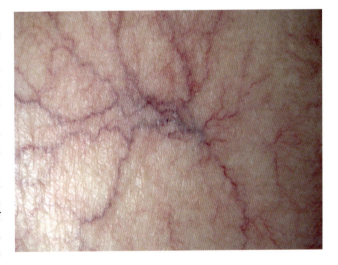

Fig. 14.181 Telangiectases due to intravascular large B-cell lymphoma. They are longer and thicker than classic idiopathic telangiectasia

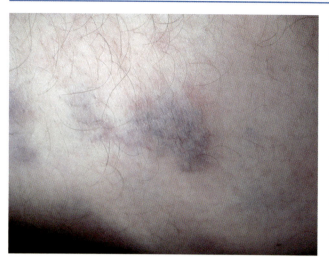

Fig. 14.182 Violaceous subcutaneous nodule with indistinct borders and overlying fine telangiectasia representing intravascular large B-cell lymphoma

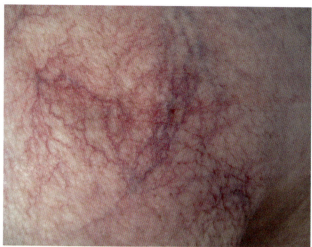

Fig. 14.184 Indurated plaque with overlying telangiectases. A punch biopsy was helpful for establishing the diagnosis of intravascular lymphoma in this case

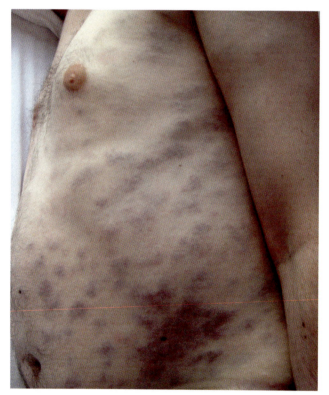

Fig. 14.183 Disseminated panniculitis-like lesions in a patient with intravascular large B-cell lymphoma. A bruise-like indurated plaque is remarkable on the flank

plastic cells. Circulating atypical cells are not seen on the peripheral blood examination.

Management. Intravascular lymphoma has a poor prognosis, especially when visceral organ involvement is present. Topical therapies have no effect and aggressive medications should be used. Multiagent chemotherapy, including anthracycline, combined with rituximab, is the most commonly used option.

14.1.3 Blastic Plasmacytoid Dendritic Cell Neoplasm

Blastic plasmacytoid dendritic cell neoplasm is a rare and distinct type of lymphoma originating from plasmacytoid dendritic cells and is associated with an aggressive course. Formerly the origin of this lymphoma was believed to be NK (natural killer) cells, and therefore it was named blastic NK-cell lymphoma. However, in the last years, plasmacytoid dendritic cell type 2 (a myeloid precursor) has been proposed as the cell of origin of this lymphoma. It is more common in middle-aged adults. The typical location of the lesions is the head and trunk, but lesions can occur anywhere on the skin, including the anogenital area and mucosal surfaces. There may be solitary, a few, or sometimes generalized lesions. Bluish-red or brownish nodules, indurated, deeply located plaques (*see* Fig. 14.185), and tumors (*see* Fig. 14.186) are observed. They may be hemorrhagic but ulceration is unusual.

Clinically, it may be difficult to distinguish this type of lymphoma from cutaneous infiltration of hematologic neoplasia. Histologically dense infiltration of medium-sized monomorphic blastoid cells extends from the dermis to the subcutis, and erythrocyte extravasation is prominent. Positive immunohistochemical reactions of CD123, Tdt, CD4, and CD56 are typical features.

The tumor has a rapid progressive course. In addition to the generalization of skin lesions, concomitant involvement of lymph nodes, bone marrow (leukemic dissemination), and other visceral organs, including the central nervous system, may develop in a short time.

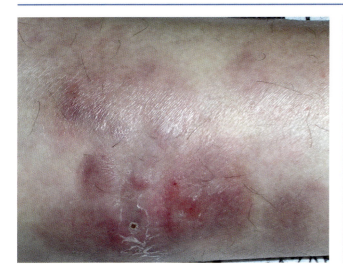

Fig. 14.185 Blastic plasmacytoid dendritic cell neoplasm presenting as bluish red-colored indurated plaques on the leg

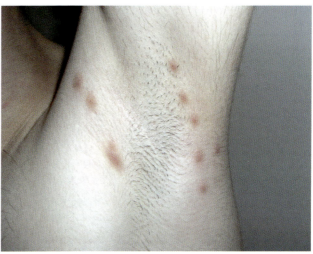

Fig. 14.187 Nodular scabies (scabies granuloma) seen as multiple round brownish-red papules on the axilla, a typical location

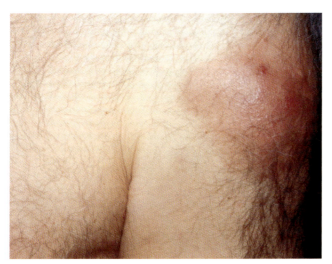

Fig. 14.186 Blastic plasmacytoid dendritic cell neoplasm shown as a large reddish-brown mass on the upper arm. The clinical presentation is nonspecific, and the diagnosis has been established by biopsy in this case

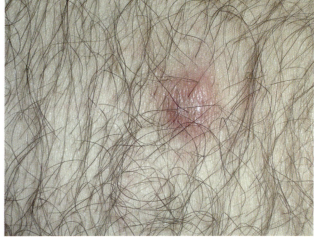

Fig. 14.188 Light brown-colored, smooth-surfaced nodule on the trunk representing nodular scabies. They are itchy

Management. Systemic chemotherapy and bone marrow transplantation are the main therapeutic options. However, an initial positive response to chemotherapy is usually followed by a relapse. Allogeneic stem cell transplantation can also been utilized.

14.2 Pseudolymphomas of the Skin

Pseudolymphomas of the skin are considered to be a group of benign reactive diseases sharing some common clinical and histopathologic features with cutaneous lymphomas. However, pseudolymphomas of the skin mostly demonstrate polyclonality with proliferation of both T and B lymphocytes. It is also possible that one lineage of a cell type may be predominant. Hence these pseudolymphomas are divided into B cell or T cell. Various entities with different etiologies and different clinical features, including actinic reticuloid, lymphomatoid contact dermatitis, and nodular scabies (*see* Figs. 14.187, 14.188, 14.189 and 14.190) are described in the spectrum of pseudolymphoma with regard to their histopathologic features. In this section lymphocytoma cutis and Jessner's lymphocytic infiltration of the skin, both of which are differential diagnostic challenges of cutaneous lymphomas, are discussed in detail.

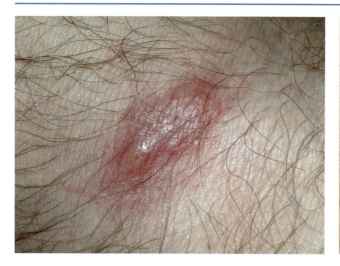

Fig. 14.189 Oval persistent nodule on the trunk histologically diagnosed as pseudolymphoma. The history of generalized pruritus in the patient and in the family members may be helpful for diagnosis of nodular scabies

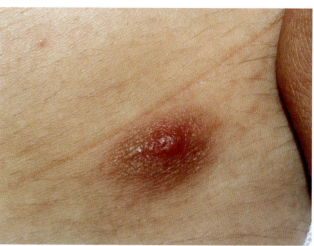

Fig. 14.191 Pseudolymphoma on the site of a thick bite

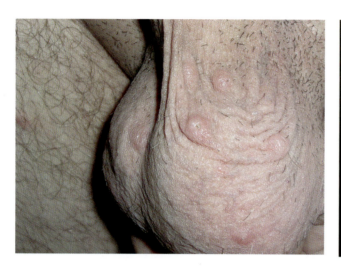

Fig. 14.190 Multiple papulonodular lesions on the scrotum of an adult with scabies; a common location of nodular scabies

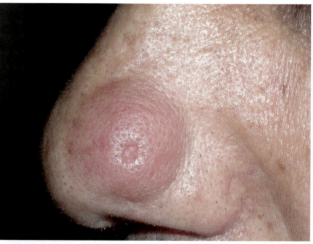

Fig. 14.192 Solitary nodular lesion of lymphocytoma cutis on the nose, a typical location

14.2.1 Lymphocytoma Cutis (Pseudolymphoma of Spiegler-Fendt)

Lymphocytoma cutis is a B-cell pseudolymphoma presenting with erythematous papulonodular lesions. It is mostly idiopathic but may also develop following tick bites (*see* Fig. 14.191), injections, foreign body reactions, tattoos, or acupuncture. Pseudolymphomas triggered by these factors are also be called the "reactive lymphoid hyperplasias" by some authors. Moreover, some systemic drugs may induce the development of pseudolymphoma, and this may be called "drug-induced pseudolymphoma." Borrelia burgdorferi infection may be a cause of lymphocytoma cutis in endemic areas. It is more common in children and young adults, but it may occur at any age. Women are more commonly affected.

The nose (*see* Fig. 14.192), cheeks (*see* Fig. 14.193), forehead, and earlobes are the most common locations of lymphocytoma cutis, but it may also be seen on the scalp, chest, nipple, arms (*see* Fig. 14.194), and large skin folds. It generally appears as a solitary lesion (*see* Figs. 14.192, 14.193, and 14.194), but in rare instances multiple (*see* Fig. 14.195), grouped, or generalized lesions may develop. Multiple lesions may be related to systemic drug use. Red-brown to red-purple, dome-shaped, firm asymptomatic papules reach 0.5 to 2 cm size in a short time and then remain usually stable. Tiny papules with a tendency to confluence and plaques may be other presentations of pseudolymphoma (*see* Fig. 14.196). Some nodules may be lobulated (*see* Fig. 14.197). The surface of lymphocytoma cutis is usually intact (*see* Fig. 14.198).

14.2 Pseudolymphomas of the Skin

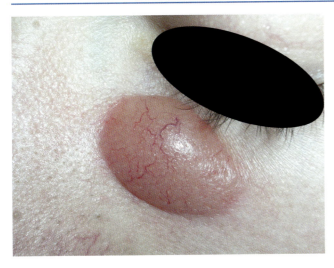

Fig. 14.193 Solitary reddish nodular lesion with smooth surface on the face seen in the figure is a typical presentation of lymphocytoma cutis, but cutaneous lymphomas should be excluded with biopsy

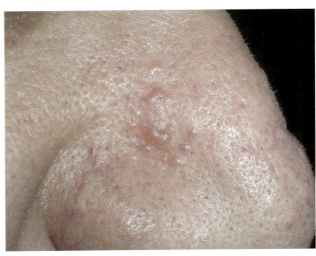

Fig. 14.196 Multiple light-brown papules restricted to the nose histologically diagnosed as pseudolymphoma; not a common presentation

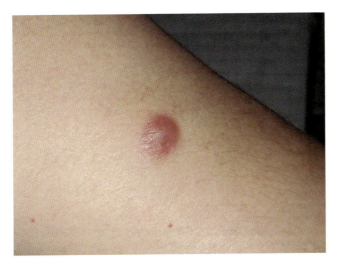

Fig. 14.194 Lymphocytoma cutis on the arm

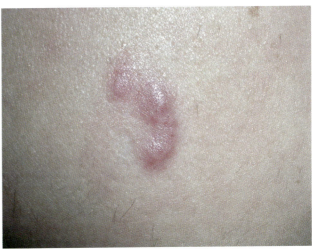

Fig. 14.197 Lymphocytoma cutis manifesting as a lobulated solitary lesion on the cheek

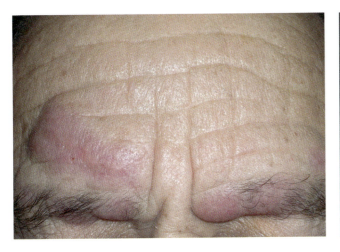

Fig. 14.195 Lymphocytoma cutis seen as a few large erythematous plaques on the forehead

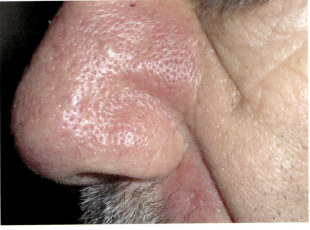

Fig. 14.198 Pseudolymphoma presenting as an erythematous plaque on the nose. The intact surface of the tumor is typical

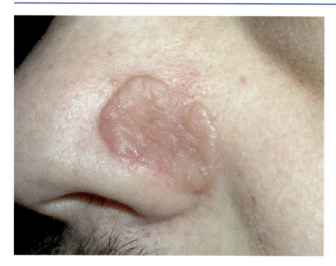

Fig. 14.199 Hypertrophic scar on the removal site of a pseudolymphoma

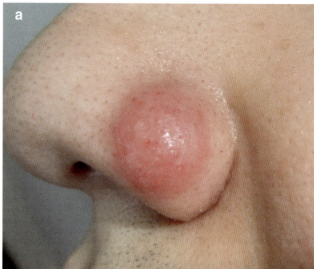
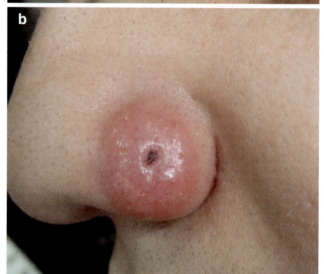
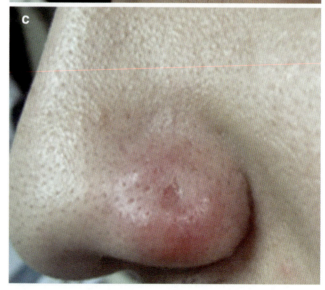

Fig. 14.200 (a) Solitary lymphocytoma cutis. (b) The same lesion during the early period of therapy with high potent topical corticosteroids. (c) Good response after 3 weeks of therapy

Clinical differentiation from primary cutaneous lymphomas such as CD4+ small/medium pleomorphic T-cell lymphoma, and marginal zone lymphoma is difficult. Granuloma faciale, nonulcerated lesions of basal cell carcinoma (see Fig. 11.27), and keloid (see Fig. 8.102) may also be considered in the differential diagnosis. In addition to basic histopathologic studies immunoprofile and molecular biological diagnostic procedures should be evaluated together to establish the correct diagnosis. Predominant lymphocytic nodular infiltration without atypia accompanied by plasma cells in the superficial dermis and intermingled eosinophils, and reactive germinal centers are the main histologic hallmarks. Infiltration sometimes invades the reticular dermis. As opposed to cutaneous lymphomas, monoclonality is absent, but staining with B-cell markers is predominant. Apart from all these, clinicopathologic correlation is very important. If suspicion of lymphoma cannot completely be eliminated, systemic examination and radiologic screening should be performed.

Management. Underlying factors, when found, should be eliminated. Systemic antibiotic therapy can be used if laboratory tests support Borrelia infection. If a systemic drug is suspected as a triggering factor, it can be stopped or switched.

The course of lymphocytoma cutis is variable. Spontaneous healing without scarring is possible, but this may occur after a long time. There is no proven risk of malignant transformation. Therefore aggressive therapies, including removal of tumors which could be associated with a risk of unsightly scars (see Fig. 14.199), should be avoided. Patients may be concerned owing to the rapid growth of the tumor; therefore they must be informed about the natural course of the disease. Topical (see Fig. 14.200a–c) or intralesional corticosteroids (see Figs. 14.201a and b, 14.202a and b, 14.203a–d) are the therapy of choice.

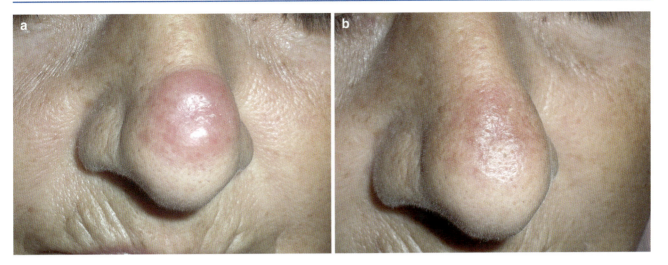

Fig. 14.201 (a) Solitary lymphocytoma cutis. (b) Good response to intralesional corticosteroid application (three sessions of triamcinolone acetonide). Note the satisfactory cosmetic result

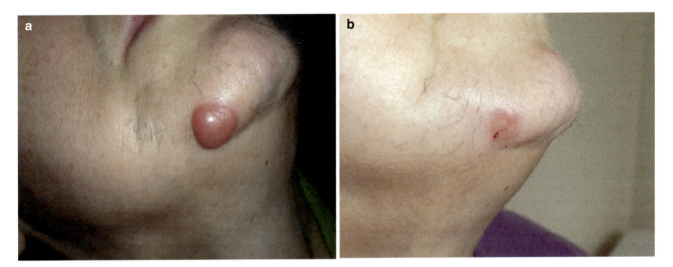

Fig. 14.202 (a) Solitary lesion of lymphocytoma cutis on the chin. (b) The same lesion successfully treated with intralesional corticosteroid application

However, it should be remembered that intralesional corticosteroid application is associated with a risk of atrophy. Some lesions show complete regression with intralesional corticosteroid therapy, but some cases show one or more recurrences on the same site (see Fig. 14.204) or elsewhere. Systemic corticosteroids and intralesional interferon alpha may be used for refractory lesions. Radiotherapy can be an alternative option in case of failure of other therapies.

14.2.2 Jessner's Lymphocytic Infiltration of the Skin (Jessner-Kanof Disease)

Jessner's lymphocytic infiltration of the skin is a T-cell pseudolymphoma characterized by erythematous papules and plaques predominantly located on the face. The etiology is unknown, and most patients are young adults. The cheeks and forehead are the most common locations (see Fig. 14.205), but disease may arise on other sites of the head (see Fig. 14.206), neck, trunk (see Fig. 14.207), and proximal extremities. Solitary, a few, or sometimes numerous lesions (see Fig. 14.207) may be seen. The typical presentation of Jessner lymphocytic infiltration of the skin is seen as sharply demarcated, dull or purplish-red, slightly infiltrated papules (see Fig. 14.205) and plaques (see Fig. 14.208). It is usually asymptomatic, but mild pruritus may be present.

The lesions may persist for several months. Their duration is usually longer than the lesions of polymorphic light eruption, and they do not show distinct seasonal variation. Contrary to discoid lupus erythematosus, there is no follicular hyperkeratosis, scales, or atrophy on the surface of the plaques. Slowly enlarging plaques with central clearing

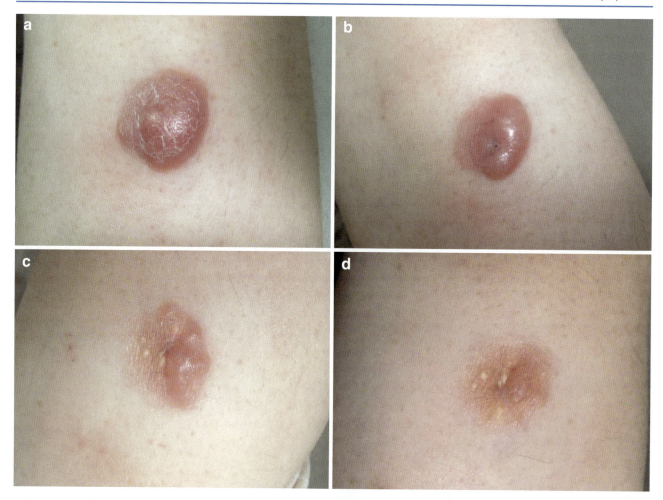

Fig. 14.203 (a) A solitary pseudolymphoma on the trunk. (b–d) The stepwise decline of the lesion's size after intralesional corticosteroid applications

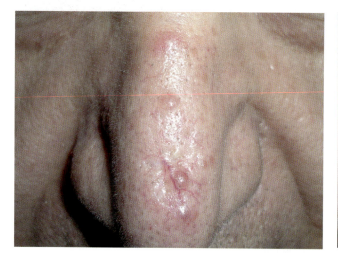

Fig. 14.204 Recurrence of pseudolymphoma, shown as small papules. The previous lesions had been treated with intralesional corticosteroids

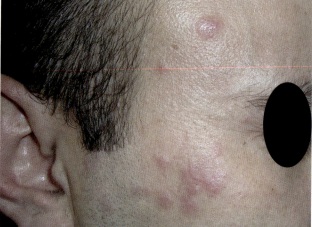

Fig. 14.205 Jessner's lymphocytic infiltration of the skin presenting as erythematous papules on the cheek, a typical location. Another lesion is also noticeable on the temple

may cause annular lesions (see Figs. 14.208 and 14.209) similar to those of subacute cutaneous lupus erythematosus and granuloma annulare. Granuloma faciale and primary cutaneous lymphomas such as marginal zone lymphoma (see Fig. 14.168) can also be considered in the differential diagnosis.

The diagnosis can be established by evaluation of both clinical and histopathologic features. The epidermis is

14.2 Pseudolymphomas of the Skin

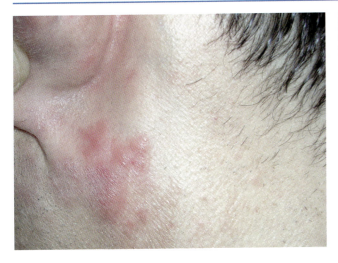

Fig. 14.206 Jessner's lymphocytic infiltration of the skin seen as erythematous plaques on the retroauricular area

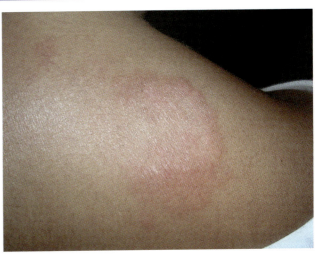

Fig. 14.209 Jessner's lymphocytic infiltration of the skin manifesting as a non-scaly, erythematous annular plaque

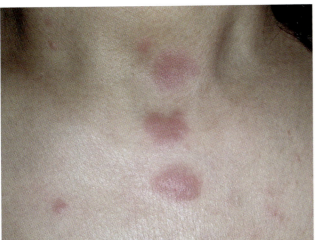

Fig. 14.207 Multiple erythematous papules and nodules on the upper trunk; a rare presentation of Jessner's lymphocytic infiltration of the skin

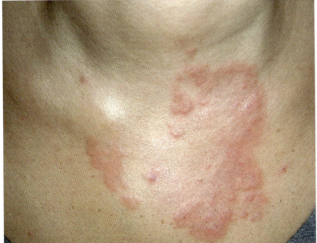

Fig. 14.208 Large annular plaque on the chest. Jessner's lymphocytic infiltration of the skin should be considered in the differential diagnosis of annular plaques

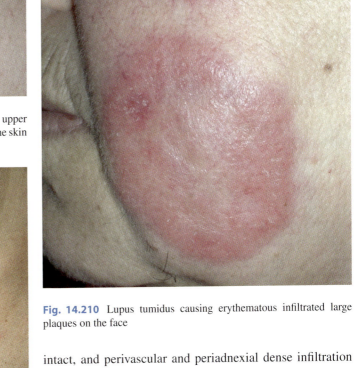

Fig. 14.210 Lupus tumidus causing erythematous infiltrated large plaques on the face

intact, and perivascular and periadnexial dense infiltration of lymphocytes without atypia is the main histopathologic feature. Dermal edema is absent as opposed to polymorphic light eruption. Immunostaining with T-cell markers is always positive, but it may also be positive with B-cell markers. Lupus tumidus (*see* Fig. 14.210), a variant of cutaneous lupus erythematosus, has some common clinical

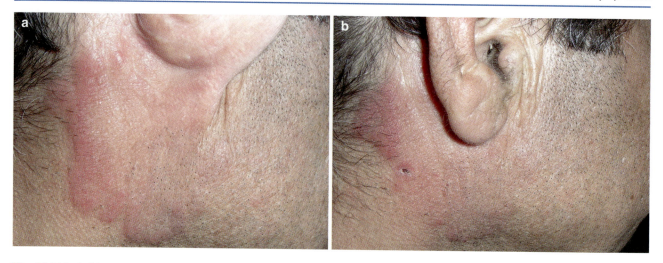

Fig. 14.211 (a–b) Annular plaque caused by Jessner's lymphocytic infiltration of the skin, which was successfully treated with topical corticosteroids

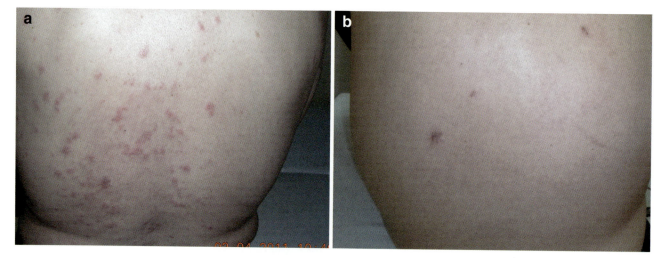

Fig. 14.212 (a) Multiple lesions of Jessner's lymphocytic infiltration of the skin on the trunk. (b) Clearance of all the lesions after short-term treatment with systemic antimalarial drugs (hydroxychloroquine)

and histopathologic features with Jessner's lymphocytic infiltration of the skin, but dermal mucin deposition is prominent in the former. On the other hand, it is suggested that both diseases are in the same spectrum.

Jessner lymphocytic infiltration of the skin is not associated with any systemic disease. Therefore further examination of these patients is not indicated.

Management. Jessner lymphocytic infiltration of the skin is not associated with malignant transformation and tends to resolve spontaneously without dyspigmentation or scarring. Therefore therapy is performed for cosmetic purposes only. Topical corticosteroids may be used for limited lesions (*see* Fig. 14.211a and b). Intralesional corticosteroids may be applied if topical use is not effective. Multiple lesions may be treated with systemic antimalarial drugs such as hydroxychloroquine. All lesions may clear after therapy (*see* Fig. 14.212a and b). However, this disease has a chronic course and may relapse after cessation of the drug.

14.3 The Skin Infiltration of Hematologic Neoplasms

Some hematologic neoplasms such as non-Hodgkin lymphomas, Hodgkin lymphoma, leukemia, and plasma cell dyscrasia (including multiple myeloma) may infiltrate the skin secondarily. The clinical appearance of these neoplastic infiltrations is not uniform and mostly not specific. Localized or widespread firm papules, nodules, plaques, and tumors may be seen in all types of these hematologic neoplasms, but different skin lesions may also be encountered. The diagnosis of systemic lymphoproliferative disease and associated systemic manifestations supported by

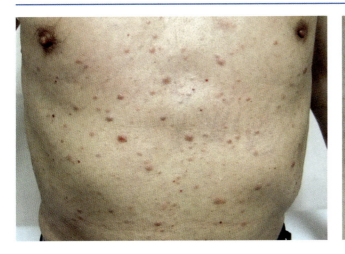

Fig. 14.213 Leukemia cutis. Disseminated erythematous papulonodular lesions in a patient with acute myeloid leukemia

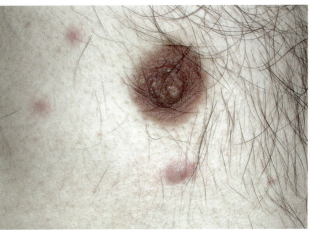

Fig. 14.214 Skin-colored firm papules representing the neoplastic infiltration of acute lymphoblastic leukemia. These lesions were a sign of recurrence of the hematologic malignancy

histopathologic, immunophenotypical, and molecular biological features is helpful in establishing the diagnosis.

14.3.1 Leukemia Cutis

Many nonspecific skin findings — including purpura, excoriations related to generalized pruritus, exaggerated arthropod bite reactions, cutaneous vasculitis, reactive neutrophilic dermatoses, opportunistic infections, and paraneoplastic pemphigus — may occur during the course of the leukemias. The skin is also among the extramedullary involvement areas of the leukemias. The migration of leukemic cells to the epidermis, dermis, and subcutis, called leukemia cutis, is usually a late finding of this neoplasm. Most of the patients have bone marrow and other organ involvement at the time of diagnosis. Rarely, skin may be the sole involved organ (aleukemic leukemia cutis), and bone marrow involvement occurs later. Sometimes skin lesions indicate the relapse of the hematologic neoplasm.

Leukemia cutis may occur in many types of leukemia, including both myeloid and lymphoid forms. It may be seen in adults and children. The ratio of skin involvement is very high in adult T-cell leukemia, which is a very rare variant. In some subtypes (M4, M5) of acute myeloid leukemia, the rate of skin involvement is high, too.

Leukemia cutis presents with a wide spectrum of lesions. Multiple erythematous or skin-colored, asymptomatic, firm papules that are 2 to 5 mm in size or sometimes nodules are the most typical presentations (see Figs. 14.213 and 14.214). Their surface may be smooth (see Fig. 14.214) or sometimes eroded and crusted (see Fig. 14.215). Disseminated lesions may rapidly develop. They are more common on the face, scalp and trunk but may occur anywhere including scar sites. Ecchymotic, hemorrhagic, or indurated plaques, figurated erythema-like lesions, diffuse infiltration of the face

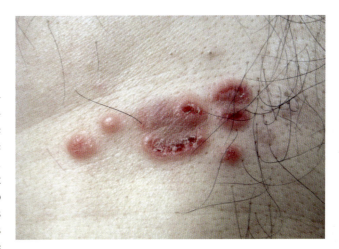

Fig. 14.215 Leukemia cutis presenting as erythematous papules on the trunk in a patient with acute myeloid leukemia. Note the eroded surface on some papules

(see Fig. 14.216a), pyoderma gangrenosum-like ulcerations, paronychia-like lesions, panniculitis-like subcutaneous lesions, erythroderma, and bullous lesions are among the other mucocutaneous signs of leukemia cutis. Gingival hyperplasia caused by neoplastic infiltration and tonsillary involvement are commonly observed in patients with acute myeloid leukemia. These lesions may cause pain, and bleeding. "Leonine facies" may occur due to infiltration of facial skin, especially in patients with chronic lymphocytic leukemia. Dermal nodules developing in patients with acute myeloid leukemia, myelodysplastic syndrome, or chronic myelogenous leukemia (which are called chloromas or granulocytic sarcomas), are characterized by a bluish-green color related to myeloperoxidase. In the latter two diseases granulocytic sarcomas indicate a blast crisis. The lesions may also develop, on other sites including soft tissue and bone.

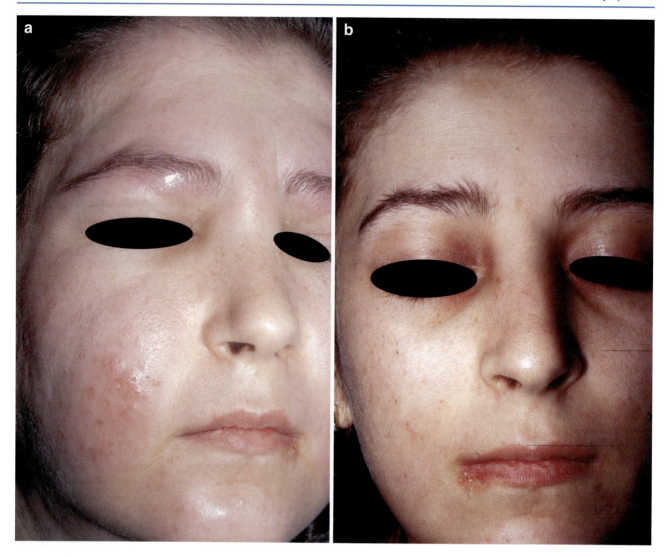

Fig. 14.216 (**a**) Diffuse leukemic infiltration of the face in a patient with acute lymphoblastic leukemia. (**b**) Clearance of the lesions after chemotherapy

Nodular cutaneous metastasis of solid cancers (*see* Fig. 16.2), skin infiltration of nodal lymphomas (*see* Fig. 14.223), graft versus host disease, urticaria pigmentosa (*see* Fig. 9.5), and disseminated Candida infection may all be considered in the differential diagnosis of papulonodular lesions of leukemia cutis. Skin biopsy generally confirms the diagnosis. Histologically, the neoplastic cells locate predominantly on perivascular and periadnexial areas but may also be dispersed among collagen bundles of the dermis. Epidermal involvement and subcutaneous invasion are also possible. Immunophenotyping targeting antigenic characteristics of the original leukemia and molecular studies may support the diagnosis. Besides hematologic findings, different systemic symptoms may be present in these patients owing to the infiltration of various organs by neoplastic cells. In cases in which the diagnosis is dubious, a complete blood count, bone marrow aspiration, and biopsy should be performed.

Management. Cutaneous infiltration is an indicator for a poor prognosis of leukemias and it may affect the therapeutic decisions. As an exception, in congenital leukemia, skin lesions do not alter the prognosis. Systemic chemotherapy is mostly efficacious for the skin lesions (*see* Fig. 14.216a and b), but recurrence is possible. In rare instances, only the skin lesions of leukemia may be refractory. Total body electron beam therapy or PUVA therapy can be added to chemotherapy in such refractory cases.

14.3.2 Cutaneous Infiltration of Hodgkin Lymphoma

Hodgkin lymphoma is a nodal lymphoma characterized by atypical cells of B-cell lineage. It may occasionally be associated with lymphomatoid papulosis and sometimes may cause nonspecific skin findings such as generalized pruritus and

14.3 The Skin Infiltration of Hematologic Neoplasms

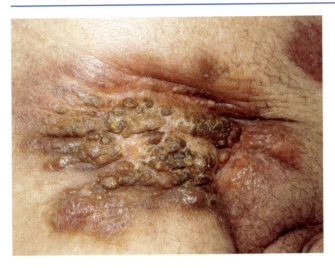

Fig. 14.217 Hodgkin lymphoma. Diffuse neoplastic infiltration of the skin around the inguinal lymph node is seen

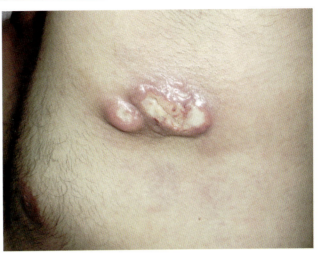

Fig. 14.219 Cutaneous infiltration of Hodgkin lymphoma presenting as an ulcerated mass on the axilla

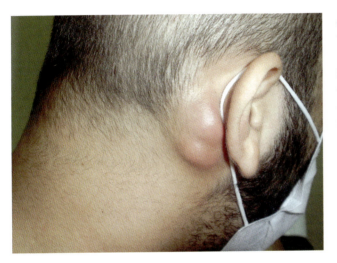

Fig. 14.218 Cutaneous infiltration of Hodgkin lymphoma shown as a subcutaneous mass on the retroauricular area

acquired ichthyosis. Skin infections including herpes zoster are seen with increased frequency in patients with this systemic lymphoma. Like many other hematologic malignancies, Hodgkin lymphoma may directly invade skin. However, after the advances in the therapy of the disease in the last decades, skin involvement, which is usually a late manifestation, is rarely encountered. On very rare occasions skin involvement may be the initial presentation of Hodgkin lymphoma. Most patients with cutaneous infiltration are adults.

Skin may be involved as a result of direct extension from the underlying lymph nodes or due to hematogenous spread. The skin lesions have an acute onset and occur typically on the distal part of the involved lymph nodes (*see* Fig. 14.217). They may be seen on the chest of patients with severe mediastinal disease. Erythematous nodules, indurated plaques (*see* Fig. 14.217), panniculitis-like lesions, and tumoral masses (*see* Fig. 14.218) may occur in a limited area or sometimes in a more generalized fashion. They may be ulcerated (*see* Fig. 14.219).

The main diagnostic challenge is the secondary cutaneous infiltration of other hematologic neoplasms. Histologically dense dermal infiltration of neoplastic cells, including characteristic Reed-Sternberg cells of nodal disease, is seen. An inflammatory infiltration including eosinophils is present. As Hodgkin lymphoma shows CD30 expression, other CD30+ diseases of the skin, especially primary cutaneous anaplastic large cell lymphoma (*see* Fig. 14.144), should be excluded.

Management. If the disease is limited to the skin, the prognosis is very good. Skin lesions representing the advanced stage of lymphoma may also heal after chemotherapy, but the prognosis is relatively worse.

14.3.3 Cutaneous Infiltration of Non-Hodgkin Lymphomas

Nodal non-Hodgkin lymphomas may infiltrate skin relatively more often than occurs in Hodgkin lymphoma. The skin involvement commonly occurs in the late stage of the disease and may be a sign of a poor prognosis. Typically patients have multiple lesions (*see* Fig. 14.220) and sometimes disseminated lesions develop in an eruptive fashion (*see* Fig. 14.221). Brownish-red, lilaceous (*see* Fig. 14.222) or skin-colored (*see* Fig. 14.223) firm nodules, infiltrated plaques, and large tumors may be seen. Most lesions have a smooth surface but eroded (*see* Fig. 14.224), ulcerated, and crusted lesions may also rarely be encountered. The history of the rapid onset of the lesions may be helpful when distinguishing this disorder from primary cutaneous lymphomas. Differentiation from leukemia cutis (*see* Fig. 14.213) is mostly established with biopsy and associated systemic and blood manifestations of both diseases. Histologically, diffuse dermal infiltration

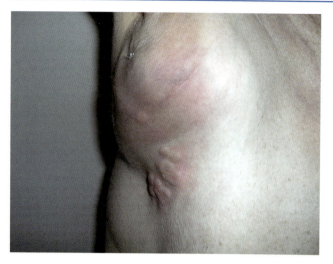

Fig. 14.220 Neoplastic skin infiltration associated with axillary lymph node involvement in a patient with nodal non-Hodgkin lymphoma

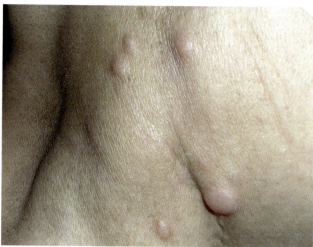

Fig. 14.223 Non-Hodgkin nodal lymphoma manifesting as skin-colored, round, scattered nodules on the trunk

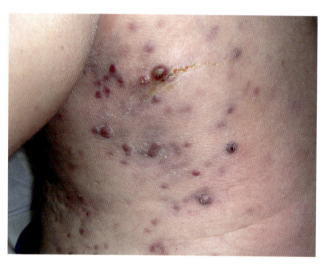

Fig. 14.221 Disseminated erythematous papules and nodules overlying diffuse neoplastic infiltration on the trunk of a patient with terminal stage systemic anaplastic large cell lymphoma

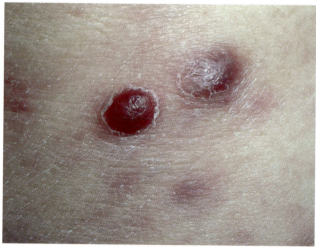

Fig. 14.224 Skin infiltration of systemic anaplastic large T-cell lymphoma. Note that one of the nodules is eroded

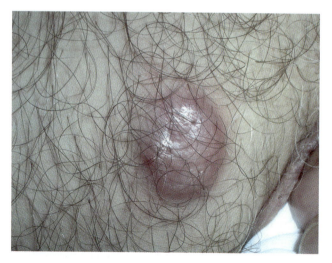

Fig. 14.222 A large erythematous nonspecific tumor on the leg which was diagnosed histopathologically as skin infiltration of non-Hodgkin nodal lymphoma

of neoplastic lymphocytes with a grenz zone below the epidermis is typical. Immunophenotyping provides determination of the subtype of systemic lymphoma. Positivity of the ALK1 stain enables the differentiation of systemic CD30+ anaplastic large cell lymphoma from its cutaneous counterpart, which nearly always lacks ALK1 expression.

Management. The cutaneous involvement of non-Hodgkin nodal lymphomas represents advanced disease and is associated with concomitant involvement of other organs. The treatment must be planned according to underlying systemic lymphoma. Systemic chemotherapy and bone marrow transplantation are usually the therapies of choice.

14.3.4 Cutaneous Infiltration of Plasma Cell Dyscrasia

Multiple myeloma and other paraproteinemias may be the underlying cause of some skin diseases, including

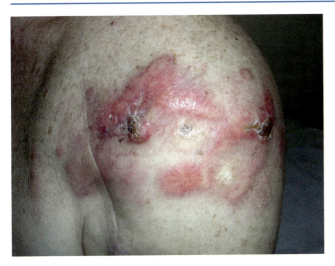

Fig. 14.225 Indurated plaques seen on the shoulder of a patient with advanced stage of a plasma cell dyscrasia

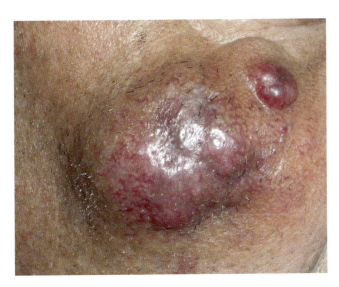

Fig. 14.226 Large erythematous mass on the face representing cutaneous infiltration of multiple myeloma

erythema elevatum diutinum, subcorneal pustular dermatosis, and reactive neutrophilic dermatoses such as Sweet syndrome and pyoderma gangrenosum. Skin infiltration of multiple myeloma, namely cutaneous plasmacytoma, and of other paraproteinemias which may be seen in advanced stages of the disease, is rare. Bluish-red dermal or subcutaneous nodules and plaques (*see* Figs. 14.225 and 14.226) may be seen. Histologic examination reveals predominant atypical plasmacytes in the diffuse dermal or subcutaneous infiltration. Diagnosis of plasma cell dyscrasia can be confirmed by peripheral blood examination and bone marrow biopsy.

Management. The prognosis of plasma cell dyscrasia associated with skin infiltration is poor. Systemic chemotherapy (melphalan) is indicated in the presence of multiple lesions or systemic disease.

Suggested Reading

Akaraphanth R, Douglass MC, Lim HW. Hypopigmented mycosis fungoides: treatment and a 6(1/2)-year follow-up of 9 patients. J Am Acad Dermatol. 2000;42:33–9.

Baykal C, Buyukbabani N, Kaymaz R. Familial mycosis fungoides. Br J Dermatol. 2002;146:1108–10.

Bekkenk MW, Geelen FA, van Voorst Vader PC, et al. Primary and secondary cutaneous CD30(+) lymphoproliferative disorders: a report from the Dutch Cutaneous Lymphoma Group on the long-term follow-up data of 219 patients and guidelines for diagnosis and treatment. Blood. 2000;95:3653–61.

Burgdorf WHC, Plewig G, Wolff HH, Landthaler M. Braun-Falco's dermatology, edn 3. Italy: Springer-Verlag; 2009.

Cerroni L, Gatter K, Kerl H. Skin lymphoma. The illustrated guide, edn 3. Singapore: Wiley-Blackwell; 2009.

Cheeley J, Sahn RE, DeLong LK, Parker SR. Acitretin for the treatment of cutaneous T-cell lymphoma. J Am Acad Dermatol. 2013;68:247–54.

de-Misra RF, Garcia M, Dorta S. Solitary oral ulceration as the first appearance of lymphomatoid papulosis: a diagnostic challange. Clin Exp Dermatol. 2010;35:165–8.

Desai A, Telang GH, Olszewski AJ. Remission of primary cutaneous anaplastic large cell lymphoma after a brief course of brentuximab vedotin. Ann Hematol. 2013;92:567–8.

de Souza A, el-Azhary RA, Camilleri MJ, et al. In search of prognostic indicators for lymphomatoid papulosis: a retrospective study of 123 patients. J Am Acad Dermatol. 2012;66:928–37.

El Shabrawi-Caelen L, Kerl H, Cerroni L. Lymphomatoid papulosis: reappraisal of clinicopathologic presentation and classification into subtypes A, B, and C. Arch Dermatol. 2004;140:441–7.

Elcin G, Duman N, Karahan S, et al. Long-term follow-up of early mycosis fungoides patients treated with narrowband ultraviolet B phototherapy. J Dermatolog Treat. 2014;25:268–73.

Fink-Puches R, Chott A, Ardigó M, et al. The spectrum of cutaneous lymphomas in patients less than 20 years of age. Pediatr Dermatol. 2004;21:525–33.

Hanna S, Walsh N, D'Intino Y, Langley RG. Mycosis fungoides presenting as pigmented purpuric dermatitis. Pediatr Dermatol. 2006;23:350–4.

Herrmann JL, Hughey LC. Recognizing large-cell transformation of mycosis fungoides. J Am Acad Dermatol. 2012;67:665–72.

Hsu YJ, Su LH, Hsu YL, et al. Localized lymphomatoid papulosis. J Am Acad Dermatol. 2010;62:353–6.

Jain S, Zain J, O'Connor O. Novel therapeutic agents for cutaneous T-Cell lymphoma. J Hematol Oncol. 2012;5:24.

James WD, Berger T, Elston D. Andrew's diseases of the skin: Clinical Dermatology, edn 11. China: Saunders Elsevier; 2011.

Kazakov DV, Burg G, Kempf W. Clinicopathological spectrum of mycosis fungoides. J Eur Acad Dermatol Venereol. 2004;18:397–415.

Kempf W, Kazakov DV, Schärer L, et al. Angioinvasive lymphomatoid papulosis: a new variant simulating aggressive lymphomas. Am J Surg Pathol. 2013;37:1–13.

Kempf W, Pfaltz K, Vermeer MH, et al. EORTC, ISCL, and USCLC consensus recommendations for the treatment of primary cutaneous CD30-positive lymphoproliferative disorders: lymphomatoid papulosis and primary cutaneous anaplastic large-cell lymphoma. Blood. 2011;118:4024–35.

Kempf W, Rozati S, Kerl K, et al. Cutaneous peripheral T-cell lymphomas, unspecified/NOS and rare subtypes: a heterogeneous group of challenging cutaneous lymphomas. G Ital Dermatol Venereol. 2012;147:553–62.

Knobler R, Berlin G, Calzavara-Pinton P, et al. Guidelines on the use of extracorporeal photopheresis. J Eur Acad Dermatol Venereol. 2014;28 (Suppl 1):1–37.

Kunishige JH, McDonald H, Alvarez G, et al. Lymphomatoid papulosis and associated lymphomas: a retrospective case series of 84 patients. Clin Exp Dermatol. 2009;34:576–81.

LeBoit PE, Burg G, Weedon D, Sarasin A. Pathology and genetics of skin tumours. World Health Organization Classification of Tumours. France; IARC Press; 2006.

Liu HL, Hoppe RT, Kohler S, et al. CD30+ cutaneous lymphoproliferative disorders: the Stanford experience in lymphomatoid papulosis and primary cutaneous anaplastic large cell lymphoma. J Am Acad Dermatol. 2003;49:1049–58.

Martorell-Calatayud A, Hernandes-Martin A, Colmenero I, et al. Lymphomatoid papulosis in children: report of 9 cases and review of the literature. Actas Dermosifiliorg. 2010;101:693–701.

Nanda A, AlSaleh QA, Al-Ajmi H, et al. Mycosis fungoides in Arab children and adolescents. A report of 36 patients from Kuwait. Pediatr Dermatol. 2010;27:607–13.

Nofal A, Abdel-Mawla MY, Assaf M, Salah E. Primary cutaneous aggressive epidermotropic CD8+ T-cell lymphoma: proposed diagnostic criteria and therapeutic evaluation. J Am Acad Dermatol. 2012;67:748–59.

Olsen E, Vonderheid E, Pimpinelli N, et al. ISCL/EORTC. Revisions to the staging and classification of mycosis fungoides and Sezary syndrome: a proposal of the International Society for Cutaneous Lymphomas (ISCL) and the cutaneous lymphoma task force of the European Organization of Research and Treatment of Cancer (EORTC). Blood. 2007; 110:1713–22.

Ozguroglu E, Buyukbabani N, Ozguroglu M, Baykal C. Generalized telangiectasia as the major manifestation of angiotropic (intravascular) lymphoma. Br J Dermatol. 1997;137:422–5.

Prince HM, Whittaker S, Hoppe RT. How I treat mycosis fungoides and Sézary syndrome. Blood. 2009;114:4337–53.

Puddu P, Ferranti G, Frezzolini A, et al. Pigmented purpura-like eruption as cutaneous sign of mycosis fungoides with autoimmune purpura. J Am Acad Dermatol. 1999;40:298–9.

Rigel DS, Robinson JK, Ross M, Friedman RJ, Corkerell CJ, Lim HW, Stockfleth HW, Kirkwood JM. Cancer of the skin. China: Saunders Elsevier; 2011.

Sokol L, Naghashpour M, Glass LF. Primary cutaneous B-cell lymphomas: recent advances in diagnosis and management. Cancer Control. 2013;19:326–44.

Swerdlow SH, Campo E, Harris NL, et al. WHO Classification of Tumours of Haematopoietic and Lymphoid Tissues, edn 4. Lyon: IARC Press; 2008.

Trautinger F, Knobler R, Willemze R, et al. EORTC consensus recommendations for the treatment of mycosis fungoides/Sézary syndrome. Eur J Cancer 2006;42:1014–30.

Vonderheid EC, Bernengo MG, Burg G, et al; ISCL. Update on erythrodermic cutaneous T-cell lymphoma: report of the International Society for Cutaneous Lymphomas. J Am Acad Dermatol. 2002; 46:95–106.

Wahie S, Dayala S, Husain A, et al. Cutaneous features of intravascular lymphoma. Clin Exp Dermatol. 2011;36:288–91.

Whittaker SJ, Foss FM. Efficacy and tolerability of currently available therapies for the mycosis fungoides and Sezary syndrome variants of cutaneous T-cell lymphoma. Cancer Treat Rev. 2007;33:146–60.

Wilcox RA. Cutaneous B-cell lymphomas: update on diagnosis, risk-stratification, and management. Am J Hematol. 2013;88:73–6.

Willemze R, Jaffe E, Burg G, et al. WHO-EORTC classification for cutaneous lymphomas. Blood. 2005;105:3768–85.

Willemze R. Primary cutaneous B-cell lymphoma: classification and treatment. Curr Opin Oncol. 2006;18:425–31.

Yazganoglu KD, Topkarci Z, Buyukbabani N, Baykal C. Childhood mycosis fungoides: a report of 20 cases from Turkey. J Eur Acad Dermatol Venereol. 2013;27:295–300.

Zackheim HS, Jones C, Leboit PE, et al. Lymphomatoid papulosis associated with mycosis fungoides: a study of 21 patients including analyses of clonality. J Am Acad Dermatol. 2003; 49:620–3.

Histiocytoses 15

Histiocytoses are classified into two main groups according to the morphologic and immunophenotypic characteristics of the cells forming the infiltrate: Langerhans cell histiocytoses, which are formed by a very precise type of cells harboring Birbeck granules, a cytoplasmic organelle, and expressing antigens like CD1a and langerin; and the non-Langerhans cell histiocytoses, in which cells of monocyte/macrophage or dendritic lineage proliferate. A clear distinction between these two groups of cells was lacking in the past. However, in the last decades it is well known that both groups of diseases have different histopathologic, immunophenotypical, and electron microscopic findings and systemic manifestations. Among the various diseases classified in the group of non-Langerhans cell histiocytoses, histopathology and immunophenotyping are sometimes not sufficient to make a precise diagnosis. Clinical features including extent, and type of the skin lesions and associated systemic findings may be crucial in establishing the proper diagnosis.

Another type of cell that can only be differentiated from Langerhans cell by the absence of Birbeck granules is known as the indeterminate cell. This cell is found in indeterminate cell histiocytosis. The variants of histiocytoses will be discussed in this chapter.

15.1 Langerhans Cell Histiocytosis

Langerhans cell histiocytosis, formerly known as histiocytosis-X, is a rare clonal disorder characterized by idiopathic monoclonal proliferation of bone marrow–derived Langerhans cells that are present in the epidermis, lymph nodes, and the respiratory tract. Langerhans cell histiocytosis predominantly involves the skin and bones, but most of the visceral organs may be affected. Different clinical types have been defined according to the severity of involvement: chronic unifocal (eosinophilic granuloma), chronic multifocal (Hand-Schüller-Christian disease), and acute disseminated type (Letterer-Siwe disease). However, clinical findings of them may overlap, thereby diminishing the importance of this classification. Currently, these types are considered to be the different ends of the spectrum of the same disease. Hashimoto-Pritzker disease (congenital self-healing reticulohistiocytosis) is a variant of Langerhans cell histiocytosis, but in this rare subtype, lesions are confined to the skin since birth or neonatal period.

Langerhans cell histiocytosis occurs mostly sporadically, but familial cases are also occasionally seen. The etiology is unknown. The disease typically starts in childhood, generally between the ages of 1 and 3. However, in rare cases, lesions may appear later. In adults, it may be associated with secondary hematologic malignancies. Mucocutaneous lesions may not be found in all patients, but their presence is helpful in confirming the diagnosis. In addition to the involvement of skin, and oral and genital mucosae, the nails may also be affected.

The chronic unifocal type is mostly noticed as a swelling on the long or flat bones. Radiologic examinations reveal the osteolytic lesions. Spontaneous fractures may develop. Mandibular and maxillary lesions may cause premature loss of teeth. There may sometimes be noduloulcerative lesions on the palate and gingivae. Cutaneous lesions may be seen as yellowish nodules that are sometimes ulcerated.

The chronic multifocal type is characterized by bone lesions, diabetes insipidus, exophthalmos, and mucocutaneous lesions. Cranial bones, especially the temporoparietal part, are more commonly involved. Exophthalmus may be unilateral or bilateral. Mucocutaneous lesions may be found in less than half of the patients starting from early childhood. Papules, nodules, plaques, and xanthoma-like cutaneous lesions may be located on the trunk, scalp, face, axillae, perineum, and groin.

The acute disseminated type is characterized by the early occurrence of multisystemic involvement along with widespread mucocutaneous lesions. Lesions usually start in early childhood or sometimes in young adulthood. Onset in the older population is rare. Men are more commonly affected than women. This type of Langerhans cell histiocytosis has a very rich spectrum of dermatologic manifestations. The trunk (see Fig. 15.1), scalp (see Fig. 15.2), face (see Fig. 15.3), and intertriginous sites such as the axillae (see Fig. 15.4), groin, and retroauricular area are more commonly involved. Lesions

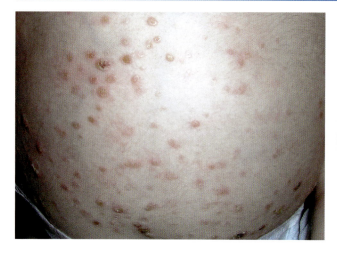

Fig. 15.1 Langerhans cell histiocytosis presenting as irregularly distributed small papulosquamous lesions on the trunk of a child

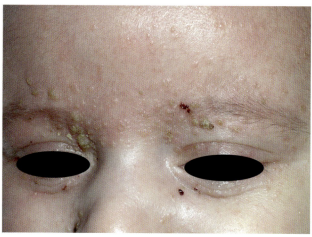

Fig. 15.3 Langerhans cell histiocytosis causing persistent scales and crusts on the face

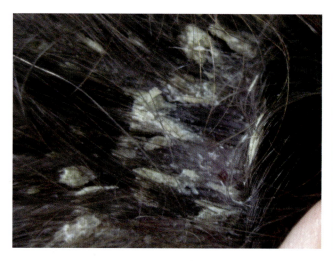

Fig. 15.2 Thick scales on the scalp that are refractory to symptomatic therapies should be alarming for Langerhans cell histiocytosis. Scalp biopsy was diagnostic in this case

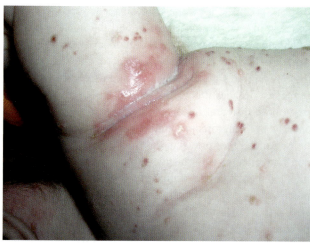

Fig. 15.4 Intertrigo-like dermatitis on the axillary fold associated with discrete papulovesicular lesions in a patient with Langerhans cell histiocytosis

may also be found on the external ear and palmoplantar area. Tiny, pinkish or yellowish-brown, slightly raised discrete papules covered with crusts or scales irregularly scattered on the body is the typical presentation (see Figs. 15.1, 15.5, and 15.6). Eroded, exudative, or ulcerated nodules may sometimes be predominant (see Fig. 15.7). Papules and nodules may show confluence on the trunk and on rare occasions cover the entire body (see Figs. 15.8 and 15.9).

Some patients present with lesions that are confined to the intertriginous areas that mainly have an eroded surface (see Figs. 15.10 and 15.11). Eroded or ulcerated lesions with a persistent course may be malodorous. Vesicles, pustules, and purpura (see Fig. 15.12) may develop in the course of the disease. In the palmoplantar area a papulovesicular or vesiculopustular eruption may sometimes occur (see Fig. 15.13). Palmar or plantar petechiae (see Fig. 15.14) are also typical for Langerhans cell histiocytosis and are among the signs of

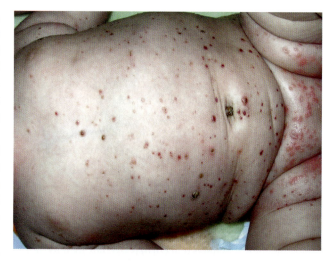

Fig. 15.5 Disseminated lesions of Langerhans cell histiocytosis with typical distribution on the trunk and inguinal folds

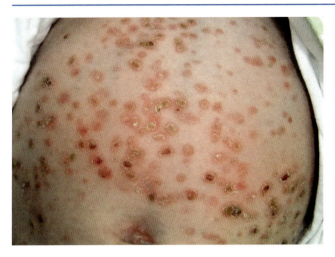

Fig. 15.6 Discrete papules covered with thick crusts seen in a child with Langerhans cell histiocytosis

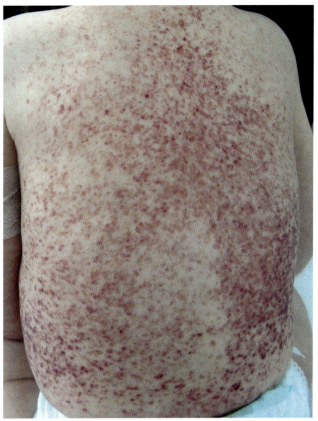

Fig. 15.8 Papulosquamous lesions showing a tendency to confluence and covering nearly the entire back of a child with Langerhans cell histiocytosis

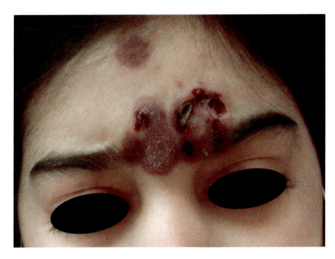

Fig. 15.7 Large erythematous nodule on the midface; an unusual presentation of Langerhans cell histiocytosis. Note also the associated purpura on the forehead

a poor prognosis. Intertriginous, facial, or scalp lesions with papulovesicles, erosions, and fine scaling (*see* Fig. 15.3) can lead to a misdiagnosis of seborrheic dermatitis, especially in infants. But therapy-resistant seborrheic dermatitis-like lesions on intertriginous locations intermingled with purpura must always be a red flag for Langerhans cell histiocytosis. Bacterial intertrigo, candidiasis, atopic dermatitis, scabies, Darier disease, and chickenpox are among the other diseases frequently considered in the differential diagnosis.

Oral mucosal lesions with erosion and ulceration are predominantly seen on the gingivae (*see* Fig. 15.15) and may cause gingival bleeding. Genital lesions are not uncommon. Necrotic and ulcerated lesions (*see* Fig. 15.16) may develop, and they may be associated with genital discharge. A solitary persistent nodule or chronic ulcer on the genitalia may be a sign of Langerhans cell histiocytosis and can be mistaken for extramammary Paget disease (*see* Fig. 2.79), squamous cell carcinoma (*see* Fig. 11.141), malignant melanoma or Behçet disease. Other

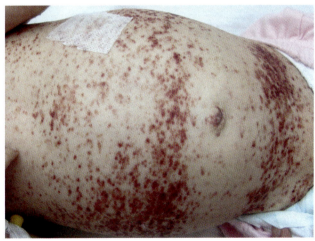

Fig. 15.9 Disseminated papular lesions associated with purpura. Two major clinical features of Langerhans cell histiocytosis are seen concomitantly on the trunk

findings of Langerhans cell histiocytosis include nail changes such as paronychia (*see* Fig. 15.17), onycholysis, subungual hyperkeratosis, nail dystrophy (*see* Fig. 15.18) and purpuric streaks on the nailbed. Nail involvement is also a poor prognostic sign of the disease.

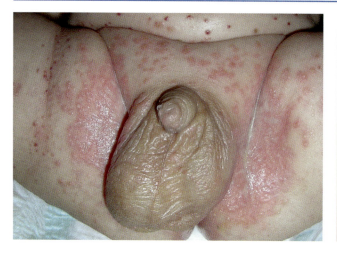

Fig. 15.10 Intertriginous dermatitis on the inguinal folds of a child caused by Langerhans cell histiocytosis. This appearance can easily be mistaken for seborrheic dermatitis

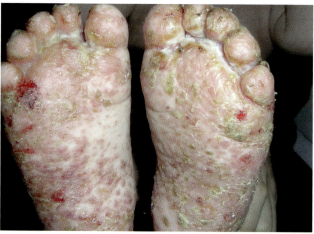

Fig. 15.13 Vesiculopustular eruption showing erosion and crusting on the soles of the feet in a patient with Langerhans cell histiocytosis

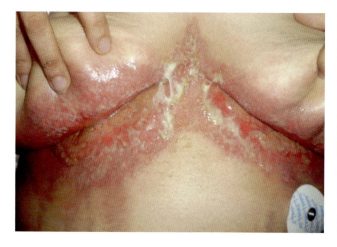

Fig. 15.11 Severe intertriginous dermatitis with pronounced erosion in an adult woman attributable to Langerhans cell histiocytosis. In this case, the lesions were secondarily infected

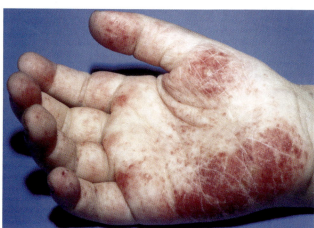

Fig. 15.14 Palmar purpura owing to Langerhans cell histiocytosis

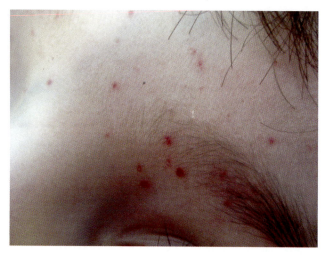

Fig. 15.12 Petechiae on the face of a child with Langerhans cell histiocytosis

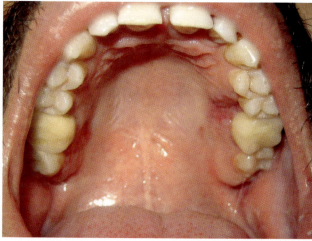

Fig. 15.15 Langerhans cell histiocytosis may involve the oral mucosa, especially the gingivae as seen here

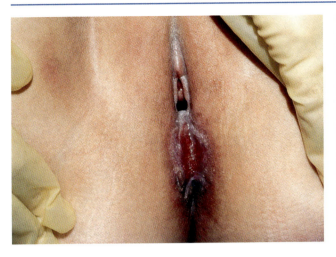

Fig. 15.16 Ulceration caused by Langerhans cell histiocytosis on the vulva of a child. Langerhans cell histiocytosis should be considered in the differential diagnosis of genital erosions and ulcerations

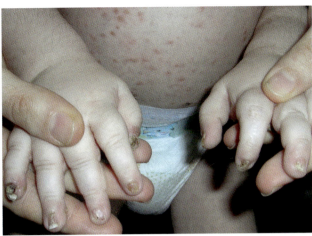

Fig. 15.18 Subungual hyperkeratosis and nail dystrophy in a child with Langerhans cell histiocytosis

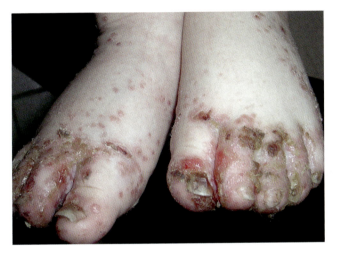

Fig. 15.17 Vesiculopustular eruption of Langerhans cell histiocytosis on the feet involving the paronychial area of the toes

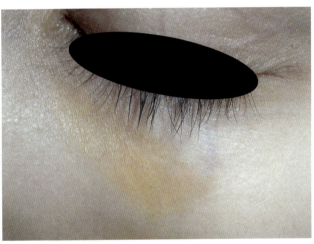

Fig. 15.19 Xanthoma-like yellow flat plaque on the face, an unusual presentation seen in the late period of Langerhans cell histiocytosis

Mucocutaneous lesions may heal spontaneously, but resolution is mostly followed by exacerbations. Especially, secondary infected lesions may result in scarring. Sometimes xanthoma-like lesions may occur secondarily during the late period of the disease (see Fig. 15.19). Furthermore, juvenile xanthogranuloma may rarely develop in patients with Langerhans cell histiocytosis.

The general health status of the patient may be compromised, and fever and weight loss may be found. Systemic involvement of various organs may be seen in the course of the disease, and sometimes it may be fatal. Dyspnea, cyanosis, and pneumothorax are among the possible findings of respiratory involvement, which may sometimes be asymptomatic. Liver involvement may lead to hepatomegaly, jaundice, and even hepatic failure. Lymphadenopathy and splenomegaly may also be seen. Osteolytic lesions of flat bones, vertebrae, and cranial bones develop in the late course and may be painful. Bone marrow involvement of Langerhans cell histiocytosis causing hematologic findings is rare. It may be followed by secondary systemic infections.

The diagnosis is always established by biopsy. Many patients have a history of being misdiagnosed and treated erroneously for an infectious or inflammatory dermatosis. The histologic appearance of involved organs, including the skin, reveals infiltration with Langerhans cells bearing lobulated reniform nuclei and abundant eosinophilic cytoplasm. Immunohistochemically these cells express S-100 protein and antigens like CD1a and langerin. The infiltration is usually seen in the upper dermis and can be epidermotropic. In the late period a granulomatous pattern or xanthomatous change in the cell cytoplasm may be seen. Detection of Birbeck (Langerhans) granules by electron microscopy may confirm the diagnosis.

Prognosis mainly depends on the extent of systemic involvement and age of the patient. Solitary or multiple papulonodular lesions seen in Hashimoto-Pritzker disease always resolve spontaneously, but recurrence may occur, thus the patients should be followed. The chronic unifocal type is associated with less organ involvement and usually heals spontaneously. On the other hand, the chronic multifocal type has a slow progressive course. Letterer-Siwe disease has a variable course. It may show a chronic course, may heal completely, or may less frequently follow a fulminant course leading to organ failure or death. Adult patients may present with localized or generalized disease, but multisystem involvement is more frequent and is associated with a poor prognosis.

Management. After confirming the diagnosis with a skin biopsy, peripheral blood examination, liver function tests, and radiologic imaging for skeletal and visceral involvement should be performed. In addition to the age of the patient, the severity of the mucocutaneous lesions and the presence of systemic involvement should be considered in determining the therapy. Localized skin lesions may heal with the use of topical corticosteroids, and aggressive therapy may not be necessary. Disseminated skin lesions may be treated with topical nitrogen mustard, systemic corticosteroids, thalidomide, isotretinoin or PUVA. Surgical intervention, intralesional corticosteroid injections, and radiotherapy are the therapeutic alternatives for bone lesions. Chemotherapy (vinblastine, chlorambucil, etoposide, cladribine) may be applied for systemic involvement, especially in organ dysfunction. Recurrence is possible even after complete response to therapy. Long-term surveillance is necessary.

15.2 Non-Langerhans Cell Histiocytoses

Non-Langerhans cell histiocytoses consist of a group of diseases with different clinical and histopathologic features. Although they are mainly described with dermatologic findings, most may show visceral involvement. Papules, nodules, and plaques are the presentations of the skin lesions. While some patients have a solitary skin lesion, others have disseminated lesions.

15.2.1 Juvenile Xanthogranuloma

Juvenile xanthogranuloma is the most common type of non-Langerhans cell histiocytoses, presenting typically as self-healing skin lesions and rarely causing visceral involvement. The etiology is unknown. It may be present at birth but it more commonly arises in the first year of life or in early childhood; it may rarely develop in older children or young adults. The head and neck are the most commonly involved areas (*see* Fig. 15.20). The upper trunk (*see* Fig. 15.21) and limbs (*see* Fig. 15.22) are also frequent sites. However, any skin site may be involved. Lesions may also appear on the oral mucosa, usually on the lateral sides of the tongue and on the hard palate.

Juvenile xanthogranuloma manifests as papules or nodules of variable number and size. Typical lesions have a yellowish to

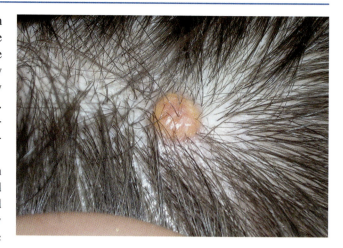

Fig. 15.20 Juvenile xanthogranuloma manifesting as an orange-colored nodule on the scalp, a common location

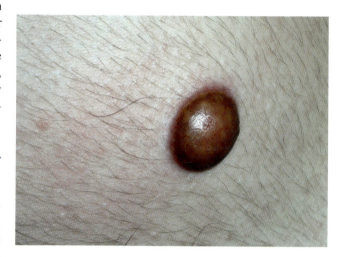

Fig. 15.21 Solitary dome-shaped, smooth-surfaced juvenile xanthogranuloma with yellowish-brown color located on the upper trunk

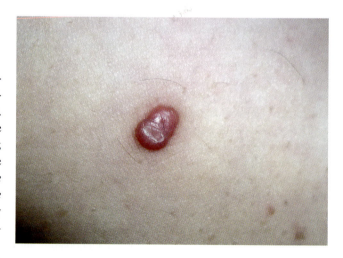

Fig. 15.22 Solitary oval-shaped juvenile xanthogranuloma located on the leg

15.2 Non-Langerhans Cell Histiocytoses

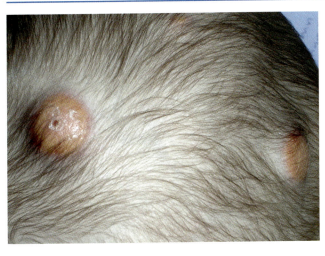

Fig. 15.23 Two orange-colored round large nodules of juvenile xanthogranuloma on the scalp of a child

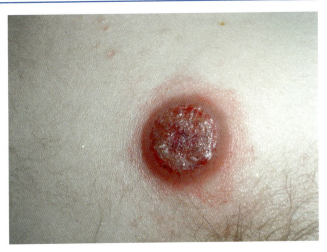

Fig. 15.25 Large nodular juvenile xanthogranuloma with crusting on the surface

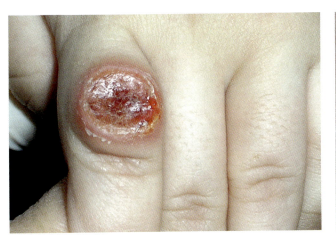

Fig. 15.24 Large nodular juvenile xanthogranuloma with eroded surface covered with crusts on the finger. Biopsy has revealed the diagnosis in this case

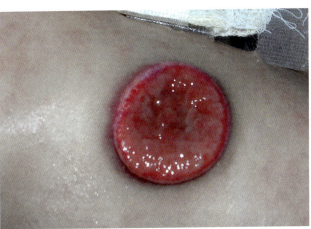

Fig. 15.26 Large nodular juvenile xanthogranuloma showing superficial ulceration

brown or orange hue, which is helpful as a differentiating feature (see Figs. 15.20 and 15.21). Skin lesions may be classified mainly as small and large nodular forms according to their size. The large nodular form is seen as a solitary or a few round or oval, sharply defined, firm asymptomatic nodules measuring 1 to 2 cm in diameter (see Figs. 15.20, 15.21, 15.22, and 15.23). The surface of the lesion is usually intact (see Fig. 15.21), but erosion and crusting (see Figs. 15.24 and 15.25), or superficial ulceration (see Fig. 15.26) may occur. Telangiectases may be observed on the surface of some lesions. Solitary, large, dome-shaped nodular lesions may be confused with Spitz nevus (see Fig. 3.218), isolated mastocytoma (see Fig. 9.19), dermatofibroma (see Fig. 8.6), and tuberous xanthoma. The small nodular form of juvenile xanthogranuloma is observed mostly on the upper trunk as multiple, irregularly scattered, dome-shaped, firm papules with a smooth surface measuring 2 to 5 mm in diameter (see Figs. 15.27 and 15.28). The clinical picture may

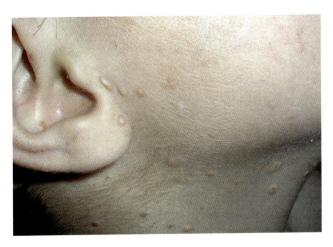

Fig. 15.27 Small nodular form of juvenile xanthogranuloma. Note the multiple small, yellow papules with a smooth surface on the earlobe, face, and neck

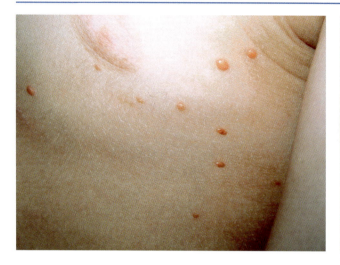

Fig. 15.28 Multiple, orange-colored discrete papules, 2 to 5 mm in diameter located on the trunk representing the small nodular form of juvenile xanthogranuloma

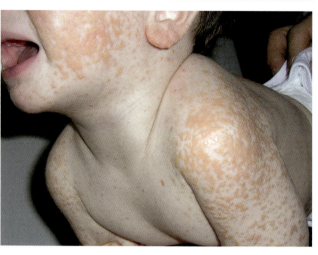

Fig. 15.30 Lichenoid papules of juvenile xanthogranuloma with a tendency to cluster and form plaques on the face and arms

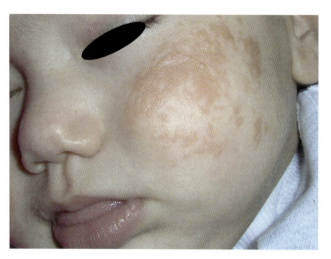

Fig. 15.29 Clustered juvenile xanthogranuloma on the cheek of a child

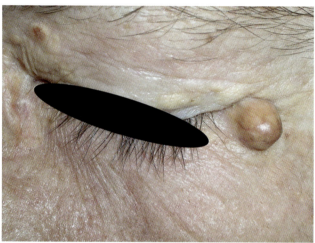

Fig. 15.31 Papules, nodules, and plaques (mixed lesions) of juvenile xanthogranuloma are seen concomitantly in an adult patient. In contrast to its name, the disease may also be seen in adults (adult xanthogranuloma)

look like eruptive xanthomas related to hyperlipidemia. However, the lipid profile of the patients is normal. Multiple small papulonodular lesions may also be mistaken for molluscum contagiosum, eruptive Spitz nevus, urticaria pigmentosa (*see* Fig. 9.6), Langerhans cell histiocytosis (*see* Fig. 15.1), and other non-Langerhans cell histiocytoses such as benign cephalic histiocytosis (*see* Fig. 15.35). In particular, benign cephalic histiocytosis may not be clinically easy to distinguish from multiple small lesions of juvenile xanthogranuloma.

Apart from the classic presentations, juvenile xanthogranuloma may also appear in different clinical pictures such as clustered, lichenoid, mixed, giant, and subcutaneous lesions. Multiple papulonodular lesions with a tendency to coalesce and form plaques are called clustered juvenile xanthogranuloma (*see* Figs. 15.29 and 15.30). Multiple, generalized, 1 to 3 mm papules may be seen in the generalized lichenoid form. Large nodules and small papules may be concurrently seen in the mixed form (*see* Fig. 15.31). Giant juvenile xanthogranuloma is a rare variant that is described as a lesion exceeding 2 cm (*see* Fig. 15.32a). The clinical appearance of a giant lesion is also variable. It is described as a flat plaque or a plaque consisting of coalesced papules or a uniform mass with discrete papules and nodules at the periphery. Lesions, especially large nodules or giant masses, may be ulcerated (*see* Fig. 15.26), and crusting may be remarkable on the surface. Giant lesions must be distinguished from dermatofibrosarcoma protuberans (*see* Fig. 13.61) and other soft tissue neoplasms. Subcutaneous lesions are mostly solitary and are difficult to diagnose clinically.

Extracutaneous involvement is not common and is mostly noted concomitantly with skin lesions but may sometimes be isolated. Any site including the eyes, lungs, kidneys, liver, and other visceral organs may be affected but among these the eye, especially the uvea, is the commonest site of involvement.

15.2 Non-Langerhans Cell Histiocytoses

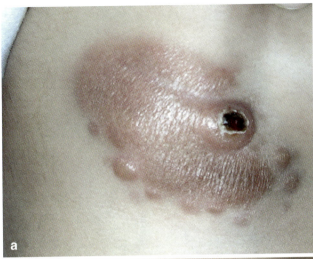
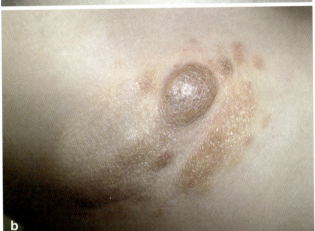
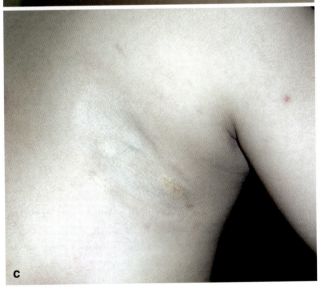

Fig. 15.32 (a) Giant solitary plaque of juvenile xanthogranuloma on the trunk. There are also papules at the periphery. (b) Partial spontaneous resolution of the lesions in nine months. (c) Complete healing of the lesions two years later. Note the atrophic scar on the lesion site

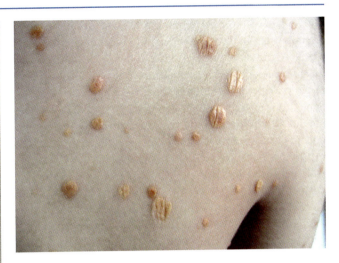

Fig. 15.33 Small nodular form of juvenile xanthogranuloma during the regression period. Note the folded surface of the flattened lesions which were soft on palpation

Eye lesions of juvenile xanthogranuloma are mostly unilateral and may cause yellowish vascular lesions or heterochromia. They tend to bleed, leading to hemorrhage of the anterior chamber of the eye and may consequently cause secondary glaucoma and vision loss. Eye involvement is mostly seen in childhood patients with multiple skin lesions. It can also appear later on after the occurrence of skin lesions. Although very rare, various other symptoms may be found according to the site of visceral involvement. Lung involvement is rarely associated with dyspnea. Lesions of the central nervous system may cause epilepsy, diplopia, or ataxia.

The diagnosis is usually established by histopathologic examination of a skin biopsy. Histopathologic features are common in all clinical forms. Dense infiltration of histiocytes with foamy, xanthomatous cytoplasm in the dermis is typical. Rarely, these cells may be spindle-shaped. Touton type giant cells are usually found. Other inflammatory cells such as eosinophils, lymphocytes, and plasma cells are intermingled with the histiocytes. As opposed to the Langerhans cell histiocytosis, the histiocytic cells do not express S100, CD1a, or langerin. In contrast, these cells are positive for CD68.

Juvenile xanthogranuloma is not associated with any lipid disorder or metabolic anomalies such as diabetes insipidus. However, it may be concomitantly seen with neurofibromatosis type I or juvenile chronic myelogenous leukemia and more rarely with other hematologic malignancies.

Skin involvement of juvenile xanthogranuloma has a benign course and is mostly associated with spontaneous regression in the childhood period. The lesions regress approximately within 6 months to 6 years. Initially tumors flatten and their hard texture diminishes in time, becoming soft with a folded surface (*see* Fig. 15.33). Larger lesions may heal with atrophy and dyspigmentation (*see* Fig. 15.32b and c).

Management. In patients with multiple skin lesions of juvenile xanthogranuloma, possible accompanying ocular involvement should be investigated. However, routine screening for visceral involvement in asymptomatic patients is not recommended. Peripheral blood examination should be performed to search for concomitant juvenile chronic myelogenous leukemia.

The age of the patient and the number of skin lesions are important in the management of juvenile xanthogranuloma. Aggressive surgery that can cause unsightly scars must be avoided, since spontaneous regression is expected in childhood. Even multiple and giant lesions show a tendency to spontaneous regression (see Fig. 15.32a–c). The parents of children should be informed about the benign course of the disease. On the other hand, lesions occurring in adulthood may be persistent. These lesions can be surgically removed or destructed by carbondioxide laser for cosmetic relief.

Like skin lesions visceral lesions of juvenile xanthogranuloma may also heal spontaneously, but those interfering with vital functions should be treated. Ocular lesions are persistent and are associated with increased risk of complications; therefore they are usually treated. Topical, intralesional, or systemic corticosteroids can be used. Radiotherapy is another option for eye involvement.

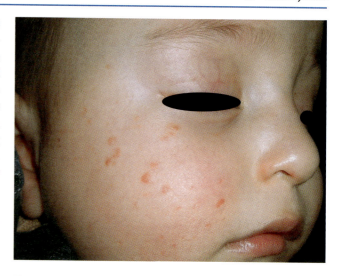

Fig. 15.34 Small papular lesions are evident on the face of a child younger than 3 years of age; this is the most typical presentation of benign cephalic histiocytosis

15.2.2 Benign Cephalic Histiocytosis

Benign cephalic histiocytosis is a rare type of non-Langerhans cell histiocytoses seen in childhood and characterized by self-healing multiple small papules limited to the skin. It is a sporadic disease and the general health of the patient is normal. The onset is mostly in the first three years of life. Lesions are typically located on the face, most commonly on the cheeks (see Fig. 15.34), eyelids, and forehead. However, the ears and other sites of the head and neck (see Fig. 15.35) may also be involved. In a subset of patients, lesions may also be observed on the trunk (see Fig. 15.36) or extremities. The number of lesions is variable, and some patients have numerous papules. The flat-topped, smooth-surfaced, asymptomatic papules are round or oval with a pink to yellowish-brown color (see Fig. 15.37). The size of the papules is between 2 and 8 mm, and they slowly increase in size (see Figs. 15.34, 15.35, 15.36, and 15.37). They are typically discrete and irregularly distributed. But confluent papules may also be observed. They are most commonly confused with the flat, skin-colored papules of verruca plana. In addition, it is not always easy to distinguish benign cephalic histiocytosis from the small nodular form of juvenile xanthogranuloma (see Fig. 15.27). The papules of benign cephalic histiocytosis are different from the ones seen in Langerhans cell histiocytosis, which are scaly or crusted (see Fig. 15.1). Urticaria pigmentosa (see Fig. 9.1) is another common clinical misinterpretation. However, Darier sign is negative in benign cephalic histiocytosis. Histopathologic examination reveals infiltration of histiocytes filling the upper dermis. These cells have oval nuclei and pale cytoplasm, which can be xanthomized in older lesions. Scattered lymphocytes

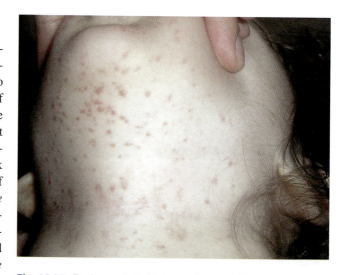

Fig. 15.35 Benign cephalic histiocytosis presenting as numerous tan to yellowish-brown persistent papules, 2 to 4 mm in diameter involving the face and neck exclusively

and occasional multinuclear giant cells can also be observed. Immunostaining with S100 protein and CD1a is negative, but CD68, Factor XIIIa, and CD11b are positive.

Management. There is no need for further examination of the patients. After a long waxing and waning period of 1 to 4 years, lesions nearly always heal spontaneously. They may fade in the order of appearance. Slight hyperpigmentation may be observed on the regression sites, but scar formation is not expected. Therefore, any destructive modality or medical therapy is not indicated. Patients or parents should be informed about the expected course of the lesions. Adequate diagnosis will prevent unnecessary interventions that can cause scarring.

15.2 Non-Langerhans Cell Histiocytoses

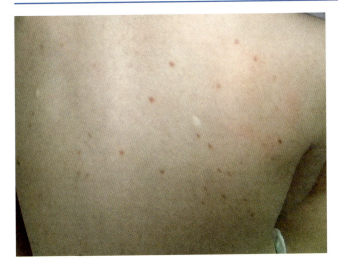

Fig. 15.36 Although they are not as common as lesions on the head, small papular lesions of benign cephalic histiocytosis may also be encountered on the trunk as seen in this child

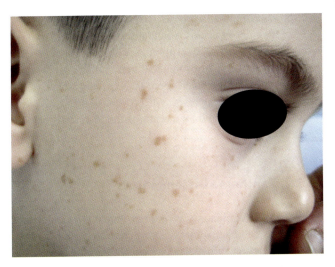

Fig. 15.37 Discrete, slightly raised, yellowish-brown papules on the cheeks of a child with benign cephalic histiocytosis. Lesions were restricted to the face in this patient

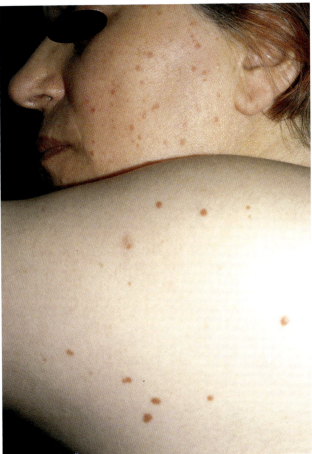

Fig. 15.38 Generalized eruptive histiocytosis presenting as a papular eruption involving the face and arms in an adult patient

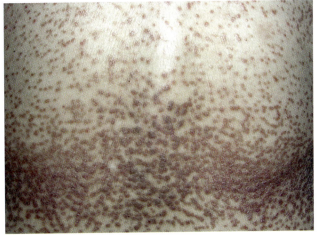

Fig. 15.39 Numerous papular lesions of generalized eruptive histiocytosis on the trunk

15.2.3 Generalized Eruptive Histiocytosis

Generalized eruptive histiocytosis is a rare type of non-Langerhans cell histiocytoses limited to skin with generalized papules. It is more common in middle-aged adults. The face (*see* Fig. 15.38), trunk (*see* Fig. 15.39), and proximal parts of the extremities are the most common sites. Oral and genital mucous membranes may rarely be involved. Round or oval, skin-colored, reddish-brown or bluish-red papules that are between 3 and 10 mm (*see* Figs. 15.40 and 15.41) are asymptomatic. The surface of the papules is smooth. They do not tend to form clusters, but they may be symmetrically arranged (*see* Fig. 15.40). New lesions tend to occur in years. In some patients hundreds of lesions distributed on the whole body may be observed (*see* Fig. 15.39). Patients are in good general health, and there are no accompanying laboratory findings.

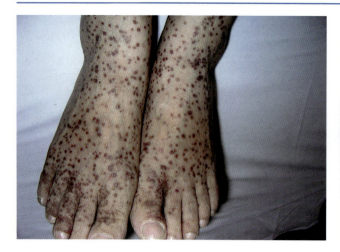

Fig. 15.40 Papular lesions of generalized eruptive histiocytosis are usually symmetrically distributed, as seen here

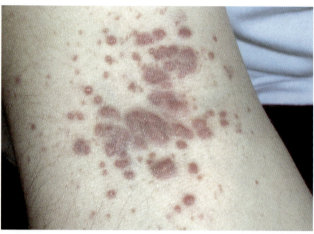

Fig. 15.42 Brownish-colored, firm papules on the antecubital fossa representing early lesions of xanthoma disseminatum. Flexural areas are often involved

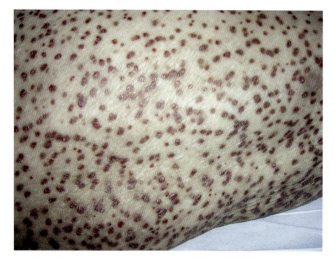

Fig. 15.41 Typical discrete papular lesions of generalized eruptive histiocytosis with reddish-brown color and smooth surface

Generalized eruptive histiocytosis can clinically be mistaken for eruptive xanthoma, adult cutaneous mastocytosis (see Fig. 9.23), sarcoidosis, and eruptive syringoma (see Fig. 5.6) in addition to other types of non-Langerhans cell histiocytoses. Benign cephalic histiocytosis causing similar papules starts in childhood and more commonly involves the head and neck area (see Fig. 15.34). The papular lesions of xanthoma disseminatum are more yellowish and tend to increase rapidly in size, leading to large nodules (see Fig. 15.42). Systemic symptoms and cervical lymphadenopathy are absent in generalized eruptive histiocytosis in contrast to findings in Rosai-Dorfman disease. Arthritis accompanies patients with multicentric reticulohistiocytoses.

Histopathologic examination of generalized eruptive histiocytosis reveals dense infiltration of histiocytes in the upper and mid-dermis. Giant cells are generally absent. Immunostaining with S100 and CD1a is negative, as in other non-Langerhans cell histiocytoses, but CD68, Mac 387, and Factor XIIIa are positive. Birbeck granules are not found on electron microscopy.

Management. Lesions spontaneously heal with slight brownish pigmentation or without any pigmentation or scar. Therefore, any surgical or medical therapy is not indicated. Patients should be informed about the expected course of the lesions. Adequate diagnosis will prevent unnecessary systemic examinations and interventions that can result in scar formation.

15.2.4 Xanthoma Disseminatum

Xanthoma disseminatum is one of rarest types of non-Langerhans cell histiocytoses and is characterized by diabetes insipidus and mucocutaneous lesions that may be progressive. The etiology is unknown. It generally begins in the second or third decade, and men are more commonly affected than women. Xanthoma disseminatum occurs mostly sporadically, and it may be associated with several systemic diseases such as multiple myeloma, Waldenström macroglobulinemia, monoclonal gammopathy, and hypo- or hyperthyroidism.

The disease manifests as multiple cutaneous lesions usually located on flexural (see Fig. 15.42) and intertriginous areas. But lesions may also be found on the face, eyelids (see Fig. 15.43), trunk, fingers, and toes. Symmetrically distributed, brown, reddish or dark yellow, dome-shaped or linear, firm small papules are the typical initial lesions (see Fig. 15.42). Papules may gradually increase in number over years. Disseminated papular eruption may be confused with other non-Langerhans cell histiocytoses and eruptive xanthomas. Serum lipid levels are normal in xanthoma disseminatum. Lesions may slowly enlarge over years and tend to confluence, especially in intertriginous areas, leading to large nodules, plaques, or tumors (see Fig. 15.44). Lesions on these areas may become soft, slack, and yellow in time (see Fig. 15.45a and b).

15.2 Non-Langerhans Cell Histiocytoses

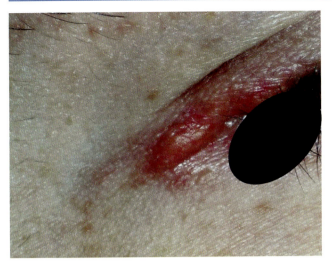

Fig. 15.43 Involvement of the eyelid in the early period of xanthoma disseminatum

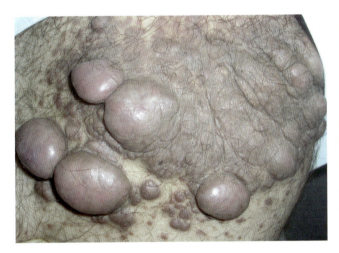

Fig. 15.44 Papules and nodules merged into large plaques on the inguinal fold in the advanced stage of xanthoma disseminatum

Even large cutaneous lesions are asymptomatic. However, large nodules and tumors are usually disfiguring. They may cause functional impairment, particularly those located on the fingers (*see* Fig. 15.46). Large plantar lesions may interfere with walking. The surface of the tumors is intact, but lesions on the plantar area may be ulcerated owing to trauma. Large nodules on the perineum may interfere with defecation.

Mucosal involvement of xanthoma disseminatum is also common. Lesions may be located on the various parts of the oral mucosa (*see* Fig. 15.47), epiglottis, and respiratory tract, including the nasal vestibule (*see* Fig. 15.48), larynx, pharynx, and trachea. Mucosal lesions of the upper respiratory tract can be life-threatening owing to respiratory obstruction. Conjunctival and corneal involvement may also be seen. Ocular lesions may even lead to blindness. Diabetes insipidus is a common finding in xanthoma disseminatum that may cause a misinterpretation of the disease as Langerhans cell histiocytosis, but visceral and bone involvement is not found.

The clinical course of xanthoma disseminatum is described in three forms. In the self-healing form, lesions regress spontaneously after several years. The persistent form is associated with continuing mucocutaneous lesions. The progressive form is associated with organ dysfunction or central nervous system involvement.

Eruptive xanthoma related with hyperlipidemia, xanthomatous lesions of Langerhans cell histiocytosis (*see* Fig. 15.19), and other non-Langerhans cell histiocytoses such as generalized eruptive histiocytosis (*see* Fig. 15.39), indeterminate cell histiocytosis (*see* Fig. 15.56), and multicentric reticulohistiocytosis (*see* Fig. 15.51) are among the differential diagnostic diseases. Histopathology reveals dermal infiltrate of histiocytes with angulated or scalloped cytoplasmic borders, intermingled with giant cells, lymphocytes, and neutrophils. The histiocytes show positive immunostaining for CD68 and Factor XIIIa and are negative for S100 and CD1a.

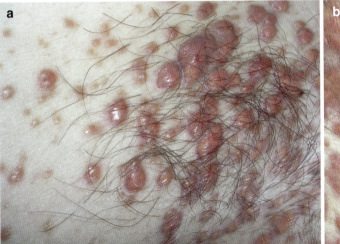
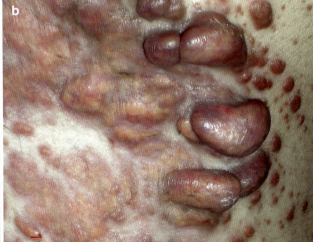

Fig. 15.45 (**a**) Pinkish firm papulonodular lesions on the axilla in the early period of xanthoma disseminatum. (**b**) Advanced stage of the disease; lesions showed remarkable enlargement and softening on palpation, became slack in appearance, and their color changed to yellow

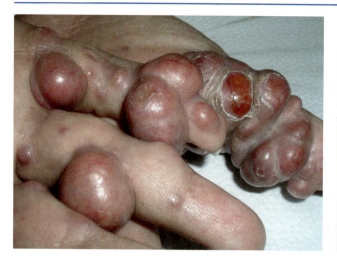

Fig. 15.46 Multiple hard papulonodular lesions forming big tumoral masses on the fingers of a patient with xanthoma disseminatum

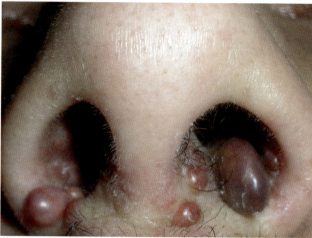

Fig. 15.48 Papulonodular lesions on the nasal mucosa due to xanthoma disseminatum. Severe involvement of the upper respiratory tract may be life-threatening as a result of obstruction

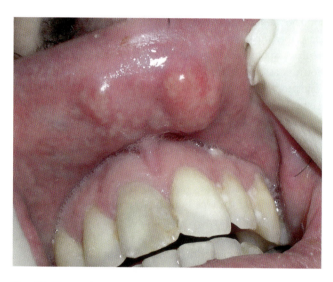

Fig. 15.47 Papulonodular lesions on the oral mucosa (upper lip in the figure), a common presentation of xanthoma disseminatum

In the presence of these histopathologic and immunohistochemical findings suggestive of a non-Langerhans cell histiocytosis, the distribution and other clinical characteristics of the mucocutaneous lesions, and accompanying diabetes insipidus support the diagnosis of xanthoma disseminatum.

Management. After confirmation of the diagnosis, patients can be examined and tested for the possible associated mucosal lesions and systemic findings related to systemic involvement. Laryngeal and tracheal involvement can be investigated with bronchoscopy. Sellar MRI may reveal changes compatible with pituitary gland involvement. Laboratory examinations, including protein electrophoresis, can be performed in order to screen the possible accompanying diseases.

The effect of any of the therapeutic modalities has not been proved. Spontaneous healing is also possible (self-healing form). Therefore a "wait and see" policy may be adopted in cases without serious mucosal involvement. Local management of skin lesions includes surgical excision, carbon dioxide laser, electrocoagulation, and cryotherapy. However, recurrence may be seen in a short time after surgical or destructive therapies and they are not routinely used.

Systemic therapy in xanthoma disseminatum is usually considered for progressive mucosal involvement and for extensive or disfiguring skin lesions. Systemic corticosteroids can be tried but are not effective in all cases. Clofibrate or fenofibrate is another alternative and can be partially effective in some cases. Cyclophosphamide, vinblastine, azathioprine, and chlorambucil alone or in combination with systemic corticosteroids have all been used with variable results. Lesions may be partially controlled with therapy but may progress after cessation of the drugs (*see* Fig. 15.49a–c). Removal of larger nodules and tumors causing functional problems may be performed for palliative purposes (*see* Fig. 15.49c and d). Local recurrence may take place even after aggressive surgery (*see* Fig. 15.49e). Diabetes insipidus should also be treated medically.

15.2.5 Reticulohistiocytosis

Two subtypes of reticulohistiocytosis exist: reticulohistiocytic granuloma and multicentric reticulohistiocytosis.

15.2.5.1 Reticulohistiocytic Granuloma (Solitary Cutaneous Histiocytosis)

Reticulohistiocytic granuloma is characterized by solitary lesions seen exclusively in adulthood. Although the etiology of the disease is unknown, trauma seems to be a triggering factor. It is not associated with any systemic findings. The

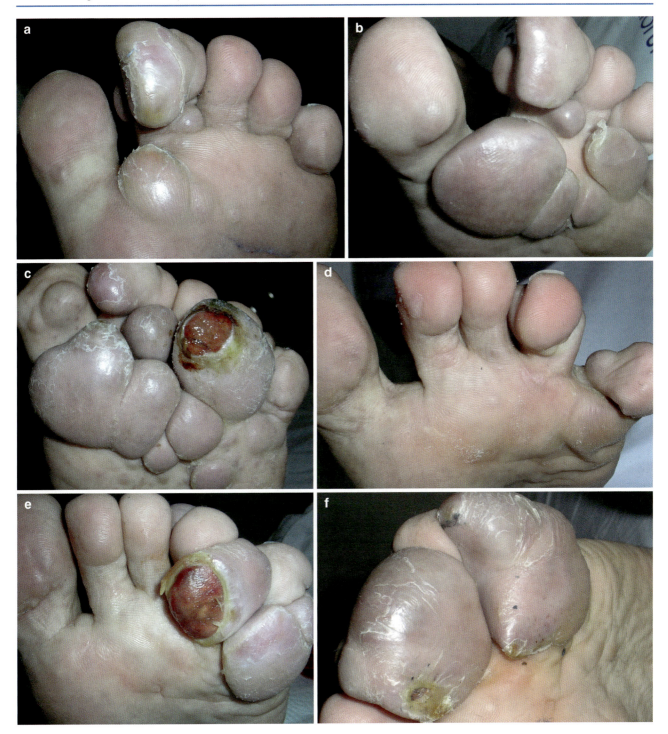

Fig. 15.49 (a) A few papulonodular lesions on the toes and sole caused by xanthoma disseminatum. (b) Although systemic therapy (cyclophosphamide, vinblastine) had been administered, plantar lesions increased in size and number (two years later). (c) Lesions enlarged and one showed ulceration under long term systemic corticosteroid therapy (three years later). (d) Lesions disappeared completely after excision. (e) Relapse of the nodules occurred one year after surgery (f) Enlargement of the nodules (two years after surgery)

solitary lesion is more commonly located in the head and neck area but may occur at any skin or mucosal sites. It grows rapidly in the beginning. Soft or firm, yellowish to red, asymptomatic papulonodular lesion is usually smaller than 2 cm (see Fig. 15.50). Spitz nevus (see Fig. 3.217), dermatofibroma (see Fig. 8.6), juvenile xanthogranuloma (see Fig. 15.23), and isolated mastocytoma (see Fig. 9.17) are among the differential diagnostic possibilities. The diagnosis depends on the histopathologic examination, which reveals upper and mid-dermal dense histiocytic infiltration

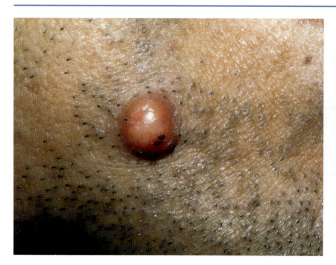

Fig. 15.50 Reticulohistiocytic granuloma presenting as a solitary dome-shaped nodule on the face

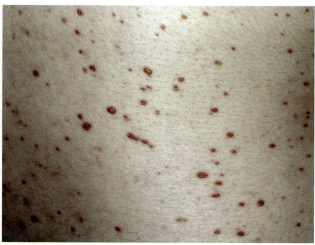

Fig. 15.51 Disseminated dome-shaped brownish papules on the trunk of a patient with multicentric reticulohistiocytosis

with deeply eosinophilic or ground-glass cytoplasm and many giant cells. Immunohistochemically these cells express CD68, HAM 56, and Factor XIIIa and are negative for CD1a. S100 is also usually negative.

Management. Reticulohistiocytic granuloma is a benign lesion that can resolve spontaneously. The solitary tumor may be removed surgically.

15.2.5.2 Multicentric Reticulohistiocytosis

Multicentric reticulohistiocytosis is a rare type of non-Langerhans histiocytoses characterized by the involvement of mucocutaneous sites, joints, and other visceral organs. The disease starts at about 30 to 40 years of age. Yellowish to brown, dome-shaped papules or large nodules may be disseminated involving the head, extremities, and trunk (*see* Figs. 15.51 and 15.52). They show a tendency to cluster, forming plaques, but they do not ulcerate. Mucosal sites including the mouth, nose, and pharynx are involved in approximately half of the patients. Secondary nail changes may be observed. Symmetric destructive polyarthritis mostly involving the fingers, wrists, and knees may be associated. The disease can occasionally affect other organs, including the muscles, eyes, heart, thyroid, and stomach. It is suggested to be a paraneoplastic marker of solid visceral cancers and sometimes lymphoproliferative malignancies.

The diagnosis is confirmed with biopsy. Histopathologic examination of skin lesions reveals dermal infiltration of mononucleated and multinucleated histiocytoses with abundant eosinophilic cytoplasm. Immunohistochemical findings include CD68, HAM56, and Factor XIIIa positivity.

Management. The prognosis is poor in cases with systemic involvement and associated malignant tumors. Methotrexate, nonsteroidal anti-inflammatory agents, systemic corticosteroids, and bisphosphonates may be

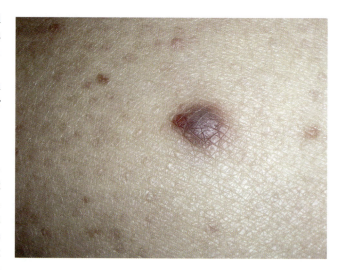

Fig. 15.52 Nodular lesion on the trunk of a patient with multicentric reticulohistiocytosis

effective in skin lesions and joint involvement but recurrence may be seen.

15.2.6 Necrobiotic Xanthogranuloma

Necrobiotic xanthogranuloma is a very rare multisystem disease that typically affects the periorbital skin. It is more commonly seen in adults after middle age. Reddish-yellow, slowly growing, indurated firm periorbital nodules that tend to coalesce into larger plaques are typical lesions (*see* Figs. 15.53 and 15.54). They may invade the subcutis, leading to local tissue destruction. Some lesions may be ulcerated. The trunk (*see* Fig. 15.55) and extremities may also be involved. The disease has a chronic progressive course. Secondary ocular complications such as proptosis and

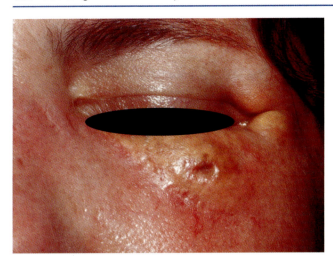

Fig. 15.53 Necrobiotic xanthogranuloma presenting as an indurated yellow plaque around the eye, a distinctive location

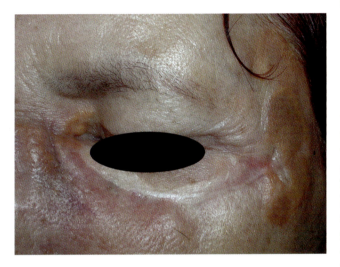

Fig. 15.54 Yellow plaques around the eye and temple resembling xanthelasma in a patient with necrobiotic xanthogranuloma

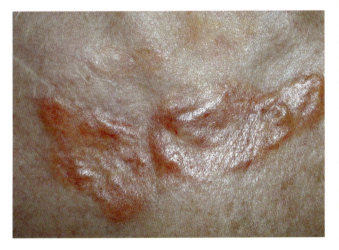

Fig. 15.55 Sharply demarcated yellow indurated plaque on the chest histopathologically diagnosed as necrobiotic xanthogranuloma

restriction of ocular motility may occur. Rarely, extracutaneous involvement, including the heart, kidney, ovaries, intestine, and pharynx may be associated. Periorbital lesions can be confused with xanthelasma, diffuse normolipemic plane xanthoma, and xanthoma disseminatum (*see* Fig. 15.43). Histopathologic findings reveal necrobiosis of dermal collagen and a mixed infiltration composed of giant cells of Touton and foreign body type, lymphocytes, and plasma cells in the dermis and subcutis. Necrobiotic xanthogranuloma may be associated with monoclonal gammopathies.

Management. Patients should be screened and followed for possible accompanying paraproteinemias. Because facial lesions are disfiguring, patients usually seek therapy. However, a standard therapeutic regimen does not exist. Intralesional corticosteroids can be applied for cutaneous lesions. Systemic corticosteroids and chlorambucil are among the systemic drug alternatives. Surgical intervention may improve cosmetic appearance.

15.2.7 Sinus Histiocytosis With Massive Lymphadenopathy (Rosai-Dorfman Disease)

Sinus histiocytosis with massive lymphadenopathy is a rare type of histiocytosis characterized by persistent bilateral cervical lymphadenopathy, but it may also involve other lymph nodes, the skin, tongue, upper respiratory tract, eye, and bones. It is more common in children and young adults. Massive painless cervical lymphadenopathy associated with fever, weight loss, and elevated erythrocyte sedimentation rate may simulate a systemic lymphoma. Skin involvement is only seen in a small percentage of patients. Reddish-brown macules or firm indurated papules, nodules, and rarely tumors may occur simultaneously with lymph node involvement or sometimes are the initial manifestations of the disease. Disseminated skin lesions associated with massive lymphadenopathy are helpful for the diagnosis. Histologically, a mixed infiltration in the dermis, including histiocytes with abundant lightly eosinophilic cytoplasm, is observed. Scattered multinucleate cells and Touton type giant cells may be seen. Plasma cells and lymphocytes are also found. Another feature helpful for diagnosis, known as emperipolesis, is the phagocytosis of lymphocytes and plasma cells by the histiocytes. Histiocytic cells express monocyte/macrophage markers and S100, while CD1a is negative.

The disease has a protracted course with episodes of exacerbations and remissions. Most cases show spontaneous resolution; however, the disease may rarely be fatal.

Management. Since cutaneous lesions of Rosai-Dorfman disease heal spontaneously, treatment is not necessary. However, in the presence of involvement of vital organs and nodal lesions causing serious complications, therapy may be

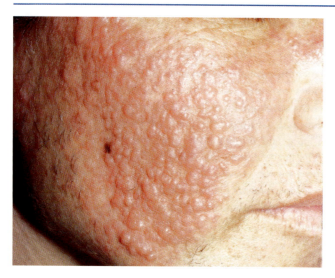

Fig. 15.56 Indeterminate cell histiocytosis presenting as confluent papulonodular lesions on the face

required. Various systemic chemotherapeutic agents have been used with variable success. Systemic corticosteroids may be effective, but recurrence is common after cessation of therapy. Surgery may be used for lesions causing compression of vital organs.

15.3 Indeterminate Cell Histiocytosis

Indeterminate cell histiocytosis is a very rare disease characterized by cutaneous infiltration of dendritic indeterminate cells that morphologically resemble Langerhans cells but do not contain Birbeck granules in the cytoplasm. The onset is usually in adulthood and there are variable numbers of skin lesions. Various sites of the skin may be involved but not the mucous membranes. Firm, dome-shaped, dull red or brown papules and nodules vary in size between 0.2 and 1 cm. The surface of the papules is usually smooth with no scales or crusting, although on occasion nodules may be ulcerated. Plaques may appear as a result of the confluence of multiple papules (*see* Fig. 15.56). Hundreds of lesions may arise suddenly in a subset of patients. Multiple lesions are not easy to distinguish clinically from the lesions of non-Langerhans cell histiocytoses such as generalized eruptive histiocytosis (*see* Fig. 15.38), multicentric reticulohistiocytosis (*see* Fig. 15.51), or xanthoma disseminatum (*see* Fig. 15.42). Moreover, solitary lesions may be confused with juvenile xanthogranuloma (*see* Fig. 15.21). The diagnosis is always confirmed with biopsy and additionally with electron microscopy, as it is mandatory to document the absence of Birbeck granules which are present in Langerhans cells. Hence, Langerhans cell histiocytosis can be eliminated. There is a dermal infiltration of histiocytes, and the typical reniform nuclei, seen also in Langerhans cells, may be visible. But the epidermal involvement usually present in Langerhans cell histiocytosis is absent. Immunostaining with Langerhans cell markers, namely S100 and CD1a, is positive, as are macrophage markers. Laboratory examinations are normal.

Management. The disease is among the types of histiocytoses with a good prognosis. Systemic involvement and serious complications are not expected. Patients can be followed without any therapeutic intervention.

Suggested Reading

Black A, Bershow A, Allen PS, Crowson AN. Seventy-nine-years-old man with Langerhans cell histiocytosis treated with cladribine. J Am Acad Dermatol. 2011;65:681–3.

Bolognia JL, Jorizzo JL, Schaffer JV. Dermatology, edn 3. London: Mosby; 2012.

Calonje JE, Brenn T, Lazar AJ, McKee PH. McKee's pathology of the skin, edn 4. China: Elsevier; 2012.

Caputo R. Text atlas of histiocytic syndromes. London: Martin Dunitz; 1998.

Caputo R, Veraldi S, Grimalt R, et al. The various clinical patterns of xanthoma disseminatum. Considerations on seven cases and review of the literature. Dermatology. 1995;190:19–24.

Chang MW. Update on juvenile xanthogranuloma: unusual cutaneous and systemic variants. Semin Cutan Med Surg. 1999;18:195–205.

Edelbroek JR, Vermeer MH, Jansen PM, et al. Langerhans cell histiocytosis first presenting in the skin in adults: frequent association with a second haematological malignancy. Br J Dermatol. 2012;167:1287–94.

Hasegawa S, Deguchi M, Chiba-Okada S, Aiba S. Japanese case of benign cephalic histiocytosis. J Dermatol. 2009;36:69–71.

Hernandez-Martin A, Baselga E, Drolet BA, et al. Juvenile xanthogranuloma. J Am Acad Dermatol. 1997;36:355–67.

Jih DM, Salcedo SL, Jaworsky C. Benign cephalic histiocytosis: a case report and review. J Am Acad Dermatol. 2002;47:908–13.

LeBoit PE, Burg G, Weedon D, Sarasin A. Pathology and genetics of skin tumours. World Health Organization Classification of Tumours. France; IARC Press; 2006.

Lindahl LM, Fenger-Grøn M, Iversen L. Topical nitrogen mustard therapy in patients with Langerhans cell histiocytosis. Br J Dermatol. 2012;166:642–5.

Oka M, Oniki S, Komatsu M, et al. Xanthoma disseminatum with intracranial involvement: case report and literature review. Int J Dermatol. 2010;49:193–9.

Pruvost C, Picard-Dahan C, Bonnefond B, et al. Vinblastine treatment for extensive non-X histiocytosis (xanthoma disseminatum). Ann Dermatol Venereol. 2004;131:271–3.

Seaton ED, Pillai GJ, Chu AC. Treatment of xanthoma disseminatum with cyclophosphamide. Br J Dermatol. 2004;150:346–9.

Sharath Kumar BC, Nandini AS, Niveditha SR, et al. Generalized eruptive histiocytosis mimicking leprocy. Indian J Dermatol Venereol Leprol. 2011;77:498–502.

Tirumalae R, Rout P, Jayaseelan E, et al. Paraneoplastic multicentric reticulohistiocytosis: a clinicopathologic challenge. Indian J Dermatol Venereol Leprol. 2011;77:318–20.

Weedon D. Weedon's skin pathology, edn 3. China: Elsevier; 2010.

Yazganoglu KD, Erdem Y, Buyukbabani N, Baykal C. A giant congenital plaque. Pediatr Dermatol. 2012;29:217–8.

Cutaneous Metastasis

Different kinds of tumors may cause metastatic spread to the skin. In this chapter, cutaneous metastasis of solid visceral cancers will be discussed. Some skin malignancies may also cause hematogenous metastasis to distant skin sites. Cutaneous metastasis of malignant melanoma, which has different features, is discussed in detail in the relevant chapter. Furthermore, Paget disease, which is mainly considered an intraepidermic metastasis, is discussed in the chapter about precancerous lesions and in situ malignancies. Metastases (skin infiltration) of hematologic neoplasms have different clinical features from cutaneous metastasis of solid tumors, thus discussed in the chapter about cutaneous lymphomas.

Metastatic carcinoma of the skin is not a very rare problem. It occurs nearly in 3 to 10 percent of patients with solid neoplasia. It is mostly a late manifestation of visceral malignancies, and many patients also have concurrent metastases of lymph nodes or other organs. Most patients with cutaneous metastasis have a previously identified primary tumor. While cutaneous metastasis may be a sign of recurrence, in rare cases it may be the initial presentation of a visceral malignancy. Like the metastasis of visceral organs, skin metastasis is usually a sign of poor prognosis. The major impact of skin metastasis is on the treatment plan of the primary tumor.

Cutaneous metastasis may occur in proximity to the primary tumor but also on any area distant from it. It reaches the skin in different ways. Direct extension from underlying structures may be the cause of nearby lesions. This kind of extension is more common in oral cancer (*see* Fig. 11.135) and breast cancer. Metastatic skin lesions may also occur from direct invasion of lymph node metastasis (*see* Fig. 16.1). Implantation of neoplastic cells during a needle biopsy or surgery of visceral cancer may be a rare etiologic factor of cutaneous metastasis. Metastatic dissemination through the lymphatics or the bloodstream is a common cause of cutaneous metastasis in areas distant from the primary tumor. Breast, lung, and kidney cancers may cause metastases on the scalp via hematogenous spread.

Nearly all visceral cancers may show metastasis to the skin in variable frequency. The frequency of cutaneous metastasis is mainly related to the frequency of the primary tumor. The main causes of cutaneous metastasis are breast cancer in women and lung cancer followed by colon cancer in men. This correlates with the frequent types of primary malignancy seen in the general population. In contrast, some frequent malignancies such as prostate cancer rarely metastasize to the skin. Malignant melanoma is a significant cause of cutaneous metastasis in both sexes. Since solid cancers are mostly seen in adults, cutaneous metastases are also encountered in those adults older than 40 to 50 years. In children, skin infiltration of hematologic neoplasms as well as cutaneous metastases of neuroblastoma and rhabdomyosarcoma may be seen.

Cutaneous metastasis of solid cancers shows a wide spectrum of clinical features. Several clinical types have been described. In general, the clinical appearance of skin metastasis is not pathognomonic for the underlying cancer type but some features are seen in distinct tumor types. More than one clinical pattern of cutaneous metastasis may be seen concomitantly.

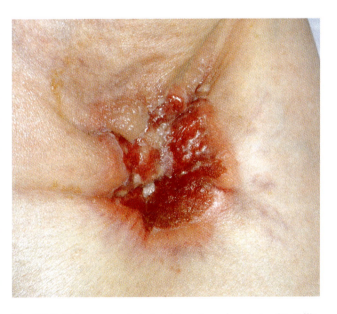

Fig. 16.1 Cutaneous metastasis of breast carcinoma on the axilla. Ulcerated tumoral lesion was related to axillary lymph node metastasis

16.1 Nodular Cutaneous Metastasis

This is the most common presentation of cutaneous metastasis and can be observed as multiple tiny papules (*see* Fig. 16.2), nodules (*see* Fig. 16.3), or large plaques (*see* Fig. 16.4). Solitary nodular metastatic lesions may also be seen (*see* Fig. 16.5). Lesions appear suddenly and then may enlarge slowly or rapidly. In the case of hematogenous spread, any cutaneous site of the body may be involved, but the oral mucosa is a rare location (*see* Fig. 16.6). Some patients have irregularly distributed multiple lesions (*see* Fig. 16.7). The firm to hard nodules are skin-colored (*see* Figs. 16.2 and 16.8), reddish (*see* Fig. 16.5), violaceous (*see* Fig. 16.9) or brownish, and they may be elevated or deeply located. Cutaneous metastases of malignant melanoma may be black (*see* Fig. 12.69), bluish, or skin-colored (amelanotic) (*see* Fig. 12.73). Metastasis of breast carcinoma may sometimes be hyperpigmented (*see* Figs. 16.10 and 16.11). Metastasis of neuroblastoma shows a bluish tinge. A hemangioma-like vascular appearance may be seen typically in cutaneous metastasis of renal cell carcinoma but also rarely in other carcinomas (*see* Fig. 16.12). Nodular metastatic lesions are usually asymptomatic but sometimes they may be painful. The surface of the metastatic skin lesions is usually intact but may become ulcerated and covered with necrotic crusts (*see* Figs. 16.13 and 16.14). Ulcerated lesions are prone to secondary infections. A solitary ulcerated metastatic nodule (*see* Fig. 16.15) may resemble a basal cell carcinoma or squamous cell carcinoma.

The most common involved area of nodular cutaneous metastasis is the skin in proximity to the primary cancer. Breast and lung carcinomas are very common malignancies that typically metastasize to the chest wall as a neighboring area (*see* Fig. 16.16). The abdomen, back, scalp (*see* Fig. 16.17), and face are other locations of cutaneous metastasis of lung carcinoma. Distant metastases of breast carcinoma such as on the limbs are not very common. Oral squamous cell carcinoma may metastasize to nearby skin areas including the head, neck, and chest. Cancers of the uterus may spread to the skin of the genitalia and pubic area (*see* Fig. 16.18). On the other hand, renal cell carcinoma may metastasize to distant skin sites, especially to the head and neck. Cutaneous metastasis restricted to the extremities is rare and is mostly seen in relation to malignant melanoma (*see* Fig. 12.66). Bladder carcinoma may cause distant cutaneous metastases, including the extremities (*see* Fig. 16.19). Nodular cutaneous metastasis of the lower abdomen and pelvic region is usually related to gastrointestinal and genitourinary malignancies (*see* Figs. 16.20, 16.21, and 16.22). Colorectal cancers may cause cutaneous metastasis anywhere on the body, including the perineum (*see* Fig. 16.23), extremities, and scalp. Stomach cancer is an uncommon cause of cutaneous metastasis involving the skin of the abdomen, rarely spreading to distant areas, including the face (*see* Fig. 16.24). Signet-ring cell carcinoma of the bowel may appear in different clinical presentations on different skin sites (*see* Fig. 16.25).

Nodular types of cutaneous metastasis may sometimes be arranged linearly (*see* Fig. 16.26) or in a dermatomal (zosteriform) pattern. This latter rare presentation is mostly seen in breast, lung, prostate, ovary, uterus, kidney, and colon carcinomas.

Nodular cutaneous metastasis on the umbilicus is called Sister Mary Joseph nodule (*see* Fig. 16.27) and is mostly originated from stomach, colon, uterine, ovarian, and pancreatic carcinomas. The hard, fixed nodule may be ulcerated and may cause discharge. Pyogenic granuloma, seborrheic keratosis, endometriosis, and primary malignant neoplasms of the periumbilical area may sometimes be challenging in the differential diagnosis of this type of metastasis.

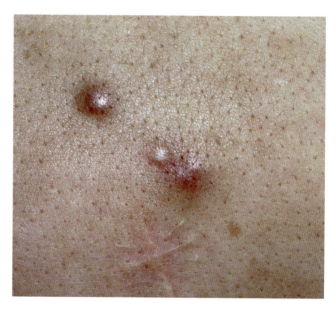

Fig. 16.2 Nodular cutaneous metastasis on the trunk of a patient with breast carcinoma. Note a few skin-colored papulonodular lesions

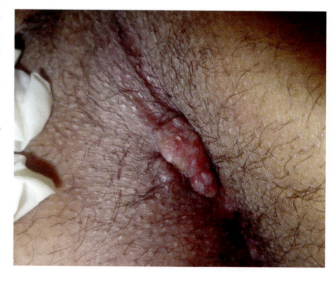

Fig. 16.3 Nodular cutaneous metastasis presenting as large perianal nodules in a patient with colorectal carcinoma

16.1 Nodular Cutaneous Metastasis

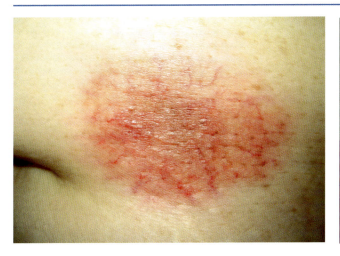

Fig. 16.4 Nodular cutaneous metastasis seen as a plaque with telangiectasia on the surface

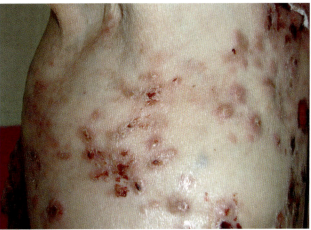

Fig. 16.7 Multiple irregularly distributed nodular lesions of cutaneous metastasis of breast carcinoma. Note that some lesions are ulcerated and crusted

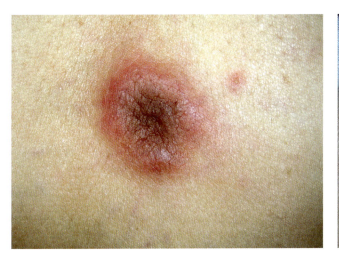

Fig. 16.5 Reddish solitary lesion of nodular cutaneous metastasis

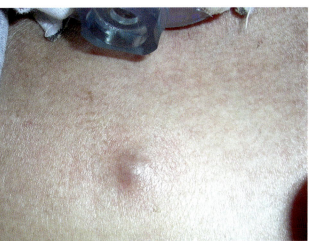

Fig. 16.8 Skin-colored metastatic nodule of esophageal carcinoma on the neck

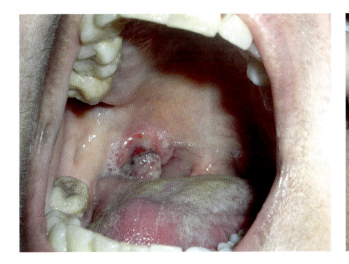

Fig. 16.6 Mucosal metastatic lesion showing ulceration. Oral mucosa is an uncommon site of metastasis

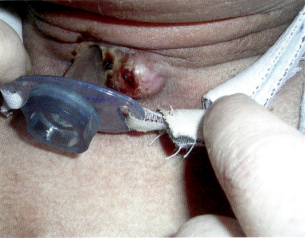

Fig. 16.9 Ulcerated violaceous metastatic nodule of esophageal carcinoma located adjacent to the tracheostomy site

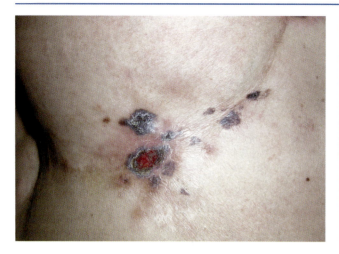

Fig. 16.10 Multiple hyperpigmented lesions of cutaneous metastasis on the mastectomy site in a patient with breast carcinoma

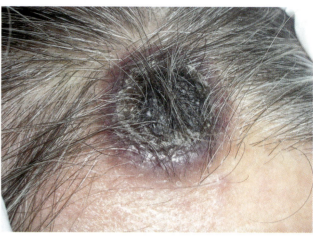

Fig. 16.13 Ulcerated nodular cutaneous metastasis on the scalp

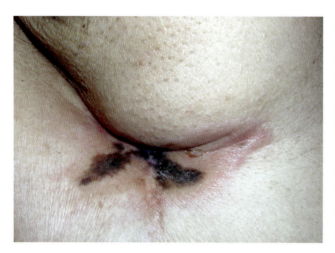

Fig. 16.11 Hyperpigmented nodular cutaneous metastasis on the axilla of a patient with breast carcinoma. Individual lesions look clinically suggestive of malignant melanoma

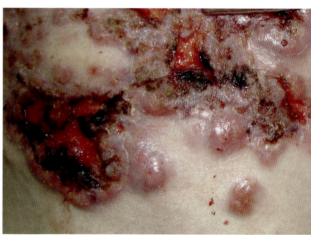

Fig. 16.14 Confluent lesions of nodular cutaneous metastasis involving a large area. Broad ulcerations are noticeable in this patient with breast carcinoma

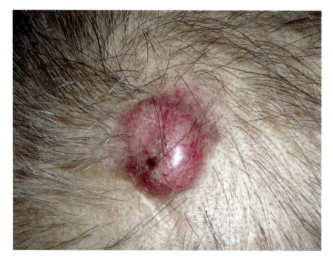

Fig. 16.12 A reddish, hemangioma-like nodular cutaneous metastasis on the scalp in a patient with lung carcinoma

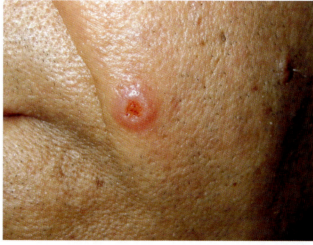

Fig. 16.15 Ulcerated nodule of cutaneous metastasis resembling non-melanoma skin cancer. Metastatic lesions are firm on palpation

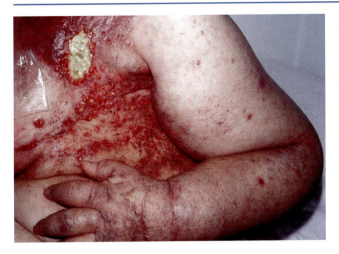

Fig. 16.16 Cutaneous metastases of breast carcinoma around the mastectomy site, axilla and arm associated with lymphedema of the hand and arm

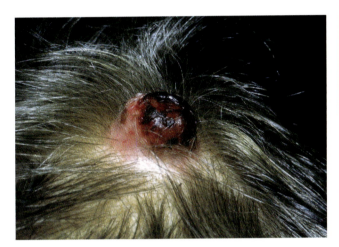

Fig. 16.17 Nodular cutaneous metastasis on the scalp caused by lung carcinoma

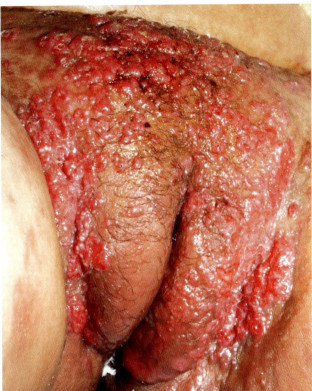

Fig 16.18 Cutaneous metastasis as multiple papulonodular lesions on the vulva and pubic area were caused by carcinoma of the uterus

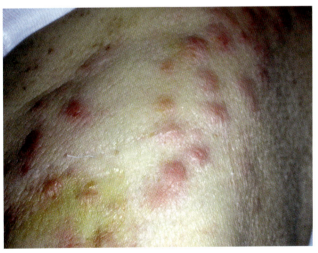

Fig. 16.19 Cutaneous metastasis of bladder carcinoma presenting as multiple erythematous nodules on the thigh

16.2 Carcinoma Erysipeloides

Carcinoma erysipeloides is the second most common type of cutaneous metastasis. It occurs by lymphatic spread of solid visceral cancers and clinically looks like an inflammatory lesion such as erysipelas or cellulitis. Typical lesions are erythematous, sharply demarcated patches or slightly raised plaques measuring 5 to 20 cm in diameter (*see* Fig. 16.28). Larger lesions may also be found (*see* Fig. 16.29). Some lesions are ill-defined (*see* Fig. 16.30). They are mostly asymptomatic but may sometimes be tender. Lesions are warm to touch. In contrast to erysipelas, systemic symptoms like fever and chills are not usual, and there is no response to antibiotic therapy. Since breast carcinoma is the most frequent cause of carcinoma erysipeloides, the lesions are typically localized on the cancerous breast (*see* Fig. 16.28) or on neighboring areas such as the other breast, upper back (*see* Fig. 16.30), and upper arm. They may also appear on the site of mastectomy (*see* Fig. 16.29), indicating the recurrence of the primary tumor.

Moreover, metastasis from other organs, including the gastrointestinal system, genitourinary system, pancreas, larynx, tonsils, parotid gland, bladder, and lung, may cause carcinoma erysipeloides in different locations. Carcinoma erysipeloides caused by bladder or ovary cancers may be seen on the skin of abdominal and pelvic regions (*see* Fig. 16.31). The patches and plaques of this special type of skin metastasis are persistent and may become yellowish and fibrotic in time.

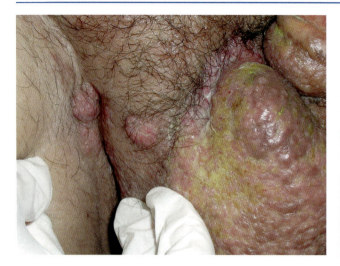

Fig. 16.20 Cutaneous metastasis presenting as multiple nodules and indurated plaques on the male genitalia and inguinal area. Colon carcinoma was the underlying cause

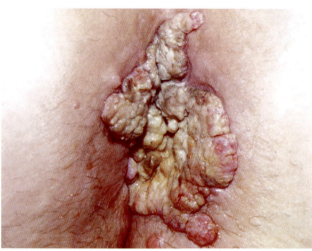

Fig. 16.23 A vegetating mass on the perianal area resulting from the metastasis of colorectal cancer

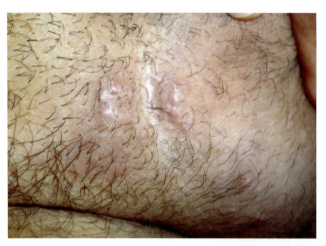

Fig. 16.21 Cutaneous metastasis of colon carcinoma seen as indurated plaques on the lower abdomen

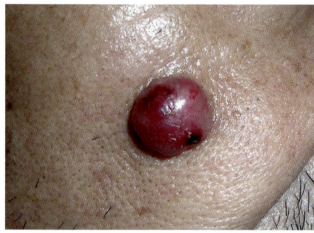

Fig. 16.24 Metastatic nodule on the face; a rare presentation of stomach cancer

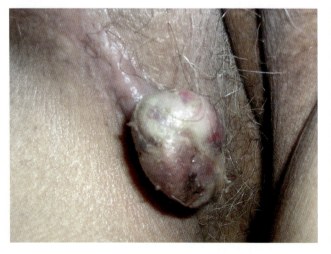

Fig. 16.22 A polypoid nodule on the inguinal area caused by the metastasis of stomach cancer

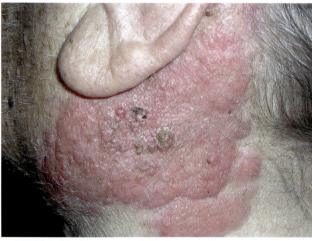

Fig. 16.25 Large erythematous indurated plaques on the neck and retroauricular area caused by metastasis of signet-ring cell carcinoma of the bowel

16.2 Carcinoma Erysipeloides

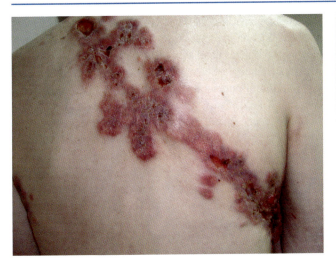

Fig. 16.26 Linearly arranged nodules and plaques representing cutaneous metastasis of the breast

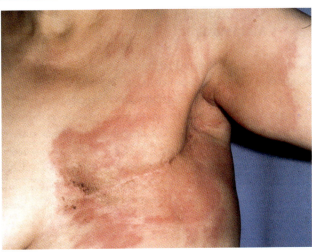

Fig. 16.29 Ill-defined large plaque of carcinoma erysipeloides on the mastectomy area and upper arm indicating the relapse of breast cancer

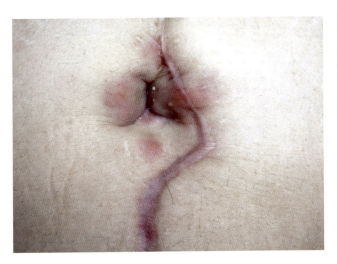

Fig. 16.27 Nodular metastasis at the umbilicus (Sister Mary Joseph nodule) in a patient with stomach cancer

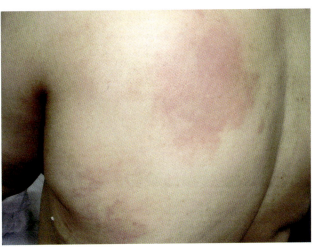

Fig. 16.30 Carcinoma erysipeloides located on the upper back of a patient with breast carcinoma. Lesions are ill-defined in this case

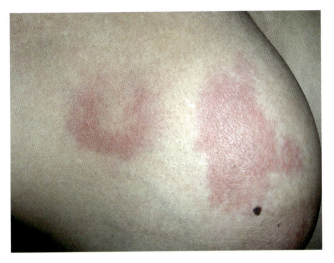

Fig. 16.28 Persistent erythematous patches on the breast. A distinctive presentation of cutaneous metastasis called carcinoma erysipeloides was caused by breast carcinoma in this case

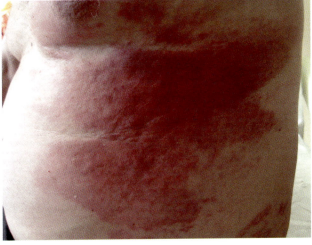

Fig. 16.31 Carcinoma erysipeloides on the lower abdomen attributable to bladder cancer

16.3 Scleroderma-like Cutaneous Metastasis

Scleroderma-like cutaneous metastasis (carcinome en cuirasse) is characterized by morphea-like indurated areas (see Figs. 16.32 and 16.33) due to fibrosis and may cause diagnostic difficulty in the early stages. Ill-defined lesions that occur mostly on the trunk may be slightly erythematous or reddish-purple. Their surface may be folded or verrucous (see Fig. 16.34). This type of cutaneous metastasis extends slowly. Overlying nodules and ulcers may also appear in the late stage. Various malignancies including the breast, head and neck, gastrointestinal (see Fig. 16.33) and genitourinary cancers (see Figs. 16.32 and 16.34) may present with scleroderma-like metastatic skin lesions. They may cause functional problems in relation to their location.

Alopecia neoplastica caused by dermal sclerosis is a rare presentation of cutaneous metastasis occurring on the scalp (see Fig. 16.35). Since it occurs via hematogenous spread, various cancers, including lung, breast, kidney, prostate, and colon, may be the underlying causes. Indurated alopecic plaques may clinically be misdiagnosed as cicatricial alopecia, pseudopelade, morphea, or trichilemmal cyst (see Fig. 4.43). Primary adenoid cystic carcinoma is another differential diagnostic challenge on the scalp.

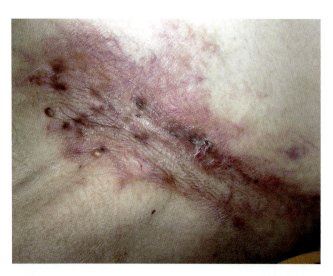

Fig. 16.32 Scleroderma-like cutaneous metastasis (carcinome en cuirasse) presenting as a morphea-like well-defined plaque on the trunk. Bladder cancer was the underlying cause

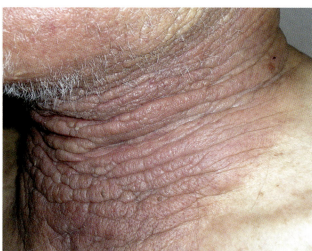

Fig. 16.34 Scleroderma-like cutaneous metastasis with a folded surface on the chest and neck of a patient with bladder cancer

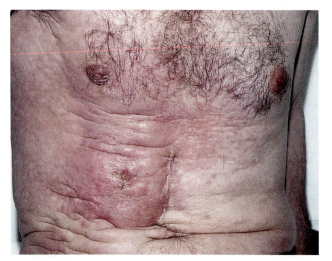

Fig. 16.33 Scleroderma-like cutaneous metastasis causing diffuse induration on a large area of the trunk in a patient with stomach cancer

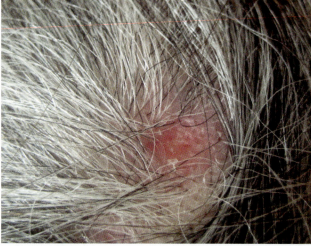

Fig. 16.35 Alopecia neoplastica seen as a localized firm plaque on the scalp of a patient with lung carcinoma. Such lesions may be confused with other causes of alopecia

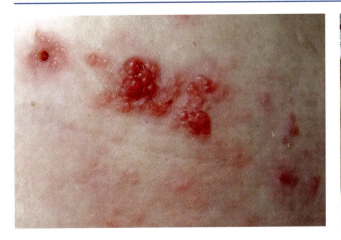

Fig. 16.36 Grouped telangiectatic papules representing carcinoma telangiectoides in a patient with breast carcinoma

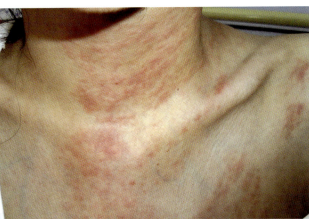

Fig. 16.38 Erythematous annular plaques: a rare presentation of cutaneous metastasis. In this case, the underlying tumor was a signet-ring cell carcinoma of gastrointestinal origin

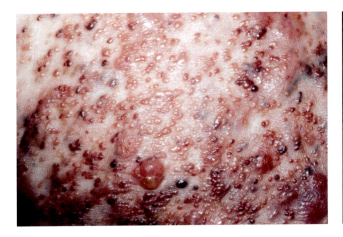

Fig. 16.37 Carcinoma telangiectoides manifesting as numerous telangiectatic papules on the trunk of a patient with breast carcinoma. Note some of them show tendency to confluence

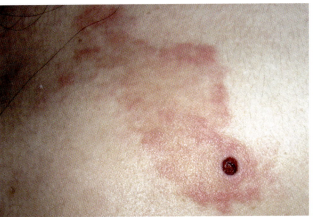

Fig. 16.39 Erythema annulare centrifugum-like cutaneous metastasis in a patient with signet-ring cell carcinoma of gastrointestinal origin (The ulceration on the erythematous plaque was caused by punch biopsy)

16.4 Telangiectatic Metastatic Carcinoma

Telangiectatic metastatic carcinoma (carcinoma telangiectoides) is another rare type of cutaneous metastasis mostly seen in patients with breast and prostate carcinomas. Violaceous telangiectatic papules (*see* Figs. 16.36 and 16.37) may resemble lesions of lymphangioma circumscriptum (pseudovesicles) (*see* Figs. 6.195 and 6.196), but metastatic papules are harder and do not contain fluid.

16.5 Erythema Annulare Centrifugum-like Metastasis

Erythema annulare centrifugum-like metastasis is an unusual presentation of cutaneous metastasis with erythematous annular persistent plaques. Signet-ring cell carcinoma of gastrointestinal origin is among the causes of this type of cutaneous metastasis (*see* Figs. 16.38 and 16.39).

As we have stated, cutaneous metastases have different clinical presentations and therefore may be difficult to diagnose in some cases. On the other hand, it should be kept in mind that various clinical types of cutaneus metastasis may occur concurrently due to the same tumor and cause a polymorphic appearance (*see* Figs. 16.40 and 16.41). A history of a primary identified malignancy supports the clinical diagnosis. However, the diagnosis should be confirmed by biopsy. A secondary tumoral infiltration resembling the primary neoplasm is mostly detected by histopathologic examination, but a specific histologic appearance determining the exact type of the tumor may not be always seen. When the origin of the primary malignancy is unknown, the role of histopathologic examination becomes more prominent. In these cases, immunohistochemistry may be helpful in determining the origin of the visceral cancer and sometimes may help to exclude a

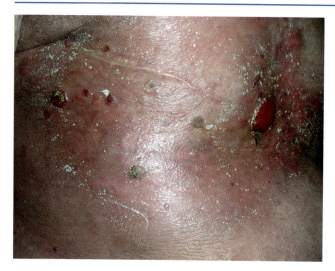

Fig. 16.40 Nodular cutaneous metastasis (ulcerated elevated nodules) overlie scleroderma-like cutaneous metastasis (diffuse induration) in a patient with breast carcinoma

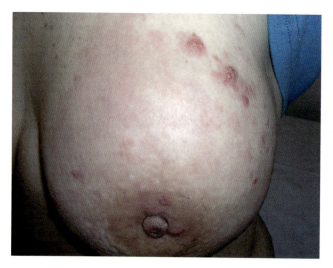

Fig. 16.41 Carcinoma erysipeloides (erythematous patches) and carcinoma telangiectodes (grouped reddish papules) seen concomitantly in a patient with breast carcinoma

primary skin tumor. On the other hand, the histopathologic features of cutaneous metastasis are related to the clinical type. Neoplastic cells may be located in the dermis, subcutis, or blood vessels, including the lymphatics. The nodular type of cutaneous metastasis shows dense infiltration of neoplastic cells in the dermis and subcutis. Tightly packed neoplastic cells are seen in superficial and deep dermal lymphatics without a marked inflammatory infiltration in carcinoma erysipeloides. While neoplastic cells are located around fibrosing collagen bundles in carcinome en cuirasse, they are found in ectatic lymphatics of the superficial dermis in carcinoma telangiectoides.

Management. Cutaneous metastasis is commonly seen together with visceral metastasis. Therefore this is usually a signal of poor prognosis in cancer. In general, systemic chemotherapy for the primary tumor is the main therapeutic option. The general health of the patient, type of skin metastasis, and location and number of lesions play an additional role in determining the treatment. Surgery or intralesional chemotherapy can be used in patients who have solitary or a few nodular lesions and are otherwise relatively in good health. Radiotherapy is another option and may be combined with excision. On the other hand, surgery is not feasible for carcinoma erysipeloides and scleroderma-like cutaneous metastasis. Even radical mastectomy may not be effective in cases of carcinoma erysipeloides with breast carcinoma. Systemic chemotherapy is the single alternative method in these types of cutaneous metastasis and for disseminated nodular lesions. However, some lesions may be therapy-resistant or may relapse after cessation of chemotherapy. Supportive care for ulceration and secondary infection may be helpful. On the other hand, there are visceral malignancies that have relatively good prognosis despite skin involvement. Cutaneous metastasis of neuroblastoma seen in infants may show spontaneous regression.

Suggested Reading

Elder DE, Elenitsas R, Johnson BL, Murphy GF, Xu X. Lever's histopathology of the skin, edn 10. Philadelphia: Lippincott Williams and Wilkins; 2008.

Lin JY, Lee Jy, Chao SC, Tsao CJ. Telangiectatic metastatic breast carcinoma preceded by en cuirasse metastatic breast carcinoma. Br J Dermatol. 2004;151:523–4.

Nava G, Greer K, Patterson J, Lin KY. Metastatic cutaneous breast carcinoma. A case report and review of the literature. Can J Plast Surg. 2009;17:25–7.

Poiares-Baptista A, De Vasconcelos AA. Cutaneous pigmented metastasis from breast carcinoma simulating malignant melanoma. Int J Dermatol. 1988;27:124–5.

Reichel M, Wheelond RG. Inflammatory carcinoma masquerading as erythema annulare centrifigum. Acta Derm Venereol. 1993;73:138–40.

Rigel DS, Robinson JK, Ross M, Friedman RJ, Corkerell CJ, Lim HW, Stockfleth HW, Kirkwood JM. Cancer of the skin. China: Saunders Elsevier; 2011.

Schwartz RA. Cutaneous metastatic disease. J Am Acad Dermatol. 1995;33:161–82.

Schwartz RA. Skin cancer: recognition and management, edn 2. Singapore: Blackwell Publishing; 2008.

Part III

Regional Differential Diagnosis of Skin Tumors

Predilection Sites of Skin Tumors

Most skin tumors have a well-known predilection for specific sites. Sometimes their subtypes also have preferential areas of involvement. Therefore, knowing the specific locations of the tumors is always helpful in clinical diagnosis.

All skin tumors are listed in this part of the atlas according to their predilections for distinct areas. The figure numbers of the tumors depicted in this book are also cited according to their locations for convenience. Some figures in the book represent rare locations of the tumors, but to make a comprehensive list of possible regional diagnostic considerations, all these rare presentations are included.

So, this practical index is planned as a guide to facilitate the clinical diagnosis of benign and malignant skin tumors depending on location. Precancerous lesions are listed among benign tumors.

SCALP (Benign)
    Seborrheic keratosis (Figs. 1.7, 1.10, 1.14, 1.15, 1.22, 1.36 and 1.59)
    Inverted follicular keratosis
    Epidermal nevus
    Nevus sebaceus (Figs. 1.93, 1.94, 1.95, 1.96, 1.97, 1.99, 1.100, 1.106, 1.108, 5.28, 5.42 and 11.11)
    Nevus comedonicus (Fig. 1.120)
    Actinic keratosis (Figs. 2.4, 2.6, 2.10 and 2.17a)
    Cutaneous horn (Fig. 2.54)
    Keratoacanthoma
    Café-au-lait macule (Fig. 3.37)
    Blue nevus (Fig. 3.62)
    Compound nevus (Fig. 3.101)
    Intradermal nevus (Figs. 3.109, 3.110 and 3.123)
    Papillomatous nevus
    Congenital melanocytic nevus (Figs. 3.144, 3.174, 3.179 and 3.181)
    Halo nevus (Fig. 3.202)
    Trichilemmal cyst (Figs. 4.40, 4.42 and 4.43)
    Proliferating trichilemmal cyst (Fig. 4.46)
    Steatocystoma multiplex
    Syringoma
    Poroid hidradenoma (Fig. 5.18)
    Tubulopapillary hidradenoma (Fig. 5.20)
    Cylindroma (Figs. 5.21, 5.22, 5.28, 5.29 and 5.33)
    Syringocystadenoma papilliferum
    Trichofolliculoma
    Trichoepithelioma (Fig. 5.39)
    Trichoblastoma (Figs. 5.42 and 5.43)
    Infantile hemangioma (Fig. 6.30)
    Pyogenic granuloma
    Senile angioma (Fig. 6.70)
    Angiolymphoid hyperplasia with eosinophilia (Fig. 6.78)
    Kimura disease
    Masson hemangioma (Fig 6.83)
    Salmon patch (Figs. 6.85 and 6.86)
    Port-wine stain (Figs. 6.87, 6.89, 6.92 and 6.93)
    Arteriovenous malformation
    Neurofibroma (Figs. 7.14 and 7.27)
    Schwannoma (Fig. 7.37)
    Perifollicular fibroma
    Juvenile hyaline fibromatosis (Fig. 8.62)
    Connective tissue nevus (Fig. 8.90)
    Infantile myofibromatosis
    Urticaria pigmentosa (Fig. 9.2)
    Diffuse cutaneous mastocytosis (Fig. 9.14)
    Isolated mastocytoma (Fig. 9.17)
    Lipoma

SCALP (Malignant)
    Basal cell carcinoma (Figs. 5.33, 11.3, 11.11, 11.12, 11.13, 11.76 and 11.77)
    Squamous cell carcinoma (Figs. 11.106 and 11.124)
    Sebaceous carcinoma (Fig. 11.160)
    Primary cutaneous adenoid cystic carcinoma
    Merkel cell carcinoma
    Lentigo maligna melanoma (Fig. 12.3)
    Superficial spreading melanoma (Fig. 12.25)
    Nodular melanoma (Figs. 12.44 and 12.46)
    Desmoplastic melanoma

Cutaneous angiosarcoma (Figs. 13.48, 13.50, 13.51, 13.52, 13.53 and 13.56)
Atypical fibroxanthoma
Mycosis fungoides (tumoral stage) (Fig. 14.31)
Folliculotropic mycosis fungoides (Figs. 14.58 and 14.60)
Sézary syndrome (Figs. 14.102 and 14.103)
Primary cutaneous follicle center lymphoma
Leukemia cutis
Langerhans cell histiocytosis (Fig. 15.2)
Juvenile xanthogranuloma (Figs. 15.20 and 15.23)
Cutaneous metastasis (Figs. 11.161, 16.12, 16.13, 16.17 and 16.35)

FOREHEAD (Benign)
Seborrheic keratosis (Figs. 1. 21, 1.38, 1.51 and 1.58)
Dermatosis papulosa nigra
Verrucal keratosis (Fig. 1.66)
Epidermal nevus (Fig. 1.76)
Nevus sebaceus (Fig. 1.87)
Actinic keratosis (Figs. 2.1, 2.7 and 2.16a)
Bowen disease (Fig. 2.21)
Cutaneous horn
Keratoacanthoma
Ephelides
Nevus of Ito (Figs. 3.45 and 3.46)
Intradermal nevus (Fig. 3.114)
Congenital melanocytic nevus
Halo nevus (Fig. 3.205)
Epidermoid cyst (Fig. 4.14)
Trichilemmal cyst (Fig. 4.41)
Steatocystoma multiplex (Figs. 4.49, 4.50 and 4.52)
Eruptive vellus hair cyst (Fig. 4.54)
Syringoma
Eccrine hidrocystoma (Fig. 5.14)
Cylindroma (Fig. 5.23)
Spiradenocylindroma (Fig. 5.27)
Syringocystadenoma papilliferum (Fig. 5.30)
Desmoplastic trichoepithelioma
Trichoepithelioma (Fig. 5.41)
Pilomatricoma
Senile sebaceous hyperplasia (Figs. 5.61 and 5.66)
Infantile hemangioma (Fig. 6.2)
Salmon patch (Fig. 6.84)
Port-wine-stain (Figs. 6.87, 6.89 and 6.107)
Angiolymphoid hyperplasia with eosinophilia
Spider angioma (Fig. 6.146)
Unilateral nevoid telangiectasia
Neurofibroma
Neurothekoma (Fig. 7.45)
Angiofibroma
Forehead plaque (tuberous sclerosis) (Figs. 8.89 and 8.90)
Milium (Fig. 11.97)

FOREHEAD (Malignant)
Basal cell carcinoma (Figs. 11.19, 11.22, 11.51, 11.62, 11.63, 11.64, 11.66, 11.68, 11.75 and 11.81)
Squamous cell carcinoma (Figs. 11.113 and 11.117)
Primary cutaneous adenoid cystic carcinoma (Fig. 11.162)
Lentigo maligna melanoma (Fig. 12.7)
Nodular melanoma
Kaposi sarcoma (AIDS-Kaposi)
Cutaneous angiosarcoma (Fig. 13.49)
Atypical fibroxanthoma
Mycosis fungoides (Figs. 14.30, 14.54 and 14.57)
Mycosis fungoides (tumoral stage) (Figs. 14.34 and 14.35)
Lymphomatoid papulosis
Primary cutaneous diffuse large B-cell lymphoma, other
Pseudolymphoma (nodular scabies)
Lymphocytoma cutis (Fig. 14.195)
Jessner's lymphocytic infiltration of the skin
Leukemia cutis (Fig. 14.216)
Langerhans cell histiocytosis (Figs. 15.3 and 15.7)

EYELID-PERIORBITAL AREA (Benign)
Seborrheic keratosis (Figs. 1.6 and 1.17)
Verrucal keratosis
Epidermal nevus (Fig. 1.76)
Nevus sebaceus (Fig. 1.87)
Actinic keratosis (Fig. 2.8)
Cutaneous horn
Keratoacanthoma (Fig. 2.73a)
Extramammary Paget disease
Lentigo simlex
Nevus of Ota (Figs. 3.45, 3.49 and 3.51)
Blue nevus (Fig. 3.66)
Intradermal nevus (Figs. 3.112 and 3.138)
Congenital melanocytic nevus (devided nevus) (Fig. 3.141)
Epidermoid cyst (Figs. 4.12 and 4.16)
Eruptive vellus hair cyst
Milium (Figs. 4.36 and 11.96)
Syringoma (Figs. 5.1, 5.2, 5.3, 5.4 and 5.5)
Apocrine hidrocystoma (Figs. 5.11 and 5.12)
Eccrine hidrocystoma (Fig. 5.36)
Eccrine acrospiroma
Spiradenoma
Cylindroma
Pilomatricoma
Trichoepithelioma (Fig. 5.40)
Trichofolliculoma
Trichilemmoma (Fig. 5.45)
Sebaceous adenoma
Infantile hemangioma (Figs. 6.16, 6.17 and 6.20)
Pyogenic granuloma (Fig. 6.53)
Senile angioma (Fig. 6.64)
Kimura disease

Salmon patch (Fig. 6.84)
Port-wine stain (Fig. 6.107)
Telangiectasia
Lymphangioma circumscriptum
Hemangioendothelioma
Palisaded encapsulated neuroma
Neurofibroma (Fig. 7.2)
Multiple mucosal neuroma (Fig. 7.39)
Angiofibroma (tuberous sclerosis) (Fig. 8.27)
Acrochordon (Fig. 8.75)
Keloid
Lipoma
Nevus lipomatosis superficialis (Fig. 10.10)

EYELID-PERIORBITAL AREA (Malignant)
Basal cell carcinoma (Figs. 11.5, 11.9, 11.10, 11.30, 11.36, 11.80 and 11.85)
Squamous cell carcinoma (Figs. 11.121 and 11.137)
Microcystic adnexal carcinoma
Sebaceous carcinoma (Fig. 11.159)
Lentigo maligna melanoma (Figs. 12.12 and 12.77)
Kaposi sarcoma (Fig. 13.38)
Cutaneous angiosarcoma (Figs. 13.49 and 13.53)
Mycosis fungoides (Figs. 14.18, 14.49 and 14.59)
Sezary syndrome (Fig. 14.99)
Lymphomatoid papulosis
Leukemia cutis (Fig. 14.216)
Langerhans cell histiocytosis (Figs. 15.3, 15.12 and 15.19)
Juvenile xanthogranuloma (Fig. 15.31)
Xanthoma disseminatum (Fig. 15.43)
Necrobiotic xanthogranuloma (Figs. 15.53 and 15.54)
Hashimoto-Pritzker disease
Sea blue histiocytosis
Cutaneous metastasis

NOSE (Benign)
Seborrheic keratosis (Figs. 1.24, 1.41 and 1.55)
Nevus sebaceus (Fig. 1.87)
Actinic keratosis (Figs. 2.3, 2.9, 2.11 and 2.13)
Cutaneous horn
Keratoacanthoma (Figs. 2.71a and 2.74)
Ephelides (Fig. 3.1)
Lentigo simplex
Nevus of Ota (Fig. 3.45)
Blue nevus (Fig. 3.68)
Intradermal nevus (Fig. 3.106)
Congenital melanocytic nevus
Spitz nevus
Epidermoid cyst (Fig. 4.7)
Milium (Figs. 4.30 and 4.34)
Trichilemmoma
Syringoma
Chondroid syringoma (Fig. 5.8)
Eccrine hydrocystoma (Figs. 5.9, 5.11 and 5.13)

Cylindroma
Trichofolliculoma
Trichoepithelioma (Figs. 5.40 and 5.41)
Desmoplastic trichoepithelioma
Senile sebaceous hyperplasia (Fig. 5.58)
Sebaceous adenoma (Figs. 5.62 and 5.63)
Infantile hemangioma (Figs. 6.18 and 6.19)
Pyogenic granuloma (Figs. 6.45 and 6.48)
Senile angioma
Salmon patch
Port-wine stain (Figs. 6.108, 6.111 and 6.121)
Telangiectasia (Fig. 6.128)
Spider angioma (Fig. 6.148)
Venous lake (Fig. 6.187)
Spindle cell hemangioendothelioma
Arteriovenous malformation
Neurofibroma
Schwannoma
Palisaded encapsulated neuroma
Fibrous papule of the nose (Figs. 8.16, 8.17, 8.18 and 8.19)
Angiofibroma (tuberous sclerosis) (Figs. 8.22, 8.24 and 8.26)
Perifollicular fibroma (Figs. 8.39, 8.40 and 8.42)
Juvenile hyaline fibromatosis
Keloid

NOSE (Malignant)
Malignant pilomatricoma (Fig. 5.54)
Basal cell carcinoma (Figs. 11.14, 11.24, 11.25, 11.26, 11.27, 11.31, 11.33, 11.34, 11.38, 11.40, 11.47, 11.49, 11.59 and 11.78)
Squamous cell carcinoma (Figs. 11.114, 11.118, 11.119 and 11.136)
Microcystic adnexal carcinoma
Sebaceous carcinoma
Lentigo maligna melanoma
Nodular melanoma
Desmoplastic melanoma
Kaposi sarcoma (Fig. 13.27)
Cutaneous angiosarcoma
Mycosis fungoides (Fig. 14.35)
Lymphomatoid papulosis
Extranodal NK/T-cell lymphoma, nasal type (Figs. 14.159 and 14.160)
Primary cutaneous marginal zone lymphoma (Fig. 14.170)
Lymphocytoma cutis (Figs. 14.192, 14.193, 14.196, 14.198, 14.199, 14.200 and 14.201a)
Primary cutaneous CD4+ small/medium (pleomorphic) T-cell lymphoma
Leukemia cutis
Juvenile xanthogranuloma
Xanthoma disseminatum (Fig. 15.50)
Rosai-Dorfmann disease
Cutaneous metastasis
Olfactory neuroblastoma

EAR (Benign)
Seborrheic keratosis (Figs. 1.18 and 1.20)
Nevus sebaceus (Figs. 1.103, 1.104 and 1.109)
Actinic keratosis (Fig. 2.12)
Cutaneous horn (Fig. 2.59)
Keratoacanthoma (Fig. 2.68)
Extramammary Paget disease
Lentigo simplex (Fig. 3.7)
Nevus of Ota (Fig. 3.47)
Blue nevus
Intradermal nevus (Figs. 3.119 and 3.122)
Spitz nevus
Reed nevus (Fig. 3.220)
Deep penetrating nevus (Fig. 3.224)
Congenital melanocytic nevus
Epidermoid cyst (Figs. 4.6, 4.11 and 4.25)
Milium (Figs. 4.32, 4.37, 4.38 and 4.39)
Eruptive vellus hair cyst
Auricular pseudocyst (Fig. 4.66)
Preauricular cyst (Figs. 4.67 and 4.68)
Cylindroma (Fig. 5.21)
Syringocystadenoma papilliferum (Fig. 5.31)
Trichilemmoma (Fig. 5.46)
Trichoepithelioma
Pilomatricoma
Senile sebaceous hyperplasia (Fig. 5.59)
Salmon patch
Infantile hemangioma (Fig. 6.30)
Diffuse neonatal hemangiomatosis (Figs. 6.33 and 6.37a)
Pyogenic granuloma
Angiolymphoid hyperplasia with eosinophilia (Figs. 6.76, 6.77, 6.79 and 6.82a)
Port-wine stain (Figs. 6.89, 6.90 and 6.102)
Telangiectasia (Fig. 6.133)
Spider angioma
Osler-Weber-Rendu syndrome (Fig. 6.141)
Solitary angiokeratoma (Fig. 6.155)
Arteriovenous malformation (Figs. 6.223, 6.224 and 6.225)
Neurofibroma
Cutaneous neuroma
Angiofibroma (Figs. 8.29 and 8.30)
Perifollicular fibroma (Figs. 8.39, 8.40 and 8.42)
Juvenile hyaline fibromatosis (Fig. 8.60)
Keloid (Figs. 8.102, 8.103, 8.104 and 8.105)
Weathering nodules of the ear (Fig. 8.111)
Angiomyolipoma (Fig. 10.8)

EAR (Malignant)
Basal cell carcinoma (Figs. 11.37, 11.48, 11.52 and 11.74)
Squamous cell carcinoma (Figs. 11.105, 11.125, 11.126 and 11.152)
Lentigo maligna melanoma (Fig. 12.10)
Nodular melanoma (Fig. 12.49)
Kaposi sarcoma (Fig. 13.8)
Cutaneous angiosarcoma (Fig. 13.56a)
Atypical fibroxanthoma (Fig. 13.64)
Mycosis fungoides (Figs. 14.8 and 14.53)
Juvenile xanthogranuloma

CHEEK/CHIN (Benign)
Seborrheic keratosis (Figs. 1.2, 1.3, 1.21, 1.34, 1.35 and 1.54)
Dermatosis papulosa nigra (Fig. 1.59)
Inverted follicular keratosis
Verrucal keratosis (Fig. 1.67)
Epidermal nevus (Fig. 1.75)
Nevus sebaceus (Figs. 1.98, 1.101, 1.102 and 1.105)
Nevus comedonicus
Actinic keratosis (Figs. 2.2, 2.5, 2.10 and 11.98)
Cutaneous horn (Fig. 2.55)
Keratoacanthoma (Figs. 2.64 and 2.66)
Ephelides (Fig. 3.1)
Lentigo simplex (Fig. 3.10)
Segmental lentiginosis (Fig. 3.15)
Lentigines (xeroderma pigmentosum) (Fig. 3.28)
Blue nevus (Fig. 3.63)
Intradermal nevus (Figs. 3.107 and 3.108)
Congenital melanocytic nevus (Fig. 3.157)
Spitz nevus
Reed nevus (Fig. 3.222)
Halo nevus
Deep penetrating nevus
Epidermoid cyst (Figs. 4.1, 4.2 and 4.27)
Milium (Fig. 4.35)
Steatocystoma multiplex (Fig. 4.55)
Syringoma (Fig. 5.2)
Eccrine hidrocystoma (Figs. 5.9, 5.10 and 5.11)
Tubulopapillary hidradenoma (Fig. 5.19)
Syringocystadenoma papilliferum
Apocrine hydrocystoma
Trichoepithelioma (Figs. 5.38 and 5.41)
Trichofolliculoma
Pilomatricoma (Figs. 5.47, 5.48 and 5.51)
Trichilemmoma
Senile sebaceous hyperplasia (Figs. 5.56, 5.57 and 5.60)
Infantile hemangioma (Figs. 6.1, 6.6, 6.7, 6.10, 6.12, 6.16, 6.17 and 6.31a)
Pyogenic granuloma (Fig. 6.48)
Port-wine stain (Figs. 6.89, 6.90, 6.100, 6.101, 6.108 and 6.111)
Telangiectasia (Fig. 6.129)
Ataxia-telangiectasia (Fig. 6.136)
Osler-Weber-Rendu syndrome (Fig. 6.140)
Unilateral nevoid telangiectasia (Fig. 6.142)
Spider angioma (Fig. 6.147)
Neurofibroma
Palisaded encapsulated neuroma (Fig. 7.41)
Fibrous papule of the nose (Fig. 8.20)
Angiofibroma (tuberous sclerosis) (Figs. 8.23, 8.24, 8.25 and 8.28)

Perifollicular fibroma (Fig. 8.42)
Lipoma (Fig. 10.2)

CHEEK/CHIN (Malignant)
Basal cell carcinoma (Figs. 1.54, 11.1, 11.2, 11.18, 11.20, 11.21, 11.22, 11.23, 11.71 and 11.93)
Squamous cell carcinoma (Figs. 11.98, 11.103, 11.116 and 11.123)
Primary cutaneous adenoid cystic carcinoma
Microcystic adnexal carcinoma
Eccrine porocarcinoma
Sebaceous carcinoma
Merkel cell carcinoma
Lentigo maligna melanoma (Figs. 12.8, 12.9, 12.11 and 12.13)
Nodular melanoma (Fig. 12.42)
Amelanotic melanoma (Fig. 12.56)
Desmoplastic melanoma (Fig. 12.60)
Kaposi sarcoma
Cutaneous angiosarcoma (Figs. 13.49, 13.53 and 13.56c)
Atypical fibroxanthoma (Fig. 13.63)
Mycosis fungoides (Figs. 14.50 and 14.83)
Lymphomatoid papulosis (Figs. 14.118 and 14.140a)
Primary cutaneous anaplastic large cell lymphoma (Fig. 14.148)
Primary cutaneous CD8+ aggressive epidermotropic cytotoxic T-cell lymphoma (Fig. 14.156)
Extranodal NK/T-cell lymphoma, nasal type (Fig. 14.160a)
Primary cutaneous CD4+ small medium pleomorphic T-cell lymphoma
Primary cutaneous marginal zone lymphoma (Figs. 14.166a and 14.171)
Primary cutaneous follicle center lymphoma
Pseudolymphoma (nodular scabies)
Lymphocytoma cutis (Figs. 14.193, 14.197 and 14.202a)
Jessner's lymphocytic infiltration of the skin (Fig. 14.205)
Lupus tumidus (Fig. 14.210)
Leukemia cutis (Fig. 14.216a)
Cutaneous infiltration of multiple myeloma (Fig. 14.226)
Langerhans cell histiocytosis
Juvenile xanthogranuloma (Figs. 15.27, 15.29 and 15.30)
Benign cephalic histiocytosis (Figs. 15.34 and 15.37)
Generalized eruptive histiocytosis (Fig. 15.38)
Reticulohistiocytic granuloma (Fig. 15.50)
Xanthoma disseminatum
Necrobiotic xanthogranuloma (Fig. 15.54)
Indeterminate cell histiocytosis (Fig. 15.56)
Cutaneous metastasis (Figs. 16.4 and 16.24)

ORAL CAVITY (Benign)
White sponge nevus (Figs. 1.136, 1.137, 1.138 and 1.139)
Leukoplakia (Figs. 2.35, 2.36, 2.37, 2.38, 2.39, 2.40, 2.41, 2.42, 2.43, 2.44, 2.45, 2.46, 2.47, 2.48 and 11.101)
Actinic cheilitis (Figs. 2.49, 2.50, 2.51, 2.52, 2.53 and 11.100)
Keratoacanthoma
Labial melanotic macule (Figs. 3.4 and 3.5)
Ephelides
Lentigo simplex (Figs. 3.11 and 3.12)
Nevus of Ota (Fig. 3.52)
Blue nevus (Fig. 3.67)
Melanocytic nevus (Fig. 3.135)
Mucocele (Figs. 4.64 and 4.65)
Fordyce spots (Figs. 5.64, 5.65 and 5.66)
Infantile hemangioma (Figs. 6.13, 6.14, 6.16, 6.24 and 6.25)
Pyogenic granuloma (Figs. 6.43, 6.44, 6.52, 6.54 and 6.55)
Port-wine stain (Figs. 6.95, 6.103, 6.109, 6.108, 6.106 and 6.110)
Telangiectasia (Figs. 6.130, 6.131 and 6.165)
Osler-Weber-Rendu syndrome (Figs. 6.138 and 6.139)
Venous lake (Figs. 6.179, 6.181, 6.184 and 6.185)
Lymphangioma circumscriptum (Fig. 6.203)
Neurofibroma (Figs. 7.19, 7.20 and 7.32)
Multiple mucosal neuroma (Fig. 7.38)
Granular cell tumor (Fig. 7.46)
Gingival fibromatosis (Fig. 8.21)
Oral fibroma (Figs. 8.45, 8.46 and 8.47)
Juvenile hyalin fibromatosis (Fig. 8.62)

ORAL CAVITY (Malignant)
Basal cell carcinoma (secondary infiltration) (Fig. 11.7)
Squamous cell carcinoma (Figs. 2.40, 11.100, 11.101, 11.102, 11.127, 11.128, 11.129, 11.130, 11.131, 11.132, 11.133, 11.134 and 11.135)
Oral florid papillomatosis (Figs. 11.153 and 11.154)
Adenoid cystic carcinoma
Malignant melanoma (Figs. 12.51 and 12.52)
Kaposi sarcoma (Figs. 13.39, 13.40 and 13.41)
Mycosis fungoides (tumoral stage)
Lymphomatoid papulosis (Fig. 14.134)
Extranodal NK/T-cell lymphoma, nasal type (Fig. 14.161)
Langerhans cell histiocytosis (Fig. 15.15)
Xanthoma disseminatum (Fig. 15.47)
Cutaneous metastasis (Fig. 16.6)

NECK (Benign)
Seborrheic keratosis (Fig. 1.3)
Verrucal keratosis
Epidermal nevus (Fig. 1.84)
Nevus sebaceus
Nevus comedonicus (Fig. 1.120)
Actinic keratosis
Keratoacanthoma
Lentigo simplex (Peutz-Jeghers syndrome)
Lentigo simplex (xeroderma pigmentosum) (Fig. 3.29)

Café-au-lait macule (Fig. 3.33)
Nevus of Ito (Figs. 3.53 and 3.55)
Blue nevus
Intradermal nevus (Fig. 3.115)
Congenital melanocytic nevus (Fig. 3.173)
Halo nevus (Fig. 3.210)
Spitz nevus
Nevus spilus (Fig. 3.228)
Epidermoid cyst (Figs. 4.20 and 4.24a)
Steatocystoma multiplex
Syringoma
Eccrine hidrocystoma
Trichoepithelioma
Trichoblastoma
Trichofolliculoma
Trichilemmoma
Senile sebaceous hyperplasia
Infantile hemangioma (Figs. 6.19 and 6.30a)
Pyogenic granuloma (Fig. 6.47)
Tufted angioma
Kimura disease
Salmon patch
Port-wine stain (Figs. 6.92, 6.93 and 6.104)
Maffucci syndrome (Fig. 6.178)
Spider angioma
Venous lake (Fig. 6.183)
Neurofibroma (Figs. 7.7 and 7.25)
Perifollicular fibroma (Fig. 8.44)
Acrochordon (Figs. 8.44, 8.67, 8.68, 8.69 and 8.82)
Urticaria pigmentosa (Fig. 9.4)
Adult mastocytosis (Fig. 9.27)
Lipoma

NECK (Malignant)
Basal cell carcinoma (Figs. 11.82 and 11.86)
Squamous cell carcinoma
Merkel cell carcinoma
Lentigo maligna melanoma (Fig. 12.5)
Nodular melanoma (Fig. 12.41)
Desmoplastic melanoma
Kaposi sarcoma
Cutaneous angiosarcoma
Dermatofibrosarcoma protuberans
Atypical fibroxanthoma
Mycosis fungoides (Figs. 14.16 and 14.22)
Lymphomatoid papulosis (Fig. 14.127)
Primary cutaneous CD8+ aggressive epidermotropic cytotoxic T-cell lymphoma (Fig. 14.156)
Primary cutaneous CD4+ small/medium T-cell lymphoma
Primary cutaneous follicle center lymphoma
Jessner lymphocytic infiltration of the skin (Figs. 14.209 and 14.211a)

Leukemia cutis
Cutaneous Hodgkin lymphoma (Fig. 14.218)
Juvenile xanthogranuloma (Fig. 15.27)
Benign cephalic histiocytosis (Fig. 15.35)
Necrobiotic xanthogranuloma (Fig. 15.55)
Cutaneous metastasis (Figs. 16.8, 16.9, 16.25, 16.34 and 16.38)

TRUNK and BUTTOCKS (Benign)
Seborrheic keratosis (Figs. 1.9, 1.11, 1.25, 1.43, 1.48, 1.49, 1.50, 1.53 and 1.89)
Verrucal keratosis
Nevus comedonicus (Figs. 1.123 and 1.124)
Becker nevus (Figs. 1.125, 1.126, 1.127, 1.128, 1.129, 1.130 and 1.131)
Epidermal nevus (Figs. 1.73, 1.74, 1.81, 1.82, 1.83, 1.84 and 1.85)
Bowen disease (Figs. 2.18, 2.20 and 11.99)
PUVA lentigines (Figs. 2.18 and 3.25)
Chronic radiodermatitis (Figs. 2.62 and 2.63)
Ephelides (Fig. 3.2)
Café-au-lait macule (Figs. 3.34 and 7.1)
Lentigo simplex (Fig. 3.9)
Actinic lentigo (Figs. 3.17, 3.20, 3.21 and 3.22)
Mongolian spot (Figs. 3.40 and 3.44)
Congenital dermal melanocytosis (Fig. 3.56)
Nevus of Ito (Figs. 3.53 and 3.54)
Blue nevus (Figs. 3.76 and 3.79)
Junctional nevus (Fig. 3.82)
Compound nevus (Figs. 3.94, 3.95, 3.96, 3.97, 3.98, 3.99 and 3.100)
Papillomatous nevus (Figs. 3.126, 3.128 and 3.130)
Intradermal nevus (Fig. 3.129)
Agminated nevus (Figs. 3.133 and 3.134)
Congenital melanocytic nevus (Figs. 3.140, 3.153, 3.158, 3.166, 3.167, 3.168, 3.169, 3.170, 3.171, 3.172 and 3.180)
Dysplastic nevus (Figs. 3.190, 3.197 and 3.200)
Halo nevus (Figs. 3.203, 3.207 and 3.209)
Spitz nevus (Fig. 3.215 and 3.216)
Nevus spilus (Figs. 3.227 and 3.229)
Meyerson nevus (Figs. 3.232 and 3.233a)
Pseudomelanoma (Fig. 3.237)
Epidermoid cyst (Figs. 4.3, 4.15, 4.17, 4.19, 4.21)
Trichilemmal cyst (Fig. 4.44)
Steatocystoma multiplex (Figs. 4.47 and 4.51)
Eruptive vellus hair cyst
Syringoma (eruptive type) (Figs. 5.6 and 5.7)
Chondroid syringoma
Tubulopapillary hidradenoma
Cylindroma (Fig. 5.24)
Spiradenoma (Fig. 5.25)

Syringocystadenoma papilliferum (Fig. 5.32)
Apocrine hidrocystoma (Fig. 5.35)
Trichoepithelioma
Pilomatricoma (Fig. 5.52)
Leiomyoma (Figs. 5.59 and 5.72)
Congenital smooth muscle hamartoma
Infantile hemangioma (Figs. 6.4a, 6.23 and 6.28)
Diffuse neonatal angiomatosis (Fig. 6.32)
Congenital hemangioma (Figs. 6.39 and 6.40)
Tufted angioma
Pyogenic granuloma (Figs. 6.47, 6.51 and 6.62)
Senile angioma (Figs. 6.63, 6.65, 6.66, 6.67, 6.68 and 6.69)
Targetoid hemosiderotic hemangioma (Fig. 6.71)
Glomeruloid hemangioma (Fig. 6.72)
Port-wine stain (Figs. 6.91, 6.96, 6.97, 6.98, 6.111, 6.117, 6.124 and 6.127)
Generalized essential telangiectasia (Fig. 6.143)
Unilateral nevoid telangiectasia
Nevus anemicus (Fig. 6.149)
Solitary angiokeratoma (Figs. 6.152, 6.157, 6.158a, 6.167, 6.168, 6.169 and 6.170)
Fabry disease
Venous lake (Fig. 6.186)
Spider angioma
Blue rubber bleb nevus syndrome
Lymphangioma circumscriptum (Figs. 6.195, 6.196, 6.197, 6.204a and 6.206)
Cystic higroma (Fig. 6.207)
Neurofibroma (Figs. 7.1, 7.3, 7.5, 7.6, 7.8, 7.9, 7.10, 7.11, 7.18 and 7.23)
Schwannoma (Fig. 7.35)
Cutaneous neuroma (Fig. 7.40)
Dermatofibroma (Figs. 8.6 and 8.14)
Epitheliod cell histiocytoma
Perifollicular fibroma (Figs. 8.43 and 8.44)
Acrochordon (Figs. 8.71, 8.72, 8.73, 8.74, 8.76, 8.77, 8.80 and 8.81)
Connective tissue nevus (Figs. 8.83, 8.86, 8.91, 8.94 and 8.95)
Papular elastorrhexis (Fig. 8.96)
Keloid (Figs. 8.97 and 8.100)
Juvenile hyaline fibromatosis
Urticaria pigmentosa (Figs. 9.1, 9.3 and 9.5)
Diffuse cutaneous mastocytosis (Figs. 9.10 and 9.13)
Isolated mastocytoma (Figs. 9.16, 9.19 and 9.22)
Adult mastocytosis (Figs. 9.23 and 9.28)
Telangiectasia macularis eruptiva perstans
Lipoma
Nevus lipomatosis superficialis (Figs. 10.9, 10.11 and 10.12)

TRUNK and BUTTOCKS (Malignant)
Basal cell carcinoma (Figs. 11.16, 11.17, 11.29, 11.32, 11.54, 11.55, 11.56, 11.57, 11.58, 11.59, 11.60, 11.61, 11.82, 11.83, 11.86 and 11.87)
Squamous cell carcinoma (Fig. 11.99)
Hidradenocarcinoma (Figs. 11.163 and 11.164)
Eccrine porocarcinoma (Fig. 11.165)
Merkel cell carcinoma
Superficial spreading melanoma (Figs. 12.1, 12.16, 12.17, 12.18, 12.19, 12.20, 12.21, 12.22, 12.23, 12.26 and 12.27)
Nodular melanoma (Figs. 12.45, 12.47 and 12.48)
Amelanotic melanoma (Figs. 12.55, 12.57 and 12.59)
Malignant blue nevus (Fig. 12.62)
Metastatic melanoma (Figs. 12.68, 12.69, 12.70, 12.71, 12.72, 12.73, 12.74, 12.80 and 12.82)
Kaposi sarcoma (Figs. 13.31, 13.22, 13.35, 13.42a, 13.45a, 13.58, 13.60 and 13.61)
Dermatofibrosarcoma protuberans (Fig. 13.59)
Liposarcoma
Malignant fibrous histiocytoma (Fig. 13.65)
Leiomyosarcoma (Fig. 13.70)
Mycosis fungoides (patch, plaque stage) (Figs. 14.1, 14.3, 14.4, 14.6, 14.10, 14.15, 14.21, 14.51, 14.65 and 14.71)
Mycosis fungoides (tumoral stage) (Figs. 14.27, 14.29 and 14.43)
Digitate parapsoriasis (Figs. 14.45, 14.46, 14.47 and 14.48)
Poikiloderma vasculare atrophicans (Figs. 14.75 and 14.76)
Lymphomatoid papulosis (Figs. 14.117, 14.129, 14.130, 14.138 and 14.139)
Primary cutaneous anaplastic large cell lymphoma (Figs. 14.141, 14.142 and 14.148c)
Primary cutaneous CD4+ small/medium pleomorphic T-cell lymphoma
Primary cutaneous CD8+ aggressive epidermotropic cytotoxic T-cell lymphoma (Figs. 14.151 and 14.152)
Extranodal NK/T-cell lymphoma (Figs. 14.162 and 14.163)
Primary cutaneous marginal zone lymphoma (Figs. 14.167 and 14.169)
Primary cutaneous follicle center lymphoma (Figs. 14.172, 14.173, 14.174, 14.175 and 14.176a)
Primary cutaneous diffuse large B cell lymphoma, other (Fig. 14.179a)
Intravascular lymphoma (Figs. 14.180, 14.181, 14.182, 14.183 and 14.184)
Lymphocytoma cutis (Figs. 14.191 and 14.194)
Jessner's lymphocytic infiltration of the skin (Figs. 14.208 and 14.212a)

Leukemia cutis (Figs. 14.213, 14.214 and 14.215)
Cutaneous Hodgkin lymphoma (Fig. 14.219)
Cutaneous infiltration of non-Hodgkin lymphomas (Figs. 14.221, 14.223 and 14.224)
Cutaneous infiltration of multiple myeloma (Fig. 14.225)
Langerhans cell histiocytosis (Figs. 15.1, 15.5, 15.6, 15.8, 15.9 and 15.18)
Juvenile xanthogranuloma (Figs. 15.21, 15.22, 15.25, 15.26, 15.28, 15.32a and 15.33)
Benign cephalic histiocytosis (Fig. 15.36)
Generalized eruptive histiocytosis (Fig. 15.38)
Xanthoma disseminatum
Multicentric reticulohistiocytosis (Fig. 15.51)
Carcinoma erysipeloides (Figs. 16.28, 16.29, 16.30, 16.31 and 16.32)
Cutaneous metastasis (Figs. 16.2, 16.7, 16.10, 16.14, 16.26, 16.38 and 16.40)

NIPPLE/AREOLA (Benign)
Seborrheic keratosis (Fig. 1.37)
Nevoid hyperkeratosis of the nipple and areola (Figs. 1.61 and 1.64)
Paget disease of the breast (Figs. 2.75, 2.76, 2.77 and 2.78)
Epidermoid cyst (Figs. 4.4 and 4.23)
Erosive adenomatosis of the nipple (Fig. 5.37)
Montgomery tubercules (Fig. 5.67)
Dartoic leiomyoma
Neurofibroma (Figs. 7.15 and 7.16)
Acrochordon (Figs. 8.71 and 8.72)

NIPPLE/AREOLA (Malignant)
Cutaneous metastasis (Fig. 16.41)

UMBILICUS (Benign)
Seborrheic keratosis
Congenital melanocytic nevus
Pyogenic granuloma

UMBILICUS (Malignant)
Sister Marry Joseph nodule (Fig. 16.27)

ANOGENITAL AREA (Benign)
Seborrheic keratosis
Cutaneous horn
Bowen disease (Figs. 2.26, 2.29a, 2.30, 2.31 and 2.33a)
Bowenoid papulosis (Figs. 2.27 and 2.28)
Erytroplasia of Queyrat (Fig. 2.34)
Extramammary Paget disease (Figs. 2.79 and 2.80)
Penile melanotic macule
Vulvar melanosis (Fig. 3.6)
Lentigo simplex (Figs. 3.8 and 3.14)
Compound nevus (Fig. 3.136)
Congenital melanocytic nevus (Figs. 3.146 and 3.172)
Blue nevus
Epidermoid cyst (Fig. 4.10)
Median raphe cyst (Fig. 4.69)
Syringoma
Syringocystadenoma papilliferum
Dartoic leiomyoma
Montgomery tubercules (Fig. 5.68)
Infantile hemangioma (Figs. 6.23 and 6.27)
Port-wine stain (Fig. 6.114)
Fordyce angiokeratoma (Figs. 6.159, 6.160 and 6.161)
Lymphangioma circumscriptum (Figs. 6.199, 6.200, 6.201 and 6.205)
Lymphangiectasia (Fig. 6.222)
Peyronie disease

ANOGENITAL AREA (Malignant)
Basal cell carcinoma (Figs. 11.6 and 11.73)
Squamous cell carcinoma (Figs. 11.107, 11.138, 11.139, 11.140, 11.141 and 11.143)
Buschke-Löwenstein tumor (Figs. 11.155 and 11.158)
Malignant melanoma (Figs. 12.53 and 12.54)
Kaposi sarcoma (Fig. 13.9)
Leiomyosarcoma (Fig. 13.70)
Epitheliod sarcoma
Pseudolymphoma (nodular scabies) (Fig. 14.190)
Langerhans cell histiocytosis (Figs. 15.10 and 15.16)
Xanthoma disseminatum
Cutaneous metastasis (Figs. 16.3, 16.18, 16.20 and 16.23)

ARM (Benign)
Seborrheic keratosis
Verrucal keratosis
Epidermal nevus (Figs. 1.85 and 1.91)
ILVEN (Fig. 1.86)
Nevus comedonicus
Becker nevus (Figs. 1.125, 1.133, 1.134 and 1.135)
Smooth nuscle hamartoma (Fig. 1.135)
Bowen disease
Cutaneous horn (Figs. 2.56 and 2.57)
Keratoacanthoma
Ephelides (Fig. 3.3)
PUVA lentigines (Fig. 3.23)
Lentigines (xeroderma pigmentosum) (Figs. 3.27 and 12.4)
Ectopic Mongolian spot (Fig. 3.42)
Nevus of Ito (Fig. 3.53)
Congenital dermal melanocytosis (Fig. 3.56)
Acquired dermal melanocytosis (Fig. 3.60)
Blue nevus (Fig. 3.72)
Actinic lentigo
Café-au-lait macule

Compound nevus
Junctional nevus (Fig. 3.81)
Dysplastic nevus
Spitz nevus
Reed nevus
Congenital melanocytic nevus (Figs. 3.156, 3.165, 3.170 and 3.175)
Epidermolysis bullosa nevus (Fig. 3.224)
Nevus spilus (Fig. 3.226)
Meyerson nevus (Fig. 3.231)
Epidermoid cyst (Fig. 4.13)
Trichilemmal cyst (Fig. 4.45)
Eruptive vellus hair cyst (Figs. 4.53 and 4.56)
Chondroid syringoma
Tubulopapillary hidradenoma
Spiradenoma
Syringocystadenoma papilliferum
Pilomatricoma (Figs. 5.50 and 5.53)
Leiomyoma
Infantile hemangioma (Fig. 6.15)
Senile angioma
Glomeruloid hemangioma (Fig. 6.73)
Angiolymphoid hyperplasia with eosinophilia (Fig. 6.81)
Port-wine-stain (Figs. 6.96, 6.97, 6.98, 6.99, 6.100, 6.101, 6.102, 6.103, 6.104, 6.105, 6.106, 6.107, 6.108, 6.109, 6.110, 6.111, 6.112, 6.113, 6.114, 6.115, 6.116, 6.117, 6.118, 6.119 and 6.120)
Generalized essential telangiectasia
Angioma serpiginosum
Spider angioma
Solitary angiokeratoma (Figs. 6.144 and 6.153)
Angiokeratoma circumscriptum
Angiokeratoma Mibelli (Fig. 6.162)
Blue rubber bleb nevus syndrome (Fig. 6.174)
Maffucci syndrome (Fig. 6.176b)
Lymphangioma circumscriptum
Schwannoma
Neurofibroma (Figs. 7.24, 7.28 and 7.33)
Dermatofibroma (Figs. 8.4, 8.5 and 8.6)
Acquired digital fibrokeratoma (Fig. 8.50)
Epitheliod cell histiocytoma (Fig. 8.58)
Urticaria pigmentosa (Fig. 9.5)
Diffuse cutaneous mastocytosis
Isolated mastocytoma (Fig. 9.17)
Lipoma (Figs. 10.2 and 10.3)

ARM (Malignant)
Basal cell carcinoma (Fig. 11.42)
Squamous cell carcinoma (Figs. 11.104, 11.112 and 11.115)
Merkel cell carcinoma
Lentigo maligna melanoma (Figs. 12.4 and 12.6)
Superficial spreading melanoma
Nodular melanoma (Fig. 12.43)
Kaposi sarcoma (Figs. 13.23 and 13.31)
Cutaneous angiosarcoma (Figs. 13.54 and 13.55)
Dermatofibrosarcoma protuberans (Fig. 13.62)
Fibrosarcoma
Epithelioid sarcoma (Fig. 13.72)
Mycosis fungoides (Figs. 14.36, 14.44, 14.69 and 14.82)
Lymphomatoid papulosis (Figs. 14.132, 14.137 and 14.140d)
Primary cutaneous anaplastic large cell lymphoma (Figs. 14.144, 14.146 and 14.150a)
Primary cutaneous CD8+ aggressive epidermotropic cytotoxic T-cell lymphoma (Figs. 14.153 and 14.158a)
Primary cutaneous marginal zone lymphoma
Blastic plasmacytoid dendritic cell neoplasm (Fig. 14.186)
Lymphocytoma cutis (Fig. 14.203a)
Langerhans cell histiocytosis (Fig. 15.4)
Juvenile xanthogranuloma (Fig. 15.30)
Generalized eruptive histiocytosis (Fig. 15.38)
Xanthoma disseminatum (Fig. 15.42)
Cutaneous metastasis (Fig. 16.16)

HAND (Benign)
Seborrheic keratosis (flat type) (Figs. 1.40 and 1.44)
Epidermal nevus
Becker nevus (Fig. 1.132)
Actinic keratosis (Figs. 2.14 and 2.15)
Bowen's disease (Figs. 2.22 and 2.23)
Chronic radiodermatitis (Fig. 2.61)
Keratoacanthoma (Figs. 2.67, 2.69 and 2.70)
Actinic lentigo (Figs. 3.18 and 3.19)
Blue nevus (Fig. 3.71)
Congenital melanocytic nevus (Figs. 3.145 and 3.162)
Spitz nevus (Fig. 3.218)
Epidermoid cyst (Fig. 4.9)
Digital mucous cyst
Poroma
Infantile hemangioma (Figs. 6.3 and 6.9)
Pyogenic granuloma (Figs. 6.41, 6.46 and 6.56)
Osler-Weber-Rendu syndrome
Angiolymphoid hyperplasia with eosinophilia (Fig. 6.80)
Port-wine stain (Figs. 6.96, 6.105 and 6.120)
Glomeruloid hemangioma
Glomus tumor
Angioma serpiginosum (Fig. 6.145)
Angiokeratoma Mibelli
Blue rubber bleb nevus syndrome (Fig. 6.173)
Maffucci syndrome (Fig. 6.176b)
Angioma serpiginosum
Glomulovenous malformation
Neurofibroma (Figs. 7.4 and 7.7)
Amputation neuroma (Figs. 7.43 and 7.44)

Neurothekeoma
Dermatofibroma (Fig. 8.3)
Acquired digital fibrokeratoma (Figs. 8.48 and 8.56)
Infantile digital fibromatosis (Fig. 8.59a)
Knuckle pads (Fig. 8.66)
Calcifieng aponeurotic fibroma
Connective tissue nevus (Fig. 8.88)
Giant cell tumor of the tendon sheath (Figs. 8.109 and 8.110)
Isolated mastocytoma (Fig. 9.15)
Adult mastocytosis (Fig. 9.25)

HAND (Malignant)
Basal cell carcinoma (Figs. 11.4 and 11.43)
Squamous cell carcinoma (Figs. 11.111, 11.220, 11.142, 11.144, 11.145 and 11.150)
Merkel cell carcinoma (Fig. 11.167)
Lentigo maligna melanoma
Acral lentiginous melanoma
Nodular melanoma
Kaposi sarcoma (Figs. 13.12, 13.16 and 13.22)
Atypical fibroxanthoma
Fibrosarcoma
Epitheliod sarcoma
Mycosis fungoides (Fig. 14.20)
Lymphomatoid papulosis (Figs. 14.120, 14.124 and 14.137)
Juvenile xanthogranuloma (Fig. 15.24)
Xanthoma disseminatum (Fig. 15.46)
Multicentric reticulohistiocytosis

LEG (Benign)
Seborrheic keratosis
Stucco keratosis (Fig. 1.60)
Clear cell acanthoma
Epidermal nevus
ILVEN
Becker nevus
Bowen disease (Fig. 2.11)
Keratoacanthoma (Fig. 2.65)
PUVA lentigines (Figs. 3.24 and 14.109)
Café-au-lait macule (Figs. 3.64 and 3.74)
Compound nevus
Papillomatous nevus (Fig. 3.127)
Congenital melanocytic nevus (Figs. 3.148, 3.149, 3.166, 3.170, 3.171, 3.177 and 3.184)
Dysplastic nevus (Fig. 3.191)
Spitz nevus (Fig. 3.217)
Reed nevus
Nevus spilus
Epidermoid cyst
Eruptive vellus hair cyst
Chondroid syringoma
Eccrine hidrocystoma

Tubulopapillary hidradenoma
Spiradenoma
Syringocystadenoma papilliferum
Pilomatricoma (Fig. 5.49)
Leiomyoma (Fig. 5.73)
Infantile hemangioma (Figs. 6.11 and 6.30a)
Diffuse neonatal hemangiomatosis (Fig. 6.34)
Senile angioma
Congenital hemangioma
Port-wine stain (Figs. 6.94 and 6.113)
Cutis marmorata telangiectatica congenita (Figs. 6.150 and 6.151)
Solitary angiokeratoma (Fig. 6.154)
Angiokeratoma circumscriptum (Figs. 6.163 and 6.164)
Blue rubber bleb nevus syndrome (Figs. 6.172 and 6.175)
Maffucci syndrome
Glomus tumor (Figs. 6.188 and 6.192)
Lymphangioma circumscriptum
Neurofibroma (Figs. 7.29 and 7.30)
Schwannoma (Fig. 7.36)
Palisaded ancapsulated neuroma (Fig. 7.42)
Neurothekeoma
Dermatofibroma (Figs. 8.1, 8.2, 8.9 and 8.15)
Acquired digital fibrokeratoma (Fig. 8.51)
Epithelioid cell histiocytoma
Connective tissue nevus (Fig. 8.87)
Keloid (Figs. 8.99 and 8.107a)
Urticaria pigmentosa
Lipoma (Figs. 10.5 and 10.7)

LEG (Malignant)
Basal cell carcinoma (Fig. 11.84)
Squamous cell carcinoma (Figs. 11.108, 11.109, 11.147 and 11.149)
Carcinoma erysipeloides (Fig. 11.166)
Superficial spreading melanoma
Nodular melanoma
Metastatic malignant melanoma (Figs. 12.66, 12.67, 12.68 and 12.81)
Kaposi sarcoma (Figs. 13.3, 13.13, 13.14, 13.15, 13.27, 13.34, 13.36 and 13.44a)
Cutaneous angiosarcoma
Dermatofibrosarcoma protuberans
Malignant fibrous histiocytoma
Fibrosarcoma (Fig. 13.66)
Liposarcoma (Fig. 13.68)
Epitheliod sarcoma
Mycosis fungoides (patch, plaque stages) (Figs. 14.2, 14.5, 14.7, 14.11, 14.12, 14.13, 14.23, 14.55, 14.61, 14.66, 14.70, 14.73 and 14.74)
Mycosis fungoides (tumoral stage) (Fig. 14.39)
Lymphomatoid papulosis (Figs. 14.115, 14.116, 14.128, 14.131, 14.133, 14.136a and 14.137)

Primary cutaneous anaplastic large cell lymphoma (Figs. 14.143, 14.147 and 14.149a)
Primary cutaneous CD8+ aggressive epidermotropic cytotoxic T-cell lymphoma
Primary cutaneous gamma/delta T-cell lymphoma (Figs. 14.164 and 14.165)
Primary cutaneous marginal zone lymphoma (Fig. 14.168)
Primary cutaneous diffuse large B cell lymphoma, leg type (Fig. 14.177)
Intravascular lymphoma
Extranodal NK/T-cell lymphoma (Fig. 14.185)
Nodular scabies (Figs. 14.188 and 14.189)
Cutaneous infiltration of non-Hodgkin lymphomas (Fig. 14.222)
Generalized eruptive histiocytosis (Fig. 15.41)
Xanthoma disseminatum (Fig. 15.44)
Cutaneous metastasis (Fig. 16.19)

FOOT (Benign)
Stucco keratoses (Fig. 1.60)
Arsenical keratosis (Fig. 2.60)
Blue nevus (Fig. 3.61)
Junctional nevus (Fig. 3.86)
Compound nevus
Congenital melanocytic nevus (Fig. 3.176)
Epidermolysis bullosa nevus (Fig. 3.225)
Ganglion cyst (Fig. 4.58)
Digital mucous cyst (Figs. 4.59, 4.62a and 4.63a)
Poroma (Fig. 5.17)
Eccrine spiradenoma (Fig. 5.26)
Pyogenic granuloma (Fig. 6.57)
Port-wine stain (Figs. 6.88 and 6.115)
Blue rubber bleb nevus syndrome (Fig. 6.173)
Maffucci syndrome
Angiokeratoma Mibelli
Lymphangioma circumscriptum (Fig. 6.198)
Dermatofibroma (Fig. 8.13)
Acquired digital fibrokeratoma (Figs. 8.54 and 8.55)
Infantile digital fibromatosis
Calcifying aponeurotic fibroma
Isolated mastocytoma (Fig. 9.17)

FOOT (Malignant)
Squamous cell carcinoma
Cutaneous verrucous carcinoma (Fig. 11.152)
Eccrine porocarcinoma
Acral lentiginous melanoma (Fig. 12.31)
Nodular melanoma
Metastatic melanoma (Fig. 12.40b)
Kaposi sarcoma (Figs. 13.1, 13.6, 13.7, 13.10, 13.11, 13.15, 13.20, 13.26, 13.28 and 13.30)
Cutaneous angiosarcoma

Fibrosarcoma (Fig. 13.67)
Liposarcoma
Epitheliod sarcoma
Mycosis fungoides
Lymphomatoid papulosis
Primary cutaneous CD8+ aggressive epidermotropic cytotoxic T-cell lymphoma (Figs. 14.151 and 14.154)
Langerhans cell histiocytosis (Fig. 15.17)
Generalized eruptive histiocytosis (Fig. 15.40)
Xanthoma disseminatum (Fig. 14.59b)

PALMOPLANTAR AREA (Benign)
Epidermal nevus (Figs. 1.78 and 1.79)
Nevus comedonicus
Bowen disease (Figs. 2.19 and 2.24)
Lentigo simplex (Peutz-Jeghers syndrome) (Fig. 3.13)
Congenital dermal melanocytosis (Fig. 3.58)
Junctional nevus (Figs. 3.83 and 3.84)
Compound nevus (Figs. 3.92 and 3.93)
Intradermal nevus (Fig. 3.113)
Epidermolysis bullosa nevus (Fig. 3.225)
Epidermoid cyst (Figs. 4.5, 4.8 and 11.91)
Ganglion cyst (Fig. 4.57)
Poroma (Fig. 5.15)
Diffuse neonatal hemangiomatosis (Fig. 6.35)
Pyogenic granuloma (Figs. 6.49 and 6.59)
Glomeruloid hemangioma (Fig. 6.73)
Port-wine stain (Figs. 6.94, 6.96 and 6.122)
Intravascular papillary endothelial hyperplasia
Telangiectasia (CREST syndrome) (Fig. 6.134)
Blue rubber bleb nevus syndrome (Fig. 6.174)
Maffucci syndrome (Fig. 6.177)
Neurofibroma
Dermatofibroma
Acquired digital fibrokeratoma (Figs. 8.49 and 8.53)
Calcifieng aponeurotic fibroma (Fig. 8.63)
Dupuytren contracture (Fig. 8.64)
Plantar fibromatosis (Fig. 8.65)
Connective tissue nevus (Proteus syndrome) (Figs. 8.92 and 8.93)
Keloid (Fig. 8.101)

PALMOPLANTAR AREA (Malignant)
Squamous cell carcinoma (Fig. 11.146)
Carcinoma cuniculatum (Figs. 11.156 and 11.157)
Acral lentiginous melanoma (Figs. 12.29, 12.30, 12.32, 12.33, 12.34 and 12.65)
Amelanotic melanoma (Fig. 12.58)
Kaposi sarcoma (Figs. 13.1, 13.2, 13.4, 13.5, 13.11, 13.18, 13.24, 13.25, 13.29, 13.33, 13.34 and 13.43)
Mycosis fungoides (tumoral stage) (Figs. 14.32, 14.33, 14.40 and 14.114a)
Sézary syndrome (Figs. 14.88, 14.97 and 14.98)

Pagetoid reticulosis (Fig. 14.110)
Lymphomatoid papulosis (Fig. 14.119)
Primary cutaneous agressive epidermotropic CD8+ cytotoxic T-cell lymphoma (Fig. 14.157a)
Langerhans cell histiocytosis (Figs. 15.13 and 15.14)
Xanthoma disseminatum (Figs. 15.46 and 15.49c)

NAIL (Benign)
Bowen disease (Fig. 2.19)
Keratoacanthoma (Fig. 2.72)
Junctional nevus (melanonychia striata) (Figs. 3.87, 3.88 and 3.89)
Digital mucous cyst (Figs. 4.60 and 4.61)
Poroma (Fig. 5.16)
Pyogenic granuloma (Figs. 6.58a, 6.60 and 6.61a)
Glomus tumor (Figs. 6.189, 6.190 and 6.191)
Periungual fibroma (Figs. 8.37 and 8.38)
Periungual fibrokeratoma (Fig. 8.57)

NAIL (Malignant)
Squamous cell carcinoma (Fig. 11.143)
Acral lentiginous melanoma (Figs. 12.35, 12.38 and 12.40a)
Amelanotic melanoma (Fig. 12.39)
Kaposi sarcoma (Fig. 13.46a)

Epitheliod hemangioendothelioma (Fig. 13.57)
Langerhans cell histiocytosis (Figs. 15.17 and 15.18)

FLEXOR/INTERTRIGINOUS AREAS (Benign)
Seborrheic keratosis (Figs. 1.4 and 1.5)
Verrucal keratosis (Fig. 1.65)
Epidermal nevus (Figs. 1.77 and 1.80)
Extramammary Paget disease
Axillary freckling (Figs. 3.38 and 3.39)
Compound nevus
Steatocystoma multiplex (Fig. 4.48)
Syringoma
Acrochordon (Figs. 8.68 and 8.70)

FLEXOR/INTERTRIGINOUS AREAS (Malignant)
Basal cell carcinoma (Gorlin syndrome) (Fig. 11.86)
Granulomatous slack skin (Fig. 14.63)
Poikilodermatous mycosis fungoides (Fig. 14.80)
Pseudolymphoma (nodular scabies) (Fig. 14.187)
Cutaneous Hodgkin disease (Figs. 14.217 and 14.220)
Langerhans cell histiocytosis (Figs. 15.4, 15.10 and 15.11)
Xanthoma disseminatum (Figs. 15.44 and 15.45a)
Cutaneous metastasis (Figs. 16.1 and 16.11)

Index

A
ABCDE criteria, 95, 341, 342
Acanthosis nigricans, 262–263
Acebutolol, 177
Acitretine, 409
Acne vulgaris, 270, 272
Acoustic neuroma, 239
Acquired dermal melanocytosis, 80
Acquired digital fibrokeratoma, 257–258
Acquired epidermolysis bullosa, 312
Acquired immunodeficiency syndrome (AIDS)–related Kaposi sarcoma, 365–366
Acral lentiginous melanoma, 342–344
Acrochordon, 250, 254, 262–266
Acrocynosis, 213
Acrokeratosis verruciformis of Hopf, 15
Actinic cheilitis, 51–52
Actinic keratosis, 37–41, 69, 337
Actinic lentigo, 11, 69, 70, 316
Actinic reticuloid, 435
Adenoid cystic parotid gland carcinoma, 331
Adenoma sebaceum symmetricum, 250
Adiposis dolorosa, 286–287
Adult T-cell leukemia, 403
Adult fibrosarcoma, 376
Adult systemic mastocytosis, 281–282
Aerodigestive verrucous carcinoma, 328–329. *See also* Oral florid papillomatosis
African Kaposi sarcoma, 368–370
Aggressive digital papillary adenoma, 150
Agminated nevus, 92, 95
Agminated spitz nevus, 116
Alemtuzumab, 410
Aleukemic leukemia cutis, 443
Alopecia, 392, 395, 403, 405
Alopecia neoplastica, 474
Alport syndrome, 167
Amelanotic melanoma, 349–350
Amitriptilin, 167
Amputation neuroma, 242
Angiofibroma, 250
Angiokeratoma, 201–202, 211–216
    angiokeratoma circumscriptum, 213–214
    angiokeratoma of Fordyce, 211–213
    angiokeratoma of Mibelli, 213–214
    Fabry disease, 214–215
    solitary angiokeratoma, 211
Angioleiomyoma, 166–167
Angiolipoleiomyoma, 287
Angiolipoma, 287
Angiolymphoid hyperplasia with eosinophilia, 190–193

Angioma serpiginosum, 208–209
Angiomatous dermatofibroma, 247–248
Angora hair nevus, 20
    syndrome, 22
Anhidrosis, 215
Anhidrotic ectodermal dysplasia, 138
Apocrine hidrocystoma, 155–156
Apocrine mixed tumor, 147
Arsenical keratosis, 54
Arteriovenous malformation, 229–230
Ataxia telangiectasia, 206–207
Atenolol, 177
Atrophic dermatofibroma, 247, 248
Atypical fibroxanthoma, 375
Atypical genital melanocytic nevus, 96
Atypical mole syndrome, 109
Atypical spitzoid melanocytic neoplasm, 117
Auricular pseudocyst, 142
Axillary freckling, 64, 74, 232

B
Bacillary angiomatosis, 185, 365
Balanitis xerotica obliterans, 324
Bannayan-Zonana syndrome, 287
Bart-Pumphrey syndrome, 262
Basal cell carcinoma
    basosquamous carcinoma, 308–309
    chronic arsenic exposure, 294, 296
    cystic type, 303
    fibroepithelial type (Pinkus tumor), 308
    hereditary tumor syndromes
        Bazex-Dupré-Christol syndrome, 315–316
        Gorlin syndrome, 311–315
    metastatic, 310–311
    morphoeic (sclerosing) type, 305–307
    noduloulcerative (nodular) type, 298–303
    pigmented type, 307–308
    polypoid, 294, 295
    recurrent type, 309–310
    superficial type, 303–306
    with albinism, 298
    with xeroderma pigmentosum, 297, 307
Basaloid follicular hamartoma, 31
Basosquamous carcinoma, 308–309
Bathing trunk nevus, 102, 105
Bazex-Dupré-Christol syndrome, 132, 297, 315, 316
Becker nevus, 32–34, 119
    syndrome, 23, 34
Benign cephalic histiocytosis, 458–460

Benign epidermal tumors
   hamartomas
      Becker nevus, 32–35
      epidermal nevus, 18–24
      nevus comedonicus, 30–32
      nevus sebaceus, 24, 30
   keratinocytic tumors
      clear cell acanthoma, 13, 18, 42, 182, 302, 349
      nevoid hyperkeratosis, 9, 10, 15–17, 60
      seborrheic keratosis, 3–15
      verrucal keratosis, 17
   white sponge nevus, 35–36
Benign epithelial melanosis, 96
Benign fibrohistiocytic tumors. *See* Fibrohistiocytic tumors
Benign neonatal hemangiomatosis, 178, 179
Benign symmetric lipomatosis, 286
Benign vascular tumors
   angiolymphoid hyperplasia with eosinophilia, 190–193
   congenital hemangioma, 179–181
   description, 169
   glomeruloid hemangioma, 189–190
   infantile hemangioma, 169–179
   intravascular papillary endothelial hyperplasia, 193
   kaposiform hemangioendothelioma, 181–182
   Kimura disease, 192–193
   pyogenic granuloma, 182–186
   senile angioma, 186–189
   targetoid hemosiderotic hemangioma, 189
   tufted angioma, 182
Bexarotene, 406, 409, 410
Birbeck granules, 453
Birt-Hogg-Dubé syndrome, 254–255
Blackhead-like punctum, 126, 129
Blastic NK-cell lymphoma, 434
Blastic plasmacytoid dendritic cell neoplasm, 434–435
Bleomycin, 59, 272
Bloom syndrome, 206
Blue nevus
   agminated, 83
   Carney syndrome, 68
   cellular, 82
   classic 80, 81
   hypochromic variant, 83
   nevus of Ota, 76
   plaque-like lesion, 83
Blue rubber bleb nevus syndrome, 216–217
Bonnet-Dechaume-Blanc syndrome, 230
Borrelia burgdorferi infection, 436
Bortezomib, 410
Botulinum toxin, 149, 167
Bowen disease, 42–48, 54, 70, 71, 316, 325
Bowenoid papulosis, 43–44
Branchio-oto-renal syndrome, 143
Brentuximab vedotin, 420
Breslow thickness, 336
Brooke-Spiegler syndrome, 132, 151–153, 156, 297
Bullous mastocytosis, 278, 279
Bullous mycosis fungoides, 405
Buschke-Löwenstein tumor, 329
Buschke-Ollendorff syndrome, 267, 268
Buttonhole sign, 232

C
Café-au-lait macule
   McCune Albright syndrome, 72, 74
   neurofibromatosis, 73, 74

Calcifying aponeurotic fibroma, 261
Calcinosis cutis, 130
Capillary hemangioma. *See* Infantile hemangioma
Capillary malformations
   angiokeratoma, 211–216
   nevus flammeus, 193–204
   telangiectasia, 204–211
Capillaro-lymphaticovenous malformation, 193, 201
Carcinoma cuniculatum, 329–330
Carcinoma erysipeloides, 471, 473, 476
Carcinoma telangiectoides. *See* Telangiectatic metastatic carcinoma
Carmustine, 408
Carney syndrome, 65–68, 82, 239
Castello syndrome, 147
Castleman disease, 190
Cavernous hemangioma, 170
Cavernous lymphangioma, 222
Cellular blue nevus, 82–84
Cellular neurothekeoma, 242–243
Cellulitis, 223, 225–228
Cerebriform collagen nevus, 203, 268
Cetuximab, 186
Cherry angioma. *See* Senile angioma
Chilblains, 213
CHILD syndrome, 22, 23
Chloroma, 443
Chondrodermatitis nodularis helicis, 273
Chondroid syringoma, 147
Chondrosarcoma, 217
Chronic radiodermatitis, 54–55, 316–317
Chronic radiation keratosis, 55
Cladribine, 283
Classic Kaposi sarcoma, 360–365
Clear cell acanthoma, 13, 18, 42, 182, 302, 349
Clonal nevus, 119
CLOVES syndrome, 203
Clustered juvenile xanthogranuloma, 456
Cobb syndrome, 199, 202
Collagenoma. *See* Connective tissue nevus
Combined hemangioma, 171
Common acquired melanocytic nevus
   compound nevus, 86–90
   intradermal (dermal) nevus, 86, 87, 90–93
   junctional nevus, 84–86
   melanonychia striata, 86–87
   papillomatous nevus, 92, 94, 95, 101
   with Turner syndrome, 84
Compound nevus, 86–90
Congenital dermal melanocytosis, 79–80
Congenital follicular melanocytic nevus, 102, 103
Congenital hemangioma, 179–181
Congenital melanocytic nevus, 98–108, 119
Congenital smooth muscle hamartoma, 104, 167
Connective tissue nevus
   Buschke-Ollendorff syndrome, 267–268
   eruptive collagenoma, 268–269
   familial cutaneous collagenoma, 268
   papular elastorrhexis, 269
   Proteus syndrome, 267–268
   tuberous sclerosis, 266–267
Cornea verticillata, 215
Cornu cutaneum. *See* Cutaneous horn
Cowden syndrome, 159
CREST syndrome, 206
Crosti lymphoma, 431
Crowe sign, 72, 74
Crow-Fukase syndrome, 190

Index

Cutaneous angiosarcoma, 370–372
Cutaneous B-cell lymphomas, 426
    intravascular large B-cell lymphoma, 433–434
    primary cutaneous diffuse large B-cell lymphoma, 431–433
    primary cutaneous follicle center lymphoma, 430–432
    primary cutaneous marginal zone lymphoma, 428–431
Cutaneous cysts
    auricular pseudocyst, 142
    digital mucous cyst, 139–141
    epidermoid cyst, 125–131
    eruptive vellus hair cyst, 137–138
    median raphe cyst, 143
    mucocele, 140–142
    preauricular cyst, 142–143
    steatocystoma multiplex, 136–137
    trichilemmal cyst, 134–136
Cutaneous horn, 9, 10, 38, 47, 52–53, 324, 327
Cutaneous lymphomas
    hematologic neoplasms, skin infiltration of, 442–447
    primary
        blastic plasmacytoid dendritic cell neoplasm, 434–435
        cutaneous B-cell lymphomas, 426–434
        cutaneous T-cell lymphomas, 381–426
    pseudolymphomas of skin, 435–442
    skin infiltration of hematologic neoplasms, 442–447
Cutaneous malignant melanoma. See Malignant melanoma
Cutaneous mastocytosis
    diffuse cutaneous mastocytosis, 278–279
    isolated mastocytoma, 279–280
    telangiectasia macularis eruptiva perstans, 281
    urticaria pigmentosa, 275–277
Cutaneous meningospinal angiomatosis, 202
Cutaneous metastasis
    carcinoma erysipeloides, 471, 473
    erythema annulare centrifugum-like metastasis, 475–476
    malignant melanoma, 467
    nodular cutaneous metastasis, 468–471
    scleroderma-like cutaneous metastasis, 474
    telangiectatic metastatic carcinoma, 475
Cutaneous neuroma, 240
Cutaneous plasmocytoma, 447
Cutaneous sarcomas
    atypical fibroxanthoma, 375
    cutaneous angiosarcoma, 370–373
    dermatofibrosarcoma protuberans, 373–375
    epithelioid hemangioendothelioma, 372–373
    epithelioid sarcoma, 378
    fibrosarcoma, 376–377
    Kaposi sarcoma, 365–370
    leiomyosarcoma, 377–378
    liposarcoma, 376–377
    malignant fibrous histiocytoma, 375–376
    malignant peripheral nerve sheath tumor, 378–379
Cutaneous T-cell lymphomas, 381, 426
Cutaneous verrucous carcinoma, 328
Cutis marmorata telangiectatica congenita, 203, 210–211
Cylindroma, 151–152
Cylosporine, 39
Cyrano nose, 173
Cystadenoma, 155–156
Cystic basal cell carcinoma, 303
Cystic higroma, 224–225

D
Dabrafenib, 356
Dacarbazine, 356

Darier sign, 276, 277, 279
Dartoic leiomyoma, 166
Dazosin, 167
Deep penetrating nevus, 118–119
Denileukin diftitox, 410
Dercum disease. See Adiposis dolorosa
Dermal leiomyosarcoma, 377
Dermal melanocytic tumors
    blue nevus, 80–83
    congenital dermal melanocytosis, 79–80
    Mongolian spot, 74, 76
    nevus of Ito, 78–79
    nevus of Ota, 76–78
Dermal neurofibroma, 231–232
Dermatofibroma, 245–247
Dermatofibrosarcoma protuberans, 373–375
Dermatofibrosis lenticularis disseminate, 267
Dermatopathic lymphadenopathy, 403
Dermatosis papulosa nigra, 15
Dermoscopy
    angiokeratoma, 211
    actinic lentigo, 70
    blue nevus, 82
    dermatofibroma, 247
    dysplastic nevus, 110
    melanocytic nevi, 92
    pigmented basal cell carcinoma, 308
    Reed nevus, 117
    seborrheic keratosis, 8
    venous lake, 219
Desmoplastic melanoma, 336, 350
Desmoplastic Spitz nevus, 116–117
Desmoplastic trichoepithelioma, 157–158
Diabetes insipidus, 460
Diascopy, 210, 219
Diclofenac, 41
Diffuse cutaneous mastocytosis, 278–279
Diffuse lipomatosis, 286
Diffuse neonatal hemangiomatosis, 178–179
Digital mucous cyst, 139–141
Digitate parapsoriasis, 391–392
Dimple sign, 247
Discoid lupus erythematosus, 50, 316, 317
Divided nevus of the eyelid, 96
Divided nevus of the penis, 96
Down syndrome, 147
Drug-induced pseudolymphoma, 436
Dupuytren contracture, 262, 378
Dyskeratosis congenita, 36, 47
Dysplastic nevus, 109–112, 335
    syndrome, 109–110

E
Eccrine hidrocystoma, 145, 147–149
Eccrine mixed tumor, 147
Eccrine porocarcinoma, 333
Eccrine spiradenoma, 152–153. See also Spiradenoma
Ectopic Mongolian spot, 75
Ectropion, 366, 403–404
Eczema, 121
Elephantiasis nostras verrucosa, 226
Embolization, 230
Emperipolesis, 465
Encephalotrigeminal angiomatosis, 199–200
Enchondroma, 212
Endemic Kaposi sarcoma, 368–369

Eosinophilic granuloma, 449
Ephelides, 63–64, 339
Epidermal inclusion cyst, 125
Epidermal melanocytic tumors
    actinic lentigo, 68–72
    café-au-lait macule, 72–74
    lentigo simplex, 65–67
    segmental lentiginosis, 68
Epidermal nevus
    ichthyosis hystrix, 20–22
    inflammatory linear verrucous epidermal nevus, 22
    nevus unius lateris, 18–20
    nevus verrucosus, 8, 18–19, 69
    seborrheic keratosis, 9, 19
    syndromes, 18, 22–24
Epidermal precancerous lesions
    actinic cheilitis, 51–52
    actinic keratosis, 37–41, 69, 337
    arsenical keratosis, 54
    Bowen disease, 42–46
    chronic radiodermatitis, 54–55
    cutaneous horn, 52–53
    erythroplasia of Queyrat, 46–47
    extramammary Paget disease, 61–62
    keratoacanthoma, 55–60
    leukoplakia, 47–51
    Paget disease of the breast, 59–61
Epidermoid cyst, 125–131, 160, 314
Epidermolysis bullosa, 121–122, 132, 327
Epidermolysis bullosa nevus, 121–122
Epidermolytic palmoplantar keratoderma, 262
Epinephrine, 282, 283
Epithelioid cell histiocytoma, 258–259
Epithelioid hemangioendothelioma, 372–373
Epithelioid sarcoma, 378
Erlotinib, 186
Erosive adenomatosis of the nipple, 156
Eruptive collagenoma, 268–269
Eruptive syringoma, 146
Eruptive vellus hair cyst, 31, 137–138
Erythema ab igne, 327
Erythema annulare centrifugum-like metastasis, 475–476
Erythroderma, 13
Erythrodermic mycosis fungoides, 400–403
Erytroleukoplakia, 50
Erythroplasia of Queyrat, 46–47
Extramammary Paget disease, 61–62
Extracorporeal photochemoterapy, 409
Extraocular sebaceous carcinoma, 331
Extranodal NK/T-cell lymphoma, nasal type, 421, 426–428

F
Fabry disease, 214–216
Familial cutaneous collagenoma, 268
Familial cylindromatosis, 151, 152
Familial multiple lipomatosis, 286
Familial presenile sebaceous hyperplasia, 162
Fanconi anemia, 72
Ferguson-Smith type multiple eruptive keratoacanthoma
Fibroepithelial basal cell carcinoma, 308
Fibro-fatty residual tissue, 170–171
Fibrofolliculoma, 254
Fibrohistiocytic tumors
    acquired digital fibrokeratoma, 256–258
    acrochordon, 262–263
    angiofibroma, 249–252
    Birt-Hogg-Dubé syndrome, 254–255
    calcifying aponeurotic fibroma, 261
    connective tissue nevus, 267–269
    dermatofibroma, 245–247
    epithelioid cell histiocytoma, 258–259
    fibromatoses, 261–262
    fibrous papule of the nose, 248–249
    giant cell tumor of tendon sheath, 273
    infantile digital fibromatosis, 259–260
    infantile myofibromatosis, 260
    juvenile hyaline fibromatosis, 260–261
    keloid and hypertrophic scar, 269–271
    oral fibroma, 255–256
    perifollicular fibroma, 254–255
    periungual fibroma, 252–254
    weathering nodules of the ear, 273
Fibromatoses, 261–262
Fibrosarcoma, 217, 376–377
Fibrous papule of the nose, 248–249
Filariasis, 226
Flat seborrheic keratosis, 10, 11, 70
5-Fluorouracil, 41, 46, 52, 59, 259, 272, 310
Flushing, 279
Follicular atrophoderma, 315
Folliculitis, 104
Folliculotropic mycosis fungoides, 392–395, 408
Forehead plaque, 250, 266–267
Freckles, 459–460. *See also* Ephelides
Frictional keratosis, 50
Fucosidosis, 214

G
Gabapentin, 167
Ganglion cyst, 139
Gardner syndrome, 287
Generalized dermal melanosis, 70
Generalized eruptive histiocytosis, 459–460
Generalized essential telangiectasia, 208
Genital leiomyoma, 167
Giant cell tumor of the tendon sheath, 273, 378
Giant comedo, 126, 129
Gingival fibromatosis, 250
Gingival hyperplasia, 443
Gingival hypertrophy, 261
Glaucoma, 76, 457
Glomangioma, 220–221
Glomangiomyoma, 220
Glomus tumor, 220–222
Glomuvenous malformation, 220–222
Glomeruloid hemangioma, 189–190
Gorlin syndrome, 125, 127, 132, 297, 311–314
Granular cell tumor, 243
Granulocytic sarcoma, 443
Granulomatous mycosis fungoides, 394–396
Granulomatous slack skin, 394–396
Grybowski type generalized eruptive
    keratoacanthoma, 58

H
Hair follicle tumors
    pilomatricoma, 160–162
    trichilemmoma, 159
    trichoblastoma, 158
    trichoepithelioma, 156–158
    trichofolliculoma, 158

Index

Hairless congenital melanocytic nevus, 98
Halo nevus, 112–115
Hamartomas of epidermis
    Becker nevus, 32–35
    epidermal nevus, 18–24
    nevus comedonicus, 30–32
    nevus sebaceus, 24–30
Hand-Schüller-Christian disease, 449
Hashimoto-Pritzker disease, 449, 453–454
Hematologic neoplasms, skin infiltration of, 442
    Hodgkin lymphoma, 444–445
    leukemia cutis, 443
    non-Hodgkin lymphomas, 445–446
    plasma cell dyscrasia, 446–447
Hemophagocytic syndrome, 421, 422
Hereditary benign intraepithelial dyskeratosis, 36
Hereditary hemorrhagic telangiectasia, 207–208
Hereditary leiomyomatosis and renal cell cancer (HLRCC) syndrome, 167
Hereditary tumor syndromes
    Bazex-Dupré-Christol syndrome, 311–316
    Gorlin syndrome, 311–314
Hereditary trichodysplasia, 132
Hidradenitis suppurativa, 325, 326
Hidradenocarcinoma, 332
Hidradenoma papilliferum, 156
Hidroacanthoma simplex, 150
Hidrotic ectodermal dysplasia, 138
Highly activated antiretroviral therapy, 365
Histiocytosis
    indeterminate cell histiocytosis, 466
    Langerhans cell histiocytosis, 449–454
    non-Langerhans cell histiocytosis, 454–466
Histiocytosis-X. See Langerhans cell histiocytosis
HIV infection, 245, 287, 365
Hobnail hemangioma, 189
Hodgkin disease, 407, 444–445
Hoffman-Zurhalle nevus, 288
Horn cyst, 8–9
Howel-Evans syndrome, 36, 47
Huriez syndrome, 325, 326
Hybrid cyst, 137
Hyperpigmentation
    Becker nevus, 32–33
    café-au-lait macules, 74
    ephelides, 63–64
    mycosis fungoides, 397–398
    nevus of Ota, 76–77
    Sézary syndrome, 403
Hypertrophic granulation tissue, 185
Hypertrophic scar, 271–272
Hypohidrosis, 215
Hypohidrotic ectodermal displasia, 315
Hypopigmented mycosis fungoides, 396–398

I
Iatrogenic Kaposi sarcoma, 366–368
Ichthyosis hystrix, 20–22
ILVEN. See Inflammatory linear verrucous epidermal nevus
Imatinib, 193, 283, 374
Imiquimod, 41, 46, 52, 62, 173, 186, 310, 417
Incontinentia pigmenti, 20
Indeterminate cell histiocytosis, 449, 466
Indolent systemic mastocytosis, 281
Infantile digital fibromatosis, 259–260
Infantile fibrosarcoma, 376
Infantile hemangioma, 169–179
Infantile myofibromatosis, 260
Inflamed epidermoid cyst, 130–131
Inflammatory linear verrucous epidermal nevus (ILVEN), 22
Infundibular cyst. See Epidermoid cyst
Ingenol mebutate, 41
Interferon alfa, 176, 177, 181, 192, 272, 283, 406, 408
Intertriginous dermatitis, 450, 452
Intertrigo-like dermatitis, 449, 450
Intradermal (dermal) nevus, 86, 87, 90–93
Intravascular large B-cell lymphoma, 206, 433–434
Intravascular papillary endothelial hyperplasia, 193
Inverted follicular keratosis
    nevus sebaceus, 28–29
    seborrheic keratosis, 15
Ipilimumab, 356
Irritated seborrheic keratosis, 11, 12
Irritation fibroma, 255–256
Isolated collagenoma, 268
Isolated mastocytoma, 279–280
Isotretinoin, 137, 138, 163

J
Jessner's lymphocytic infiltration, 439–441
Junctional nevus, 84–86
Juvenile aponeurotic fibroma, 261
Juvenile hyaline fibromatosis, 260–261
Juvenile melanoma, 114
Juvenile xanthogranuloma, 453, 455–458

K
Kaposiform hemangioendothelioma, 173, 181–182
Kaposi sarcoma
    AIDS-related, 365–366
    classic, 359–365
    endemic, 368–370
    iatrogenic, 366–368
Kasabach-Merritt syndrome, 181, 182
Keloid, 269–271
Keratinocytic tumors
    clear cell acanthoma, 13, 18, 42, 182, 302, 349
    nevoid hyperkeratosis, 9, 10, 15–17, 60
    seborrheic keratosis, 3–15
    verrucal keratosis, 17
Keratinocytic epidermal nevus. See Epidermal nevus
Keratoacanthoma, 55–60
Keratoacanthoma centrifigum marginatum, 57
Ketron-Goodman disease, 392, 420
Kimura disease, 192–193
Kindler syndrome, 47
Klippel-Trenaunay syndrome, 175, 199–202, 225
Knuckle pads, 262
Koenen tumor, 252–254, 258

L
Labial melanotic macule, 64, 65
LAMB syndrome. See Carney syndrome
Lambrolizumab, 356
Langerhans cell histiocytosis, 449–454
    acute disseminated type, 449
    chronic multifocal type, 449
    chronic unifocal type, 449
    Hashimoto-Pritzker disease, 453–454
Large congenital melanocytic nevus, 33, 102–107
Laugier-Hunziker syndrome, 67

Ledderhose disease, 262
Leiomyoma, 166–167
Leiomyosarcoma, 377–378
Lentigo maligna, 10, 70, 72, 338
Lentigo maligna melanoma, 336–338
Lentigo profusa, 65–67
Lentigo simplex
    Carney syndrome, 67, 68
    genital lentigines, 65, 66
    lentigo profusa, 65–67
    LEOPARD syndrome, 66
    Peutz-Jeghers syndrome, 66–67
Leonine facies, 443
LEOPARD syndrome, 65–67
Leptomenengeal melanoma, 108
Leser-Trélat sign, 13
Lethal midline granuloma. See Extranodal NK/T-cell lymphoma, nasal type
Letterer-Siwe disease, 449
Leukonychia, 190
Leukoplakia
    Howel-Evans syndrome, 47
    Kindler syndrome, 47–48
    oral hairy, 50
    pachyonychia congenita, 47–48
    squamous cell carcinoma, 316–317
Lichen planus, 50, 318, 324
Lichen sclerosus et atrophicus, 65, 325
Lipoma
    adiposis dolorosa, 286
    angiolipoleiomyoma, 287
    angiolipoma, 287
    Bannayan-Zonana syndrome, 287
    benign symmetric lipomatosis, 286
    Gardner syndrome, 287
    intramuscular lipoma, 287
    Proteus syndrome, 203
    spinal dysraphism, 203
    spindle cell lipoma, 287
Liposarcoma, 286, 376–377
Lish nodules, 237
Louis-Bar syndrome, 206
Lupus tumidus, 441–442
Lymphangiectasia, 229
Lymphangioma circumscriptum, 202, 222–224
Lymphangiosarcoma, 217, 227
Lymphedema, 201, 215, 224–227, 364, 370
    lymphedema-distichiasis syndrome, 225
    lymphedema praecox, 225
    lymphedema tarda, 225
Lymphocytoma cutis, 422, 436–440
Lymphomatoid contact dermatitis, 435
Lymphomatoid papulosis
    and mycosis fungoides, 417
    and primary cutaneous anaplastic large cell lymphoma, 417
    clinical features, 411–416
    regional, 414
    type A, 416
    type B, 417
    type C, 416–417
    type D, 417
    type E, 417
Lupus vulgaris, 316, 317

M
Macrocystic lymphatic malformation, 222, 224
Macroglossia, 223

Maculopapular cutaneous mastocytosis, 275–277
Madelung disease. See Benign symmetric lipomatosis
Maffucci syndrome, 175, 217–218
Malignant adnexal tumors
    eccrine porocarcinoma, 333
    hidradenocarcinoma, 332
    malignant pilomatricoma, 162
    microcystic adnexal carcinoma, 332–333
    primary cutaneous adenoid cystic carcinoma, 331–332
    sebaceous carcinoma, 330–331
Malignant blue nevus, 351
Malignant chondroid syringoma, 147
Malignant cylindroma, 152
Malignant eccrine poroma. See Porocarcinoma
Malignant epithelial tumors
    basal cell carcinoma, 293–314
    malignant adnexal tumors, 330–333
    squamous cell carcinoma, 315–328
    verrucous carcinoma, 328–330
Malignant fibrous histiocytoma, 375–376
Malignant granular cell tumor, 243
Malignant melanoma
    characteristics, 335
    congenital melanocytic nevus, 108
    macrosatellites, 347–351
    metastatic, 351–357, 467
    primary cutaneous
        acral lentiginous melanoma, 342–345
        amelanotic melanoma, 349–350
        desmoplastic melanoma, 350
        lentigo maligna melanoma, 336–339
        malignant blue nevus, 351
        mucosal melanoma, 348
        nodular malignant melanoma, 345–348
        spitzoid melanoma, 350
        superficial spreading melanoma, 339–342
Malignant peripheral nerve sheath tumor, 236, 239, 378–379
Malignant pilomatricoma, 161
Malignant schwannoma. See Malignant peripheral nerve sheath tumor
Marfanoid habitus, 240
Maria-Unna hypotrichosis, 132
Marjolin ulcer, 325, 326
Masson hemangioma, 193
Mastocytosis
    adult systemic mastocytosis, 281–283
    cutaneous mastocytosis, 275–281
McCune Albright syndrome, 72, 74
Median raphe cyst, 143
Mees lines, 54
Meige disease, 225
Melanoacanthoma, 9
Melanocytic nevus. See also Nevus cell nevus
    common acquired melanocytic nevus, 84–95
    congenital melanocytic nevus, 97–108
    deep penetrating nevus, 118–119
    dysplastic nevus, 109–112, 335
    epidermolysis bullosa nevus, 121–122
    halo nevus, 112–115
    Meyerson nevus, 121
    mucosal melanocytic nevi, 96–97
    nevus spilus, 119–120
    pseudomelanoma, 122–123
    Reed nevus, 117–118
    Spitz nevus, 114–117
Melanocytic tumors
    dermal, 76–84
    epidermal, 68–74

Melanonychia striata, 45, 65, 86, 87, 95
   junctional nevus, 87
Melanoerythroderma, 403
Melanotic lesions
   ephelides, 63, 64
   labial melanotic macule, 64, 65
   penile melanotic macule, 65
   vulvar melanosis, 65
Merkel cell carcinoma, 333–334
Metastatic basal cell carcinoma, 310–311
Metastatic malignant melanoma
   in-transit metastasis, 351, 352
   macrosatellites, 351
   papulonodular, 351–353
   soft tissue, 351
Methotrexate, 59, 409, 420
Meyerson nevus, 121
Microcystic adnexal carcinoma, 332–333
Microcystic lymphatic malformation, 222
Miescher nevus, 87
Milia en plaque, 133
Milium, 131–134, 151, 314–316
Milium-like cyst, 392, 393
Milroy disease, 225, 226, 228
Mole. See Melanocytic nevus
Molluscum contagiosum, 56
Mongolian spot, 74–76
Montgomery tubercules, 165
Montelukast, 283
Morphoeic (sclerosing) basal cell carcinoma, 305–307
Mucinorrhea, 392
Mucocele, 140–142, 256
Mucoid cyst. See Digital mucous cyst
Mucosal melanocytic nevi, 95–97, 348
Mucosal melanoma, 348
Mucosal neuromas, 240
Mucous cyst of oral mucosa. See Mucocele
Mucous retention cyst, 141
Muir-Torre syndrome, 58, 163, 164, 297, 331
Multicentric reticulohistiocytosis, 464
Multinodular keratoacanthoma, 57
Multiple endocrine neoplasia type 1 (MEN 1), 249
Multiple endocrine neoplasia type 2B (MEN-2B), 240
Multiple familial trichoepithelioma, 156
Multiple hamartoma syndrome, 159
Multiple mucosal neuroma, 240
Multiple myeloma, 446–447, 460
Mycosis fungoides
   classic, 382–391
   digitate parapsoriasis, 391–392
   erythrodermic, 400–403
   folliculotropic, 392–395
   granulomatous slack skin, 394, 396
   hyperpigmented, 397, 398
   hypopigmented, 396–398
   pagetoid reticulosis, 392
   poikilodermatous, 399–400
   purpuric, 397–398
   Sézary syndrome, 402–405
Myotonic dystrophy, 160
Myxoid cyst. See Digital mucous cyst

N
NAME syndrome. See Carney syndrome
Norrowband UVB, 406
Necrobiotic xanthogranuloma, 464–465
Neural skin tumors
   granular cell tumor, 243
   neurofibroma, 231–299
   neuromas, 240–242
   neurothekeoma, 242–243
   schwannoma, 237–239
Neurilemmoma, 237–239. See also Schwannoma
Neurocutaneous (leptomeningeal) melanocytosis, 108
Neurofibroma
   dermal, 231–232
   plexiform, 232–239
   neurofibromatosis, 103, 231–237
Neurofibrosarcoma. See Malignant peripheral nerve sheath tumor
Neuromas
   cutaneous, 240
   multiple mucosal, 240
   palisaded encapsulated, 241
   traumatic, 241–242
Neurothekeoma, 242–243
Nevoid basal cell carcinoma. See Gorlin syndrome
Nevoid hyperkeratosis of the nipple and areola, 9, 16
Nevomelanocytic benign tumors
   dermal melanocytic tumors, 76–84
   epidermal melanocytic tumors, 68–74
   melanocytic nevi, 84–123
   melanotic lesions, 63–65
Nevus anemicus, 210
Nevus araneus, 209–210
Nevus cell nevus. See Melanocytic nevus
Nevus comedonicus, 30–31
Nevus comedonicus syndrome, 23, 31
Nevus en cocarde, 87
Nevus flammeus
   Cobb syndrome, 202
   Klippel-Trenaunay syndrome, 200–202
   phakomatosis pigmentovascularis, 203
   port-wine stain, 194–199
   Proteus syndrome, 203
   salmon patch, 194
   spinal dysraphism, 203–204
   Sturge-Weber syndrome, 199–200
Nevus fuscoceruleus ophthalmomaxillaris, 76–78.
   See also Nevus of Ota
Nevus lipomatosus superficialis, 285–288
Nevus of Ito, 78–79
Nevus of Ota, 76–78, 96
Nevus sebaceus
   apocrine hydrocytoma, 155
   characteristics, 24–27
   inverted follicular keratosis, 28–29
   phakomatosis pigmentokeratotica, 27
   pigmented basal cell carcinoma, 29–30
   polypoid basal cell carcinoma, 29–30
   seborrheic keratosis, 28–29
   syndrome, 22
   syringocystadenoma papilliferum, 28, 153–154
   trichoblastoma, 28, 158
   viral wart, 28–29
Nerve sheath myxoma, 242
Nevus spilus, 27, 119–120, 203
Nevus unius lateris, 18–20
Nevus verrucosus, 8, 18–19, 69
Nicolau-Ballus syndrome, 147
Nifedipine, 167, 283
Nitrogen mustard, 408
Nivolumab, 356
Nodular cutaneous metastasis, 468–473
Nodular malignant melanoma, 345–348
Nodular plexiform neurofibroma, 236

Noduloulcerative (nodular) basal cell carcinoma, 298–303
Non-identical attached nevus, 87, 89
Nonivoluting congenital hemangioma, 179, 181
Non-Langerhans cell histiocytosis
    benign cephalic histiocytosis, 458–459
    generalized eruptive histiocytosis, 459–460
    juvenile xanthogranuloma, 454–458
    multicentric reticulohistiocytosis, 464
    necrobiotic xanthogranuloma, 464–465
    reticulohistiocytic granuloma, 462–464
    reticulohistiocytosis, 462–464
    sinus histiocytosis with massive lymphadenopathy, 465–466
    xanthoma disseminatum, 460–462
Noonan syndrome, 147, 225

O

Ocular sebaceous carcinoma, 331
Oral facial digital syndrome type I, 132
Oral fibroma, 255–256
Oral florid papillomatosis, 328–329
Oral hairy leukoplakia, 50
Oral hemangioma, 175
Oral melanotic macule, 64. See also Labial melanotic macule
Oral melanocytic nevi, 95–96. See also Mucosal melanocytic nevi
Oral mucosal melanoma, 348
Organoid nevus. See Nevus sebaceus
Osler-Weber-Rendu syndrome, 207–208
Osteoma cutis, 161
Osteopoikilosis, 267
Osteosarcoma, 217

P

Pachyonychia, 47
Pachyonychia congenita, 125, 136, 137
Paget disease of the breast, 16, 59–61
Pagetoid reticulosis, 392, 408
Palisaded encapsulated neuroma, 241
Palmar fibromatosis, 261, 262
Palmar purpura, 450, 452
Palmoplantar pits, 312–314
Papillary adenoma of the nipple, 156
Papillary eccrine adenoma, 150–151
Papillomatous nevus, 92, 94–95, 101, 114, 115
Papular elastorrhexis, 269
Parkes-Weber syndrome, 201–202
Partial unilateral lentiginosis, 68. See also Segmental lentiginosis
Pegylated liposomal doxorubicin, 410
Penile fibromatosis, 262
Penile melanotic macule, 65
Periungual fibrokeratoma, 256
Periungual fibroma, 252–254
Peutz-Jeghers syndrome, 65–67
Peyronie disease, 262
PHACES syndrome, 172
Phakomatosis pigmentokeratotica, 22, 23, 27, 119–120
Phakomatosis pigmentovascularis, 75, 76, 119–120, 199, 203, 210
Pharmacologic nevus, 210
Phenoxybenzamine, 167
Phlebectasia, 218–220
Photodynamic therapy, 310
Pigmented actinic keratosis, 10, 40
Pigmented basal cell carcinoma, 29, 30, 307–308
Pigmented Paget disease, 60, 61
Pigmented purpura-like mycosis fungoides, 397
Pigmented spindle cell nevus, 117–118. See also Reed nevus
Pigmented trichoblastoma, 158

Pilar cyst. See Trichilemmal cyst
Piloleiomyoma, 166–167
Pilomatrical carcinoma, 161
Pilomatricoma, 160–162, 285
Plantar fibromatosis, 262
Plasma cell dyscrasia, cutaneous infiltration of, 446–447
Pleomorphic adenoma, 147
Plexiform neurofibroma, 232, 237, 238
Plexiform Spitz nevus, 118
POEMS syndrome, 189, 190
Poikiloderma, 204
Poikilodermatous mycosis fungoides, 399–400
Poikiloderma vasculare atrophicans. See Poikilodermatous mycosis fungoides
Polydactyly, 201
Polydactylous Bowen disease, 45
Polypoid basal cell carcinoma, 29–30, 294, 295
Poroid hidradenoma, 150
Poroma, 149, 150
Porocarcinoma, 29
Porokeratosis Mibelli, 327
Poromatosis, 149
Port-wine stain, 75, 194–202
Postinflammatory hypopigmentation, 15
Preauricular cyst, 142–143
Preauricular sinus. See Preauricular cyst
Premature sebaceous hyperplasia, 162
Primary acquired melanosis, 96–97
Primary cutaneous adenoid cystic carcinoma, 331–332
Primary cutaneous anaplastic large cell lymphoma, 417–423
Primary cutaneous CD4+ small/medium T-cell lymphoma, 422, 426
Primary cutaneous CD8+ aggressive epidermotropic cytotoxic T-cell lymphoma, 392, 420, 424–426
Primary cutaneous CD30+ lymphoproliferative disorders
    lymphomatoid papulosis, 411–417
    primary cutaneous anaplastic large cell lymphoma, 417–423
Primary cutaneous diffuse large B-cell lymphoma, 431–433
Primary cutaneous follicle center lymphoma, 430–432
Primary cutaneous gamma/delta T-cell lymphoma, 422, 428
Primary cutaneous marginal zone lymphoma, 428–431
Proliferating trichilemmal cyst, 135–136
Proliferative verrucous leukoplakia, 50
Propranolol, 177, 179
Proteus syndrome, 22, 199, 203, 267–268
Psammomatous melanotic schwannoma, 239
Pseudo-Darier sign, 167
Pseudo-Hutchinson sign, 86
Pseudo-Kaposi sarcoma, 363
Pseudolymphomas, of skin
    Jessner's lymphocytic infiltration, 439, 442
    lymphocytoma cutis, 436–440
    nodular scabies, 435
Pseudomelanoma, 122–123
Pseudoxanthomatous mastocytosis, 279
Purpuric mycosis fungoides, 397–398
Pustular mycosis fungoides, 405
PUVA (psoralen + ultraviolet A) therapy, 42, 70, 71, 86, 315, 406–408
PUVA lentigines 407, 408
Pyoderma gangrenosum, 420
Pyogenic granuloma, 182–187, 364
Pyogenic granuloma-like exophytic Kaposi sarcoma, 363, 364

R

Ranula, 141–142
Rapamycin, 252, 368
Rapidly involuting congenital hemangioma, 179, 206
Reactive lymphoid hyperplasia, 436

Recurrent basal cell carcinoma, 309–310
Reed nevus, 117–118
Reed-Sternberg cells, 445
Reed syndrome, 167
Resiquimod, 39
Reticulohistiocytosis, 462
Reticulohistiocytic granuloma, 462–464
Retinoic acid, topical, 17
Rituximab, 432–434
Rodent ulcer, 298
Rombo syndrome, 132, 156, 297, 310, 314
Romidepsin, 410
Rosai-Dorfman disease, 460. See also Sinus histiocytosis with massive lymphadenopathy
Rubinstein-Taybi syndrome, 160
Rudimentary digit, 242, 258

S
Salmon patch, 194
Scabies granuloma, 435. See also Nodular scabies
Sarcomatoid squamous cell carcinoma, 375
Satellite congenital melanocytic nevus, 98, 100
Satellite piyogenic granuloma, 186, 187
Schimmelpenning-Feurstein-Mims syndrome, 22, 23, 26
Schöpf-Schulz-Passarge syndrome, 156, 297
Schwannoma, 237, 239
Schwannomatosis, 239
Scleroderma-like cutaneous metastasis, 474
Sclerosing sweat duct carcinoma, 332, 333. See also Microcystic adnexal carcinoma
Sclerotherapy, 140, 218, 219
Sebaceoma, 163
Sebaceous adenoma, 28, 163–164
Sebaceous carcinoma, 29, 164, 330–331
Sebaceous epithelioma, 28, 163–164
Sebaceous gland tumors
    Fordyce spots, 164–165
    sebaceous adenoma and epithelioma, 163–164
    senile sebaceous hyperplasia, 162–163
Sebaceous trichofolliculoma, 158
Seborrheic keratosis
    actinic lentigo, 70
    basal cell carcinoma, 12, 296
    characteristics, 3–11
    cutaneus horn, 9–10
    dermatosis papulosa nigra, 15
    inflammatory, 12–13
    inverted follicular keratosis, 15
    lentigo maligna, 10, 337
    Leser-Trélat sign, 13
    nevoid hyperkeratosis of the nipple and areola, 9, 16
    nevus sebaceus, 28–29
    pigmented actinic keratosis, 10, 40
    stucco keratosis, 15
Segmental lentiginosis, 68
Senile angioma, 186–189
Senile sebaceous hyperplasia, 162–163
Sessile neurofibroma, 233, 235
Sézary syndrome
    characteristics, 400–405
    ectropion, 403, 404
    melanoerythroderma, 403
    secondary pseudomonas infection, 405, 406
Shagreen patch, 250, 266–267
Sialidosis, 214
Silver nitrate, 186
Silver-Russel syndrome, 72

Sinus histiocytosis with massive lymphadenopathy, 465–466
Sirolimus, 182, 252, 368
Sister Marry Joseph nodule, 468, 473
Skin appendage tumors, benign
    hair follicle tumors, 156–162
    sebaceous gland tumors, 162–165
    smooth muscle tumors, 166–167
    sweat gland tumors, 147–156
Skin tag. See Acrochordon
Smooth muscle hamartoma, 34
Sodium cromoglycate, 182
Solar elastosis, 338
Solar keratosis. See Actinic keratosis
Solitary angiokeratoma, 211
Solitary circumscribed neuroma, 241
Solitary cutaneous histiocytosis. See Reticulohistiocytic granuloma
Solitary mastocytoma. See Isolated mastocytoma
Speckled lentiginous nevus, 27
Spider angioma, 209–210
Spiegler-Fendt pseudolymphoma. See Lymphocytoma cutis
Spinal dysraphism, 203–204
Spindle cell lipoma, 287
Spiradenocylindroma, 153
Spiradenoma, 28, 152–153
Spitz nevus, 114–117
Spitzoid melanoma, 117, 350
Squamous cell carcinoma
    actinic cheilitis, 316
    actinic keratosis, 316
    Bowen disease, 45, 316
    charactheristics, 315–326
    chronic fistula, 316, 318, 325, 326
    chronic radiodermatitis, 316, 318
    cutaneous horn
    discoid lupus erythematosus, 316, 317
    epidermolysis bullosa, 327
    hypertrophic lichen planus, 316, 318
    keratoacanthoma, 320
    leukoplakia, 50, 316, 317
    lupus vulgaris, 316, 317
    metastatic, 327–328
    organ transplant recipient, 316, 318
    scleroatrophy, 325, 326
    xeroderma pigmentosum, 316, 317
Steatocystoma multiplex, 136–137
Stevens-Johnson syndrome, 122
Stewart-Treves syndrome, 227–228, 370–372
Strawberry hemangioma, 170
Stucco keratosis, 15
Sturge-Weber syndrome, 175, 199–200
Subcutaneous leiomyosarcoma, 377, 378
Subungual fibroma, 252–254
Subungual keratoacanthoma, 58
Superficial basal cell carcinoma, 54, 303–305
Superficial mucocele, 140
Superficial plantar fibromatosis, 262
Superficial spreading melanoma, 339–342
Sutton nevus, 112–114. See also Halo nevus
Sweat gland tumors, benign
    apocrine hidrocystoma, 155–156
    chondroid syringoma, 147
    cylindroma, 151–152
    eccrine hidrocystoma, 147–149
    erosive adenomatosis of the nipple, 156
    hidradenoma papilliferum, 156
    poroid hidradenoma, 150
    poroma, 149–150
    spiradenoma, 152–153

Sweat gland tumors, benign (*Cont.*)
    syringocystadenoma papilliferum, 153–155
    syringoma, 145–147
    tubulopapillary hidradenoma, 150–151
Syndactyly, 201
Syringocystadenoma papilliferum, 28, 153–155
Syringocystadenocarcinoma papilliferum, 155
Syringoma, 146–147
Syringotropic mycosis fungoides, 392
Systemic anaplastic large T-cell lymphoma, skin infiltration of, 417, 419, 445, 446
Systemic lupus eritematosus, 245

T

T4 endonuclease V in liposome, 41
Targetoid hemosiderotic hemangioma, 189, 211
Telangiectasia
    angioma serpiginosum, 208–209
    ataxia telangiectasia, 206–207
    charachteristics, 204–206
    cutis marmorata telangiectatica congenita, 210–211
    generalized essential telangiectasia, 208
    nevus anemicus, 210
    Osler-Weber-Rendu syndrome, 207–208
    spider angioma, 209–210
    unilateral nevoid telangiectasia, 208
Telangiectasia macularis eruptiva perstans, 206, 281
Telangiectatic metastatic carcinoma, 475
Temozolamide, 356
Thrombosed angiokeratoma, 189
Timolol, 177
Total body electron beam therapy, 408, 409
Trametinib, 356
Transformed mycosis fungoides, 417
Transplantation keratosis. *See* Verrucal keratosis
Traumatic neuroma, 241–242
Treacher-Collins syndrome, 143
Trichilemmal cyst, 126, 134–135, 285
Trichilemmoma, 28, 52, 159
Trichoblastoma, 28, 158
Trichoblastic carcinoma, 158
Trichodiscoma, 254
Trichoepithelioma, 156–158
Trichofolliculoma, 158
Trisomy 22 mosaicism, 143
Tryptase, 277, 279, 281
Tuberous sclerosis, 250–252, 262, 266–267
Tubular apocrine adenoma, 150
Tubulopapillary hidradenoma, 28, 150–151
Tufted angioma, 182
Turban tumor, 151
Turner syndrome, 84, 113, 160, 225
Tyndal effect, 74
Type II segmental Cowden disease, 22

U

Unilateral nevoid telangiectasia, 208
Unna nevus. *See* Papillomatous nevus
Urticaria pigmentosa, 275–277, 458

V

Vascular malformations
    arteriovenous malformation, 229–230
    capillary malformations, 204–216
    glomus tumor and glomuvenous malformations, 220–222
    lymphatic malformations, 224–228
    venous malformations, 216–220
Vemurafenib, 55, 319, 356
Venous lake, 218–220
Verapamil, 272
Verruca anogenitalis, 146
Verruca filiformis, 52, 53
Verruca plana, 145
Verruca plantaris, 329
Verruca vulgaris, 150, 159, 258
Verrucal keratosis, 17
Verrucous carcinoma
    Buschke-Löwenstein tumor, 329
    carcinoma cuniculatum, 329–330
    cutaneous verrucous carcinoma, 228
    oral florid papillomatosis, 328–329
Verrucous hemangioma, 214
Vinblastine, 192, 369
Vincristine, 176, 177, 182, 369
Viral wart, 28–29
Vismodegib, 310
Vitiligo, 113, 115
von Recklinghausen disease, 72, 231
Vorinostat, 410
Vulvar melanosis, 65

W

Waldenström macroglobulinemia, 460
Weathering nodules of the ear, 273
Werner syndrome, 297
Westerhof syndrome, 72
White sponge nevus, 35–36
Wood lamp examination, 210, 336
Woringer-Kolopp disease, 392. *See also* Pagetoid reticulosis
Wrestler's ear, 142

Y

Yellow nail syndrome, 226

X

Xanthelasma, 146
Xanthoma disseminatum, 460–462
Xanthomatosis and chylous lymphedema, 227, 228
Xeroderma pigmentosum
    actinic lentigo, 70–72
    basal cell carcinoma, 297, 307
    ephelides, 64
    keratoacanthoma, 58
    lentigo maligna melanoma, 336
    squamous cell carcinoma, 317

Z

Zanolimumab, 410